# SALVAGE

# *Laser Beams in the Atmosphere*

# Laser Beams in the Atmosphere

## V. E. Zuev

Director, Institute of Atmospheric Optics
Siberian Branch, Academy of Sciences of the USSR
Tomsk, USSR

Translated from Russian by

James S. Wood

CONSULTANTS BUREAU • NEW YORK AND LONDON

Library of Congress Cataloging in Publication Data

Zuev, V. E. (Vladimir Evseevich)
    Laser beams in the atmosphere.

    Bibliography: p.
    Includes indexes.
    1. Atmosphere — Laser observations. I. Title.
QC975.9.A1Z8                   551.5′028                  81-19508
ISBN 0-306-10967-0                                        AACR2


Luch lazera v atmosfere

This translation is published under an agreement with the Copyright Agency of the USSR (VAAP).



Printed in the United States of America

# *Preface*

Although scarcely 20 years have passed since the creation of the first laser, laser engineering has enjoyed a variety of applications in science and in practice. Among these applications, a special place is held by those related to the propagation of laser radiation in the atmosphere. Some, such as laser communication and information-transmission systems, locating and telemetering systems, and mapping and navigation systems, require access to quantitative data on the effects of the atmosphere on the parameters of the laser beam serving as the carrier of useful information, since the efficacy of any such system depends significantly on the influence of the atmosphere.

Another set of laser applications associated with the propagation of coherent radiation in the atmosphere requires the solution of both direct and inverse problems related to this complex subject. The kind of application in question is the use of lasers for long-range monitoring of various physical parameters of the atmosphere—a new and highly promising direction in science and engineering.

Finally, lasers are being used extensively in the development of ultra-high-resolution spectroscopic methods that will permit the spectra of substances in the gaseous phase to be obtained with practically 100% resolution and virtually undistorted by the slit function of the spectrometer. This consideration has direct bearing on the problem of quantitative estimation of the absorption of laser radiation by atmospheric gases; such estimates are obtainable from the experimental data only in the event that the absorption spectra recorded by the instrument are free of distortions.

Moreover, in light of the highly monochromatic nature of laser radiation, it is clear that a complete set of data on its propagation in the atmosphere would prove immensely useful for the solution of many problems unrelated to laser applications. Typical of such problems are: assessment of the radiation term in weather-prediction equations, the solution of inverse problems in satellite meteorology, the determination of the heat balance of the Earth as a planet, and the liberation of astronomical observation data from the aggravating influence of the atmosphere.

The propagation of laser radiation in the atmosphere is accompanied by an enormous set of linear and nonlinear interaction phenomena. None of these phenomena ever manifests itself in isolation. They may be classified into the following main groups on the basis of purely qualitative criteria: (1) refraction of rays by a laser beam; (2) absorption of laser energy by atmospheric gases; (3) dissipation of laser energy by aerosol particles, by air-density fluctuations, etc.; (4) fluctuations of the parameters of laser beams due to atmospheric turbulence.

Each of the aforementioned groups of phenomena of interaction of laser radiation with the atmosphere can emerge both in the realm of linear optics and in the realm of nonlinear optics. On the other hand, each group has clear-cut specific characteristics, which must be taken into consideration in related theoretical and experimental studies.

High monochromaticity, spatial confinement, and the possibility of generating laser pulses with large power, high energy, and very small pulsewidths levy stringent demands on the planning and conduct of theoretical and experimental investigations of the propagation of laser radiation in the atmosphere. It turns out in the majority of cases that the information acquired in many years of research on the propagation of optical waves in the atmosphere is patently unsuited to the kinds of quantitative estimates needed for lasers.

The broad-based development of a multidisciplinary research program on the propagation of laser radiation in the atmosphere has not only contributed substantially to the advancement of the problem itself, but has also stimulated the advent of new directions in science and technology, not the least of which are those directions associated with methods of long-range laser monitoring of the atmosphere and ultrahigh-resolution laser spectroscopy. Nonlinear atmospheric optics, which has emerged and taken shape in the last 10 or 12 years, holds a rightful place among these new directions of science.

The progress achieved in the solution of the problem of propagation of laser radiation in the atmosphere is currently mirrored in many thousands of articles published in various periodicals, dozens of surveys, and several complete books devoted to individual aspects of this multifaceted program. It seems most timely in this connection to undertake a generalization of the total problem in monograph form. Such is the objective of the present book.

The material in this book is grouped into seven chapters. The first chapter discusses the problems of refraction of laser radiation propagating both in the ground layer of the atmosphere (geodesic refraction) and along inclined paths (astronomical refraction). The second chapter is devoted to a systematic presentation of the problems of absorption of laser radiation by atmospheric gases. The laws of scattering of laser radiation by atmospheric aerosols (clouds, fogs, hazes, etc.) and hydrometeors, along with molecular scattering, are described in the third chapter. The fourth chapter generalizes the results of theoretical and experimental studies of the propagation of laser radiation in a turbulent atmosphere.

The fundamental results of research on various nonlinear effects accompanying the propagation of laser radiation in the atmosphere are analyzed in the fifth chapter. Thus, the first five chapters of the book cover all of the main aspects of the subject from the standpoint of the solution of direct atmospheric–optical problems associated with the study of the influence of the atmosphere on a laser beam propagating in it and, conversely, the influence of a beam on the atmosphere.

The sixth chapter summarizes data on the interference attributable to laser radiation propagating in the atmosphere. Although this chapter is of a secondary nature, it can be coordinated with the first five chapters to obtain, in the final analysis, information on the signal-to-noise ratios and, hence, to provide quantitative estimates of the operating efficiency of particular laser systems in the atmosphere under various conditions of propagation (with specific reference to various conditions in the atmosphere and various ray-propagation geometries).

The seventh and last chapter describes methods of long-range monitoring of various physical parameters of the atmosphere and the use of lasers for quantitative diagnostics of the gaseous components of the atmosphere by laser-spectroscopic methods. Both of these topics have vital bearing on the solution of many present-day problems, and for that reason considerable attention is devoted to their discussion. In particular, they are called upon to solve the problem of developing modern high-sensitivity and real-time methods for monitoring the state and dynamics of environmental pollution.

The fundamental results of theoretical and experimental work in progress both in the Soviet Union and abroad are generalized in every chapter of the book. A major portion of the materials included in the book have been obtained by the author and his many students and colleagues at the Institute of Optics of the Atmosphere of the Siberian Branch of the Academy of Sciences of the USSR.

The author is extremely pleased to acknowledge his deepest gratitude to his colleagues, A. B. Antipov, Yu. S. Balin, O. K. Voitsekhovskaya, V. N. Genin, I. I. Ippolitov, B. V. Kaul', G. M. Krekov, A. V. Kuzikovskii, V. P. Lukin, G. G. Matvienko, I. É. Naats, L. I. Nesmelova, A. A. Pershin, V. V. Pokasov, I. V. Samokhvalov, V. A. Sapozhnikova, S. D. Tvorogov, and V. V. Fomin for their resourceful assistance in preparation of the manuscript. The author extends special thanks to Yu. F. Arshinov, M. V. Kabanov, Yu. D. Kopytin, Yu. S. Makushkin, and V. L. Mironov for their effective aid in the preparation of a number of materials and their constructive criticism of pertinent chapters of the manuscript; their efforts have contributed greatly to improving the quality of the book.

V. E. Zuev

# Contents

# 1

# *Refraction of Light Rays in the Atmosphere*

## *1.0. Introduction*

Optical refraction in the earth's atmosphere (usually called terrestrial refraction) is a physical phenomenon with a research history spanning many centuries. Extensive bibliographies on the subject may be found in [1–4]. By no means, however, has the problem seen its final solution, particularly when one considers the stringent demands imposed on the accuracy of determination of the refraction corrections associated with practical applications of highly directional laser beams.

In this chapter we briefly sketch the present status of the problem of light refraction in the earth's atmosphere, with special emphasis on the error analysis of various expressions for determining the angles of terrestrial refraction.

Objects whose observation requires the application of refraction corrections may be classified into three main groups according to their positions relative to earth:

1. objects situated at great distances outside the earth's atmosphere (stars, planets, and other astronomical bodies), i.e., the case of astronomical refraction, whose investigation boasts the longest history;

2. objects close to or inside the earth's atmosphere (but beyond the atmospheric ground layer), where allowance must be made for the finite distance to the object, astronomical refraction data are not directly applicable, and the refraction process is properly called terrestrial;

3. objects close to or on the actual surface of the earth (within the limits of the ground layer), where we have the special case of terrestrial refraction known as geodesic refraction, whose analysis and correction exhibit very specific attributes.

It is presumed in all three cases that the observer is situated on the earth's surface or close to it. When the receiving optical system is located in or beyond the atmosphere and the observed object is on the earth's surface, the resulting refraction is called photogrammetric. The treatment of this type of refraction does not differ in principle from the three cases listed above.

Besides the indicated types of refraction, another classification scheme identifies optical refraction as regular and random (stochastic, statistical). Regular refraction is interpreted as the average angle of refraction, which depends on meteorological conditions. Random refraction refers to the comparatively low-frequency fluctuations of the refraction angle at a frequency around 0.01 Hz or lower. More rapid variations of the refraction (at frequencies of 0.1–100 Hz) are called quivering of the optical image. The theory and methods of correcting for this effect are most rigorously formulated on the basis of the theory of optical wave propagation in a turbulent atmosphere (see Chap. 4).

Finally, in addition to vertical refraction, which is the main topic of discussion below, it is sometimes necessary to investigate side refraction induced by horizontal inhomogeneity of the refractive index. Published estimates indicate that this refraction component can result in appreciable corrections for the vertical refraction as well.

## 1.1. Slant-Path Terrestrial Refraction

The physical cause of the curvature of a light beam (refraction) in the earth's atmosphere is inhomogeneity of the refractive index. For this reason, the optical refraction equations are derived on the basis of Snell's law of refraction, which follows from the Fermat principle.

Let us consider two elementary layers of the atmosphere at a certain height $z$ from the surface of the earth (Fig. 1.1), with refractive indices $n(z)$ and $n(z)+dn(z)$. The angles of the incident and emergent beams at the interface between the two layers are related by the following equation, consistent with the refraction law:

$$n(z)\sin \xi(z)=\left[n(z)+dn(z)\right]\sin\left[\xi(z)+d\xi(z)\right] \tag{1.1}$$

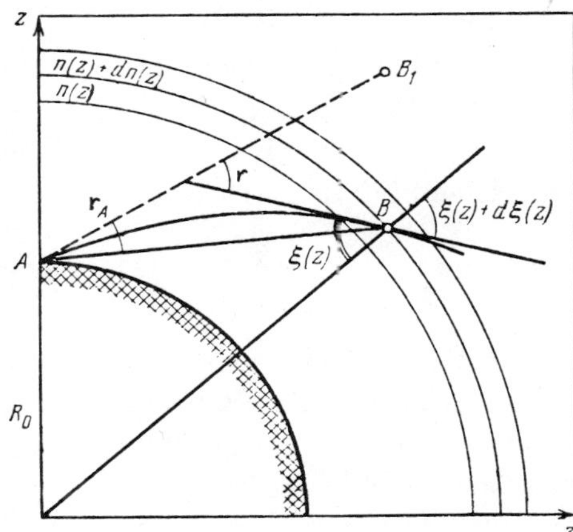


Fig. 1.1. Geometrical diagram for calculation of terrestrial refraction angles.

Expanding the sine of the sum of the angles in (1.1) and making use of the relations $\cos d\xi(z)=1$ and $\sin d\xi(z)=d\xi(z)$, we obtain

$$n(z)\sin\xi(z)=[n(z)+dn(z)][\sin\xi(z)+\cos\xi(z)\,d\xi(z)] \qquad (1.2)$$

From (1.2) we immediately deduce the elementary angle in question:

$$d\xi(z)=-\tan\xi(z)\frac{dn(z)}{n(z)} \qquad (1.3)$$

where $[n(z)+dn(z)]$ is approximated by $n(z)$ in the denominator.

Expression (1.3) is the fundamental equation of refraction theory. For horizontal paths the total angle of refraction is determined by subsequent transformations of this equation subject to particular assumptions and constraints. In the case of inclined paths it is necessary to perform integration with respect to the height. Accordingly, for the total angle of terrestrial refraction along slant paths (i.e., for the angle between the tangents to the ray at the observation point and at the object point) we have

$$r=-\int_{n(0)}^{n(z)}\frac{\tan\xi(z)}{n(z)}\,dn(z) \qquad (1.4)$$

so that the complete angle of terrestrial refraction is uniquely determined by the profile of the refractive index in the atmosphere.

In the practice of geodesic, radar, and other measurements, however, our primary concern is not the total angle of terrestrial refraction given by the integral (1.4), but the angle $r_A$ between the true zenith distance of the object and its apparent zenith distance; we refer to this angle simply as the "terrestrial refraction angle."

Existing refraction theories differ from one another in their hypotheses concerning the parameters of the atmosphere at different heights and the corresponding methods for computation of the integral (1.4). The dependence of the refractive index on the parameters of the atmosphere in the visible and infrared wavelength intervals has the form [1]

$$n-1=C_\lambda \frac{P}{T}\left(1-0.132\frac{e}{P}\right) \tag{1.5}$$

where $C_\lambda$ is a coefficient depending on the wavelength. For the part of the spectrum in the vicinity of $\lambda=0.6\ \mu$m, we have $C_\lambda=1.0485\times10^{-4}$ when the pressure $P$ and the absolute humidity $e$ are measured in mm Hg and the temperature $T$ in degrees Kelvin. Estimates according to (1.5) indicate that the maximum humidity variations induce at most a 0.5% variation of the refractive index. This weak influence of the humidity is usually neglected. Instead of the pressure and temperature dependence of the refractive index, it is customary to use its dependence on the gas density, which is uniquely expressed in terms of $P$ and $T$ by the familiar equation of state for an ideal gas.

Two basic approaches are employed for computation of the integral (1.4). The first approach is to obtain approximate relations based on a series of simplifying assumptions. The second involves numerical computations for special models of the atmosphere. An illustrative example of the first approach is the approximate expression obtained from (1.4), under rather crude assumptions, for calculation of the total angle of terrestrial refraction. If we introduce the parameters

$$\alpha=\frac{n_0^2-1}{2n_0^2};\quad s=\frac{H}{R_0+H};\quad \eta=\frac{2s\sin^2\xi-2\alpha(1-x)}{\cos^2\xi} \tag{1.6}$$

where $n_0$ is the refractive index at the earth's surface ("ground-level index"), $H$ is the height of the object (maximum value of $z$), and $R_0$ is the radius of the earth; and, if we neglect small terms containing $s^2$, $\eta^2$, and $\alpha^2$ in the series expansion of the integrand in (1.4), we obtain the following expression, assuming that the atmospheric layers are plane parallel [2]:

$$r(\xi,H)\simeq\alpha[1-x(H)]\tan\xi \tag{1.7}$$

which goes over into the approximate expression for astronomical refraction in the case of zero relative density of the atmosphere at height $H$: $x(H)=0$.

As is apparent from (1.7), under the given assumptions the refraction angle depends only on the density values at the observer and object levels.

Calculations show [2] that the use of this expression yields maximum errors of 1.5% in comparison with calculations based on the inclusion of higher-order terms, provided that $\xi \leqslant 75°$. The computational error for expression (1.7) increases rapidly for large zenith angles. More accurate approximate expressions can be obtained on the basis of specific models of the atmosphere (for the pressure and temperature profiles) [1–4]. The following expression for the terrestrial refraction angle $r_A$, derived under the same assumptions as (1.7), is given by Numerova [5]:

$$r_A = \frac{n_0 - 1}{n_0} \tan \xi \, \frac{1}{H} \int_0^H \left[ 1 - x(z) \right] dz \qquad (1.8)$$

Estimates show that expression (1.8) ensures error limits of 10 angular seconds in the calculation of $r_A$ and provides a simple means for estimation of the relative value of this quantity in comparison with astronomical refraction. In particular, for an object at a height of 1 km the value of $r_A$ amounts to 5% of the astronomical refraction, at a height of 10 km it is 38%, at 100 km it is 92%, and at 300 km it is 97%.

A rather large number of tables has been compiled to date on the basis of numerical computations of terrestrial refraction according to particular models of the atmosphere. For example, the results of calculations of the total terrestrial refraction for object zenith angles in the vicinity of 85° to 90° and for observation stations at various heights above the ground level in the case of a standard atmosphere were published in 1940 [6]. Calculated refraction data obtained for horizontal ray paths ($\xi = 90°$) at various geographic latitudes on the basis of monthly mean aerological measurements of the density of the atmosphere during the International Geophysical Year (IGY) have been tabulated by Link and Neuzil [7].

Kushtin [8] has obtained nomograms for calculation of the photogrammetric refraction angle (with the observer above and the observed object below, using an aerial-photographic optical system).

A series of tables is also available for determining the astronomical refraction angles. Tables of calculations of the terrestrial refraction angle $r_A$ for a standard atmosphere with $\xi \leqslant 85°$ and $H \leqslant 15$ km are given in [5], together with tables of approximate corrections for fluctuations of the initial conditions. Kolchinskii [2] has carried out precise detailed calculations of the terrestrial refraction angles for the 1960 temporal standard atmosphere (TSA-60) [9]. The results of astronomical refraction observations ($H = \infty$) spanning many years may be found in the Pulkovo Observatory refraction tables [10].

Tabulated data as well as data calculated according to approximate expressions (with allowance for ground-level conditions) are better suited to estimates for typical, rather than concrete, atmospheric conditions. Abundant, albeit nonsystematic (with respect to time and geographic locale), measurements of the refraction angles and a comparison of the results of these measurements with the calculated values indicate that, while good agreement is obtained in the majority of cases, sizable discrepancies (as high as several minutes) are also frequently observed [2]. These discrepancies are particularly large for large zenith angles, in which case they attain tens of minutes. Such instances, which are usually referred to as anomalous refraction, certainly detract from the reliability of refraction estimates under concrete meteorological conditions. Accordingly, for the solution of many practical problems it is exceedingly important to have access to reliable ongoing quantitative information about the atmospheric parameters affecting refraction in order to be able to incorporate appropriate corrections. For example, Fannin and Jehn [11] have proposed a procedure for determining the difference between the angles under standard atmospheric conditions and those under conditions consistent with the time of observation at ground level. The corresponding expression for the angular difference $\Delta r_A$ between the observed and true directions to the object has the form

$$\Delta r_A = (n_0 - n_0') - \frac{1}{y} \int_0^y (n - n')\, dy \tag{1.9}$$

where $n_0$ and $n_0'$ are the values of the refractive index under standard and nonstandard conditions at ground level, $n$ and $n'$ are the corresponding profiles of the refractive indices obtained from aerological probe results, $y$ is a parameter related nonlinearly to the object height $H$ and the observed positional angle $h$ of the object by the equation

$$y = R_0 \sin h \left[ \left( \sin^2 h + \frac{R_0 + H}{R_0} - 1 \right)^{1/2} - \sin h \right] \tag{1.10}$$

in which $R_0$ is the radius of the earth. A weak link in the proposed procedure is the use of aerological data, which require considerable time for their acquisition (roughly 1 h). Significantly more promising are procedures based on real-time data acquisition by laser probing (monitoring) of the atmosphere [12–14]. A detailed description of methods for the laser monitoring of various parameters of the atmosphere is given in Chap. 7.

## 1.2. Horizontal-Path Terrestrial Refraction

The angle of terrestrial refraction along horizontal paths (geodesic refraction angle) under the condition of a homogeneous underlying surface and a layered atmosphere is related to the physical parameters of the atmosphere by elementary expressions [1]. The refraction for horizontal paths is normally characterized by the coefficient of terrestrial refraction (CTR) $K$, which is defined as the ratio of the earth's radius to the radius of curvature of a ray refracted by the atmosphere and treated as a circular arc. The latter assumption (in the definition of the CTR) enables us to deduce the following obvious relation between the terrestrial refraction angle (angle between the observed and true directions to an object) and the CTR:

$$r_h = \tfrac{1}{2}KL \tag{1.11}$$

where $L$ is the distance to the observed object along the earth's surface in angular minutes (nautical-mile equivalent). If $r_h$ is measured in minutes and $L$ in kilometers, the numerical coefficient in (1.11) should be 0.926 instead of $1/2$.

To determine the dependence of the CTR on the state of the atmosphere, we make use of the fact that the radius of curvature of the ray is $R = dz/\cos\xi(z)\cdot d\xi(z)$, where $dz$ is the thickness of the elementary refracting layer. Thus, using expression (1.3) for $d\xi(z)$, we obtain for an inclined ray in the general case

$$K_\angle(z) = \frac{R_0 + z}{R} = -(R_0 + z)\frac{dn(z)}{dz}\sin\xi(z) = K(z)\sin\xi(z) \tag{1.12}$$

where $K(z)$ is the CTR of a horizontal ray at height $z$. It is evident from (1.12) that the CTR is uniquely determined by the gradient of the refractive index along the ray path. The relationship of the CTR to the other parameters of the atmosphere (in terms of the refractive index) can be deduced on the basis of expression (1.5), from which it follows that

$$\frac{dn(z)}{dz} = -\eta\left[-\frac{T}{P}\frac{dP(z)}{dz} + \frac{dT(z)}{dz}\left(1 - 0.132\frac{e}{P}\right) + 0.132\frac{T}{P}\cdot\frac{de(z)}{dz}\right]$$

$$\tag{1.13}$$

where the parameter $\eta = C_\lambda P/T^2$. The dependence on the humidity in (1.13), as mentioned, is inconsequential. The influence of $de/dz$ is even smaller. The pressure gradient in the earth's atmosphere is practically constant. In the ground layer of air $dP(z)/dz = -0.095$ mm Hg/m. Thus, the main physical parameters affecting the value of the CTR are the air temperature and the pressure, as well as the temperature gradient along the ray path. For a given temperature gradient the variations of the CTR with the meteorological conditions are also governed by the parameter $\eta$. It is readily estimated that the CTR experiences at most a twofold variation due to $\eta$ over the entire range of possible temperature and pressure variations in the ground layer.

It is assumed in the derivation of the foregoing CTR expressions that the atmosphere is homogeneous and has a regular structure along the ray path. It is reasonable to expect that such assumptions will not always be justified under real conditions. This fact can induce significant deviations of the measured CTR from the value calculated according to data on the meteorological parameters of the atmosphere. For example, it follows from an analysis of the results of a comparison of optical and meteorological data [15] that the disparities between the calculated and measured values of the CTR can attain 30 or 40% in many cases, even in meteorological observations at both ends of a specific ray path. Such disparities have a number of characteristics in common within the boundaries of large geographical regions and can be taken into account through the use of empirical relations [16]. In many situations it is necessary to take more precise account of the disparities for each specific path. It is significant in this regard that the disparity between the calculated and measured values of the CTR tend to diminish with increasing path length as a result of averaging of local topographical and ground-soil features [16].

Another factor limiting the applicability of expressions (1.12) and (1.13) for real paths lies in the temporal variability of the atmospheric conditions. In a number of cases this variability in conjunction with the features of a given locale (profile of the path, microclimate, etc.) produces so-called anomalous refraction of a more or less persistent nature, where, for example, the inclination of the apparent horizon can vary by several tens of minutes or even by 1 or 2°. More often the temporal variability of the atmospheric conditions induces appreciable temporal variations of the refraction angles (i.e., random refraction). This effect will be discussed in closer detail below.

Thus, only a rather crude estimate of the CTR can be obtained from the expressions relating the CTR to the physical parameters of the atmosphere. For concrete real conditions such an estimate can be improved either on the basis of preliminary statistical data relating to the spatial and temporal variations of the physical parameters of the atmosphere along an investigated path or on the basis of real-time information about the profiles of the corresponding physical parameters, as obtained, for example, by the methods of laser monitoring of the atmosphere.

## 1.3. Random Refraction

Rapid deviations of a light ray due to moving inhomogeneities of the air represent random refraction, which in many cases, without additional monitoring, can diminish the steering accuracy of radar systems or the accuracy of determination of the coordinates of an observed object as well as lower the efficiency of operation of data-transmission systems using optical channels. These considerations place far greater practical significance on random refraction than in the earlier treatment of practical astronomical and geodesic problems.

The fundamental problems of astronomical and geodesic observations have elicited the greatest interest in systematic refraction measurements for the purpose of selecting and recommending the most favorable time for observations. In the course of investigation, of course, rapid variations of the refraction angle have also been observed. Thus, on the basis of many years of astronomical refraction observations, Krat [17] identifies four types of rapid oscillations of the image of the edge of the solar disk in a telescope (refraction angle): (1) oscillations with a constant frequency of 0.5–1 Hz and a random amplitude; (2) "irregular" image quivering of a random nature with amplitudes attaining several seconds of arc and with a mean frequency of 0.1 and 0.2 Hz. The other two types of oscillations have higher frequencies (10 Hz and higher) and result in blurring of the image. (A quantitative description of these types of oscillations is presented in Chap. 4.)

Beckmann [18] and Hodara [19] have observed random refraction along horizontal paths, noting slow drifting of a laser beam over paths of 5–15 km at a rate of several angular seconds per hour. More systematic observations of low-frequency temporal beam fluctuations have been carried out for thermal radiation sources with the extraction of spectral intervals at wavelengths of 0.856, 0.943, and 1.03 $\mu$m [20]. The results of these observations for a 10-km path reveal the existence of periods of beam-direction fluctuations lasting roughly 1 and 4 to 5 h. Estimates of the probable optical inhomogeneities of the atmosphere due to such fluctuations yield scales of approximately 10 and 40 km. The fluctuations of the beam direction in these observations attained an amplitude of 15 angular sec.

## 1.4. Spectral Behavior of Optical Refraction

The spectral dependence of optical refraction is determined by the dispersion properties of the air, which are quantitatively characterized by the wavelength dependence of $C_\lambda$ in expression (1.5). Knowing that the influence of humidity on $C_\lambda$ in the optical wavelength range is negligible, we can make the transition from the refractivity $N_0 = (n-1) \cdot 10^{-6}$ for certain initial values $P_0$ and $T_0$ to the refractivity for arbitrary $P$ and $T$ on the basis of the relation $N = N_0 P T_0 / T P_0$. The refractivity for dry air in the visible region of the spectrum at a temperature $T = 273.15°$K and pressure $P = 760$ mm Hg can be calculated according to the equation [21]

$$N = C_\lambda \frac{P}{T} = \left( 103.38 + \frac{0.5854}{\lambda^4} \right) \frac{P}{T} \tag{1.14}$$

The numerical values of $N$ in the spectral interval from 0.2 to 20 $\mu$m at a pressure of 760 mm Hg and at temperatures of $\pm 30$, $\pm 15$, and 0°C may be found in the *Geophysics Handbook* [22].

Link and Sekera [6] have investigated the spectral dependence of the optical refraction along slant paths for dry air in the visible region of the spectrum. The wavelength dependence of the refraction angle for horizontal paths is discussed in [23], from which it follows that the refraction angle varies within 6% limits in the wavelength range from 0.4 to 11 $\mu$m if the complex valuedness of the refractive index of air is disregarded.

In the infrared spectral region, which is saturated with the absorption bands for atmospheric gases, it is necessary to take the complexity of the refractive index into account. It is essential to note, however, that in the event of a large value of the imaginary part of the refractive index (absorption index) a light ray suffers large absorption to the extent that its influence is on a par with the (real) refraction [24]. The problem of refraction with partial absorption (for a very small value of the absorption index) has not been adequately studied to date, despite its timeliness in connection with the need for relevant data over the entire range of electromagnetic wavelengths. In regard to research in this area, we cite the work of

Rozenberg and Mel'nikova [25], who have shown that in the case of refraction with partial absorption it is necessary to be aware of the emergence of effects that set the stage for the hypothetical possibility of spatial selection of mutually incoherent components of a light ray according to their polarization states. Also of definite interest here is a method proposed by Khvostikov back in 1946 [26] for determining refraction on the basis of measurements at two wavelengths; the two-wavelength method has been elaborated in recent times in specialized developments [27].

In the large-wavelength limit, optical refraction is identical to radio-wave refraction. The latter has two principal features that distinguish it from optical refraction. First, the wavelength dependence of the refractive index can be completely neglected in the radio range [28]. This dependence is already insignificant in the long-wave optical range.

The second important distinction of radio-wave refraction is the more important role of humidity in this range. Figure 1.2 gives the results of calculations of standard radio refraction (i.e., for the standard atmosphere with respect to pressure and temperature) at 100 and 0% humidity, as well as for various heights and zenith angles of the observed objects [29]. It is evident from the figure that the humidity correction to the angle of radio refraction can attain 5′ for observations along a horizontal path (90° zenith angle).

Some of the problems associated with radio refraction, including practical computational techniques, are discussed in [28–30]. We note that the radio refraction angles are greater than the optical refraction angles under the identical most typical atmospheric conditions. Whereas the curvature of the path of an optical beam in a horizontal direction under these condition attains a radius of curvature $R \simeq 50{,}000$ km, the maximum for radio waves is $R = 25{,}000$ km [28]. The difference between the optical and radio refraction angles along different lines of sight is mainly attributable to the moisture content of the atmosphere and can therefore be corrected when the humidity profile is known.

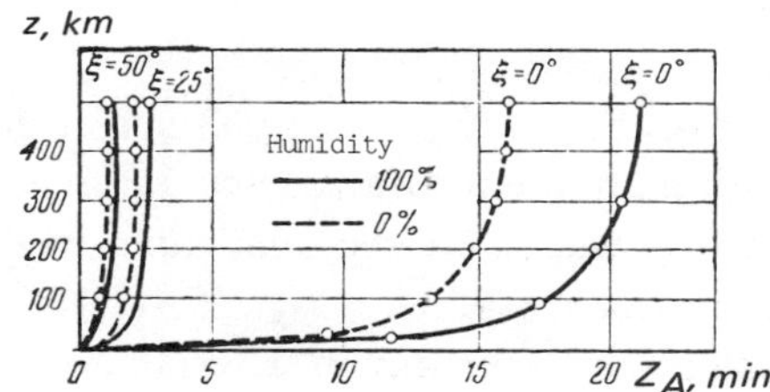


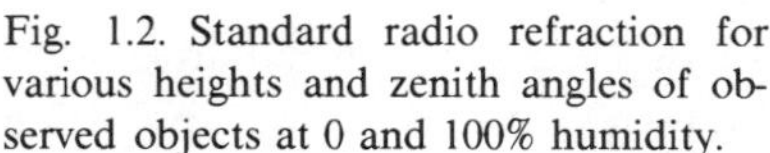
Fig. 1.2. Standard radio refraction for various heights and zenith angles of observed objects at 0 and 100% humidity.

## 1.5. Influence of the Error of Determination of Various Parameters on the Error of Calculation of the Terrestrial Refraction Angles

The most common method of determining terrestrial refraction in practice is based on numerical integration of the exact refraction equation. It is assumed in this connection that all the parameters involved in this equation are precisely known. This is hardly the case, however, and so it is important to ascertain how the errors of measurement of particular parameters affect the results of quantitative determination of the angle of terrestrial refraction. The corresponding calculations have been carried out by Genin and Nelyubin [31], whose work we shall follow.

The terrestrial refraction angle $r$ for an object situated at height $H$ is written in the form [2]

$$r = \zeta - \xi = \tan^{-1} \frac{\sin \theta}{\cos \theta - \gamma} - \xi \tag{1.15}$$

where

$$\theta = R_0 n_0 \sin \xi \int_{R_0}^{R_0 + H} \frac{dR}{R\left[ (Rn)^2 - (R_0 n_0 \sin \beta)^2 \right]^{1/2}} \tag{1.16}$$

$\gamma = R_0 / (R_0 + H)$, $R_0$ is the radius of the earth at the site of the measuring apparatus, $R = R_0 + z$, $z$ is the height variable along the path of the light ray, $\xi$ and $\zeta$ are the apparent and true zenith distances to the observed object, and $n_0$ and $n(z)$ are the refractive indices at the observation site and at height $z$. The latter index is expressed in terms of the meteorological parameters in the general case according to the equation

$$n = 1 + C'_\lambda = 1 - \frac{C_\lambda \rho}{\rho_0} = 1 + C_\lambda \frac{T_0}{P_0} \frac{P}{T} \tag{1.17}$$

in which $C_\lambda = C'_\lambda \rho_0$ is a coefficient depending on the wavelength $\lambda$; $P$, $T$, and $\rho$ are the pressure, temperature, and density of the air at height $z$; and $P_0$, $T_0$, and $\rho_0$ are the same quantities at the observation point.

From expressions (1.15)–(1.17) we readily deduce an equation for calculating the error of determination of the terrestrial refraction angle due to errors in the determination of the refractive index profile or of the temperature and pressure profiles [see (1.17)]:

$$\sigma_r(P,T)=\frac{C_\lambda n_0 T_0 F}{P_0}\int_{R_0}^{R_0+H}\left[\sigma^2(P)+\left(\frac{P}{T}\right)^2\sigma^2(T)\right]^{1/2}\frac{W}{T}\,dR \qquad (1.18)$$

where

$$F=\frac{(1-\gamma\cos\theta)R_0\sin\xi}{1-2\gamma\cos\theta+\gamma^2}$$

$$W=\frac{Rn}{\left[(Rn)^2-(R_0 n_0\sin\xi)^2\right]^{3/2}} \qquad (1.19)$$

and $\sigma(P)$ and $\sigma(T)$ are the root-mean-square (rms) errors of determination of the pressure and temperature; according to radiosonde data [32], these errors have values of 0.6–0.1 mbar and 2.0–0.5°C, depending on the height.

The results of calculations of $\sigma_r(P,T)$ in angular seconds according to (1.18) for the above-indicated errors of determination of the profiles $P(z)$ and $T(z)$ and for various values of $H$ and the zenith distance are summarized in Table 1.1.

Expressions for the error of determination of the terrestrial refraction angle due to temperature and pressure measurement errors at the site of the measuring apparatus are deduced from (1.15) and (1.16) and have the form

$$\sigma_r(T_0)=\frac{C_\lambda F\sigma(T)}{T_0}\int_{R_0}^{R_0+H}nW\,dR \qquad (1.20)$$

$$\sigma_r(P_0)=\frac{C_\lambda F\sigma(P_0)}{P_0}\int_{R_0}^{R_0+H}nW\,dR \qquad (1.21)$$

Table 1.2 gives the results of calculations of $\sigma_r(T_0)$ in angular seconds according to (1.20) for various heights $H$ and zenith distances in the case

Table 1.1. Values of $\sigma_r(P,T)$ in Angular Seconds (″) for Pressure and Temperature Errors $\sigma(P)=0.6$–0.1 mbar and $\sigma(T)=2.0$–0.5°C

| | Zenith distance, deg | | | | | | |
|---|---|---|---|---|---|---|---|
| $H$, km | 45 | 70 | 80 | 85 | 88 | 89 | 90 |
|---|---|---|---|---|---|---|---|
| 5 | 0.09 | 0.24 | 0.49 | 0.99 | 2.48 | 4.99 | 177.0 |
| 10 | 0.08 | 0.20 | 0.43 | 0.94 | 2.42 | 4.90 | 179.0 |
| 50 | 0.04 | 0.10 | 0.24 | 0.61 | 2.10 | 4.75 | 183.0 |
| ∞ | 0.01 | 0.01 | 0.05 | 0.27 | 1.60 | 4.29 | 193.0 |

Table 1.2. Values of $\sigma_r(T_0)$ in Angular Seconds ($''$) for $\sigma(T)=0.1°C$

| $H$, km | Zenith distance, deg | | | | | | |
|---|---|---|---|---|---|---|---|
| | 45 | 70 | 80 | 85 | 88 | 89 | 90 |
| 5 | 0.04 | 0.10 | 0.20 | 0.41 | 1.06 | 2.24 | 42.7 |
| 10 | 0.03 | 0.08 | 0.18 | 0.38 | 1.01 | 2.18 | 43.1 |
| 50 | 0.02 | 0.06 | 0.14 | 0.30 | 0.90 | 2.07 | 44.3 |
| $\infty$ | 0.02 | 0.05 | 0.12 | 0.26 | 0.83 | 2.02 | 47.1 |

$\sigma(T)=0.1°C$. It follows from expressions (1.20) and (1.21) that $\sigma_r(P_0)=\sigma_r(T_0)[\sigma(P_0)/\sigma(T_0)](T_0/P_0)$, so that the data of Table 1.2 and the latter equation can be used to determine $\sigma_r(P_0)$.

Genin and Nelyubin [31] have also calculated the error of determination of the terrestrial refraction angle due to inaccurate knowledge of the air humidity; the results show that it is fully justified to neglect the humidity in the optical wavelength range, whereas in the radio range the humidity contribution is significant.

Tables 1.3 through 1.5 summarize the results of calculations of the errors induced in the terrestrial refraction angle by errors in the determination of the height $z_0$ of the measuring apparatus, the object height $H$, and the radiation wavelength [31].

The accuracy of calculation of the terrestrial refraction angle is strongly influenced by errors in the determination of the inclination of equal-density layers. It is assumed in the derivation of expression (1.4) that the equal-density layers comprise spheres concentric with each other and with the surface of the earth. In reality, irregularities of the earth's surface create temperature and pressure gradients and, hence, gradients of the refractive index, which impart angles of inclination to the equal-density layers.

The inclination of the layers at height $z$ is described by the expression [33]

$$\Delta i(z)=0''.389\frac{G(z)}{\rho(z)}-1''.116\Gamma(z) \tag{1.22}$$

where $\Delta i(z)$ is the inclination of the layers in minutes, $G(z)$ and $\Gamma(z)$ are the horizontal pressure and temperature gradients in millibars and degrees Kelvin per degree of latitude, and $\rho(z)$ is the air density in kilograms per cubic meter.

Using (1.22) in conjunction with the expression derived from (1.1) and (1.2) for calculation of the errors of determination of the terrestrial refrac-

**Table 1.3.** Values of $\sigma_r(z_0)$ in Angular Seconds ($''$) for Initial-Height Error $\sigma(z_0)=10$ m

| $H$, km | Zenith distance, deg | | | | | | |
|---|---|---|---|---|---|---|---|
| | 45 | 70 | 80 | 85 | 88 | 89 | 90 |
| 5 | 0.12 | 0.32 | 0.66 | 1.30 | 2.80 | 4.15 | 6.80 |
| 10 | 0.27 | 0.74 | 1.50 | 2.85 | 5.50 | 7.33 | 10.14 |
| 50 | 0.55 | 1.45 | 2.93 | 5.42 | 9.96 | 13.03 | 16.32 |
| $\infty$ | 0.81 | 2.10 | 3.80 | 6.54 | 12.40 | 16.60 | 21.04 |

tion angle $\sigma_r(\Delta i)$ due to inclination of the equal-density layers [31]

$$\sigma_r(\Delta i)=\frac{F}{R_0\sin\xi}\frac{1}{\rho'}\int_{R_0}^{R_0+H}\frac{Rn^2\Delta i(z)\,dR}{R^2n^2-R_0^2n^2\sin^2\xi} \qquad (1.23)$$

we can readily calculate the values of $\sigma_r(\Delta i)$ for a specified value of $\Delta i(z)$. If $\Delta i(z)$ is measured in angular minutes, we have $\rho'=3438$ in Eq. (1.23).

The results of calculations of $\sigma_r(\Delta i)$ for a layer situated at a height $z=1$ km having an inclination $\Delta i=1'$ are given in Table 1.6.

It is clear from Table 1.6 that the inclination of the layers can have a profound influence on the error of determination of the terrestrial refraction angle, particularly in the bottom 100-m layer of the atmosphere, where the gradients of the refractive index are most pronounced.

Nelyubin [34] has conducted detailed numerical experiments to determine the terrestrial refraction angle errors originating from space–time fluctuations of the atmospheric parameters. The experiments were based on simple empirical relations:

$$\sigma^2(t)=\sigma_1^2 t \qquad (1.24)$$

$$\sigma^2(L)=\sigma^2(L_1)L \qquad (1.25)$$

where $\sigma(t)$ is the rms fluctuation of the meteorological parameter in time

**Table 1.4.** Values of $\sigma_r(H)$ in Angular Seconds ($''$) for Object-Height Error $\sigma(H)=1$ km

| $H$, km | Zenith distance, deg | | | | | | |
|---|---|---|---|---|---|---|---|
| | 45 | 70 | 80 | 85 | 88 | 89 | 90 |
| 5 | 2.25 | 5.79 | 11.81 | 22.41 | 42.32 | 53.42 | 68.81 |
| 10 | 1.65 | 4.42 | 8.86 | 16.10 | 26.90 | 31.74 | 38.58 |
| 50 | 0.19 | 0.51 | 1.00 | 1.72 | 2.88 | 3.64 | 4.60 |
| 100 | 0.01 | 0.13 | 0.26 | 0.47 | 0.89 | 1.21 | 1.64 |

Table 1.5. Values of $\sigma_r(\lambda)$ in Angular Seconds (″) for Wavelength Error $\sigma(\lambda)=0.1\ \mu$m (Ruby Laser, $\lambda=0.69\ \mu$m)

| $H$, km | \multicolumn{7}{c}{Zenith distance, deg} | | | | | | |
|---|---|---|---|---|---|---|---|
|  | 45 | 70 | 80 | 85 | 88 | 89 | 90 |
| 5 | 0.04 | 0.12 | 0.24 | 0.47 | 1.03 | 1.58 | 2.70 |
| 10 | 0.07 | 0.21 | 0.42 | 0.81 | 1.66 | 2.35 | 3.35 |
| 50 | 0.17 | 0.45 | 0.91 | 1.66 | 3.02 | 3.98 | 5.30 |
| $\infty$ | 0.20 | 0.54 | 1.10 | 2.05 | 3.85 | 5.19 | 6.04 |

interval $t$, $\sigma_1$ is the same in unit time interval, $\sigma(L)$ is the rms fluctuation of the meteorological parameter over a distance $L$, and $\sigma(L_1)$ is the same over unit distance $L_1$. It has been shown [32, 35, 36] that expression (1.24) is valid for $t\leqslant 12$ h, and expression (1.25) up to $L\lesssim 700$–$1000$ km. The calculations were carried out for summer and winter seasonal conditions, for time intervals of 6, 12, and 24 h, for heights $H=5$, 10, 25, 50, and 100 km, and for values of $s=100$, 300, 500, and 1000 km. The local seasonal model for the European Territory of the USSR (ET USSR) was used in the calculations for various values of $s$.

The results of the calculations indicate that the observed anomalies of astronomical and terrestrial refraction [37–41] can be completely explained by space–time fluctuations of the atmosphere or by differences between the true profile of the refractive index at the measurement site and the particular model used as the basis for compilation of the corresponding tables for determination of the refractive indices.

Figure 1.3, which is borrowed from [42], illustrates the material discussed above from the standpoint of the error of determination of the angular distance to a distant object situated at a height of 10 km. Curve a corresponds to complete neglect of refraction; curve b is plotted on the basis of the standard model of the atmosphere; curve c characterizes the errors of determination of the angular distances with terrestrial refraction taken into account in the local model of the atmosphere for ET USSR; and, finally,

Table 1.6. Values of $\sigma_r(\Delta i)$ in Angular Seconds (″) for Layer at Height $z=1$ km with Inclination $\Delta i=1'$

| $H$, km | \multicolumn{7}{c}{Zenith distance, deg} | | | | | | |
|---|---|---|---|---|---|---|---|
|  | 45 | 70 | 80 | 85 | 88 | 89 | 90 |
| 5 | 6.20 | 6.23 | 6.36 | 6.86 | 13.70 | 15.28 | 34.71 |
| 10 | 3.10 | 3.14 | 3.29 | 3.84 | 6.92 | 13.04 | 26.94 |
| 50 | 0.62 | 0.68 | 0.84 | 1.41 | 5.51 | 10.87 | 26.50 |
| $\infty$ | 0.01 | 0.05 | 0.17 | 0.65 | 3.48 | 9.78 | 27.41 |

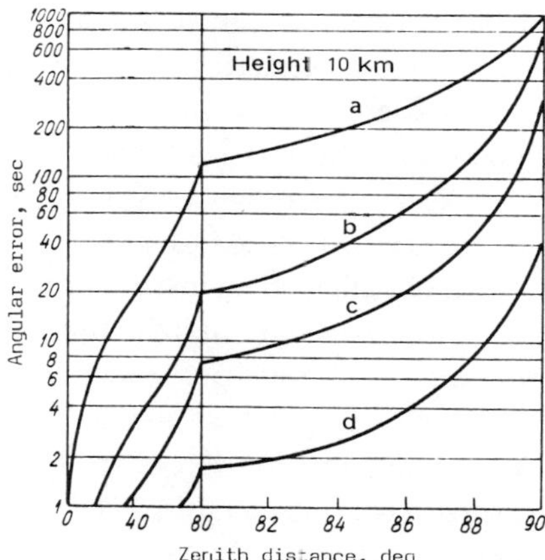


Fig. 1.3. Errors of determination of refraction angles for various initial data on the parameters of the atmosphere.

curve d is plotted with regard for the real distribution of the meteorological parameters and, hence, for the profile of the refractive index according to radiosonde data. Curve d gives a notion of the theoretical error limits in the determination of the distance to an object at a height of 10 km when the primary information about the meteorological parameters is obtained from a single radiosonde ascent in the atmosphere. The accuracy of determination of the terrestrial refractive index can be improved over the data of curve d by increasing the accuracy and speed of access to measurements of the meteorological parameters or by means of extremely complex and costly indirect experimental measurements.

Considering the insufficient speed of the radiosonde method for measuring the meteorological parameters and, in a number of instances, the complete lack of radiosonde data in the region of determination of the terrestrial refraction angle, several authors have proposed various algorithms and nomograms for determining that angle on the basis of more nearly real-time temperature and pressure measurements in the immediate vicinity of the refraction observation point [43–45]. The optimum distribution of nodes of the numerical integration grid for minimization of the refraction-angle error has been calculated in [46].

## 1.6. Experimental Studies of Geodesic Refraction

Pronounced inhomogeneities of the refractive-index field in the ground layer of the atmosphere essentially preclude the possibility of any accurate determination of the refractive index on the basis of tabulated data and measurements of the temperature and pressure at the observation point. Accordingly, geodesic refraction data meeting practical requirements can be obtained either from measurements of the meteorological parameters along the given path or by indirect experimental measurements.

As an example of experimental work on geodesic refraction, we examine the work of Alekseev and others [47], who have acquired and analyzed exhaustive instrument data over measurement paths extending 39.6 and 14.9 km in the atmosphere above the flat plains region. The measurements were performed with a transit instrument, whose height, like the heights of the first and second sources and the distance between them, was determined by third-class trigonometric leveling. The indicated heights turned out to be equal to 371.7, 453.7, and 379.2 m, respectively. They were used to calculate the true zenith angles of the first and second sources within $\pm 1''$ error limits; the indicated angles turned out to be equal to $90°03'37''.6$ and $90°02'15''$.

The difference between the true and observed zenith distances was used to find the vertical refraction angle $r$, from which the coefficient of refraction $K$ was determined according to the equation

$$K = \frac{2r}{L} \qquad (1.26)$$

in which $L$ is the distance to the observed object, expressed in angular units ($1' = 1852$ m); it values for the first and second sources were $21'23''$ and $8'01''$. Simultaneously, the meteorological parameters at heights of 1 and 4 m near the observation site were measured, and the windspeed and temperature gradients were determined, along with the Richardson number Ri [48]:

$$\mathrm{Ri} = \frac{g}{T}(\gamma - \gamma_a)\left(\frac{dU}{dz}\right)^{-2} \qquad (1.27)$$

where $g$ is the acceleration due to the force of gravity, $T$ is the air temperature in degrees Kelvin, $\gamma = dT/dz$ is the vertical temperature gradient, $\gamma_a = 0.01°K/m$, and $dU/dz$ is the windspeed gradient.

The coefficient of refraction was calculated from the meteorological parameters of the atmosphere according to the equation

$$K = 504 \frac{P}{T^2}(0.0342 - \gamma) + K_e \qquad (1.28)$$

where $P$ is the pressure in millibars and $K_e$ is a correction for the air humidity.

The measurements of the coefficient $K$ for the second source ($K_2$) were carried out in different seasons, once per hour, continuously over a period of several days. For the first source $K_1$ was determined only during the dark time in connection with the visibility conditions. A total of about 70 simultaneous measurements of $K_1$ and $K_2$ and approximately 900 measurements of $K_2$ alone were performed.

Figure 1.4 gives the results of the simultaneous measurements of $K_1$ and $K_2$. In order to determine the correlation between $K_1$ and $K_2$, the correlation coefficient $\rho_{K_1 K_2}$ was calculated according to the equation [49]

$$\rho_{K_1 K_2} = \frac{\sum_{i=1}^{n} (K_{1i} - \langle K_1 \rangle)(K_{2i} - \langle K_2 \rangle)}{\left[ \sum_{i=1}^{n} (K_{1i} - \langle K_1 \rangle)^2 \sum_{i=1}^{n} (K_{2i} - \langle K_2 \rangle)^2 \right]^{1/2}} \tag{1.29}$$

It turned out that $\rho_{K_1 K_2} = 0.83$ for $K_2 < 0.6$ and $\rho_{K_1 K_2} = 0.37$ for $K_2 > 0.6$.

The values of $K$, measured ($K_{\text{meas}}$) and calculated ($K_{\text{calc}}$) according to expression (1.28), were compared for three sets of measurement conditions in terms of the Richardson number: (1) $\text{Ri} > 0.1$; (2) $0 < \text{Ri} < 0.1$; (3) $\text{Ri} < 0$. For $\text{Ri} > 0.1$ the values of $K_{\text{meas}}$ and $K_{\text{calc}}$ are uncorrelated; in the second case $\rho_{K_{\text{meas}} K_{\text{calc}}} = 0.29$; and for $\text{Ri} < 0$ the correlation is strong: $\rho_{K_{\text{meas}} K_{\text{calc}}} = 0.97$. On the basis of these results, the authors of [47] arrive at the preliminary conclusion that (1.28) is applicable only under convection conditions ($\text{Ri} < 0$). The same conjecture is supported by a comparison between $K$ and $\text{Ri}$ (for $\text{Ri} < 0$ the correlation coefficient $\rho_{K, \text{Ri}} = 0.74$).

The 24-h variation of the coefficient $K$ is shown in Figs. 1.5 and 1.6. The values of $K$ in the first of these figures were obtained during 1974 and 1975 under roughly identical meteorological conditions in corresponding measurement periods. The second figure illustrates the 24-h variation of $K$

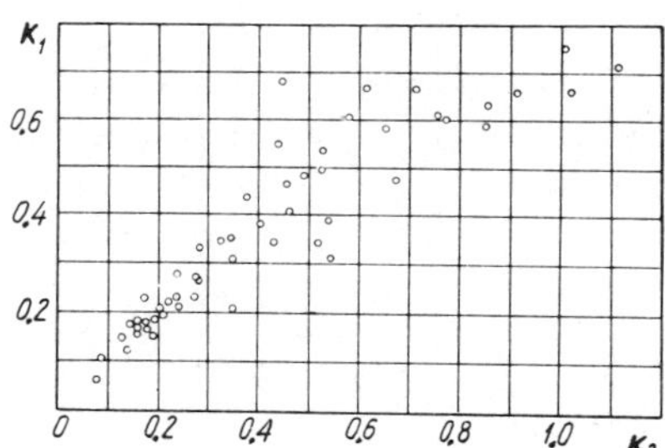

Fig. 1.4. Comparison of refraction coefficients measured at stations 1 and 2.

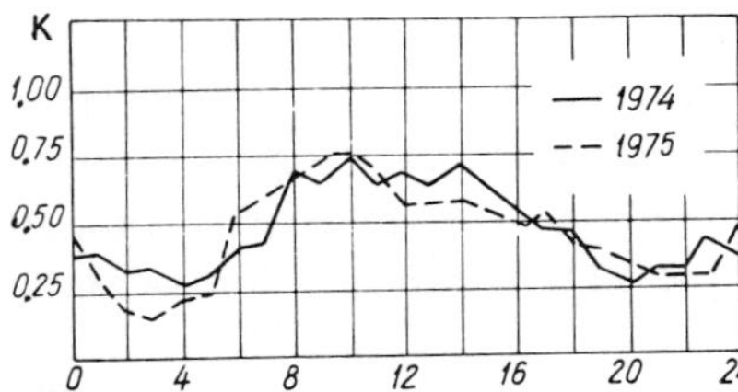

Fig. 1.5. Comparison of 24-h variations of geodesic refraction coefficient obtained in 1974 and 1975.

in certain months. It is seen that the 24-h variation of $K$ exhibits significant changes throughout the year.

Several authors [50–52] have conducted experimental investigations of geodesic refraction over water surfaces. Gabrielyan and Manucharyan [50] performed measurements over a 15-km path above the high-mountain Lake Sevan at altitudes of 6–16 m. Maslich and others [51] report the results of studies over reservoirs [53] and above extensive territories of the midlatitude and polar shelves [54–56]. Alekseev [52] has published data from measurements of the refraction coefficient in the coastal region of the Black Sea along an 8-km path at heights of 3.8–9.5 m above the water surface.

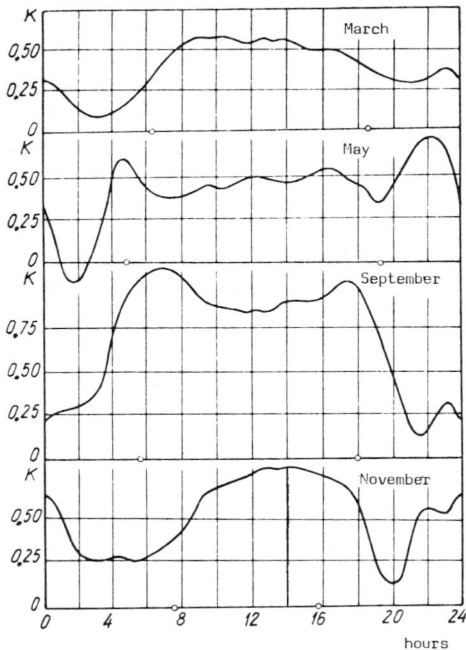


Fig. 1.6. Average 24-h variation of geodesic refraction coefficient during certain months. The circles on the time axis indicate the times of sunrise and sunset.

The results of the Lake Sevan measurements [50] indicate that the vertical refraction coefficient can fluctuate within 1-min limits during a summer day, with predominantly upward convexity of the ray trajectory. Measurements of the horizontal refractive index over a 1-yr period disclose variations within limits of three angular seconds.

The average values of the refraction coefficient obtained in the Black Sea measurements at opposite ends of the given path were found to differ, indicating the presence of corresponding inhomogeneities of the meteorological parameters of the atmosphere along the path.

Detailed refraction studies in the shelf regions [52, 54–56] led the authors to a number of important conclusions: In the atmospheric layer next to the water in the coastal region there are sizable vertical temperature gradients, which attain values of 0.4°K/m; they diminish with height according to a logarithmic law, irrespective of the type of stratification.

The overwater layer of the atmosphere in the midlatitude shelf regions has normal stratification in the morning hours, whereas around noon and in the evening hours it is stratified with inversion layers. The overwater layer in the polar shelf regions generally has inversion stratification.

Quantitative data on the refraction angles for a 5-km path under shelf conditions are summarized in Table 1.7.

The daytime behavior of the vertical refraction coefficient under shelf conditions differs sharply from its corresponding behavior under continental conditions. This difference also applies to the fluctuations of the absolute values of the given coefficient. For example, under midlatitude and polar shelf conditions its values fluctuate from $-2.09$ to $+1.66$ and from $-0.05$ to $+0.81$, respectively.

The bottom 5-m overwater layer of the atmosphere is capable of creating conditions for the superrefraction of light rays (mirages), which can be disregarded in practice.

**Table 1.7.** Extreme Values of Refraction Angle in Shelf Region

| Overwater layer, m | Refraction angle | | 24-h variation of zenith distance |
|---|---|---|---|
| | negative | positive | |
| 0–4 | $-137''$ | $+219''$ | $5'56''$ |
| 4–8 | $-58''$ | $+98''$ | $2'36''$ |
| 8–12 | $-33''$ | $+45''$ | $1'18''$ |
| 12–16 | $-17''$ | $+28''$ | $0'45''$ |
| 16–20 | $-8''$ | $+23''$ | $0'31''$ |

## 1.7. Conclusion

The foregoing discussions indicate that, despite the relative simplicity of the theoretical determination of the coefficients of terrestrial refraction, only with real-time access to information on the distributions of the meteorological parameters along the measurement path is it feasible to attain the kind of accuracy demanded in present-day practice. The smaller the errors of measurement of the meteorological parameters, the more precisely the refraction coefficient will be determined. The number of points at which the meteorological parameters are measured depends significantly on the nature of the inhomogeneities. Thus, a method that actually yields continuous profiles of the atmospheric parameters would satisfy all the requirements expected of data on the meteorological parameters. These requirements are met by the methods of long-distance laser monitoring of the atmosphere, the details of which are discussed in Chap. 7.

The accuracy demands for measurements of the meteorological parameters are especially critical in the ground layer of the atmosphere and at large zenith distances, because in either case one is dealing with the maximum inhomogeneity of the refractive-index field of the atmosphere.

An analysis of the content of the present chapter indicates that the future treatment of atmospheric refraction problems must be geared to the perfection of methods for the acquisition of quantitative information on the distribution functions of the atmospheric parameters affecting refraction, consistent with current demands of time and space. No less crucial is the development of experimental methods for the investigation of terrestrial refraction, particularly in the ground layer and at large zenith distances.

# 2

# Absorption of Laser Radiation by Atmospheric Gases

## 2.0. Introduction

The high monochromaticity of laser radiation, coupled with the sharp selectivity of its absorption by atmospheric gases, imposes rigorous demands on the accuracy of determination of both the laser spectra and the absorption spectra of atmospheric gases.

The problem of quantitative assessment of the absorption of laser radiation in the atmosphere could not have been solved on the basis of the previously accumulated store of knowledge about the absorption spectra of atmospheric gases, because the latter had been acquired without sufficient resolution for these purposes. The stated problem required the development of a more precise theory and new experimental methods. The major achievements in both respects have been made in the last 8 to 10 yr and were therefore not covered in the author's previous book [1].

## 2.1. Fundamental Definitions

### 2.1.1. Absorption Coefficient; Optical Thickness; Spectral Transmittance (Absorptance)

We assume that Bouguer's law is valid for the absorbing medium. Then the absorption coefficient $k(v)$ of the medium for radiation of frequency $v$ is defined as the proportionality factor in the differential expression for Bouguer's law [1]:

$$dI(v) = -k(v)I(v)\,dl \tag{2.1}$$

where $dI(\nu)$ is the attenuation of directional radiation of intensity $I(\nu)$ transmitted through a layer of the medium of thickness $dl$.

In the case of a homogeneous medium, the integration of (2.1) with respect to the layer thickness $l$ yields the familiar elementary expression for Bouguer's law

$$I(\nu)=I_0(\nu)e^{-k(\nu)l} \tag{2.2}$$

in which $I_0(\nu)$ and $I(\nu)$ are the radiation intensities before and after transmission through the layer of the medium of thickness $l$.

The exponent in Eq. (2.2) is customarily called the optical thickness of the medium:

$$\tau=k(\nu)l \tag{2.3}$$

Quite often, the expression for the optical thickness of the medium is formulated in terms of the column number density of the medium $w$, rather than the geometrical thickness $l$, where $w$ is the product of the gas concentration and the geometrical thickness. In this case,

$$\tau=k'(\nu)w \tag{2.4}$$

Of course, the factors $k(\nu)$ and $k'(\nu)$ in expressions (2.2) and (2.4) have different physical dimensions.

The quantities

$$T(\nu)=\frac{I(\nu)}{I_0(\nu)}=\exp\left[-k'(\nu)w\right] \quad \text{and}$$

$$A(\nu)=\frac{I_0(\nu)-I(\nu)}{I_0(\nu)}=1-\exp\left[-k'(\nu)w\right] \tag{2.5}$$

are called the spectral transmittance and spectral absorptance, respectively. It is clear that the spectral transmittance characterizes the fraction of directional light radiation of frequency $\nu$ transmitted through a given layer of the medium. Similarly, the spectral absorptance is the fraction of radiation of frequency $\nu$ absorbed by the given layer. It is also apparent that

$$T(\nu)=1-A(\nu) \tag{2.6}$$

It is evident from expressions (2.1)–(2.4) that the absorption coefficient $k(\nu)$ is a characteristic of the absorptive properties of the medium, and its known value is sufficient for quantitative estimation of the fraction of monochromatic radiation absorbed (transmitted) by the given layer of the medium.

## 2.1.2. Transmission (Absorption) Function; Total Absorption

The transmission and absorption functions characterize the fractions of radiation in the spectral interval $\Delta\nu = \nu_2 - \nu_1$ that are transmitted through a given layer of the medium and absorbed by it. Thus, they are the analogs of the spectral transmittance and spectral absorptance for the case of non-monochromatic radiation. In accordance with this definition, we write [1]

$$T = \frac{\int_{\nu_1}^{\nu_2} I(\nu)\, d\nu}{\int_{\nu_1}^{\nu_2} I_0(\nu)\, d\nu}; \qquad A = \frac{\int_{\nu_1}^{\nu_2} \left[ I_0(\nu) - I(\nu) \right] d\nu}{\int_{\nu_1}^{\nu_2} I_0(\nu)\, d\nu} \tag{2.7}$$

On the basis of (2.5), using expressions (2.7) for the transmission ($T$) and absorption ($A$) functions, we obtain

$$T = \frac{\int_{\nu_1}^{\nu_2} I_0(\nu) T(\nu)\, d\nu}{\int_{\nu_1}^{\nu_2} I_0(\nu)\, d\nu}; \qquad A = \frac{\int_{\nu_1}^{\nu_2} I_0(\nu) A(\nu)\, d\nu}{\int_{\nu_1}^{\nu_2} I_0(\nu)\, d\nu} \tag{2.8}$$

$$T = \frac{\int_{\nu_1}^{\nu_2} I_0(\nu) \exp\left[ -k'(\nu)w \right] d\nu}{\int_{\nu_1}^{\nu_2} I_0(\nu)\, d\nu};$$

$$A = \frac{\int_{\nu_1}^{\nu_2} I_0(\nu) \left\{ 1 - \exp\left[ -k'(\nu)w \right] \right\} d\nu}{\int_{\nu_1}^{\nu_2} I_0(\nu)\, d\nu} \tag{2.9}$$

In the special case $I_0(\nu) = \text{const}$, $\nu \in [\nu_1, \nu_2]$, we have

$$T = \frac{1}{\nu_2 - \nu_1} \int_{\nu_1}^{\nu_2} T(\nu)\, d\nu; \qquad A = \frac{1}{\nu_2 - \nu_1} \int_{\nu_1}^{\nu_2} A(\nu)\, d\nu \tag{2.10}$$

or, on the basis of (2.5),

$$T = \frac{1}{\nu_2 - \nu_1} \int_{\nu_1}^{\nu_2} \exp\left[-k'(\nu)w\right] d\nu;$$

$$A = \frac{1}{\nu_2 - \nu_1} \int_{\nu_1}^{\nu_2} \left\{1 - \exp\left[-k'(\nu)w\right]\right\} d\nu \qquad (2.11)$$

We stress the fact that expressions (2.10) and (2.11) are valid only in the special case where the intensity of the radiation incident on the absorbing layer is independent of the radiation frequency within the analyzed spectral interval $\Delta\nu = \nu_2 - \nu_1$. This fact is not always acknowledged in the literature.

It is evident from (2.7) and (2.9) that the transmission and absorption functions depend not only on the absorptive properties of the medium, but also on the emission spectrum of the source in the investigated frequency interval. Accordingly, to characterize the absorptive properties of the medium in a given spectral interval apart from the influence of the emitting source, we introduce the concept of the total (or integral) absorption, defining it as follows:

$$B = \int_{\nu_1}^{\nu_2} A(\nu) \, d\nu \qquad (2.12)$$

It attains its maximum value for $A(\nu) = 1$ over the entire spectral interval $\Delta\nu = \nu_2 - \nu_1$. The total absorption is expressed in frequency units, and its magnitude may be regarded as the width of a certain spectral interval in which $A(\nu) = 1$. In this sense, the total absorption is referred to as the equivalent width of the given spectral interval.

Expressions (2.1)–(2.12) are all written for the case in which the frequency $\nu$ is taken as the spectral coordinate. The same expressions are applicable when the spectral coordinate is the wavelength $\lambda$. It must be realized, however, that expressions (2.7) and (2.9) yield the same values of the transmission and absorption functions, irrespective of which spectral coordinate is adopted, whereas expressions (2.10) and (2.11) written in terms of the coordinates $\nu$ and $\lambda$ are not equivalent, i.e.,

$$\frac{1}{\nu_2 - \nu_1} \int_{\nu_1}^{\nu_2} T(\nu) \, d\nu \neq \frac{1}{\lambda_2 - \lambda_1} \int_{\lambda_1}^{\lambda_2} T(\lambda) \, d\lambda \qquad (2.13)$$

$$\frac{1}{\nu_2 - \nu_1} \int_{\nu_1}^{\nu_2} A(\nu) \, d\nu \neq \frac{1}{\lambda_2 - \lambda_1} \int_{\lambda_1}^{\lambda_2} A(\lambda) \, d\lambda \qquad (2.14)$$

$$\frac{1}{\nu_2 - \nu_1} \int_{\nu_1}^{\nu_2} e^{-k(\nu)w}\, d\nu \neq \frac{1}{\lambda_2 - \lambda_1} \int_{\lambda_1}^{\lambda_2} e^{-k(\lambda)w}\, d\lambda \qquad (2.15)$$

$$\frac{1}{\nu_2 - \nu_1} \int_{\nu_1}^{\nu_2} (1 - e^{-k(\nu)w})\, d\nu \neq \frac{1}{\lambda_2 - \lambda_1} \int_{\lambda_1}^{\lambda_2} (1 - e^{-k(\lambda)w})\, d\lambda \qquad (2.16)$$

All of the foregoing expressions are valid for the case in which Bouguer's law is applicable to the description of the attenuation of radiation propagating in an absorbing medium. The limits of applicability of this law will be discussed in a separate section. It follows from the given equations that the energy attenuation of monochromatic and nonmonochromatic radiation is uniquely determined, within the limits of validity of Bouguer's law, by the values of the absorption coefficients. In this chapter, therefore, our attention is devoted mainly to problems relating to the determination of the absorption coefficients.

## 2.1.3. Applicability of Expressions for Estimation of the Absorption of Laser Radiation in the Atmosphere

The laser energy losses due to absorption of laser radiation by atmospheric gases can be estimated [2] by means of expressions (2.5) or (2.7)–(2.9), depending on the monochromaticity of the laser radiation and the selectivity of absorption by atmospheric gases in the corresponding spectral region.

Expressions (2.5) can be used in situations where the absorption coefficients can be considered to be independent of the frequency (wavelength) within the limits of the laser emission spectrum. This state of affairs is realized, for example, in regions that are free of absorption lines, in which case we speak of continuous absorption associated with the wings of the lines. This situation is, in fact, the most important one in practice, where the absorption coefficients assume their minimum values, and the associated spectral intervals themselves are called atmospheric windows.

When the narrow laser emission line coincides with the middle part of the broader absorption line, it is again permissible to neglect the frequency dependence of the absorption coefficient within the limits of the laser line and, hence, to use expressions (2.5), which describe exponential decay of the radiation with distance or the absorbing mass of the gas, as characterized by its column number density.

In all cases where it is impossible to neglect the frequency dependence of the absorption coefficient within the limits of the laser spectrum, the absorption of laser radiation by atmospheric gases must be estimated on the basis of the expressions (2.7)–(2.9) for the transmission and absorption functions. Now the decay of the radiation with distance or with the column number density of the gas is no longer described by an exponential law. This kind of absorption occurs in situations where the laser emission spectrum comprises a set of lines, each of which is such that the absorption coefficients are invariant within its spectral width, but has different values for different emission lines of the spectrum.

Whereas it is sufficient in connection with (2.5) to know one value of the absorption coefficient in order to predict the absorption of laser radiation for any layer thickness in the medium or for any value of the column number density of the gas, in the case of expressions (2.7)–(2.9) it is necessary to know the set of values of the absorption coefficient within the limits of the laser emission spectrum before it is possible to determine, by numerical integration, the transmission (absorption) function for each layer thickness or each value of the settled layer of gas.

When expressions (2.5) are applicable for the experimental determination of the laser energy absorbed by atmospheric gases, it suffices to obtain an accurate measurement for one layer of the medium in order to solve the problem for any other layer of the same medium. When expressions (2.5) are inapplicable, the transmission (absorption) functions must be measured for a wide interval of values of the column number density of the gas before it is possible to determine the required values for a given intermediate layer by a suitable interpolation method.

Finally, expressions (2.10) and (2.11) describe the case in which, for one reason or another, it is necessary to know the transmission (absorption) function for a part of the laser spectrum in which $I_0(\nu) = \text{const}$. Such is the case for the relative broad emission spectra dye lasers or lasers whose spectrum is specially formed in such a way as to permit neglect of the frequency dependence of the intensity.

## 2.2. Absorption at an Individual Line

The molecular absorption spectrum represents a set of individual spectral lines, each of which broadens independently of the others and is characterized by its center position, intensity, and line shape. The spectral line is therefore the basic element of such a spectrum. For this reason, we begin our discussion of the problems of laser absorption by atmospheric gases with considerations of the absorption laws for the individual line. These problems have been the topic of a great many studies, the results of which have been generalized in several books and surveys (see, e.g., [3–9]). The center position and intensity of the line are completely determined by the quantum structure of the molecule, and the line contour evolves under the action of a number of factors, which are discussed briefly below.

## 2.2.1. Shape of the Spectral Line

Under the conditions of the earth's atmosphere, the line contour is determined by: (1) radiation decay processes; (2) the Doppler effect; (3) molecular collision effects.

### 2.2.1.1. Natural Linewidth

Radiative or natural broadening of the spectral line is caused by interaction of the quantum system with zero-point oscillations of the electromagnetic field. The intensity distribution in the line is described by the expression

$$k(\nu) \sim \frac{1}{\pi} \frac{\gamma_{\mathfrak{N}}}{(\nu-\nu_0)^2+\gamma_{\mathfrak{N}}^2}, \qquad \gamma_{\mathfrak{N}} = \frac{1}{2\pi\tau_i} + \frac{1}{2\pi\tau_f} \tag{2.17}$$

where $\nu_0$ is the center frequency of the line, $\tau_{i(f)}$ is the lifetime of the initial (final) transition state, and $2\gamma_{\mathfrak{N}}$ is the natural linewidth, which is equal to the spectral interval between points of the line contour $\nu_1$ and $\nu_2$ (Fig. 2.1) specified by the condition

$$k(\nu_1)=k(\nu_2)=\tfrac{1}{2}k(\nu_0) \tag{2.18}$$

For atmospheric gases, the quantity $\gamma_{\mathfrak{N}}$ is negligible in comparison with the linewidths associated with Doppler and collision effects.

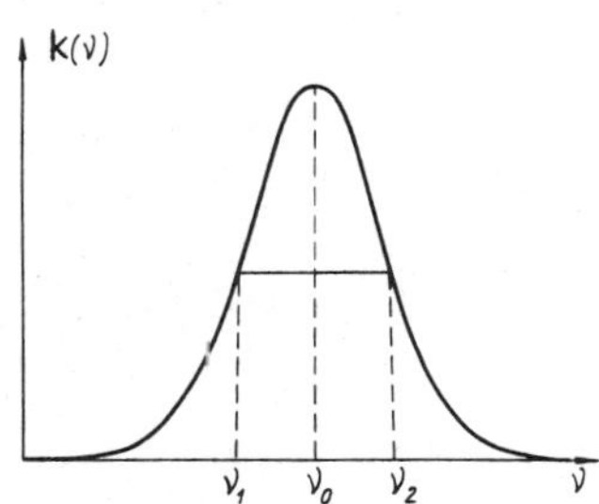


Fig. 2.1. Contour of absorption line.

### 2.2.1.2. *Doppler Broadening*

In the case of thermodynamic equilibrium for translational molecular degrees of freedom, such that the molecules have a Maxwell velocity distribution, the contour of the spectral line subjected only to Doppler broadening has the form

$$k(\nu) = \frac{S(\ln 2)^{1/2}}{\pi^{\frac{1}{2}}\gamma_{\mathscr{D}}} \exp\left[-\left(\frac{\nu-\nu_0}{\gamma_{\mathscr{D}}}\right)^2\right] \tag{2.19}$$

where

$$\gamma_{\mathscr{D}} = \frac{\nu_0}{c}\left(\frac{2kT}{m}\right)^{1/2} \tag{2.20}$$

is the Doppler half-width of the line, $T$ is the absolute temperature, $m$ is the mass of the molecule, $c$ is the speed of light, $k$ is the Boltzmann constant, and

$$S = \int_0^\infty k(\nu)\,d\nu \tag{2.21}$$

is the line intensity, which will be discussed separately.

It is evident from (2.20) that the Doppler half-width of the line depends most strongly on the center frequency of the line. The temperature in the troposphere and stratosphere at heights where the main mass of the absorbing gases is concentrated exhibits roughly a 1.5-fold variation. Consequently, for the given spectral line in this case, $\gamma_{\mathscr{D}}$ can vary approximately $\pm 15\%$ from the mean value corresponding to the mean temperature.

At a temperature $T = 300°K$, the Doppler width for the atomic oxygen line ($\lambda = 5577$ Å) is equal to $3.3 \times 10^{-2}$ cm$^{-1}$ [10]. The lines of water vapor in the region of the indicated part of the spectrum have close to this value of $\gamma_{\mathscr{D}}$. The values of $\gamma_{\mathscr{D}}$ for the lines in other parts of the spectrum and for other absorbing gases can be estimated without difficulty.

### 2.2.1.3. *Collision Broadening*

The theories of Lorentz and Anderson are most commonly used to describe the effects of spectral line broadening due to collisions of atmospheric gas molecules in the visible and infrared regions of the spectrum.

According to Lorentz [11], the contour of the absorption line is expressed by the familiar equation

$$k(\nu) = \frac{S}{\pi}\frac{\gamma_{\mathscr{L}}}{(\nu-\nu_0)^2 + \gamma_{\mathscr{L}}^2} \tag{2.22}$$

which is often called the dispersion contour in the literature. In Eq. (2.22), $S$ is the line intensity [see (2.21)], $\nu_0$ is the center frequency of the line,

$$\gamma_{\mathcal{L}} = \frac{1}{4\pi\tau(v)} \tag{2.23}$$

is the line half-width, and $\tau(v)$ is the lifetime of the absorbing molecule in the excited state; this lifetime depends on the collision velocity of the molecule $v$.

If we adopt the value of $\gamma_{\mathcal{L}}$ corresponding to the mean value of $\tau(v)$, we obtain the following expression for $\gamma_{\mathcal{L}}$ from the kinetic theory of gases in this case:

$$\gamma_{\mathcal{L}} = \sum_i n_i \sigma_i^2 \left[ \frac{2kT}{\pi} \left( \frac{1}{m} + \frac{1}{m_i} \right) \right]^{1/2} \tag{2.24}$$

where $n_i$ is the density of molecules of the $i$th species, $\sigma_i$ is the effective distance between the absorbing molecule and molecule of the $i$th species, and $m, m_i$ are the masses of these molecules. Here the term "effective" refers to the distance at which molecular interaction takes place, resulting in broadening of the spectral line.

Thus, according to the kinetic theory of gases, the line half-width $\gamma_{\mathcal{L}}$ is proportional to the pressure. This is an extremely important dependence, because the pressure in the atmosphere varies over a very great range. The dependence of $\gamma_{\mathcal{L}}$ on $\sigma_i$ is also significant, because $\sigma_i$ depends both on the types of pairs of colliding molecules and on the corresponding energy levels, or on the rotational quantum number $j$. The temperature dependence of $\gamma_{\mathcal{L}}$ is of the same nature as in the case of line broadening due to the Doppler effect.

A comparatively simple expression is obtained for $\gamma_{\mathcal{L}}$ in the case of a two-component gas mixture:

$$\gamma_{\mathcal{L}} = \left( \frac{2kT}{\pi} \right)^{1/2} \left[ n_a \sigma_{aa}^2 \left( \frac{2}{m_a} \right)^{1/2} + n_b \sigma_{ab}^2 \left( \frac{1}{m_a} + \frac{1}{m_b} \right)^{1/2} \right] \tag{2.25}$$

where the subscripts $a$ and $b$ refer to the absorbing and nonabsorbing molecules; $\sigma_{aa}$ and $\sigma_{ab}$ are, respectively, the effective radii of optical collisions of absorbing molecules with each other and with molecules of the impurity gas.

For a fixed value of the temperature, the expression for $\gamma_{\mathcal{L}}$ can be written in the form

$$\gamma_{\mathcal{L}} = \gamma_{\mathcal{L}}^0 (P_b + \sigma P_a) \tag{2.26}$$

which lends itself very well to interpretation of the role of the types of molecules in the broadening of the lines. In expression (2.26), $\gamma_\varrho^0$ is the line half-width under standard conditions, $P_a$ and $P_b$ are the partial pressures of the absorbing and nonabsorbing gases, and $\sigma$ is the relative efficiency of optical molecular collisions $a \to a$ and $a \to b$. The quantity $\sigma$ indicates how efficiently the absorbing molecules collide with one another from the point of view of broadening of the spectral line relative to their collisions with nonabsorbing molecules. The values of $\sigma$ depend on the species of molecules $a$ and $b$. Its values will be discussed in the section of the chapter devoted to the description of the absorption spectra of atmospheric gases.

Introducing the notation

$$P_b + \sigma P_a = P_{\text{eff}} \tag{2.27}$$

where $P_{\text{eff}}$ is the "effective" pressure, we can write a simple expression for $\gamma_\varrho$ with regard for the temperature dependence of $\gamma_\varrho$:

$$\gamma_\varrho = \gamma_\varrho^0 \frac{P_{\text{eff}}}{P_0} \left( \frac{T_0}{T} \right)^{1/2} \tag{2.28}$$

where $P_0$ and $T_0$ are the pressure and temperature corresponding to standard conditions.

In the real atmosphere, $P_{\text{eff}}$ can be replaced in many cases by the total pressure $P$ since the pressure $P_b$ of the nonabsorbing gases is significantly greater than the product $\sigma P_a$. In these cases,

$$\gamma_\varrho = \gamma_\varrho^0 \frac{P}{P_0} \left( \frac{T_0}{T} \right)^{1/2} \tag{2.29}$$

The quantum-mechanical theory developed by Anderson [12] for the pressure broadening of spectral lines is based on the fact that energy transitions can take place in both molecules of a colliding pair. Expression (2.24) is taken as the initial equation for $\gamma_\varrho$, but the effective distances are specified with regard for possible energy transitions in the colliding molecules. The following expression is obtained for $\gamma_\varrho$ in this case:

$$\gamma_\varrho^{ij} = \sum_{j_2} \left[ \frac{2kT}{\pi} \left( \frac{1}{m} + \frac{1}{m_0} \right) \right]^{1/2} n(j_2) \sigma^2(i, j, j_2)$$

where $n(j_2)$ is the concentration of perturbing molecules,

$$\sigma(i, j, j_2) = \sum_{j_2', i'} \sigma(i, i'; j_2, j_2'; j) + \sum_{j_2', j'} \sigma(i; j_2, j_2'; j, j') \qquad (2.30)$$

$i, i'$; $j, j'$ are indices characterizing the state of the absorbing molecule for which the transition $i \to j$ takes place without interaction with a perturbing molecule, and $j_2$, $j_2'$ are indices characterizing the state of the perturbing molecule. Molecular collision induces transitions $i \to i'$ and $j \to j'$ in the absorbing molecule and $j_2 \to j_2'$ in the perturbing molecule.

The available results of calculations of the line half-widths for atmospheric gases and the results of corresponding experimental studies show that $\gamma_\mathcal{L}$ has values of the order of $10^{-2}$ to $10^{-1}$ cm$^{-1}$ in the ground layer of the atmosphere [1].


### 2.2.1.4. Combined Action of Doppler and Molecular Collision Effects

Doppler and collision effects operate concurrently in the atmosphere, but their role differs substantially at different heights because the half-widths associated with the Doppler effect do not depend on the pressure, whereas $\gamma_\mathcal{L}$ depends linearly on the pressure. In the ground layer, the broadening of the majority of the absorption lines for atmospheric gases in the infrared region and all lines in the visible is mainly attributable to molecular collisions. The Doppler effect is customarily ignored under these conditions. Together with the pressure, the half-width $\gamma_\mathcal{L}$ decreases with the height, so that for each absorption line of any atmospheric gas there must be a height at which $\gamma_\mathcal{L} = \gamma_\mathcal{D}$. For lines having the same value of $\gamma_\mathcal{L}$, this height will be greater the lower the center frequency $\nu_0$ of the line. For different values of $\gamma_\mathcal{L}$ and a fixed value of $\nu_0$, the given height will be greater for broad lines and lower for narrow lines.

Consider as an example $\gamma_\mathcal{L} = 0.08$ cm$^{-1}$, which is the most probable value for atmospheric gases in the ground layer; let us compare it with the value of $\gamma_\mathcal{D}$ for the atomic oxygen line ($\lambda = 5577$ Å) at $T = 300°$K: $\gamma_\mathcal{D} = 3.3 \times 10^{-2}$ cm$^{-1}$. It turns out that the height at which $\gamma_\mathcal{L} = \gamma_\mathcal{D}$ is equal to 7 km in this case. Naturally, this height will be greater for broader lines in the given part of the spectrum and smaller for narrower lines. It is evident from the example that it may be necessary to take the combined Doppler and collision effects into account even at tropospheric heights for the visible region of the spectrum.

The combined analysis of both line-broadening effects yields the following expression for the absorption coefficient:

$$k(\nu) = \frac{k_0 y}{\pi} \int_{-\infty}^{\infty} \frac{\exp(-t^2)}{y^2 + (x-t)^2} dt \qquad (2.31)$$

where

$$k_0 = \frac{S}{\gamma_{\mathfrak{D}}} (\ln 2/\pi)^{1/2}; \qquad y = \frac{\gamma_{\mathfrak{L}}}{\gamma_{\mathfrak{D}}} (\ln 2)^{1/2}; \qquad x = \frac{\nu - \nu_0}{\gamma_{\mathfrak{D}}} (\ln 2)^{1/2}$$

$$(2.32)$$

A comparison of expressions (2.19) and (2.22), which describe the contours of the absorption lines due to Doppler and molecular collision effects, shows that the values of the absorption coefficients in the wings of the line decay more rapidly in the case of the first effect than in the case of the dispersion contour. This effect is illustrated in Fig. 2.2 by the corresponding curves plotted for the case of equal intensities and half-widths. It must be emphasized, however, that the question of whether the dispersion contour correctly describes the behavior of the wings requires special consideration, to which a separate section of the chapter is devoted. The inception of the Doppler effect at the molecular frequency $\omega_0$ is limited by the condition $1/\tau \ll \omega_0 \bar{v}/c = \kappa \bar{v}$, where $\kappa = 2\pi/\lambda$, $\tau$ is the time between collisions, and $\bar{v}$ is the mean thermal velocity; this condition can be rewritten in the form $2\pi l \gg \lambda$ $(\kappa l \gg 1)$, where $l = \bar{v}\tau$ is the mean free path and $\lambda = 2\pi c/\omega_0$ is the optical wavelength.

If the number of collisions is such that $\kappa l \ll 1$, then the collision perturbations of the energy states of the molecules (phase shift and amplitude variation of stationary states) and the resulting decrease of the lifetime

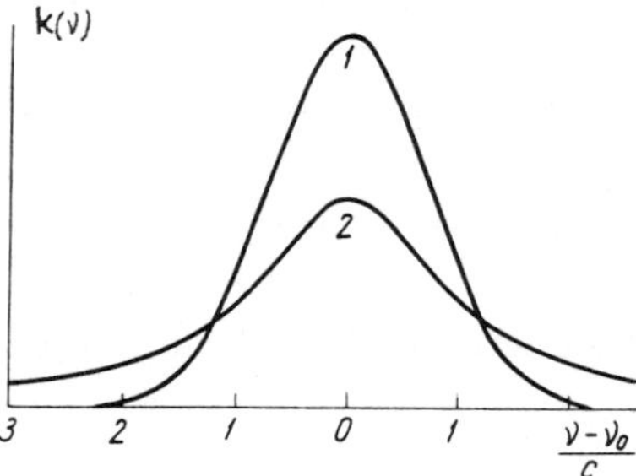


Fig. 2.2. Line contours associated with Doppler broadening (1) and with collision or radiation-extinction broadening (2) for equal intensities and linewidths.

of molecules in the excited state and, accordingly, broadening of the line contour can be joined by variations in the shape and parameters of the line contours due to collision limiting or slowing of molecular motion at a distance $\lambda/2\pi$. In the radio range, where limiting or slowing of the translational motion of a molecule to $l \leqslant \lambda/2\pi$ is possible at low pressures such that phase shifting and, hence, uniform broadening is slight, the evolution of the line contour acquires a diffusion mechanism, namely collision narrowing and deformation of the Doppler into a dispersion contour (Dicke effect [14]). In linear optical spectroscopy, the observation of contour deformation is clearly possible at transitions corresponding to large values of the rotational quantum number $J$, for which the collision broadening factor is small ($B_{br} \leqslant 0.1$ MHz/Torr), and under the condition $l \leqslant \lambda/2\pi$ collision broadening does not mask the inception of the diffusion contour-shaping mechanism.

Specific cases of the inception of diffusion narrowing of the Doppler contour of atomic spectral lines have been investigated in a number of theoretical papers [9, 13, 15–19]. Even in the event of statistical independence of the phase shift of states and variation of $\bar{v}$ due to collision of an absorbing with a perturbing molecule, the results of a calculation of the line contour within the context of the semiclassical approach indicate that the convolution of the profiles of the Doppler and dispersion contours is a first approximation of the real contour. The results of a theoretical analysis of particular cases of statistical interdependence of both parameters show that the effect is stronger for the middle part of the contour than for the wings of the line [13].

Armstrong [20] has calculated the influence of this effect on the value of the molecular extinction in the atmosphere for the slant-path propagation of radiation from a $CO_2$ laser. For $\lambda = 10.6$ $\mu$m the influence of collision narrowing along paths $L = 10$ km with $\alpha = 85°$ induces a 20% error in the prediction of atmospheric extinction. The literature does not contain any experimental data on the inception of the diffusion contour-formation mechanism for atmospheric gases, unless one considers investigations of the spontaneous Raman scattering spectra for $N_2$ and $CO$ [21].

## 2.2.2. Line Intensity

As mentioned [see Eq. (2.21)], the spectral line intensity represents the integral of the absorption coefficient describing the line contour.

Quantum mechanics yields the following expression for the line intensity associated with the transition of a molecule from the $j$th to the $i$th state

[10]:

$$S_{ij} = \frac{n_j}{g_i n} \frac{8\pi^3 \nu_{i,j} |R_{i,j}|^2}{3hc} \left[ 1 - \exp\left( \frac{-h\nu_{i,j}}{kT} \right) \right] \tag{2.33}$$

where $n_j$ is the concentration of molecules in the lowest state, $n$ is the concentration of all molecules, $g_i$ is the statistical weight of the $i$th state, $\nu_{i,j}$ is the transition frequency, $|R_{i,j}|^2$ is the square of the $ij$th matrix element of the dipole moment, $T$ is the absolute temperature, $h$ and $k$ are the Planck and Boltzmann constants, and $c$ is the speed of light.

The matrix element of the dipole moment $\mathbf{M}$ is expressed in terms of the wave function of molecular states $\Psi_i$ and $\Psi_j$:

$$R_{i,j} = \int \Psi_i^* \mathbf{M} \Psi_j \, dv \tag{2.34}$$

[The wave functions are the solutions of the Schrödinger equation. The integration in (2.34) is carried out over the entire configuration space; $dv$ is an element of that space.]

The wave functions obey the well-known orthogonality relation

$$\int \Psi_i^* \Psi_j \, dv = 0 \ (i \neq j) \tag{2.35}$$

from which we arrive at the important conclusion that the matrix element $R_{i,j}$ is equal to zero in the case of a constant dipole moment. Thus, if the dipole moment of the molecule remains invariant in transition, the corresponding oscillatory process is optically inactive, and its corresponding absorption line is absent in the spectrum.

We note that dipole interaction of an electromagnetic field with matter is not the only factor responsible for light absorption. Spectral lines can also appear in connection with variations of the magnetic dipole as well as the electric and magnetic multipoles, with concomitant energy transitions. However, the intensities of these lines are very small. Thus, transitions associated with variation of the molecular electric dipole moment yield line intensities $10^5$ to $10^8$ times greater in order of magnitude than in the case of variations of the magnetic dipole and electric quadrupole moments.

The matrix elements $R_{i,j}$ are related to the well-known Einstein coefficients $A_{i,j}$ characterizing the probability of stimulated emission and absorption between the $i$th and $j$th molecular levels:

$$A_{i,j} = \frac{64\pi^4 \nu_{i,j}^3}{3hg_i c} |R_{i,j}|^2 \tag{2.36}$$

The coefficient $A_{i,j}$ for electric dipole emission has values of the order of $10^8$, 10, and 1 $\sec^{-1}$ for electron, vibrational, and rotational transitions, respectively.

The most difficult problem in calculating the line intensities is the determination of the squares of the matrix elements $|R_{i,j}|^2$ of the transition dipole moment. We shall return to this problem in discussing methods for the determination of the absorption coefficients.

## 2.3. Shape of the Far Wings

The problem of the shape of the far wings has lately taken on exceptional significance. On the one hand, the significance is in connection with the fact that all existing experimental data on continuous absorption in the atmospheric windows conflict both with one another and with the predictions of existing theories, while, on the other hand, precise quantitative data on the coefficients of continuous absorption in the far wings are urgently needed for the solution of inverse problems in satellite meteorology, where the distribution curves of particular physical parameters of the atmosphere are reproduced from the results of measurements of the spectral composition of outgoing radiation.

The most successful solution of the problem of the shape of the far wings of the absorption lines and, hence, of the nature of continuous absorption in the atmospheric windows has been realized in just the last few years. The results of the corresponding theory are presented, together with a systematic description of that theory, in a book published in 1977 [22]. We now briefly summarize the theory and its implications.

### 2.3.1. Mathematical Foundation of the Theory

We consider a gas existing in thermodynamic equilibrium and isolate from it an elementary volume of such proportions that, on the one hand, the long-wave approximation and, on the other, statistical-analytic methods are applicable. Then, using the standard technique, we reduce the multiple-particle problem to the binary case and invoke the semiclassical approach, whereby molecules are quantum entities and their interaction (motion relative to their center of mass) is treated as classical. After reduction to binary collisions, we write the correlation function for the dipole moment and calculate it, including averaging over the elementary volume. We ultimately obtain the following expression for the absorption coefficient associated with the transition $\alpha \to \beta$:

$$k_{\alpha\beta}(\nu) = \frac{4\pi^2\nu}{ch}\left[1 - \exp\left(\frac{-h\nu}{kT}\right)\right]\mathfrak{N}'\mathfrak{N}''\rho_\alpha \left\langle\left\langle\left|\int_0^\infty dt\, e^{i\nu t}\langle\alpha|Q^{-1}PQ|\beta\rangle\right|^2\right\rangle\right\rangle$$

$$(2.37)$$

where $\alpha$ and $\beta$ characterize the sets of quantum numbers, $\mathfrak{N}'$ and $\mathfrak{N}''$ are the concentrations of absorbing and perturbing particles, $\rho_\alpha$ denotes elements of the probability density matrix for the absorbing molecule, $P$ is the dipole moment of the absorbing molecule, the brackets $\langle\langle\ \rangle\rangle$ signify the operation of averaging over states of the perturbing molecule and over the elementary volume, and $Q$ is the evolution operator.

Next we pose the problem of obtaining expressions in a form suitable for further analysis. We use the following approximations: (1) an adiabatic approximation that enables us to separate intramolecular motions and to represent the wave function of the unperturbed molecule by the product of the electron, vibrational, and rotational parts; (2) an adiabatic approximation for solution of the equations for the evolution operator $Q$, assuming that transitions between different vibrational and rotational states are not induced by intermolecular collisions; (3) an approximation associated with representation of the perturbation due to molecular collisions, where this approximation is expressed in the form of an expansion in multiples:

$$U_b = \sum_m A_m / R^m \tag{2.38}$$

where $R$ is the intermolecular spacing and the trajectories of the molecules are assumed to be rectilinear; (4) asymptotic methods for the estimation of integrals in regard to computation of the time integral.

Applying the indicated approximations and averaging over the elementary volume, we obtain the following expressions for the absorption coefficients:

$$k(\nu) = \sum_{\alpha,\beta} k_{\alpha\beta}(\nu) \tag{2.39}$$

$$k_{\alpha\beta}(\nu) = S_{\alpha\beta}\gamma_{\alpha\beta}(\nu)F_{\alpha\beta}(\nu)\Phi_{\alpha\beta}(\nu)M_{\alpha\beta}(\nu) \tag{2.40}$$

where $k(\nu)$ is the absorption coefficient at frequency $\nu$, representing the sum of the absorption coefficients of different lines with center frequencies $\nu_{\alpha\beta}$,

$S_{\alpha\beta}$ is the integral line intensity,

$$\gamma_{\alpha\beta} = \frac{\nu}{\nu_{\alpha\beta}} \times \frac{1 - \exp(-h\nu/kT)}{1 - \exp(-h\nu_{\alpha\beta}/kT)} \tag{2.41}$$

$$F_{\alpha\beta} = \frac{1}{R_{\alpha\beta}} \int_0^{R_{\alpha\beta}} \frac{R \exp[-V(R)/kT]}{\left(R_{\alpha\beta}^2 - R^2\right)^{1/2}} dR \tag{2.42}$$

$$\Phi_{\alpha\beta}(\nu) = \exp\left[-\mathcal{D}\tau_{\alpha\beta,\nu}\frac{\nu^2}{c^2}\right] \tag{2.43}$$

$$\tau_{\alpha\beta,\nu} = \left\{2\pi\upsilon \int_0^{R_{\alpha\beta}} R \exp\left[\frac{-V(R)}{kT}\right] dR\right\}^{-1} \tag{2.44}$$

$V(R)$ is the energy of molecular interaction, $\upsilon$ is the relative velocity of the colliding molecules, and $\mathcal{D}$ is the diffusion coefficient. The significance of the quantity $R_{\alpha\beta}$ will be made clear later. The factor $M_{\alpha\beta}$ in (2.40) is associated with the binary collision correlation function. It will be analyzed below.

It is evident from Eq. (2.41) that the factor $\gamma_{\alpha\beta}$ grows increasingly significant the greater the difference between $\nu$ and $\nu_{\alpha\beta}$, i.e., the farther the wings of the line that are analyzed. The factor $F_{\alpha\beta}$ originates from averaging over the elementary volume and is associated with correct evaluation of the collision statistics.

The factor $\Phi_{\alpha\beta}$ is attributable to the spatial dispersion effect associated with diffusion of absorbing molecules from one elementary volume into another in the period between two collision events resulting in the resonance frequency mismatch $|\nu - \nu_{\alpha\beta}|$.

### 2.3.2. Determination of the Wings

The mathematical formulation of the condition governing the lower bound of the wing entails solving the stationary-point equation

$$h\nu = E_{\alpha\alpha'}(R) + E_{\beta\alpha'}(R) \tag{2.45}$$

in which $h\nu$ is the absorbed photon energy and $E$ is the energy of the interacting molecules characterized by the set of quantum numbers $\alpha, \beta, \alpha'$ ($\alpha'$ characterizes the state of the perturbing molecule). The given equation is used to find the stationary points, i.e., the intermolecular distances at which the system is capable of absorbing a photon of energy $h\nu$. It follows from (2.45) that these distances are a function of the frequency shift:

$$R_{s.p.} = R(\Delta\nu) \tag{2.46}$$

It turns out that different zones of the far wing of the spectral line are formed by collisions having different sets of parameters. Consequently, the evolution of the peripheral part of the line contour differs significantly from the evolution of the center of the line.

The following quantity is adopted as a large parameter in connection with asymptotic methods for estimation of the integral in (2.37):

$$t = (\nu - \nu_{\alpha\beta})\frac{R}{\nu} \gg 1 \tag{2.47}$$

The combination of (2.46) and (2.47) stipulates the lower limit $\Delta\nu_{min}$ of the wing frequencies described by the given theory:

$$|\nu - \nu_{\alpha\beta}| > \Delta\nu_{min} \tag{2.48}$$

The quantity $R(\Delta\nu)$ in (2.46) can be calculated on the basis of appropriate models of intermolecular collision processes, to be discussed later. For the time being, we merely note that order-of-magnitude estimates yield values of $\Delta\nu_{min}$ ranging from units to tens of reciprocal centimeters.

### 2.3.3. Exponential and Quasistatistical Wings

In this section, we are concerned primarily with the factor $F_{\alpha\beta}(R)$ in expression (2.40); it is significant in regard to the interpretation of the two kinds of far-wing profiles observed experimentally, namely exponential and quasistatistical, where the latter are similar in shape to the results of statistical theory.

Making use of expression (2.42) and the remarks concerning the stationary points, we infer that the function $F_{\alpha\beta}(R)$ quantitatively expresses the probability of realization of distances at which molecular interaction accounts for the shape of the wings. The function $F_{\alpha\beta}(R)$ can be calculated once the molecular interaction potential has been specified. Figure 2.3 gives the results of a calculation of this function for the Lennard–Jones (12,6) potential

$$V(R) = 4\varepsilon\left[(\sigma/R)^{12} - (\sigma/R)^{6}\right] \tag{2.49}$$

in which $\varepsilon$ and $\sigma$ are the parameters of the potential.

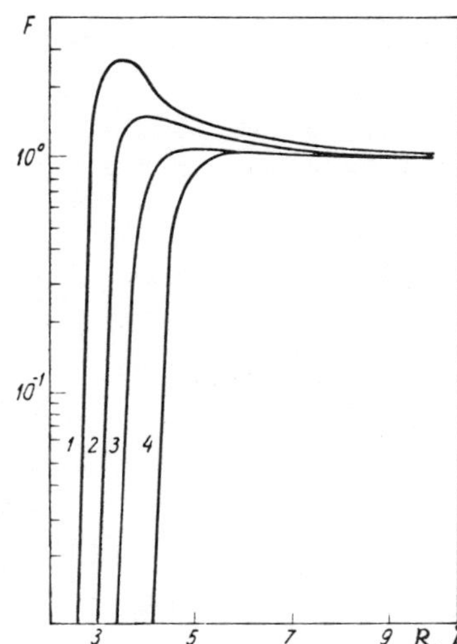


Fig. 2.3. Function $F(V(R), R)$ for the Lennard–Jones (12,6) potential. (1) $\sigma=2.7$, $\varepsilon/k=500$; (2) $\sigma=3.15$, $\varepsilon/k=360$; (3) $\sigma=3.7$, $\varepsilon/k=210$; (4) $\sigma=4.5$, $\varepsilon/k=190$.

It is seen in Fig. 2.3 that the function tends to unity for large values of $R$ and so we have the interval of frequency shifts $\Delta\nu'>\Delta\nu>\Delta\nu_{\min}$ corresponding to the condition $V(R)\ll kT$. In the second case, where $V(R)\gtrsim kT$ holds for appropriately small values of $R$ (intermolecular repulsion interval), the function $F$ exhibits an abrupt drop in the frequency interval $\Delta\nu>\Delta\nu'$. The first case corresponds to the quasistatistical zone of the periphery of the line, whereas in the second case we have exponential wings. Of course, these zones merge one into the other. We note that the occurrence of the two types of distributions has nothing to do with the need for introducing the approximation (2.38). The presence of exponential wings, observed in experiments with $CO_2$, and the correspondence between the experimental data and the calculations based on different expressions are illustrated in Fig. 2.4, which shows the region of the spectrum after the edge of the 4.3 $\mu$m band for $CO_2$. Curves 1 and 2 in this figure correspond to a dispersion contour and the contour (2.39)–(2.40) without regard for the factor $F$. Curve 3 corresponds to the empirical contour of Winter and others [23]; the crosses represent the results of a calculation according to expressions (2.39)–(2.40) with regard for $F$, and the other points represent the experimental data. We note that the empirical relation proposed in [23] well describes the given experimental data, but it is unsuitable for the description of analogous measurements in other regions of the spectrum [24]. On the other hand, as will be shown presently, the proposed theory makes it possible to interpret all the known experimental results on continuous absorption.

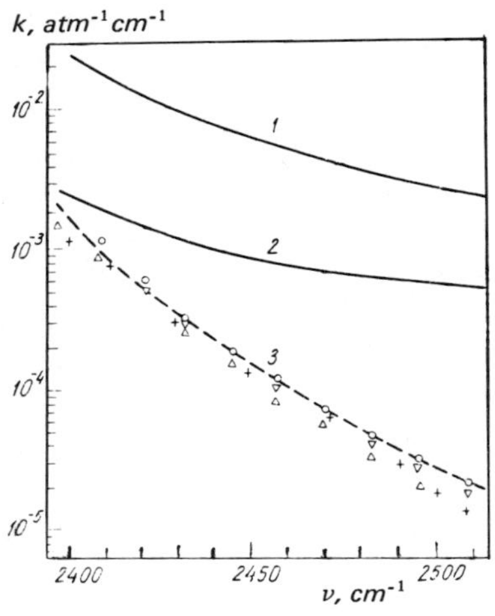



Fig. 2.4. Absorption coefficient of $CO_2$ in a mixture with $N_2$. (1) Calculated from dispersion contour; (2) calculated for $F=1$ according to (2.39) and (2.40); (3) empirical contour postulated in [23]; (I) $+$, calculated according to (2.39) and (2.40) with $F \neq 1$; (II–IV) experimental data from [23]: II, $\bigcirc$; III, $\triangle$; IV, $\triangle$.

We now examine in somewhat closer detail the problem of quasistatistical wings, in which case the factor $F_{\alpha\beta}$ can be regarded as approximately equal to unity. In this zone, the approximation of the perturbation by the multipole expansion (2.38) holds quite well, and this is important because an analysis of the results of the given theory and the existing experimental data leads to the conclusion that the spectral dispersion of multipole interactions takes place in the periphery of the line, completely accounting for the multivariety of the kinds of behavior exhibited by the absorption coefficient in the far wings.

An analysis of the possibilities for the solution of the stationary-point equation (2.45) shows that a solution can be obtained on the basis of model representations of molecular interaction in only two situations: (1) one multipole is all that remains in expression (2.38) (one-multipole approximation); (2) two terms remain in (2.38), coupled by a definite interrelationship, which results in the expression

$$\Delta\varepsilon(R) = \frac{\Delta\varepsilon_m}{R^m} + \frac{\Delta\varepsilon_{2m}}{R^{2m}} \tag{2.50}$$

(two-multipole approximation), where $\Delta\varepsilon(R)$ denotes the energy corrections to the isolated molecules due to their interaction.

We also identify two cases that are associated with the application of expression (2.50) and that depend on the signs of $\Delta\varepsilon_m$ and $\Delta\varepsilon_{2m}$:

1. constants of the same sign: $\quad \Delta\varepsilon_m > 0; \quad \Delta\varepsilon_{2m} > 0 \quad (\Delta\varepsilon_m < 0; \quad \Delta\varepsilon_{2m} < 0)$
2. constants of different signs: $\quad \Delta\varepsilon_m > 0; \quad \Delta\varepsilon_{2m} < 0 \quad (\Delta\varepsilon_m < 0; \quad \Delta\varepsilon_{2m} > 0)$

In case (1) we obtain the following expressions for the function $M_{\alpha\beta}(\nu)$ in the two-multipole approximation, neglecting the nonresonance term:

$$M_{\alpha\beta}(\nu) = \frac{4\pi N''}{(2\Delta\nu)^{1+3/m}} \left\{ \frac{\left[ \Delta\varepsilon_m + \left( \Delta\varepsilon_m^2 + 4\Delta\nu\Delta\varepsilon_{2m} \right)^{1/2} \right]^{2+3/m}}{\Delta\varepsilon_m \left[ \Delta\varepsilon_m + \left( \Delta\varepsilon_m^2 + 4\Delta\nu\Delta\varepsilon_{2m} \right)^{1/2} \right] + 4\Delta\nu\Delta\varepsilon_{2m}} \right\}$$

$$(2.51)$$

$$R_{\text{s.p.}} = \left| \frac{\Delta\varepsilon_m + \left( \Delta\varepsilon_m^2 + 4\Delta\nu\Delta\varepsilon_{2m} \right)^{1/2}}{2\Delta\nu} \right|^{1/m}$$

$$(2.52)$$

In expressions (2.50), (2.51), and below, $\Delta\nu$ and $\Delta\varepsilon$ are interpreted in the absolute-value sense.

### 2.3.4. Spectral Dispersion of Multipole Interactions

We introduce the frequency shift

$$\Delta\nu_0 = \Delta\varepsilon_m^2 / 4\Delta\varepsilon_{2m} \tag{2.53}$$

Then from expression (2.51) we obtain the following simple relations in two extreme cases:

$$M_{\alpha\beta}(\nu) \sim \frac{\Delta\varepsilon_m^{3/m}}{\Delta\nu^{1+3/m}} \qquad \text{if } \Delta\nu_0 \gg \Delta\nu \tag{2.54}$$

$$M_{\alpha\beta}(\nu) \sim \frac{\Delta\varepsilon_{2m}^{3/2m}}{\Delta\nu^{1+3/2m}} \qquad \text{if } \Delta\nu_0 \ll \Delta\nu \tag{2.55}$$

Relations (2.54) and (2.55), representing the one-multipole approximation, describe the situation in which one multipole after the other is activated with distance toward the periphery of the line, i.e., spectral dispersion of multipoles takes place at the periphery, as characterized by the fact that a higher-order multipole yields a correspondingly greater contribution to the evolution of the line contour as the frequency shift is increased.

We conclude this section by writing out an expression for the factor $M_{\alpha\beta}(\nu)$ in (2.40) in the one-multipole approximation with the nonresonance term included:

$$M_{\alpha\beta}(\nu) = \frac{4\pi N''}{m} \left\{ \frac{\delta_{\alpha\beta}}{|\nu - \nu_{\alpha\beta}|^{(3/m)+1}} + \frac{\exp(-h\nu_{\alpha\beta}/kT)\delta_{\alpha\beta}}{|\nu - \nu_{\alpha\beta}|^{(3/m)+1}} \right\} \tag{2.56}$$

where $\delta_{\alpha\beta}$ denotes the quantity $\Delta\varepsilon_m^{3/m}$ in (2.50), averaged over states of the perturbing molecule.


### 2.3.5. Comparison of Theory with Experiment

The results of a comparison of the existing experimental data on the behavior of the absorption coefficient in the far wings of the spectral lines with the corresponding results of calculations based on the given theory are described in detail in [22]. Here we concern ourselves primarily with the particular studies whose experimental data have been used for the indicated comparisons, stressing the fact that consistency between theory and experiment is obtained in every case where reference is made to the wavelength dependence of the absorption coefficient.

For the analysis we use experimental data on the absorption coefficients in the wings of the lines for molecules of ammonia [25–29], NO [30], CO [31], and water vapor [32–41]. The behavior of the absorption coefficient in the far wings differs in all these cases. The difference has been successfully interpreted with allowance for the spectral dispersion of multipole interactions. Below we highlight some of the most interesting results of comparisons between theory and experiment.

We first consider the important practical problem of the continuous absorption of water vapor in the long-wave transmission window of the atmosphere from wavelengths of 8 to 12 $\mu$m, which is widely used in satellite meteorology for remote sensing of the profiles of the atmospheric parameters on the basis of measurements of the spectral composition of outgoing radiation. The given range of wavelengths is very important in connection with the high sensitivity of the behavior of the water-vapor absorption coefficient to various factors entering into expression (2.40). This fact is illustrated by Fig. 2.5 ($H_2O$–$N_2$ mixture), in which curve 1 is obtained from the theory for $F=1, \gamma=1$, and the quantity $M$ is determined solely by the resonance term in (2.56). Curve 2 is calculated with regard for the nonresonance term in (2.56). It is seen that both curves deviate substantially from the experimental data. Allowance for the factor $\gamma$ (curve 3) increases the deviation from theoretical results. Only when all factors are taken into account, including the factor $F$ (curves 4 and 5), is satisfactory agreement of the theory with experiment obtained. It turns out in this case that the main contribution to the absorption coefficient is from high-order interactions, namely nonresonance dipole–quadrupole interaction, for which $m=8$.

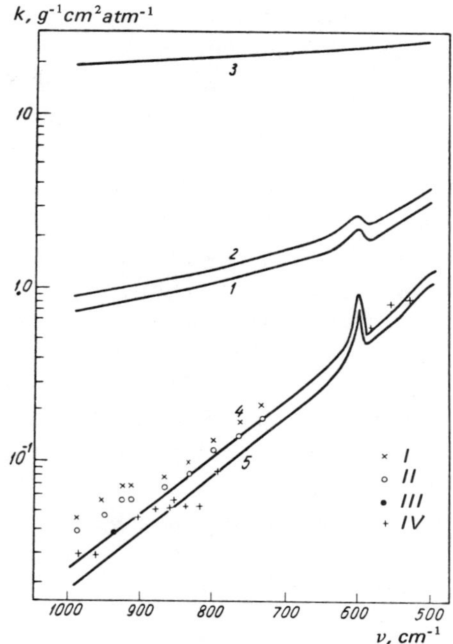



Fig. 2.5. Absorption coefficient of $H_2O$ in a mixture with $N_2$. (1) Calculated according to (2.39)–(2.40) using only the resonance term, $\gamma = F = \Phi = 1$; (2) nonresonance term included, $\gamma = F = \Phi = 1$; (3) $\gamma \neq 1$, $F = \Phi = 1$; (4, 5) calculated for $\gamma \neq 1$, $F \neq 1$ at temperatures of 300 and 320°K. Experimental results: (I), $\times$, [39], $T = 300°K$; (II), $\bigcirc$, [39], $T = 360°K$; (III), $\bullet$, [34]; (IV), $+$, [32].

The next important consideration bearing on the nature of the continuous absorption of water vapor in the atmospheric window from 8 to 12 $\mu$m involves the theoretically predicted large self-broadening factors, which attain values of the order of hundreds of units, by contrast with the middle parts of the absorption lines, where these factors are of the order of a few units. Calculations have shown that the self-broadening factor for an emission frequency of 1000 cm$^{-1}$ turns out to be equal to 180, which is consistent with the measurement results [34] obtained with a laser, where the self-broadening factor turns out to be equal to 194 at a frequency of 940 cm$^{-1}$. Another illustrative example may be found in the work of Aref'ev and others [40], in which laser measurements of $CO_2$ ($\lambda = 10.6$ $\mu$m) yield data indicating that increasing the pressure of $N_2$ from 0 to 1 atm while maintaining the same partial pressure of water vapor does not significantly alter the absorption coefficient, a fact that could account for the correspondingly large values of the self-broadening factors.

The dependence of the self-broadening factors on the frequency shift $\Delta\nu$ and their large values for large values of $\Delta\nu$ play a significant part in the interpretation of satellite measurements of outgoing radiation, which provide data on the profiles of particular atmospheric parameters. Another important implication of the given theory is the possibility of a square-law humidity dependence of the absorption coefficient in the far wings since this law normally governs absorption by dimers of water molecules or by induced bands. The same remarks are applicable to the temperature dependence of the absorption coefficient; the given theory predicts a complex nature on the part of this dependence; see expressions (2.41) and (2.44). It is impossible to extract from the corresponding experimental data an unambiguous answer to the question of the role of dimers and induced absorption bands without first performing a quantitative analysis of the influence of temperature on the absorption coefficients in the far wings.

## 2.4. Origin of the Absorption Spectra of Atmospheric Gases

### 2.4.1. Energy and Spectra of Molecules

The molecular energy may be written as follows in the general case:

$$E = E_{trans} + E_{el} + E_{vib} + E_{rot} + E_{el-vib} + E_{el-rot} + E_{vib-rot} \qquad (2.57)$$

where $E_{trans}$ is the translational, $E_{el}$ is the electron, $E_{vib}$ is the vibrational, and $E_{rot}$ is the rotational energy. The molecular translational energy can assume any values, whereas the electron, vibrational, and rotational energies can only take discrete values. The last three components of (2.57) are associated with interaction between different kinds of molecular motions. The electron energy is of the order of a few electron volts, the vibrational energy is reckoned in tenths and hundredths of 1 eV, and the rotational energy amounts to thousandths and ten-thousandths of an electron volt. Accordingly, the electron spectra of the molecules occupy the ultraviolet and visible regions of the spectra, the vibrational spectra are found in the near infrared, and the rotational spectra occupy the far-infrared and micro-wave regions.

In the event of electron transitions, the vibrational and rotational energies vary simultaneously. Thus, the electron spectrum actually represents an electron–vibration–rotation spectrum. Similarly, the vibrational spectrum comprises a set of vibration–rotation bands, and only the rotational spectrum can be recorded in its unadulterated form.

The absorption of radiation in the relevant range of the electromagnetic wave scale is mainly attributable to vibration–rotation transitions in atmospheric gas molecules. Accordingly, our focus of attention in the present section is on problems relating to the origin of the rotational and vibration–rotation spectra of these gases.

## 2.4.2. Rotational Energy and Rotational Spectra of Molecules

A rotating molecule may be envisioned as a spinning rigid body (rigid top). In this model, all molecules can be classified according to their rotational properties into four groups, depending on the ratio between the three principal moments of inertia $I_a$, $I_b$, and $I_c$ relative to the three principal axes of inertia of the molecule (Table 2.1).

### 2.4.2.1. Linear Molecules

Quantum mechanics yields the following expression for the quantized molecular rotational energy:

$$E_j = \frac{\hbar^2}{2I} j(j+1) = Bj(j+1), \qquad j=0,1,2,3,\ldots \qquad (2.58)$$

where $I$ is the moment of inertia of the molecule about the rotation axis perpendicular to the axis of the molecule through its center of mass, $B$ is the rotational constant, and $j$ is the rotational quantum number.

From (2.58) we derive an expression for the distance between two adjacent energy levels of the molecule:

$$E_{j+1} - E_j = 2B(j+1) \qquad (2.59)$$

It follows from (2.58) and (2.59) that the absolute value of $E_{j+1} - E_j$ varies inversely as the moment of inertia of the molecule. Thus, the heavier the

Table 2.1. Classification of Molecules by Their Rotational Properties

| Number | Moments of inertia | Type of molecule | Atmospheric gases associated with corresponding type of molecule |
|---|---|---|---|
| 1 | $I_a = 0,\ I_b = I_c \neq 0$ | Linear | $CO_2$, $N_2O$, $NO$, $CO$, $O_2$, $N_2$ |
| 2 | $I_a \neq 0,\ I_b = I_c \neq 0$ | Symmetrical top | None among atmospheric gases distributed on planetary scale |
| 3 | $I_a = I_b = I_c$ | Spherical top | $CH_4$ |
| 4 | $I \neq I_b \neq I_c$ | Asymmetrical top | $H_2O$, $O_3$, $HDO$ |

molecule and greater its dimensions, the longer will be the wavelengths of the region of its purely rotational spectrum.

The selection rules allow rotational transitions for

$$\Delta j = \pm 1 \tag{2.60}$$

It is evident from (2.60) and (2.58) that the frequencies of successive rotational transitions differ by $2B$, and so the rotational spectrum of a linear molecule in the rigid-top approximation consists of equidistant lines.

The rigid-top approximation postulates a constant distance between atoms in the molecule as it rotates. In reality, these distances increase more the greater the rotational energy or the higher the rotational quantum number. As the distance between nuclei of the atoms increases the rotational constant decreases, and this, in turn, decreases the distance between absorption lines on the frequency scale. The quantum-mechanical perturbation theory for the case of small centrifugal pulling forces on the molecule yields the following approximate expression for the molecular rotational energy:

$$E_j = B_j(j+1) - \mathcal{D}[j(j+1)]^2 \tag{2.61}$$

where the centrifugal distortion constant $\mathcal{D}$ has the order of magnitude $10^{-4}$ B and must be taken into account for large values of $j$.

The distribution of linear molecules by rotational levels is given by the expression

$$n_j = (2j+1)n_0 \exp\left[-\frac{Bj(j+1)}{kT}\right] \tag{2.62}$$

in which $n_0$ denotes the number of molecules in the state $j=0$ and the quantity $2j+1$ characterizes the degeneracy of the rotational levels.

### 2.4.2.2. Spherical-Top Molecules

The rotational energy levels for molecules of this configuration are determined by the same expressions (2.58) and (2.59) as in the case of linear molecules. The degree of degeneracy of the levels for these molecules differs, and so the distribution of the molecules among rotational states differs as well, viz.,

$$n_j = (2j+1)^2 n_0 \exp\left[-\frac{Bj(j+1)}{kT}\right] \tag{2.63}$$

It is apparent from a comparison of (2.63) and (2.62) that the number of molecules having a spherical-top configuration with large values of $j$ is greater than the corresponding number of linear molecules for identical values of the rotational constant and temperature.

### 2.4.2.3. Symmetrical-Top Molecule

On the planetary scale, there are no gases whose molecules could be classified as this type. We shall therefore not discuss the problem in detail. The interested reader is referred to the author's earlier monograph [1].

### 2.4.2.4. Asymmetrical-Top Molecules

Simple expressions cannot be derived for the rotational energy in this case. For example, in order to determine the energy of rotation with $j > 3$, it is necessary to solve third-, fourth-, and higher-degree equations. The corresponding calculations for the model of a rigid asymmetrical top have been carried out up to values of $j = 40$ [42].

For molecules of this configuration, a rotational level with a given $j$ splits into $2j + 1$ levels, which are designated by an index $\tau$ assuming values

$$\tau = -j, -j+1, \ldots, j-1, j \tag{2.64}$$

and are arranged in order of increasing energy from $j_{-j}$ to $j_{+j}$. The selection rules for molecules having an asymmetrical-top configuration allow transitions with a change of rotational quantum number

$$\Delta j = 0, \pm 1 \tag{2.65}$$

Transitions with $\Delta j = 0$ form the $Q$ branch, and transitions with $\Delta j = +1$ and $\Delta j = -1$ form the $R$ and $P$ branches of the given band of the absorption spectrum, respectively.

The centrifugal extension of molecules of this type induces a shift of the energy levels, which increases with the value of the rotational quantum number.

The pure rotational spectra of asymmetrical-top molecules are exceedingly complex. This result is associated primarily with the fact that to every value of $j$ there correspond $2j + 1$ distinct levels. The presence of the $Q$ branches in the absorption bands also tends to complicate the picture.

## 2.4.3. Vibrational Energy and Vibrational Spectra of Molecules

### 2.4.3.1. Vibrational Energy of Molecules

A linear molecule has $3N - 5$ vibrational degrees of freedom, and a nonlinear molecule has $3N - 6$, where $N$ is the number of atoms. The number of fundamental frequencies of molecular vibrations corresponds to the number of degrees of freedom of vibrational motion. Certain fundamental frequencies of symmetrical molecules coincide due to degeneracy.

The simplest model of vibrational motion of a molecule is the harmonic oscillator, for which quantum mechanics yields the following straightforward equation for the vibrational energy:

$$E_v = h\nu \left( v + \tfrac{1}{2} \right) \qquad (2.66)$$

where $\nu$ is the vibration frequency and $v$ is the vibrational quantum number, which takes integral values $0, 1, 2, 3, \ldots$ .

It is evident from (2.66) that the energy levels of the harmonic oscillator are equally spaced, the energy difference between adjacent levels has a value

$$E_{v+1} - E_v = h\nu \qquad (2.67)$$

Regarding the molecular vibrations as a set of vibrations of harmonic oscillators with frequencies $\nu_1, \nu_2, \nu_3, \ldots$, we write for the molecular vibrational energy

$$E_v = \left( v_1 + \tfrac{1}{2} \right) h\nu_1 + \left( v_2 + \tfrac{1}{2} \right) h\nu_2 + \left( v_3 + \tfrac{1}{2} \right) h\nu_3 + \ldots \qquad (2.68)$$

where $v_1, v_2, v_3, \ldots$ are the vibrational quantum numbers, whose set of indices designates the vibrational state of the molecule. For example, state (100) corresponds to $v_1 = 1$, $v_2 = 0$, and $v_3 = 0$. The quantities $\nu_1, \nu_2,$ and $\nu_3$ in (2.68) are customarily referred to as the fundamental vibration frequencies.

The selection rules allow transitions between energy levels of the harmonic oscillator such that the condition

$$\Delta v = \pm 1 \qquad (2.69)$$

is satisfied, only where in one of the oscillators can transition take place simultaneously for the molecule represented by a set of harmonic oscillators. Thus, the vibrational spectrum of the molecule in this case consists solely of the fundamental frequencies.

Anharmonicity of molecular vibrations injects second- and higher-order terms in the expression for the vibrational energy. For example, the following approximate expression for $E_v$ is obtained in the case of a diatomic molecule:

$$E_v = h\nu \left( v + \tfrac{1}{2} \right) - xh\nu \left( v + \tfrac{1}{2} \right)^2 + \cdots \qquad (2.70)$$

where $x$ is the anharmonicity constant.

The distances between energy levels of adjacent states in an anharmonic oscillator diminish with increasing quantum number $v$, thereby eliciting series of vibration frequencies. The selection rules for the anharmonic oscillator are considerably altered. Now all transitions satisfying the condition

$$\Delta v = 1, 2, 3, \ldots \tag{2.71}$$

are allowed, and transitions can take place simultaneously in several oscillators.

Transitions with $\Delta v = 2, 3, \ldots$ induce corresponding overtones of the fundamental frequencies, and the simultaneous variation of different vibrational quantum numbers results in the advent of combination frequencies. Finally, transitions from vibrational levels with initial values of the vibrational quantum numbers greater than or equal to unity induce "hot" vibration frequencies. The overtones are customarily denoted by $2\nu_1, 2\nu_2, 2\nu_3, \ldots, 3\nu_1, 3\nu_2, 3\nu_3, \ldots$, etc. The combination frequency formed by simultaneous variation in a three-atom nonlinear molecule, say of $v_1$ from 0 to 1, of $v_2$ from 0 to 2, and of $v_3$ from 1 to 0, is designated by the notation $\nu_1 + 2\nu_2 - \nu_3$. It occurs in the event of simultaneous absorption of the fundamental frequency $\nu_1$, absorption of the first overtone of $\nu_2$, and emission of the fundamental $\nu_3$; the change of state of the molecule in this case is denoted by (001)–(120). "Hot" frequencies are designated analogously, for example the transition (010)–(020) in a triatomic nonlinear molecule takes place with a change of only one vibrational quantum number $v_2$, the molecule going from the first to the second vibrational level, etc.

### 2.4.3.2. Vibration–Rotation Spectra of Molecules

A variation of the vibrational energy of a molecule is accompanied by a simultaneous variation of its rotational energy. The smallness of the energy of rotational quanta in comparison with the vibrational quantum energy is explained by the fact that molecular rotation does not disrupt the vibrational structure of the spectrum of the molecule. To each vibrational energy level of the molecule there corresponds a series of rotational levels, so that each vibrational transition in an ensemble of molecules goes over into a set of lines or a vibration–rotation band. Each line corresponds to the same variation of the vibrational energy and to different variations of the rotational energy. Consequently, the spectrum of vibration frequencies of a molecule forms the skeleton of its vibration–rotation spectrum, which is readily constructed by additive superposition of the vibrational and rotational transitions allowed by the selection rules if interactions between vibrations and rotations are neglected. Thus, in order to grasp the nature of the vibration–rotation spectra, it is necessary to investigate the structure of the molecular vibrational transitions. We begin the investigation with diatomic molecules as the simplest kind from the standpoint of analytical description of the spectrum interpretation problem.

We recall that the condition for the representation of any oscillatory process in a spectrum is a nonzero variation of the corresponding transition moment. We consider transitions associated with a variation of the electric dipole moments. Going over to diatomic molecules and acknowledging the stated condition, we infer at once that diatomic molecules composed of identical atoms cannot, under ordinary circumstances, have vibration–rotation spectra, because the symmetry of the molecule keeps the centers of mass of the positive and negative charges from altering their positions in the oscillatory process and so the dipole moment of the molecule does not change. The corresponding vibration frequencies constitute an example of optically inactive modes.

The spectrum of vibrational transitions of a diatomic molecule composed of unlike atoms is readily deduced from expression (2.70); thus, for the vibration frequencies $\nu_k$ we have

$$\nu_k = \nu(1-x)(v''-v') - \nu x(v''^2 - v'^2) \tag{2.72}$$

where $v''$ and $v'$ are the vibrational quantum numbers of the upper and lower states of the molecule.

It follows from (2.72) that the vibrational spectrum of a diatomic molecule consists of a set of separate series of bands, each corresponding to transitions of the molecule from a given vibrational level to neighboring levels. For example, in the case of the series beginning with the zeroth vibrational level ($v'=0$), we obtain

$$\nu_k(0, v'') = \nu(1-x)v'' - \nu x v''^2 \tag{2.73}$$

whence it is obvious that the set of vibrational frequencies and, accordingly, vibration–rotation bands is

$$\nu_1 = \nu(1-2x); \quad \nu_2 = 2\nu(1-3x); \quad \nu_3 = 3\nu(1-4x) \tag{2.74}$$

the form of which implies that the distance between adjacent lines decreases with increasing values of $v''$ and the frequency $\nu$. The lines of the series converge to a certain boundary corresponding to dissociation of the molecule. All other series have an analogous structure.

The above-described pattern of the vibration–rotation bands also applies to the case of polyatomic molecules. However, the more complex scheme of vibrational levels and the possibility of simultaneous excitation of a great many vibrational modes cause the sets of vibrational transition frequencies to overlap, and the vibration–rotation spectra of polyatomic molecules turn out to be very intricate.

We now consider the formation of fine structure within the individual vibration–rotation bands. For simplicity, we begin with diatomic molecules, whose vibration–rotation energy can be rewritten in the form

$$E'' = E_{v''} + B_{v''} j'' ( j'' + 1 ) \tag{2.75}$$

$$E' = E_{v'} + B_{v'} j' ( j' + 1 ) \tag{2.76}$$

where $E_{v''}$ and $E_{v'}$ are the vibrational energies for the two states characterized by the quantum numbers $v''$ and $v'$, as described by Eq. (2.70), and the rotational energy is written in the form $Bj( j + 1 )$. The interaction of vibrations and rotation of the molecule is accounted for in (2.75) and (2.76) by means of the rotational constant, which is a function of the vibrational quantum number $v$:

$$B_v = B_e - \alpha \left( v + \tfrac{1}{2} \right) \tag{2.77}$$

where $B_e$ is the rotational constant of the nonvibrating molecule and $\alpha$ is a constant, which amounts to not more than a few hundredths of the value of $B_e$.

From Eqs. (2.75) and (2.76) we obtain

$$E'' - E' = E_{v''} - E_{v'} + B_{v''} j'' ( j'' + 1 ) - B_{v'} j' ( j' + 1 ) \tag{2.78}$$

The quantity $E_{v''} - E_{v'} = \nu_{00}$ specifies the frequency of pure vibrational transition or the null-line frequency corresponding to $j'' = j' = 0$. The transition corresponding to the null line is forbidden by the selection rules. The position of this line is determined analytically. It is readily perceived that the position of the vibration–rotation band is determined by the null line.

Unlike pure rotational spectra, in the case of transitions described by expression (2.78) it is necessary to consider not only values of $\Delta j = j'' - j' > 0$, but also $\Delta j < 0$ and, in individual cases, $\Delta j = 0$. Transitions with $\Delta j = +1$ form the $R$ branch, whose line frequencies are greater than $\nu_{00}$. Transitions with $\Delta j = -1$ form the $P$ branch, with frequencies less than $\nu_{00}$. In this

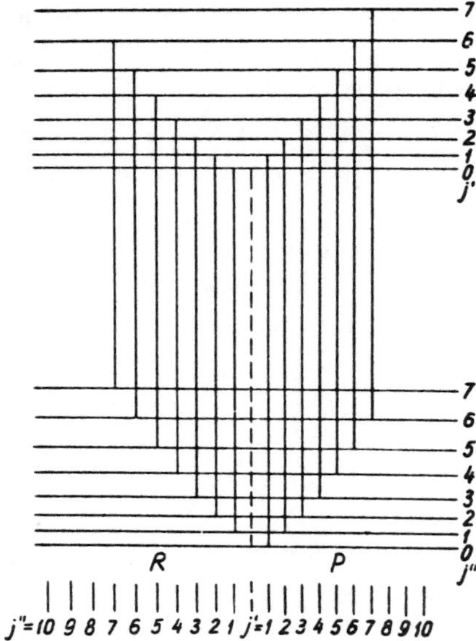



Fig. 2.6. Energy-transition diagram for vibra-tion–rotation band.

connection, the $R$ and $P$ branches of a vibration–rotation band are fre-quently referred to as the positive and negative branches, respectively. The formation of these bands is illustrated in Fig. 2.6.

Transitions with $\Delta j = 0$, forming the $Q$ branch, are allowed in diatomic molecules when the electron angular momentum is nonvanishing (as for example in the case of the NO molecule). For this branch, we obtain from (2.78)

$$E'' - E' = v_{00} + (B_{v''} - B_{v'})j(j+1) \qquad (2.79)$$

Inasmuch as the difference $B_{v''} - B_{v'}$ is very small, the distance between energy levels is likewise small, and so the lines of the $Q$ branch are very closely spaced.

We now briefly characterize the fine structure of the vibration–rotation bands of polyatomic molecules that differ according to their rotational properties, first introducing the concept of parallel and perpendicular bands, which is essential to this part of the discussion. Absorption bands that occur when the direction of the transition dipole moment coincides with the direction of the preferred symmetry axis of the molecule are called parallel. Perpendicular bands are defined analogously.

In the case of linear polyatomic molecules, the positions of the rota-tional lines within a vibration–rotation band are described by an expression analogous to (2.78), except that now the rotational constants depend on all the vibrational quantum numbers of the molecules:

$$B_{v_1, v_2, \ldots, v_k} = B_e - \sum_i \alpha_i \left( v_i + \tfrac{1}{2} g_i \right) \tag{2.80}$$

where $g_i$ is the multiplicity of degeneracy of the $i$th vibrational mode.

For perpendicular bands in this case, the selection rules allow transitions in all three ($R$, $P$, and $Q$) branches. The $Q$ branch is absent in the case of parallel bands. Both parallel and perpendicular are represented among the fundamental vibration–rotation bands of linear polyatomic molecules. Both also occur among the overtones and combination-frequency bands. We note that the type of band is readily determined from the outward appearance of its spectrum. A minimum is observed near the null line of a parallel band due to the missing $Q$ branch. In the vicinity of the null line of a perpendicular band, on the other hand, there is a maximum due to the presence of the $Q$ branch.

The positions of the rotational lines in a vibration–rotation band of molecules having a spherical-top configuration are given by the same expression as for linear polyatomic molecules. The absorption bands have $R$, $Q$, and $P$ branches. Interaction of the vibrational and rotational motions of the molecule induce splitting of threefold-degenerate vibrational modes and greatly complicate the nature of the fine structure of the vibration–rotation bands.

Molecules of the symmetrical-top type have both parallel and perpendicular bands. The nature of their vibration–rotation spectra is more complex than for linear and spherical-top molecules, particularly when the direction of the dipole moment does not coincide with the axis of the molecule. Again we point out that such molecules do not occur among the atmospheric gases encountered on a planetary scale.

Molecules of the asymmetrical-top type have the most complex pure rotational and, hence, vibration–rotation spectra. The nature of the dependence of the rotational constants on the vibrational quantum numbers is similar to (2.80). In the special case of a triatomic molecule, it has the form

$$A = A_e - \alpha_{A_1}\left( v_1 + \tfrac{1}{2} \right) - \alpha_{A_2}\left( v_2 + \tfrac{1}{2} \right) - \alpha_{A_3}\left( v_3 + \tfrac{1}{2} \right)$$

$$B = B_e - \alpha_{B_1}\left( v_1 + \tfrac{1}{2} \right) - \alpha_{B_2}\left( v_2 + \tfrac{1}{2} \right) - \alpha_{B_3}\left( v_3 + \tfrac{1}{2} \right) \tag{2.81}$$

$$C = C_e - \alpha_{C_1}\left( v_1 + \tfrac{1}{2} \right) - \alpha_{C_2}\left( v_2 + \tfrac{1}{2} \right) - \alpha_{C_3}\left( v_3 + \tfrac{1}{2} \right)$$

Here $A$, $B$, and $C$ are the rotational constants corresponding to the three principal moments of inertia of the molecule, and the constants $\alpha$ can be expressed in terms of the anharmonicity constants.

The selection rules for the given molecules depend on the particular axis along which the transition dipole moment is directed. The dipole moment for a symmetrical triatomic molecule $XY_2$ is directed along the symmetry axis of the molecule or along the axis perpendicular to it in the plane of the molecule. Both perpendicular and parallel bands can occur in this situation. In the case of water vapor, for example, the majority of the bands are perpendicular.

The nature of the vibration–rotation structure of the bands of all types of molecules, the center positions of the lines, and the shape and intensity of the latter are significantly affected by the interaction of vibrational and rotational motions of the molecules, molecular interactions in the ensemble of molecules, resonance perturbations of the levels, and the Coriolis forces. The correct description of all these effects poses an exceedingly complex and difficult problem. We shall devote an entire separate section of the chapter to it.

## 2.5. General Description of the Absorption Spectra of Atmospheric Gases

In a special section at the end of the chapter we discuss problems associated with the distribution of various gaseous components in the atmosphere. At this juncture, we merely note that our primary concern is for gases occurring in the atmosphere on a planetary scale or those most commonly occurring in the waste products of human industrial activity contaminating the atmosphere. Whereas the focus of attention in connection with the absorption functions over wide spectral intervals (as in calculations of the absorption of solar radiation in the atmosphere) is on the principal absorbing gases such as water vapor, carbon dioxide, and ozone, which are in fact the main absorbers over a wide spectral range, in the case of the laser absorption problem, on the other hand, the notion of principal absorbing gases becomes meaningless in the general sense because different gases, including the so-called small impurities, play the principal role in the absorption of radiation from different laser sources; we shall have many occasions to be convinced of this fact. And if the discussion concerns, say, water vapor as one of the principal laser-absorbing gases, it will only be in the sense that the vibration–rotation absorption spectrum of $H_2O$ occupies a very broad interval of wavelengths, is extremely abundant in lines, and is therefore typified by a large probability that the laser line will happen to be in a part of the spectrum that is not free of absorption by water vapor.

### 2.5.1. Absorption Spectrum of Water Vapor

The equilibrium positions of the nuclei in the water molecule form an isosceles triangle with the oxygen atom at its vertex (Fig. 2.7). The equilibrium angle between the O—H bonds is equal to 104° 30′, and the equilibrium length of the O—H bond is 0.958 Å. Electron transitions in the $H_2O$ molecule are associated with the interval of wavelengths less than 1860 Å (far ultraviolet), where absorption by ozone and oxygen molecules is exceptionally strong, precluding the possibility of any practical utilization of this wavelength range, at least for the transmission of any kind of information through the atmosphere.

The moments of inertia of the molecule about the three principal axes of rotation differ sharply ($I_a = 1.004 \times 10^{-40}$; $I_b = 1.929 \times 10^{-40}$; $I_c = 3.014 \times 10^{-40}$ g cm$^2$), thereby endowing the pure rotational and vibration–rotation spectra with a random and a complex structure. The absolute values of $I_a$, $I_b$, and $I_c$ are small, so that the distance between rotational lines are large and the spectra extend over a broad range of wavelengths or frequencies.

The solar spectrum exhibits absorption lines for the four isotopes of water $H_2O^{16}$, $H_2O^{18}$, $H_2O^{17}$, and $HDO^{16}$, which occur in the atmosphere in respective concentrations of 99.73, 0.2039, 0.0373, and 0.0298%. The rotational and vibrational constants of the first three isotopes differ only slightly, so the $H_2O^{17}$ lines are shifted from 1 to 11 cm$^{-1}$ relative to the corresponding $H_2O^{16}$ lines. The shift for the $H_2O^{18}$ molecule is twice as great [10]. The fundamental frequencies for the $H_2O^{16}$ and $HDO^{16}$ molecules are summarized in Table 2.2.

In addition to the three fundamental vibration–rotation bands, the vibration–rotation spectrum of $H_2O$ also contains a large number of overtone bands, combination-frequency bands, and "hot" bands, tables of which

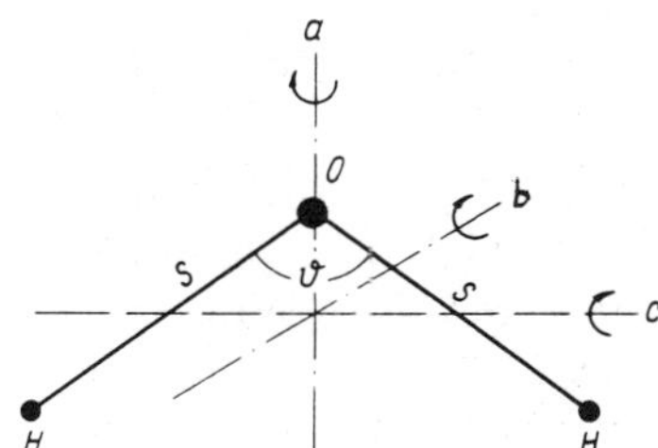


Fig. 2.7. Structural diagram of $H_2O$ molecule.

**Table 2.2.** Frequencies of Fundamental Bands of $H_2O$ Molecule [10]

| Band | Transition | Band center, $cm^{-1}$ | |
|------|-----------|-------------------|------------------|
| | | $HHO^{16}$ | $HDO^{16}$ |
| $\nu_1$ | 000–100 | 3657.05 | 2723.66 |
| $\nu_1$ | 000–010 | 1594.78 | 1403.3 |
| $\nu_3$ | 000–001 | 3755.92 | 3707.47 |

may be found in [1]. The intensity ratios between the absorption lines of the water isotopes $H_2O^{18}$ and $H_2O^{17}$ and the $H_2O^{16}$ lines correspond to the isotope concentration ratios. The HDO bands differ appreciably from the $H_2O^{16}$ bands both in their positions in the spectrum and in their line intensities.

The vibration–rotation spectrum of water vapor fills up the entire visible region as well as the near and middle infrared region approximately up to frequencies of the order of 1000 $cm^{-1}$, the visible region containing very weak combination-frequency absorption bands and the near infrared containing stronger overtone and combination-frequency bands. The strongest and broadest absorption band is the fundamental $\nu_2$ band, which has its center around a wavelength of 6.25 $\mu$m and is referred to in the literature as the 6.3 $\mu$m band. In a vertical column of the atmosphere with average humidity, this band completely absorbs solar radiation in the wavelength range from 5.5 to 7.5 $\mu$m. The center of next band in order of diminishing intensity, $\nu_3$, is situated near a wavelength of 2.66 $\mu$m. The $\nu_1$ (center near 2.74 $\mu$m) and $2\nu_2$ (center near 3.17 $\mu$m) bands together with the $\nu_3$ band are responsible for complete absorption of the solar radiation in a vertical column of the atmosphere with average humidities in the spectral region extending roughly from 2.6 to 3.3 $\mu$m. The other vibration–rotation bands of water vapor are clustered, forming absorption bands in the low-resolution (coarse-structure) spectrum with centers near 1.87, 1.38, 1.1, 0.94, and 0.81 $\mu$m, along with a series of weak bands in the visible spectrum.

The fine structure of the vibration–rotation spectrum of water vapor is extremely complex and involved. Each absorption band consists of many hundreds and even thousands of lines, the identification of which poses an exceedingly difficult task. Experimental studies have disclosed tens of thousands of absorption lines. It is safe to say that faint new lines will be detected with further improvement of the instrument resolving power. We shall cover this problem in closer detail in the section devoted to the description of methods of experimental investigation of the absorption coefficients.

The large values of the dipole moments for the $H_2O$ molecule and its isotopes are the cause of the strong rotational spectrum, which occupies a very broad spectral region extending roughly from wavelengths in the vicinity of 8 $\mu$m to several centimeters. Beginning with wavelengths of about 20 $\mu$m and extending well into the long-wave region, the pure rotational absorption spectrum of water vapor is responsible for the complete absorption of solar radiation by a vertical column of the atmosphere at all humidities. It is essential to emphasize in this connection that to speak of complete absorption by a vertical column of the atmosphere carries the implication that it is realized not only at the centers of the lines, where the absorption coefficients are a maximum, but also in the parts of the spectrum between absorption lines, where the absorption coefficients are minimal but still sufficiently strong in virtue of the contributions from the wings of nearby lines. As for the centers of the strong absorption lines, it is sufficient for the radiation to traverse very small thicknesses of the atmosphere in order to be completely absorbed at such wavelengths. These thicknesses can be reckoned in millimeters and centimeters for the strongest lines.

### 2.5.2. Absorption Spectrum of Carbon Dioxide

The linear symmetrical $CO_2$ molecule with its long C—O bond, which has a length of 1.1632 Å in the fundamental vibrational state, has four fundamental vibrational frequencies, the diagram of which is given in Fig. 2.8. Due to the symmetry of the molecule in the fundamental mode $\nu_1$, the dipole moment of the molecule is invariant, and so this frequency is optically inactive and does not appear in the absorption spectrum. The fundamental mode $\nu_2$ is twofold degenerate. In this case, it is necessary to take account of the selection rules for the vibrational quantum numbers of the vibrational angular momentum

$$\Delta l = 0, \pm 1 \qquad\qquad (2.82)$$

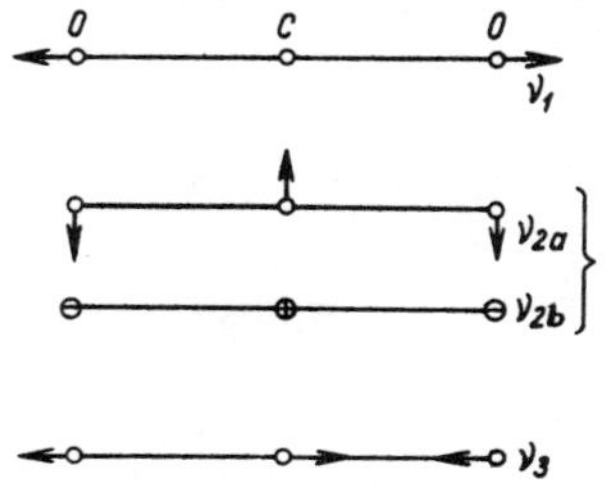

Fig. 2.8. Diagram of fundamental modes of the $CO_2$ molecule.

and the notation for the vibrational state of the molecule is furnished with an additional index for the second vibrational quantum number $v_2$.

The fundamental vibration–rotation bands active in the absorption spectrum, $v_2(00^00–01^10)$ and $v_3(00^00–00^01)$, are perpendicular and parallel, respectively. Thus, the $v_3$ band does not have a $Q$ branch.

The statistical weights of the levels of the $CO_2$ molecule with even values of the rotational quantum numbers are equal to zero. Consequently, the fine structure of the vibration–rotation bands contains only lines with odd $j$ values.

The following isotopes of the $CO_2$ molecule occur in the atmosphere: $C^{12}O_2^{16}$; $C^{13}O_2^{16}$; $C^{12}O^{16}O^{18}$; $C^{12}O^{16}O^{17}$; $C^{13}O^{16}O^{18}$; $C^{13}O^{16}O^{17}$; $C^{13}O^{18}O^{18}$, which have percentage concentrations relative to the total carbon dioxide content of the atmosphere 98.414, 1.105, 0.402, 0.073, 0.00452, 0.00082, and 0.000412%, respectively [43]. Table 2.3 gives the center positions of the $v_2$ and $v_3$ bands for the three most common isotopes of $CO_2$ in the atmosphere.

The fundamental vibration–rotation $v_2$ band with center around 15 $\mu$m along with 14 "hot" bands occupies a rather broad interval of the spectrum, roughly from 12 to 20 $\mu$m. In the central region of this band (from $\sim 13.5$ to 16.5 $\mu$m), a vertical column of the atmosphere completely absorbs solar radiation for any wavelengths in this interval. This entire set of bands is often referred to in the literature as the 15-$\mu$m band. Detailed information concerning each of these bands may be found in [1]. This region is very abundant in absorption lines. For example, Drayson [44] includes approximately 2000 lines in calculations of the absorption coefficients in the region of the 15 $\mu$m band.

The fundamental vibration–rotation absorption $v_3$ band induces very strong absorption in the atmosphere. Here also we find the combination $v_1 + v_3 - 2v_2$ $(02^00–10^01)$ band. Together these bands form what is usually called the 4.3-$\mu$m absorption band in the literature. None of the components of this band has a $Q$ branch. The intensity of the 4.3-$\mu$m band is so great that solar radiation is completely absorbed in the wavelength interval extending roughly from 4.2 to 4.4 $\mu$m in a vertical column of the atmosphere up to a height of $\sim 20$ km.

Table 2.3. Fundamental Bands $v_2$ and $v_3$ of $CO_2$ Molecule [10]

| Isotopic modification | Percentage content | Band center, cm$^{-1}$ | |
|---|---|---|---|
| | | $v_2$ | $v_3$ |
| $C^{12}O^{16}O^{16}$ | 98.420 | 667.40 | 2349.16 |
| $C^{13}O^{16}O^{16}$ | 1.108 | 648.52 | 2283.48 |
| $C^{12}O^{16}O^{18}$ | 0.408 | 662.39 | 2333 |

Besides the 15- and 4.3-$\mu$m bands discussed above, in which absorption is associated mainly with the $\nu_2$ and $\nu_3$ bands of the $C^{12}O_2^{16}$ molecule, carbon dioxide also has sets of bands clustered into complex absorption bands with centers, in order of diminishing wavelengths but not in order of intensity, at 10.4, 9.4, 5.2, 4.8, 2.7, 2.0, 1.6, and 1.4 $\mu$m, plus a number of fainter bands in the region from 1.24 to 0.78 $\mu$m. All these bands have widths of the order of 0.1 $\mu$m [1].

## 2.5.3. Absorption Spectrum of Ozone

The structure of the ozone molecule is given in Fig. 2.9. The electron transitions in the molecule form Hartley and Huggins bands in the ultraviolet region of the spectrum (wavelengths shorter than 3400 Å) as well as Chappuis bands in the region from 4500 to 7400 Å. The maximum value of the absorption coefficients in the Chappuis bands account for 7% absorption of solar radiation for an atmospheric mass equal to 2.

All three fundamental vibration–rotation absorption bands of the $O_3$ molecule are absorption-active and are situated in the infrared region of the spectrum. Their positions in the spectrum for the isotopic modifications occurring in the atmosphere are given in Table 2.4, along with the percentage contents of those isotopes.

The $\nu_1$ band overlaps the $\nu_3$ band due to the strong interaction between the corresponding energy levels. The $\nu_1$ band is considerably weaker in intensity than the $\nu_3$ band. The $\nu_2$ band overlaps the central part of the strong absorption band of $CO_2$ with center around 15 $\mu$m.

Overtones and combination frequencies form sets of vibration–rotation bands that cluster into complex absorption bands with centers around 5.75, 4.75, 3.95, 3.27, and 2.7 $\mu$m. The width of each of these bands is of the order of 0.1 $\mu$m. Their strongest member is the 4.75 $\mu$m band.

Normally in the investigation of absorption of solar radiation by the earth's atmosphere, only the absorption band with center at 9.6 $\mu$m, formed primarily by the $\nu_3$ band along with the overlapping $\nu_1$ band, is taken into consideration. These bands are situated in the center of the long-wave atmospheric window from 8 to 13 $\mu$m. Its central part with a width of about

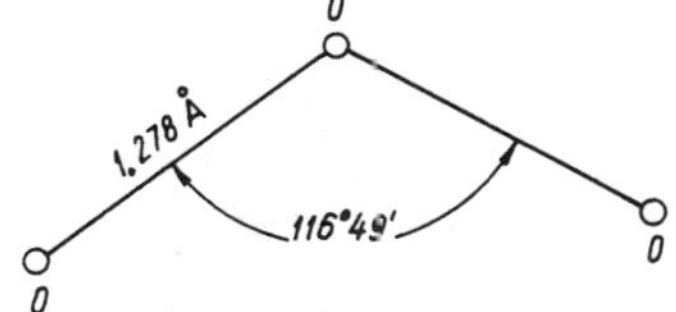


Fig. 2.9. Structure of ozone molecule.

Table 2.4. Fundamental Absorption Bands of $O_3$ Molecule [10]

| Band | $O_3^{16}$, cm$^{-1}$ | $O^{16}O^{18}O^{16}$, cm$^{-1}$ | $O^{16}O^{16}O^{18}$, cm$^{-1}$ |
|---|---|---|---|
| $\nu_1$ | 1110 | 1080 | 1095 |
| $\nu_2$ | 701.42 | 697 | 688 |
| $\nu_3$ | 1045.16 | 1008 | 1029 |
| Percentage content | 99.4 | 0.21 | 0.41 |

1 $\mu$m absorbs approximately 50% solar radiation in a vertical column of the atmosphere. It may be necessary in the quantitative assessment of the absorption of laser radiation in the atmosphere to include absorption in any of the $O_3$ bands if their lines fall within the spectral range of the laser. In particular, the very weak absorption band with center at 3.59 $\mu$m situated in the short-wave atmospheric window from 3.5 to 3.9 $\mu$m can prove quite significant.

All the absorption bands of ozone are exceedingly abundant in lines that are much more closely spaced in comparison with the lines of the vibration–rotation bands of water vapor since the ozone molecule has almost 3 times the mass of the $H_2O$ molecule, as well as a somewhat greater distance between atoms, a fact that is mirrored accordingly in the principal moments of inertia and rotational constants and, in terms of the latter, in the distances between adjacent lines of the absorption bands. A completely resolved vibration–rotation absorption band has not been obtained for the ozone molecule to date.

The strong pure rotational absorption spectrum of $O_3$ is situated in the microwave region of the spectrum, again due to the relatively great mass of that molecule.

### 2.5.4. Absorption Spectrum of Oxygen

Oxygen occurs in the atmosphere in the molecular and atomic states. Atomic oxygen is the result of dissociation of $O_2$ molecules under the action of ultraviolet radiation from the sun. The oxygen atoms produced by this dissociation, in particular, participate in the formation of ozone molecules.

Atomic oxygen in the visible and infrared regions does not have allowed electron transitions of dipole radiation. The series of forbidden transitions yields a single line with wavelength 5571 Å and a multiplet in the region from 6300 to 6364 Å. The intensities of these lines are small, but if their centers happen to coincide with the laser emission lines, then absorption of the laser radiation must certainly be taken into account.

Molecular oxygen has strong electron bands in the ultraviolet region and relatively weak ones in the red and near infrared. The eight bands in the red region occupy the spectral interval from 0.64 to 0.76 $\mu$m. The $O_2^{16}$ molecule has two discernible bands in the near infrared with centers around wavelengths of 1.0674 and 1.2683 $\mu$m. Because of the symmetry of the $O_2^{16}$ molecule, its band spectra contain only lines with alternating values of the rotational quantum number $j$. The molecule of the isotopic modification $O^{16}O^{18}$ has absorption bands situated in the red region around wavelengths of 0.6317, 0.6901, and 0.7620 $\mu$m. These bands contain lines with all values of $j$ as a result of the reduction of symmetry of this molecule in comparison with the molecule of the principal isotopic modification. Besides the molecular electron bands discussed above, oxygen also has diffuse absorption bands in the ultraviolet, visible, and near-infrared regions in connection with the presence of molecular complexes $[O_2]_2$ [45].

The intensities of all the absorption bands of $O_2$ and $[O_2]_2$ in the visible and near-infrared regions are small. Nevertheless, if any parts of them happen to coincide with the laser emission lines, it may be required to take this absorption into account.

## 2.5.5. Absorption Spectrum of Nitrogen Peroxide

The nitrogen peroxide molecule $NO_2$ is of the asymmetrical-top type. The presence of an unpaired electron in the outer electron shell of this molecule greatly complicates its spectrum as a result of spin–rotation interaction. The distance between the N and O atoms is equal to $1.19464 \pm 0.0015$ Å, and the angle at the vertex of the ONO triangle is $133.888° \pm 0.002°$ [46]. The molecule has a constant dipole moment, the magnitude of which has been estimated by various authors to lie between the limits 0.3 to 0.79 D, including the value of $0.316 \pm 0.01$ D obtained experimentally [47]. Table 2.5 gives the calculated and experimental values of the center positions of the fundamental vibration–rotation absorption bands of three isotopes of $NO_2$.

Table 2.5. Center Positions of $NO_2$ Fundamental Absorption Bands (cm$^{-1}$) [46]

| Band | $N^{14}O_2^{16}$ | | $N^{15}O_2^{16}$ | | $N^{14}O_2^{18}$ |
| | calc | exp | calc | exp | calc |
|---|---|---|---|---|---|
| $\nu_1$ | 1320.730 | 1320 | 1307.256 | 1306 | 1270.622 |
| $\nu_2$ | 749.652 | 749.650 | 740.197 | 740 | 722.787 |
| $\nu_3$ | 1616.867 | 1616.852 | 1582.147 | 1582.107 | 1587.073 |

Hardwick and Brand [46] give the center positions of 22 overtone and combination-frequency bands in the wavelength interval from 1.6 to 6.7 $\mu$m for the $NO_2$ isotopes in Table 2.5.

The electron absorption spectrum of the $NO_2$ molecule is situated in the ultraviolet region, and the pure rotational spectrum in the far-infrared region.

## 2.5.6. Absorption Spectrum of Nitrous Oxide

The nitrous oxide molecule is a linear asymmetrical molecule with strong electron bands in the far ultraviolet.

All three fundamental vibration frequencies $\nu_1 = 1285.6$ cm$^{-1}$ (7.8 $\mu$m), the twofold-degenerate $\nu_2 = 588.8$ cm$^{-1}$ (17.0 $\mu$m), and $\nu_3 = 2223.5$ cm$^{-1}$ (4.6 $\mu$m) are active in the infrared absorption spectra. In addition to the fundamental frequencies, the $N_2O$ molecule has a great many overtone, combination-frequency, and hot absorption bands. For example, 23 bands are observed in the region above 8000 cm$^{-1}$, 18 bands between 4417 and 1888 cm$^{-1}$, 14 bands between 4062 and 7431 cm$^{-1}$, and 7 bands in the interval from 2209.53 to 2798.3 cm$^{-1}$, not counting "hot" bands. The majority of these bands have low intensities, but, as in other similar cases, their role in the absorption of laser radiation must be considered separately in each instance.

The $N_2O$ molecule has 12 stable isotopes formed by combinations of $N^{14}$, $N^{15}$, $O^{16}$, $O^{17}$, and $O^{18}$ atoms. However, only the principal isotopic modification $N_2^{14}O^{16}$ has been investigated in any detail.

## 2.5.7. Absorption Spectrum of Sulfur Dioxide Gas

The gaseous sulfur dioxide molecule belongs to the class of asymmetrical tops. The equilibrium distance between the S and O atoms is equal to $1.43498 \pm 0.00015$ Å, and the vertex angle of the OSO triangle is $119.349 \pm 0.024°$ [48]. Table 2.6 gives the center positions of the fundamental vibration–rotation bands for various isotopic modifications of the $SO_2$ molecule according to experimental studies [49]. Four relatively strong absorption bands with centers around 4.0, 7.3, 8.7, and 19.3 $\mu$m are observed in the vibration–rotation spectrum of $SO_2$, where they are formed mainly by the set of fundamental bands of the isotopic modifications.

The moments of inertia $I_b$ and $I_c$ of the $SO_2$ molecule differ only slightly from one another, so it may be regarded as a symmetrical top. The

**Table 2.6.** Center Positions of $SO_2$ Fundamental Absorption Bands $(cm^{-1})$ [49]

| Isotopic modification | $\nu_1$ | $\nu_2$ | $\nu_3$ |
|---|---|---|---|
| $S^{32}O_2^{16}$ | 1156 | 522 | 1366 |
| $S^{34}O_2^{16}$ | 1147 | 518 | 1349 |
| $S^{32}O^{16}O^{18}$ | 1127 | 513 | 1346 |
| $S^{34}O^{16}O^{18}$ | 1120 | 509 | 1330 |
| $S^{32}O_2^{18}$ | 1105 | 500 | 1322 |

molecule has a constant dipole moment equal to 1.61 D [50]. The electron absorption spectrum of $SO_2$ is situated in the ultraviolet region, and the pure rotational spectrum in the far-infrared region.

## 2.5.8. Absorption Spectrum of Methane

The equilibrium configuration of the methane molecule $CH_4$ represents a tetrahedron. The molecule is of the spherical-top type. Its electron spectra are situated in the far ultraviolet (wavelengths less than 1450 Å). The high degree of symmetry of the molecule causes strong degeneracy of the vibrational energy levels. Of the nine fundamental vibration frequencies, one is twofold-degenerate, and two of them are threefold-degenerate. Thus, the molecule has altogether four distinct fundamental frequencies. The $\nu_1$ band is completely symmetrical, $\nu_2$ is twofold-degenerate, and $\nu_3$ and $\nu_4$ are threefold-degenerate. The absorption spectrum exhibits only the bands $\nu_3 = 3020.3$ cm$^{-1}$ (3.3 $\mu$m) and $\nu_4 = 1306.2$ cm$^{-1}$ (7.7 $\mu$m). The frequencies of the overtone $2\nu_2$ and the $\nu_1$ and $\nu_3$ bands are close, as are the frequencies $\nu_2$ and $\nu_4$, resulting in strong level interaction, which lifts the degeneracy of the fundamentals $\nu_3$ and $\nu_4$ and greatly complicates the structure of the vibration–rotation spectrum of methane.

Methane has a large number of overtone and combination-frequency bands, nine of which are observed in the solar spectrum in the wavelength interval from 1.6 to 3.9 $\mu$m. The fine structure of the vibration–rotation spectrum of methane has not been completely resolved to date [51–55].

## 2.5.9. Absorption Spectrum of Carbon Monoxide

The absorption spectrum of the carbon monoxide molecule has been studied in fair detail, primarily because of its structural simplicity. Electron transitions occur in the region of wavelengths shorter than 1 $\mu$m.

The fundamental vibration–rotation absorption band of the $C^{12}O^{16}$ molecule is situated near 2143.2 cm$^{-1}$ (4.67 $\mu$m). The principal overtone is centered around 4260 cm$^{-1}$. The calculated center positions of the absorption bands are (in cm$^{-1}$) 2143.2740 (0–1 band); 4260.0646 (0–2); 4207.1664 (1–3); 4154.4056 (2–4); 4101.7820 (3–5); 4049.2958 (4–6); 3996.9466 (5–7); 6350.4404 (0–3); 8414.4708 (0–4). The calculated center positions in the first two bands coincide with the experimental values to the fourth decimal place. The agreement in the next two bands is good to the second decimal place and in the next two bands to the first decimal place. The fine structure of the bands has been thoroughly investigated.

The carbon monoxide molecule has two isotopic modifications: $C^{12}O^{16}$ and $C^{13}O^{16}$, which provide a substantial contribution to the absorption of monochromatic radiation in the atmosphere.

The pure rotational spectrum of the CO molecule is situated in the far-infrared and microwave regions of the electromagnetic-wave scale.

## 2.5.10. Absorption Spectrum of Nitric Oxide

The NO molecule has a bond length equal to 1.151 Å and a constant dipole moment equal to 0.16 D.

The absorption bands of the fundamental vibrational transition (0–1) and the first overtone (0–2) are situated in the 5.3- and 2.76-$\mu$m regions. The total intensities of these bands have average values of 117 and 2.39 cm$^{-2}$atm$^{-1}$, respectively. A singular attribute of this molecule is the non-zero projection of the total electron orbital moment onto the axis of the molecule, so that each line is observed to split into two, where the intensities of the lines of the satellite bands are 4 to 5 orders of magnitude lower than for the lines of the principal bands.

## 2.5.11. Induced Spectra of Molecules

Any perturbations of absorbing molecules can cause electric dipole transitions normally forbidden by the selection rules for the isolated molecules to become allowed. The resulting absorption spectra are called induced.

The nature of the spectra comprised in the broad absorption bands in the region of the fundamental vibration frequencies of molecules is attributable to collision deformation of the molecules. The symmetry of the electron shell is reduced in this case, and an induced dipole moment sets in. Translational spectra appear in the far-infrared region at high pressures. The corresponding transitions refer to a variation of the translational energy

**Table 2.7.** Data on Induced Bands of $N_2$ and $O_2$

| Gas | Spectral interval, $cm^{-1}$ | Absorption peak, $cm^{-1}$ | Source |
|---|---|---|---|
| Fundamental band | | | |
| $N_2$ | 2190–2600 | 2300 | [56] |
| $O_2$ | 1400–1800 | 1580 | [56] |
| First overtone | | | |
| $N_2$ | 4400–4800 | 4650 | [56] |
| $O_2$ | 2900–3300 | 3100 | [56] |
| Translational spectra | | | |
| $N_2$ | 0–300 | 110 | [57] |
| $O_2$ | 0–400 | 110 | [57] |

of the interacting particles. A second modification of transitions induced in molecular interactions comprises transitions responsible for absorption at frequencies equal to the sum or difference of frequencies of vibrational or rotational transitions in each of the interacting molecules.

Data on the induced bands of $N_2$ and $O_2$ are given in Table 2.7.

## 2.6. Methods of Calculation of the Line Parameters and Absorption Coefficients of Atmospheric Gas Molecules

As we have already shown above, in order to determine the absorption coefficients it is necessary to have data on the parameters of the lines, including the center positions, intensities, and half-widths. In this section, therefore, we briefly portray the present status in regard to the calculation of those parameters. We are mainly concerned with the vibration–rotation spectra of atmospheric gas molecules, bearing in mind that they are situated in the most relevant range of the electromagnetic wave scale from the point of view of applied problems in atmospheric optics.

### 2.6.1. The Vibration–Rotation Schrödinger Equation

The vibration–rotation states of a molecule are characterized by the Schrödinger equation

$$H\Psi = E\Psi \tag{2.83}$$

The molecular vibration–rotation Hamiltonian was first obtained by Wilson and Howard [58]. This topic was subsequently investigated by several others [59–69]. Watson [70], using the properties of the inverse tensor of inertia, has recently obtained the vibration–rotation Hamiltonian in its simplest form, which has been appropriated in all subsequent papers:

$$H = \tfrac{1}{2} \sum_{\alpha\beta} \mu_{\alpha\beta} \mathcal{P}_\alpha \mathcal{P}_\beta - \sum_{\alpha\beta} \mu_{\alpha\beta} p_\alpha \mathcal{P}_\beta + \tfrac{1}{2} \sum_{\alpha\beta} \mu_{\alpha\beta} p_\alpha p_\beta + \tfrac{1}{2} \sum_{s\sigma} p_{s\sigma}^2 - \tfrac{1}{8} \sum_\alpha \mu_{\alpha\alpha} + U$$

$$(2.84)$$

Here $U$ is the potential function of the nuclear system with allowance for the effective electron field, $\mathcal{P}_\alpha$ and $p_\beta$ are the projections of the total and vibrational angular momenta onto the axis of a coordinate system fixed in the molecule $(\alpha, \beta = x, y, z)$, $\mu_{\alpha\beta}$ denotes the components of the inverse tensor of inertia, and $p_{s\sigma}$ denotes the momenta representing the conjugates of the normal coordinates $q_{s\sigma}$.

The eigenvalues and eigenfunctions of the operator (2.84) cannot be determined in closed form, so it is necessary to invoke approximation methods. The first step in this direction is the extraction from $H$ of a certain reasonable zeroth approximation and a small perturbation operator. In view of the special characteristics of the operators $\mu_{\alpha\beta}$ and $U$, the perturbation operator turns out to be inhomogeneous and can be represented by an expansion with respect to a certain small parameter. The usual small parameter adopted in the theory of vibration–rotation spectra is the ratio $\kappa = (m/M)^{1/4} \sim (B/\omega)^{1/2}$, where $B$ is the average rotational constant, $\omega$ is the average fundamental frequency, $m$ is the electron mass, $M$ is the average mass of nuclei in the molecule, and $\kappa$ is the Born–Oppenheimer parameter. An expansion of the operator $H$ in powers of the parameter $\kappa$ is obtained by expanding the operators $\mu_{\alpha\beta}$ and $U$:

$$\mu_{\alpha\beta} = \sum_{k=0} \mu_{\alpha\beta}^{(k)} = \mu_{\alpha\beta}^0 + \sum_i \mu_{\alpha\beta}^i q_i + \tfrac{1}{2} \sum_{ik} \mu_{\alpha\beta}^{ik} q_i q_k + \cdots \tag{2.85}$$

$$U = \sum_{k=0} U_k = \tfrac{1}{2} \sum_i \omega_i q_i^2 + \tfrac{1}{6} \sum_{ikl} K_{ikl} q_i q_k q_l + \cdots \tag{2.86}$$

The higher coefficients of the expansion of $\mu_{\alpha\beta}$ can be expressed in terms of $\mu_{\alpha\beta}^0$ and $\mu_{\alpha\beta}^i$ by means of simple relations. These coefficients can be calculated on the basis of recursion relations [71, 72] or direct equations [70].

The properties of the coefficients due to the symmetry properties of the molecule can prove helpful in the calculations with the use of the expansions

(2.85) and (2.86) [73, 74]. The latter generates an expansion in orders of the operator (2.84):

$$H_0 = \tfrac{1}{2} \sum_\alpha \mu_{\alpha\alpha}^0 \mathcal{P}_x^2 + \tfrac{1}{2} \sum_{s\sigma} \omega_s \left( p_{s\sigma}^2 + q_{s\sigma}^2 \right) \tag{2.87}$$

$$H_1 = \tfrac{1}{2} \sum_{\alpha\beta} \mu_{\alpha\beta}^{(1)} \mathcal{P}_\alpha \mathcal{P}_\beta - \sum_\alpha \mu_{\alpha\alpha}^0 p_\alpha \mathcal{P}_\alpha + U_1 \tag{2.88}$$

$$\cdots\cdots\cdots\cdots\cdots\cdots\cdots\cdots\cdots\cdots\cdots\cdots\cdots\cdots\cdots$$

$$H_n = \tfrac{1}{2} \sum_{\alpha\beta} \mu_{\alpha\beta}^{(n)} \mathcal{P}_\alpha \mathcal{P}_\beta - \sum_{\alpha\beta} \mu_{\alpha\beta}^{(n-1)} p_\alpha \mathcal{P}_\beta + \tfrac{1}{2} \sum_{\alpha\beta} \mu_{\alpha\beta}^{(n-2)} p_\alpha p_\beta - \tfrac{1}{8} \sum_\alpha \mu_{\alpha\alpha}^{(n-2)} + U_n \tag{2.89}$$

The Hamiltonian (2.87)–(2.89) can be simplified in specific cases by means of the symmetry relations between its coefficients, but it cannot be used for linear molecules.

Several papers have been devoted to the derivation of a vibration–rotation Hamiltonian for linear molecules [75–81]; the results may be formulated as follows. The wave functions and vibration–rotation energy levels of linear molecules can be obtained from the solution of the system of equations [78]

$$\left\{ \mu \left[ \left( \mathcal{P}_x' - p_x \right)^2 + \left( \mathcal{P}_y' - p_y \right)^2 \right] + \tfrac{1}{2} \sum_{s\sigma} \omega_{s\sigma} p_{s\sigma}^2 + U \right\} \Psi = E \Psi \tag{2.90}$$

$$\left( \mathcal{P}_z' - p_z \right) \Psi + 0 \tag{2.91}$$

$$\Psi = (2\pi) W^{-1} \Psi \tag{2.92}$$

$$W = \exp \left\{ i \left[ X' - X(\theta, \varphi) \right] p_z \right\} \tag{2.93}$$

Equation (2.83) is usually solved in the Born–Oppenheimer approximation [82] on the assumption that the motion of the nuclei takes place in a field with a certain effective potential, which is obtained from the solution of the electron problem. The total wave function of the system in this case is represented by the product of the electron and nuclear wave functions. We note that calculation in more precise approximations significantly improves the given physical quantity in certain cases of interest [83–90].

In our own papers [91–94] we have deduced, for the first time, the effective vibration–rotation Hamiltonian in infinite-series form for the electron states with regard for electron–nucleus interaction. We showed that the form of the vibration–rotation Hamiltonian depends only very slightly on the electron–nucleus interaction.

### 2.6.2. Methods of Solution of the Vibration–Rotation Schrödinger Equation

Once the zeroth approximation has been identified and the perturbation operator expanded in orders of smallness, it is possible to find the approximate eigenvalues and eigenfunctions of the operator $H$. Various methods can be used for this purpose, depending on the application. Early studies relied on the ordinary matrix theory of perturbations, which can be used up to the second order to derive an expression for the vibration–rotation energy, adequately effective for diatomic molecules as well as molecules of the symmetrical-top types.

The matrix elements of the perturbation operator are calculated only numerically in the case of asymmetrical-top molecules, the denominators containing the rotational energy differences. The summation in the perturbation formulas extends over a large number of indices, and comparison with experiment shows that higher perturbation orders must be used. In view of these difficulties, beginning with early papers, the following procedure has been used to solve the vibration–rotation Schrödinger equation.

The operator $H$ is subjected to preliminary transformation, consisting in reduction to a form $\tilde{H}$ diagonal in the basis of vibrational wave functions, so that for a fixed vibrational state the operator $\tilde{H}$ is a pure rotation operator. This procedure permits an artificial separation of the vibration and rotation problems, which can be solved independently. Various operator perturbation methods and modifications of matrix perturbation theory are used to implement the procedure described above. The most common approach is the method of contact transformations (CT).

The CT method has been developed in several papers in application to vibration–rotation spectra [95–105]. Members of the author's research group [106–115] have attempted to formulate a generalized CT method based on simultaneous utilization of the algebraic and spatial properties of the set of perturbation operators $H_n$. The mathematical foundations of this approach had already been developed in application to other branches of physics. The essence of the traditional method may be summarized as follows.

Let it be required to reduce the operator

$$H = H_0 + \sum_{n=1}^{\infty} \kappa^n H_n \tag{2.94}$$

to the form $\tilde{H} = T^+ H T$, which is diagonal in the basis of eigenfunctions of the operator $H_0$. We assume that it has been possible to extract the zeroth-approximation operator $H_0$ and the operators $H_n$ from the expansion (2.94) and that perturbation theory is applicable. The operator version of perturbation theory, for which

$$T = T_1 \times T_2 \times \cdots \times T_k \times \cdots \qquad (2.95)$$

and the transformation $T_k = \exp(-i\kappa^k S_k)$ diagonalizes the $k$th term of the Hamiltonian subjected to all previous transformations, is called the CT method. Hereinafter we use the notation [95]

$$H^{(k)} = \exp\left(i\kappa^k S_k\right) H^{(k-1)} \exp\left(-i\kappa^k S_k\right), \qquad H^{(0)} \equiv H \qquad (2.96)$$

for the $k$-fold transformed Hamiltonian

$$H^{(k)} = \sum_{n=0}^{\infty} \kappa^n H_n^{(k)} \qquad (2.97)$$

Definition (2.96) in conjunction with the Hausdorff equation makes it possible to deduce a relation between the terms of the expansion of the $k$-fold and $(k-1)$-fold transformed Hamiltonians with respect to $\kappa$:

$$H_n^{(k)} = \sum_{m=0}^{[[n/k]]} \frac{i^m}{m!} \left\{ S_k^{(m)}, H_{n-km}^{(k-1)} \right\} \qquad (2.98)$$

where $[[x]]$ denotes the integer part of $x$ and

$$\left\{ S^{(m)}, A \right\} = \underbrace{\left[ S, \left[ S, \cdots \left[ S, A \right] \cdots \right] \right]}_{m}$$

The operator $S_k$ is dictated by the requirement of diagonality of $H_k^{(k)}$ in the basis of eigenfunctions of the operator $H_0$. We note that, in accordance with the definition of the transformation $T_k$ and the operator $H_n^{(k)}$ (2.97),

$$H_n^{(k)} = H_n^{(n)} \qquad (k \geqslant n) \qquad (2.99)$$

This scheme has been used successfully for diagonalization of the vibration–rotation Hamiltonian [95–105] as well as for transformation of the dipole moment operator of diatomic molecules [116–119] and the dipole moment operator in the molecular coordinate system for polyatomic molecules [120–122]. In the theory of vibration–rotation transitions in polyatomic molecules, the above-described method is used for partial diagonalization of the total vibration–rotation Hamiltonian with respect to the vibrational quantum numbers. In this case, we once again proceed from the definition of $H^{(k)}$ (2.96), but depart from the usual scheme by replacing the diagonality condition for $H_k^k$ in the basis of eigenfunctions of the zeroth-approximation operator by the requirement of diagonality of $H_k^k$ in the basis of strictly harmonic functions.

It is essential to note in connection with the traditional CT method that its formulation is not sufficiently rigorous because the system of equations for the method is incompletely specified. A consequence of this fact is the absence of a general solution of the CT equations, along with other shortcomings.

Makushkin and Tyuterev [106–115] have formulated the following system of equations for the CT method on the basis of the Primas super-operators [123–124] acting in the space $L$ of perturbation operators $H_n$ and transformations $S_n$, the superoperator $\mathcal{D}_A$ of "inner differentiation in $L$" with respect to an Hermitian operator $A \in L$, the superoperator $\langle \cdots \rangle_{H_0}$ of extraction of a block-diagonal part with respect to $H_0$, the inverse $\mathcal{D}_A^{-1}$ of the superoperator $\mathcal{D}_A$, and the special inversion $1/\mathcal{D}_A$ of the superoperator $\mathcal{D}_A$:

$$i\mathcal{D}(S_n) = H_n^{(n-1)} - H_n^n \tag{2.100}$$

$$\langle H_n^n \rangle = H_n^{(n)} \tag{2.101}$$

The general solution of this system has the form

$$iS_n = \frac{1}{\mathcal{D}}\left(H_n^{(n-1)}\right) + \langle A \rangle \tag{2.102}$$

$$H_n^n = \langle H_n^{n-1} \rangle \tag{2.103}$$

If we put $\langle A \rangle = 0$, we can deduce the results of the traditional CT method from this system. The general solutions (2.102), (2.103) provide a basis for explaining certain properties of contract transformations not hitherto investigated in the theory of vibration–rotation interactions. In particular, Eqs. (2.102) and (2.103) are also valid for degenerate states, even though they do not produce complete diagonalization of the vibration–rotation Hamiltonian in this case. Another new aspect of the given method is the possibility of transforming to a basis formed in the space of dynamical variables by the eigenvectors of the superoperators $\langle \cdots \rangle$ and $1/\mathcal{D}$. It turns out that this possibility extremely simplifies the problem of finding the transformations $S_k$ and reduces the procedure for finding $H_n^n$ to recursion relations between the coefficients of the expansion of $H_n^k$ with respect to the basis vectors. This approach ensures the efficient utilization of a computer for obtaining the "reduced" vibration–rotation energy function.

Finally, with the aid of Mellin, Fourier, or Laplace transformations, the integral representation of the above-defined superoperators makes it possible to find the transformations $S_n$ even in cases where the traditional method proves futile.

Our important result of the given method is the confirmation of the essential multivaluedness of the effective rotational Hamiltonians in vibrational diagonalization of the total vibration–rotation Hamiltonian.

In concluding this subsection, we note that the relations between the spectroscopic constants of isotopic modifications of molecules play an important part in the investigation of molecular absorption spectra. In the literature, we find isotopic relations of the nature of rules of sums and products for powers of the squares and mixed products of harmonic vibration frequencies [125–132] as well as the rotational [133] and centrifugal [134–136] constants. Members of the author's research group have proposed [137–142] a general technique for determining the isotopic relations between spectroscopic constants, making it possible to obtain relations between the squares of the frequencies of an isotope and the principal molecule, for the vibration–rotation interaction constants, including higher orders, the anharmonicity constants, centrifugal distortion, and the resonant interaction constants.

### 2.6.3. Expressions for the Line Intensities

We write the expression for the intensity of the absorption lines due to transition between vibration–rotation states of a molecule $V'R'$ and $V''R''$ in a form suitable for further analysis:

$$S_{V'R'}^{V''R''} = \frac{8\pi^3 N_0}{2hcQ_{V''R''}} \nu_{V'R',V''R''} g_{V''R''} \exp\left(-\frac{hc}{kT}E_{V''R''}\right)$$

$$\times \left[1-\exp\left(-\frac{hc}{kT}\nu_{V'R',V''R''}\right)\right] |\langle V'R'|M_z|V''R''\rangle|^2 \quad (2.104)$$

where $\langle V'R'|$ and $\langle V''R''|$ are the wave functions, $\nu_{V'R',V''R''} = E_{V'R'} - E_{V''R''}$ is the transition frequency, $E_{V'R'}$ and $E_{V''R''}$ are the energy levels, $M_z$ is the component of the electric moment vector in the rest frame, $N_0$ is the number of absorbing particles per unit of volume, $Q_{V''R''}$ is the vibration–rotation statistical sum, $g_{V''R''}$ is the statistical weight of the lowest vibration–rotation state, $h$ is the Planck constant, $c$ is the speed of light, $k$ is the Boltzmann constant, and $T$ is the absolute temperature.

The vibration–rotation line intensity in the zeroth approximation is given by the expression

$$S_0 = S_V S_R \frac{1}{Q_R} \frac{\nu_{V'R',V''R''}}{\nu_{V'V''}} \tag{2.105}$$

in which $\nu_{V'V''}$ is the center of the vibrational band,

$$S_R = g_r \exp\left(-\frac{E_{R''}}{kT}\right) L_{R''R'}\left\{1 - \exp\left(-\frac{hc}{kT}\nu_{V'R',V''R''}\right)\right\} \tag{2.106}$$

and where

$$L_{R''R'} = 3 \sum_{m'm''} |\langle R''|\Phi(zg)|R'\rangle|^2$$

is the intensity of the rotational transition line, $m'$ and $m''$ are the magnetic quantum numbers, $\Phi(zg)$ denotes the direction cosines, and $S_V$ is the band normalization factor, which does not depend on the rotational quantum numbers.

Inasmuch as

$$\sum_{R''R'} L_{R''R'} = 1 \tag{2.107}$$

$S_V$ is the integral intensity of the vibration–roation band.

It follows from the discussion of the preceding sections that vibration–rotation interaction changes the energy levels $E_{V''R''}$, $E_{V'R'}$ and the wave functions $\langle V'R'|$, $\langle V''R''|$, and, therefore, also the statistical sum $Q_{V''R''}$, the transition frequency $\nu_{V'R',V''R''}$, and the dipole moment matrix element $\langle V'R'|M_z|V''R''\rangle$. With regard for vibration–rotation interaction, the expression for $S$ assumes the form

$$S = S_0 F \tag{2.108}$$

and $S_V$ is no longer the integral intensity of the vibrational band. Expressions for the $F$ factor are obtained by the semiclassical method [143, 144], by perturbation theory [145, 146], by the CT method [147, 148], and by the effective nonrigid-top method [149–158].

We now consider the influence of random resonances on the transition probabilities. Suppose that transition takes place between vibration–rotation states, one of which is not distorted by random resonances, while the other is distorted both by vibrational (Fermi, Lagrange–Dennison, etc.) and by vibration–rotation (Coriolis) resonances. In this case, the total $F_{li}$ factor in (2.108) can be represented in the form

$$F_{li} = F_1^{li} \cdot F_2^{li} \cdot F_3^{li}, \tag{2.109}$$

where $F_1^{li} = (1 + \Phi_{li})^2$ is the factor associated with regular vibration–rotation interaction for the transition $(l\text{–}i)$,

$$F_2^{li} = F_{li}^{\mathcal{D}\mathcal{D}} = |C_{ii}^{\mathcal{D}\mathcal{D}}|^2 \left\{ 1 + \sum_{k \neq i} \frac{C_{ik}^{\mathcal{D}\mathcal{D}}}{C_{ii}^{\mathcal{D}\mathcal{D}}} \frac{\langle k | M_z | l \rangle_0}{\langle i | M_z | l \rangle_0} \frac{(1 + \Phi_{ki})}{(1 + \Phi_{li})} \right\} \tag{2.110}$$

$$F_3^i = F_{li}^{\mathrm{cor}} |C_{ii}^{\mathrm{cor}}|^2 \left\{ 1 + \sum_{n \neq i} \frac{C_{in}^{\mathrm{cor}}}{C_{ii}^{\mathrm{cor}}} \frac{\langle n | M_z | l \rangle_0}{\langle i | M_z | l \rangle_0} \frac{(1 + \Phi_{ln})(F_{ln}^{\mathcal{D}\mathcal{D}})^{1/2}}{(1 + \Phi_{li})(F_{li}^{\mathcal{D}\mathcal{D}})^{1/2}} \right\}$$

$$\tag{2.111}$$

and $C_{ik}$ denotes the coefficients of the expansion of the wave function, with allowance for resonance, with respect to the zeroth-approximation basis functions. If a particular effect does not occur, the corresponding factor is set equal to unity.

## 2.6.4. Expressions for the Line Half-Widths and Shifts

Molecular collisions constitute the decisive factor in the evolution of the line contour in the infrared (IR) and lower-frequency regions of the spectrum under the conditions prevailing in the lower layers of the atmosphere. In analyzing the absorption in the central part of a line, it is customary to use the impact approximation, which yields a dispersion relation for the line contour as a function of the frequency with half-width and center shift determined (in the resolvent operator formalism) by, respectively, the imaginary and real parts of the diagonal matrix element of the relaxation operator $\Lambda$, which has the form

$$\Lambda = -i \eta_b \int dv \langle 1 - S S^\dagger \rangle \tag{2.112}$$

where $\eta_b$ is the density of the expanding gas acting as a thermostat, $\int dv$ is the averaging operator over the classical collision parameters, $S$ is the scattering matrix, angle brackets denote the averaging operator over quantum states of the thermostat particle:

$$\langle X \rangle = Tr^b \{ \rho^b X \} \tag{2.113}$$

and $\rho^b$ is the density matrix of the thermostat particle. In expression (2.112), the product $SS^\dagger$ is interpreted in the Liouville sense, i.e., $S$ acts on the initial state in the Liouville vector (see below) and $S^\dagger$ acts on the final state in that vector.

The operator $\Lambda$ in the form (2.13) is the initial operator in the calculation of the half-widths and shifts of the lines in impact theory. For the ensuing discussion, it is necessary to introduce some new notation. Let $H_S, |\alpha lm\rangle$ and $H_b, |\beta l\mu\rangle$ be the Hamiltonians and eigenfunctions of the absorbing molecule and the thermostat molecule, respectively. Here $J(l)$ is the quantum number corresponding to the total angular momentum of the absorbing molecule (thermostat molecule), $m(\mu)$ is the quantum number corresponding to the projection of the total momentum onto a spatially fixed axis, and $\alpha(\beta)$ is the symbolic notation for all other quantum numbers.

It has been shown [159] that the relaxation operator $\Lambda$ in an isotropic gaseous medium is invariant under the space rotation group. A consequence of this invariance is the fact that the line half-widths and shifts can be calculated without any simplifying assumptions as to the structure of the Hamiltonians $H_S$ and $H_b$ and their eigenvectors [160]. The calculation of the half-widths and shifts can be portrayed schematically as follows.

The half-width and center shift of a spectral line $\alpha_i J_i \rightarrow \alpha_f J_f$ are given by the expressions (in $cm^{-1}$)

$$\gamma_{if} = -(2\pi c)^{-1} \mathrm{Im}\, \Lambda_{if,if}; \qquad \delta_{if} = (2\pi c)^{-1} \mathrm{Re}\, \Lambda_{if,if} \tag{2.114}$$

The matrix element $\Lambda_{if,if}$ can be represented as follows on the basis of (2.112) and the Wigner–Eckart theorem:

$$\Lambda_{if,if} = -i\eta_b \int dv \sum_{\beta l} \rho_{\beta l} S(b)$$

$$S(b) = \sum_{\beta' l'} \sum_{m_i m\mu} \frac{(J_f 1 m_f M | J_i m_i)(J_f 1 m_f' M | J_i' m_i')}{(2J_i + 1)(2l + 1)}$$

$$\times \left[ 1 - \langle \alpha_i J_i m_i (\beta l\mu) | S | (\beta' l'\mu')\alpha_i J_i m_i' \rangle \langle \alpha_f J_f m_f' (\beta' l'\mu') | S^+ | (\beta l\mu)\alpha_f J_f m_f \rangle \right]$$

$$\tag{2.115}$$

where $M=0, \pm 1$ and parentheses around summation indices signify that the summation is carried out with respect to both unprimed and primed versions of those indices. The rest of the analysis is essentially similar to the work of Tsao and Curnutte [7] and, up to second-order interaction terms, yields the result

$$S_0(b)=1, \qquad S_1(b)=0$$

$$S_2(b)=S_2(b)_{\text{middle}}+S_2(b)_{\text{outer}} \tag{2.116}$$

where

$$S_2(b)_{\text{outer}}=\frac{1}{2}\left\{ \sum_{m_i\mu} \frac{\langle \alpha_i J_i m_i(\beta l\mu)|P^2|(\beta l\mu)\alpha_i J_i m_i\rangle}{(2J_i+1)(2l+1)} +(i\rightarrow f)\right\} \tag{2.117}$$

$$S_2(b)_{\text{middle}}=- \sum_{\substack{m_i m_f \mu \\ M}} \sum_{\beta' l'} \frac{(J_f 1 m_f M|J_i m_i)(J_f 1 m_f' M|J_i m_i')}{(2J_i+1)(2l+1)}$$

$$\times \langle \alpha_i J_i m_i(\beta l\mu)|P|(\beta' l'\mu')\alpha_i J_i m_i'\rangle\langle \alpha_f J_f m_f'(\beta' l'\mu')|P|(\beta l\mu)\alpha_f J_f m_f'\rangle \tag{2.118}$$

and we introduce the notation

$$P=\frac{1}{\hbar}\int_{-\infty}^{\infty}(U^0)^{-1}H_c(t')U^0\,dt' \tag{2.119}$$

The evolution operator $U^0$ obeys the equation

$$i\hbar\frac{\partial U^0}{\partial t}=(H_S+H_b)U^0 \tag{2.120}$$

The interaction Hamiltonian $H_c(t)$ can be written in the form

$$H_c(t)= \sum_{\substack{\kappa_1\kappa_2 \\ q_1 q_2}} C_{q_1 q_2}^{\kappa_1\kappa_2}(t)T_{q_1}^{\kappa_1}(t)T_{q_2}^{\kappa_2}(t) \tag{2.121}$$

where $T_q^\kappa$ is the spherical component of the $2\kappa$-pole moment tensor of the molecule, $q=0, \pm 1,\ldots, \pm\kappa$, and $C_{q_1 q_2}^{\kappa_1\kappa_2}(t)$ are coefficients depending on the distance between molecules.

Substituting (2.121) into (2.119) and then into (2.117) and (2.118), invoking the Wigner–Eckart theorem, according to which

$$\langle \alpha J m | T_q^\kappa | \alpha' J' m' \rangle = (2J+1)^{-1/2} (J'\kappa m'q | Jm)(\alpha J \| T^\kappa \| \alpha' J')$$

$$(2.122)$$

where $(\alpha J \| T^\kappa \| \alpha' J')$ is the reduced matrix element, and finally summing over the magnetic quantum numbers, we have

$$S_2(b)_{\text{outer}} = \sum_{\kappa_1 \kappa_2} \frac{C_{\kappa_1 \kappa_2}}{2\hbar^2} \sum_{\beta' l'} \left\{ \sum_{\alpha'_i J'_i} |D(\alpha_i J_i \to \alpha'_i J'_i | \kappa_1)|^2 f_{\kappa_1 \kappa_2} + (i \to f) \right\}$$

$$\times |D(\beta l \to \beta' l' | \kappa_2)|^2 \qquad (2.123)$$

$$S_2(b)_{\text{middle}} = \sum_{\kappa_1 \kappa_2} \frac{C_{\kappa_1 \kappa_2}}{\hbar^2} (-1)^{J_i + J_f + \kappa_1} [(2J_i + 1)(2J_f + 1)]^{1/2}$$

$$\times \sum_{\beta' l'} D(\alpha_i J_i \to \alpha_i J_i | \kappa_1) D(\alpha_f J_f \to \alpha_f J_f | \kappa_1)$$

$$\times |D(\beta l \to \beta' l' | \kappa_2)|^2 W(J_i J_f J_i J_f; 1\kappa_1) f_{\kappa_1 \kappa_2} \qquad (2.124)$$

where

$$D(\alpha J \to \alpha' J' | \kappa) = \frac{(\alpha J \| T^\kappa \| \alpha' J')}{[(2\kappa+1)(2J+1)]^{1/2}} \qquad (2.125)$$

$$C_{\kappa_1 \kappa_2} f_{\kappa_1 \kappa_2} = \sum_{q_1 q_2} |a_{q_1 q_2}^{\kappa_1 \kappa_2}(\omega_{mn})|^2 \qquad (2.126)$$

The coefficient $C_{\kappa_1 \kappa_2}$ can be chosen in such a way as to make the function $f_{\kappa_1 \kappa_2}$ coincide with the corresponding function $f$ in [7]:

$$\omega_{mn} = \hbar^{-1} \{ E_{\alpha J} - E_{\alpha' J'} + E_{\beta l} - E_{\beta' l'} \} \qquad (2.127)$$

the quantity $a_{q_1 q_2}^{\kappa_1 \kappa_2}$ is the result of integration of the coefficients $C_{q_1 q_2}^{\kappa_1 \kappa_2}(t)$ in (2.118) with respect to the time, and $W(abcd; ef)$ is the Racah coefficient.

Expressions (2.123) and (2.124) are the fundamental analytical equations. They enable us, in particular, to account for the influence of molecular interactions on the line half-widths and shifts. The quantity $|D(\alpha J \to$

$\alpha'J'|\kappa)|^2$ plays the role of the generalized line intensity of the $2\kappa$-pole transition between levels $\alpha J$ and $\alpha'J'$, divided by $2J+1$, and can be written in the form

$$|D(\alpha J \to \alpha'J'|\kappa)|^2 = |D^0(\alpha J \to \alpha'J'|\kappa)|^2 F(\alpha J \to \alpha'J'|\kappa) \quad (2.128)$$

The factor $F$ accounts for the influence of molecular interactions and is given by expressions of the type (2.108)–(2.111).

Up to now, we have discussed the broadening problem for an isolated spectral line. In a number of instances, however, collisions induce a special kind of relaxation coupling between lines in the spectrum. Such lines are also called overlapping in the literature [160]. The quantum-mechanical theory of the broadening of overlapping spectral lines in the impact approximation was first set down in [161, 162] and was later reconstructed on a more general basis by Fano [163]. In Fano's formalism, the absorption coefficient takes the following form after introduction of the impact approximation:

$$\alpha(\omega) = \frac{2\pi\omega\eta}{3c\hbar n_0}\left[1 - \exp(-\hbar\omega/kT)\right]\mathrm{Im}\sum_{i<f}\sum_{i'f'}\rho_{1i}P_{if}^{(1)}P_{i'f'}^{(1)}$$

$$\times\left[\left(\frac{1}{\omega - \hat{L}_S - \Lambda}\right)_{i'f',if} + \left(\frac{1}{\omega - \hat{L}_S - \Lambda}\right)_{i'f',fi}\right] \quad (2.129)$$

where $\hat{L}_S$ is the Liouville operator corresponding to the absorbing-particle Hamiltonian $H_S$ and is given by the equation

$$\hat{L}_S X = \hbar^{-1}[H_S, X]$$

for an arbitrary operator $X$, $\rho_{1i}$ is the population of the initial state, $P_{if}^{(1)}$ is the reduced matrix element of the irreducible tensor dipole moment operator for the absorbing molecule, $\eta$ is the density of the absorbing gas, and $n_0$ is the refractive index of the medium. The summation in the first sum is taken only over levels satisfying the condition $E_i < E_f$.

If the operator $\Lambda$ is diagonal, i.e., if

$$\Lambda_{if,i'f'} = \Lambda_{if,if}\delta_{ii'},\delta_{ff'}$$

then the total absorption coefficient is reducible to the simple superposition of the absorption coefficients corresponding to the individual lines, each of which broadens independently of the others and has a shape described by the Van Vleck–Weisskopf equation.

The presence of nonzero off-diagonal matrix elements on the part of the relaxation operator $\Lambda$ causes overlapping [164–165] of the corresponding lines and induces certain anomalies in the transformation of the profile of the pressure spectrum [166–168]. For example, as the pressure is increased, the overlapping lines begin to approach one another at a rate proportional to the pressure squared and then merge at the center of gravity of the spectrum, forming a single uniformly broadened line.

The anomalous broadening of overlapping spectral lines has been observed experimentally, for example, in the inversion [169–170] and rotational [171] spectra of ammonia and in the microwave spectrum of oxygen [172].

The theoretical analysis of this phenomenon is largely impeded by the lack of a systematic procedure in the literature for calculating the matrix elements of the relaxation operator $\Lambda$ in the case where it is not diagonal. This deficit was recently remedied to a certain extent by Cherkasov [173–

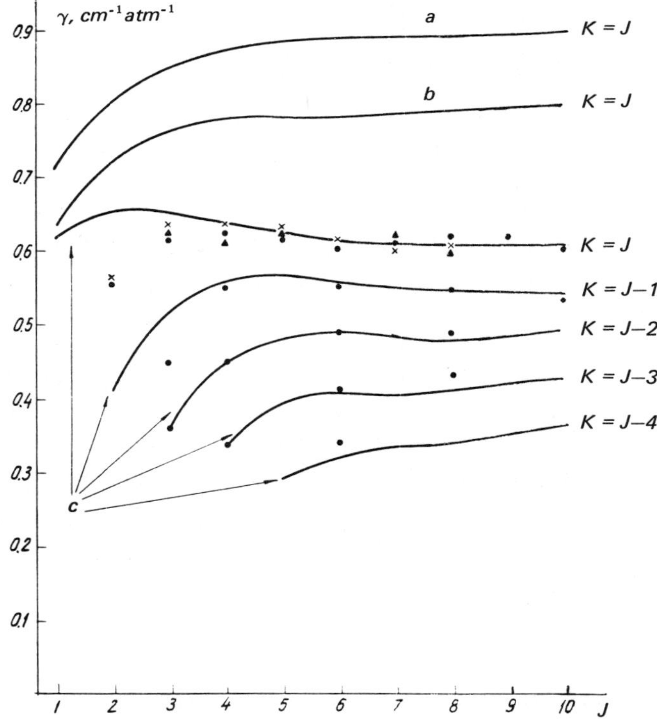


Fig. 2.10. $J$-dependence of line half-widths of the inversion spectrum of ammonia. Experimental data: (●) [177]; (▲) [178]; (×) [179].

176], who showed, in particular, that if relaxation coupling exists between spectral lines, their half-widths will always be smaller than the values that they would have if isolated in the spectrum. The indicated narrowing effect does not depend on the pressure; it is completely determined by the quantum structure of the colliding particles and their interaction potential.

The stated effect can prove quite significant in a number of cases. This is illustrated, for example, by Fig. 2.10, which gives the results of calculations of the line half-width for the inversion spectrum of ammonia in the case of self-broadening [176]. Here curve *a* corresponds to calculation by the Anderson–Tsao–Curnutte method, curve *b* to calculation in the isolated-line approximation but without the "clean break" approximation of Anderson, and curves *c* to calculation with allowance for the effect of relaxation coupling between lines. It is evident from the figure that the "clean break" approximation of Anderson yields results that are roughly 13% too large, while the invalid use of the isolated-line approximation increases the line half-width by about 30%.

The role of overlapping in atmospheric–optical problems has been totally ignored to date.

## 2.6.5. Some Results of the Theory of Vibration–Rotation Transitions in Molecules

As the foregoing discussion indicates, the calculation of the vibration–rotation energy of molecules essentially entails calculation of the vibrational energy and determination of the eigenvalues of the effective rotational Hamiltonian. The procedure for calculation of the vibration–rotation energy is best implemented with consideration for the singular characteristics of specific types of molecules because results in analytical form are obtainable in quite a few significant cases.

### 2.6.5.1. Diatomic Molecules

The given procedure is simplest for diatomic molecules. Aliev and Aleksanyan [95] have used the CT method to derive an expression for the transformed Hamiltonian:

$$\tilde{H} = \sum_{lj} X_{lj} \left( p^2 + q^2 \right)^l \wp^{2j} \tag{2.130}$$

which is the operator analog of Dunham's equation [89] for the vibration–

rotation energy:

$$E = \sum_{lj} Y_{lj}\left(V+\tfrac{1}{2}\right)J^{j}(J+1)^{j}, \qquad Y_{lj} = 2^{l}X_{lj} \tag{2.131}$$

Expressions for the first 15 coefficient $Y_{lj}$ were first obtained by Dunham. In later years, with the continued improvement of experimental accuracy, various authors have obtained expressions for other constants $Y_{lj}$. However, current experimental data (see, e.g., [180]) indicate that the expressions published in the literature fail to account for some of the experimental results. This deficit underscores the timely need for calculating the high-order vibration–rotation energy of molecules. The method proposed by the present author's research group lends itself to the application of computers for derivation of the required expressions. Results in the form of expressions for $Y_{lj}$ up to and including the tenth order are given in [112]. They are the most complete and accurate expressions available at the present time and include the previous literature data as special cases (see table 2.8).

### 2.6.5.2. Linear Molecules

Many papers have been devoted to the calculation of high orders for individual molecules. The derived expressions and numerical results account quite well for the experimental spectrum associated with rotational transitions in the fundamental vibrational state as well as in the fundamental and certain overtone bands.

General expressions for the frequencies of the rotational lines of the bands are given in [181]:

$$\left.\begin{array}{l}
1.\ V_t = V_{t'} = \cdots = 0 \\[4pt]
\left.\begin{array}{ll}
2.\ V_t = 1; & l_t = \pm 1 \\
3.\ V_t = 2; & l_t = 0, \pm 2 \\
4.\ V_t = 3; & l_t = \pm 1, \pm 3
\end{array}\right\} V_{t'}' = \cdots = 0 \\[12pt]
5.\ V_t = V_{t'} = 1 \quad \left\{\begin{array}{l} l_t = l_{t'} = \pm 1 \\ l_t = -l_{t'} = \pm 1 \end{array}\right.
\end{array}\right\} V_n, V_{n'}, \ldots \text{arbitrary}$$

$$\tag{2.132}$$

Rather than reproduce the cumbersome tables in which the results are compiled, we shall merely highlight certain results. The vibration–rotation energy for vibrational states in which only nondegenerate modes are excited has the form

$$E_{VR} = E_V + B_V J(J+1) + D_V J^2(J+1)^2 + \cdots \tag{2.133}$$

Here $E_V$ is the energy of anharmonic vibrations, and $B_V, D_V$ are the rotational and centrifugal constants.

If one twofold-degenerate mode is excited, then the levels $l = \pm 1$ split under the influence of Coriolis interaction, and

$$E_{VR}^{\pm} = E_V + B_V J(J+1) + D_V J^2(J+1)^2 \pm 2q_t^{\text{eff}} J(J+1) + \cdots$$

$$\tag{2.134}$$

where $q_t^{\text{eff}}$ is the $l$-doubling constant.

For higher vibrational states, the splitting pattern is greatly complicated by strong $l$-type rotational resonance. The expressions needed for analysis of the rotational levels may be found in Table LX of the book [181].

The practical utilization of expressions such as (2.133) and (2.134) is complicated by the cumbersomeness of the relations between the rotational and centrifugal constants and doubling constants, on the one hand, and the molecular parameters, on the other.

It has been proposed [182–185] that computers be used for the derivation of these relations. Nielsen [121] has implemented this proposition up to and including fourth order. The derived expressions have been used to analyze the spectrum of the $CO_2$ molecule.

Random vibrational resonances of the Fermi type play an important part in the spectra of linear molecules. An analysis of various manifestations of these effects is carried out in studies [185–191] based on matrix perturbation theory or numerical techniques. The method proposed by the author's group and described in Section 2.6.2 provides an effective tool for the analysis of random resonances in operator form.

### 2.6.5.3. Symmetrical Top

Specialists in atmospheric optics have lately become increasingly preoccupied with symmetrical-top type of molecule in connection with the problem of monitoring contamination of the atmosphere. We note that the focus of attention in the literature is on molecules of symmetry $C_{3v}, D_3, D_{3h}$, and $D_{3d}$ as well as considerably lower—$C_{4v}$ and $D_{2d}$.

The most complete list of general expressions for the vibration–rotation energy of the above-indicated types of molecules is given in [181] (see also the references therein). The authors of [181] have calculated the vibration–rotation energy for the following vibrational states:

$$
\left.
\begin{array}{l}
\text{1.} \quad V_t = V_{t'} = \cdots = 0 \\
\text{2.} \quad V_t = 1; \quad l_t = \pm 1 \\
\text{2.} \quad V_t = 2; \quad l_t = 0 \\
\text{4.} \quad V_t = 2; \quad l_t = \pm 2 \\
\text{5.} \quad V_t = 3; \quad l_t = \pm 1 \\
\text{6.} \quad V_t = 3; \quad l_t = \pm 3 \\
\text{7.} \quad V_t = V_{t'} = 1; \quad l_t = -l_t = \pm 1 \\
\text{8.} \quad V_t = V_{t'} = 1; \quad l_t = l_{t'} = \pm 1 \\
\left. \phantom{\text{8.} \quad V_t = V_{t'} = 1;} \right\} V_{t'} = 0
\end{array}
\right\} V_n, V_{n'}, \ldots \text{ arbitrary}
$$

$$(2.135)$$

According to the derivations of Nielsen [181], the values of the contributions of various terms of the Hamiltonian to the energy depend significantly on the values of the rotational quantum numbers $J$ and $K$. Three cases are discerned:

$$
\begin{array}{ll}
\text{A.} & J \approx K \approx 1 \\
\text{B.} & J \approx K \approx 30 \\
\text{C.} & J \approx 30, \quad K \approx 1
\end{array}
\qquad (2.136)
$$

The vibration–rotation energy expressions differ for all 24 variants. For example, in the case of variant $1A$,

$$
E_{VR} = E_V + \sigma_x^V J(J+1) + \left( \sigma_z^V - \sigma_x^V \right) K^2 - D_l^J J^2 (J+1)^2
$$

$$
- D_l^{JK} J(J+1)K^2 - D_l^K K^4 \qquad (2.137)
$$

where $\sigma_\alpha$, $D_l^J$, $D_l^{JK}$, and $D_l^K$ are the rotational and centrifugal constants. It was shown in even the earliest papers on vibration–rotation transitions for the given type of molecules that splitting is experienced by the rotational levels $|K| = 3q$ for molecules of symmetry $C_{3v}$, $D_3$, $D_{3h}$ and $|K| = 2q$ for those of symmetry $C_{4v}$, $D_{2d}$ ($K$ doubling). It turns out that in case $1C$ this effect must already be taken into account in the investigated orders ($n = 3$).

If degenerate vibrational modes are excited, the line splitting and shift pattern is enormously complicated. The corresponding expressions may be found in [181]. Closed expressions are not obtained for cases $3C$–$8C$

because it is necessary to solve higher than second-order secular equations in these variants.

As mentioned, the conventional CT method is inapplicable for calculation of the rotational energy of axisymmetrical molecules in the general case. This difficulty can be circumvented by the CT method described in Section 2.6.2. For example, in the case of molecules belonging to tetragonal symmetry groups, we have for the Hamiltonian reduced to level-shift representation

$$\tilde{H} = H_0 + U + W' + W'' + O(\varepsilon^3)$$

$$\langle \tilde{H} \rangle = \tilde{H} + O(\varepsilon^3) \tag{2.138}$$

$$W'' = -\frac{\tau^2}{2(\sigma_z - \sigma_x)}\left(\left(\mathcal{P}^2, \mathcal{P}_z\right)\right)^{[4]}\frac{\delta_+}{2 - \mathcal{P}_z} + \left(\left(\mathcal{P}^2, -\mathcal{P}_z\right)\right)^{[4]}\frac{\delta_-}{2 + \mathcal{P}_z}$$

where $H_0$ is the zeroth-approximation operator, $U + W'$ is the polynomial diagonal correction, $W''$ is the state-splitting perturbation operator, $((x, y))^{[n]}$ denotes Löwdin polynomials, and $\delta_\pm$ is a special operator.

### 2.6.5.4. Spherical Top

Vibration–rotation interaction exerts an exceedingly strong influence on the energy levels of these molecules. A vast number of papers are devoted to the analysis of these distortions [192–206].

The customary procedure for determining the vibration–rotation energy is divided into three stages:

1. partial diagonalization of the vibration–rotation energy operator with respect to vibrational quantum numbers (the transformed operator may be nondiagonal with respect to quantum numbers enumerating degenerate states);
2. symmetrization of the basis vibration–rotation wave functions;
3. diagonalization of the operator $H$, permitting determination of the fine structure of the line group with quantum number $J$.

The last stage can be done numerically, but perturbation theory is applicable in a number of cases.

As an illustration, we give approximate expressions for the vibration–rotation energy for states in which only nondegenerate modes can be excited

[207]:

$$E^{(0)}(RP) = \alpha^0 + \beta^0 R(R+1) + \gamma^0 R^2(R+1)^2 + \pi^0 R^3(R+1)^3$$

$$+ \left[(2R-3)(2R-2)\cdots(2R+5)\right]^{1/2}$$

$$\times \left[\varepsilon^0 + \rho^0 R(R+1)(-1)^R F_{APP}^{4RR}\right]$$

$$+ \left[(2R-5)(2R-4)\cdots(2R+7)\right]^{1/2}\xi^0(-1)^R F_{APP}^{6RR}$$

$$(2.139)$$

In this expression, we have introduced the effective constants $\alpha^0, \beta^0, \gamma^0, \ldots,$ which can be approximately identified with the vibrational energy and the rotational and centrifugal constants; for example, $\alpha \cong E_V$ is the vibrational energy, $\gamma/hc \simeq B_V$ is the effective rotational constant, and $\gamma/hc \simeq D$ is the centrifugal distortion constant; $F_{APP}^{4RR}$ and $F_{APP}^{6RR}$ are the Clebsch–Gordan coefficients for cubic symmetry. The symbol $P$ denotes the set of quantum numbers enumerating the symmetry types and fine-structure components of levels with given $J$.

The expressions (even approximate) for the vibration–rotation energy in vibrational states where degenerate (particularly threefold) modes are excited are extremely cumbersome. They may be found in [181, 196, 197, 208].

### 2.6.5.5. Asymmetrical Top

As mentioned earlier, the representatives of asymmetrical-top type, namely water-vapor and ozone molecules, play an extremely important part in the interaction of infrared radiation with the atmosphere. This fact accounts for the steadfast interest of researchers in the investigation of the $H_2O$ and $O_3$ spectra by theoretical as well as experimental methods. The vibration–rotation spectra of these molecules have been under investigation for more than 40 yr.

References to early papers may be found in Herzberg's work [209]. Papers published prior to 1958 are fairly completely represented in El'yashevich's book [59]. A resurgence of interest in the theoretical study of vibration–rotation transitions appeared in the midsixties. This event was motivated by the advent of high- and ultrahigh-resolution spectral instruments. It was demonstrated in this period that the satisfactory explanation of the experimental data on spectral line centers requires the inclusion of

Table 2.8. Summary of Coefficients $Y_{mj}^{(n)}$ Used in Derivation of Equations by Author's Group

| $m$ \ $j$ | 0 | 1 | 2 | 3 | 4 | 5 | 6 | 7 | 8 | 9 | 10 |
|---|---|---|---|---|---|---|---|---|---|---|---|
| 0 | $Y_{00}^{(2)}$ $Y_{00}^{(6)}$ $Y_{00}^{(10)}$ | $Y_{01}^{(0)}$ $Y_{01}^{(4)}$ $Y_{01}^{(8)}$ | $Y_{02}^{(2)}$ $Y_{02}^{(6)}$ $Y_{02}^{(10)}$ | $Y_{03}^{(4)}$ $Y_{03}^{(8)}$ | $Y_{04}^{(6)}$ $Y_{04}^{(10)}$ | $Y_{05}^{(8)}$ | $Y_{06}^{(10)}$ | $Y_{07}^{(12)}$ | $Y_{08}^{(12)}$ | $Y_{09}^{(16)}$ | $Y_{0,10}^{(18)}$ |
| 1 | $Y_{10}^{(0)}$ $Y_{10}^{(4)}$ $Y_{10}^{(8)}$ | $Y_{11}^{(2)}$ $Y_{11}^{(6)}$ $Y_{11}^{(10)}$ | $Y_{12}^{(4)}$ $Y_{12}^{(8)}$ | $Y_{13}^{(6)}$ $Y_{13}^{(10)}$ | $Y_{14}^{(8)}$ | $Y_{15}^{(10)}$ | $Y_{16}^{(12)}$ | $Y_{17}^{(14)}$ | $Y_{18}^{(16)}$ | | |
| 2 | $Y_{20}^{(2)}$ $Y_{20}^{(6)}$ $Y_{20}^{(10)}$ | $Y_{21}^{(4)}$ $Y_{21}^{(8)}$ | $Y_{22}^{(6)}$ $Y_{22}^{(10)}$ | $Y_{23}^{(8)}$ | $Y_{24}^{(10)}$ | $Y_{25}^{(12)}$ | $Y_{26}^{(14)}$ | | | | |
| 3 | $Y_{30}^{(4)}$ $Y_{30}^{(8)}$ | $Y_{31}^{(6)}$ $Y_{31}^{(10)}$ | $Y_{32}^{(8)}$ | $Y_{33}^{(10)}$ | | | | | | | |
| 4 | $Y_{40}^{(6)}$ $Y_{40}^{(10)}$ | $Y_{41}^{(8)}$ | $Y_{42}^{(10)}$ | | | | | | | | |
| 5 | $Y_{50}^{(8)}$ | $Y_{51}^{(10)}$ | | | | | | | | | |
| 6 | $Y_{60}^{(10)}$ | | | | | | | | | | |
| 7 | $Y_{70}^{(12)}$ | | | | | | | | | | |

*Key*

▨ calculated by Dunham (1932) and Tipping (1973)

▧ calculated by Woolley (1962, 1972)

▧ calculated by Thomas (1942)

▨ calculated erroneously by Woolley (1962)

twentieth-order terms with respect to $\mathscr{P}_\alpha$ in the vibration–rotation Hamiltonian (sixth perturbation approximation).

Because of serious mathematical and computational difficulties, the theoretical work in this area is of a rather hypothetical nature. The latter consideration is further emphasized by the presence of strong random perturbations.

As mentioned, to determine the vibration–rotation energy, the total Hamiltonian is first diagonalized with respect to the vibrational quantum numbers. The eigenvalues of the effective rotational energy operator are found in the general case by numerical diagonalization of the matrix of this operator in the basis of symmetrical wave functions for a rigid symmetrical top.

By contrast with the conventional CT method used in the literature, the effective nonrigid-top method developed by the author's group makes it possible to deduce general expressions for the constants in the operator $H_R^{[V]}$ and, with the aid thereof, to analyze the symmetry properties of the constants and to estimate the order of magnitude of various operators. Also, the general expressions are well suited to the synthesis of computer programs. A series of computer programs has made it possible to analyze the centrifugal distortion constants and rotational energy up to $\kappa^6$. These results provide a means for explaining the strong dependence of certain spectroscopic constants on the vibrational quantum numbers as observed experimentally for the $H_2O$ molecule. Table 2.8 lists the computer-calculated spectroscopic constants along with the spectroscopic constants calculated by other authors, including three constants calculated erroneously (crossed out in the table).

## 2.7. Experimental Methods for Determination of the Absorption Coefficients

The experimental determination of the absorption coefficients of atmospheric gases requires the acquisition of undistorted, completely resolved vibration–rotation spectra. This goal can be met if the spectral apparatus has a resolution much smaller than the width of the Doppler line contour $(\sim 10^{-3}\ cm^{-1})$ and the error of determination of the spectral absorption coefficient does not exceed a few percent.

Classical spectrometers cannot meet these requirements [210]. A resolution of $\sim 10^{-3}\ cm^{-1}$ or better can be attained with laser and Fourier spectrometers. The methods used in laser and Fourier spectroscopy for measurement of the spectral absorption coefficients are briefly analyzed below, along with their resolution, sensitivity, and applications for the solution of atmospheric problems.


## 2.7.1. Laser Spectroscopy

In linear laser spectroscopy (where the intensity of the emitted radiation is much smaller than the intensity corresponding to the onset of nonlinear effects in the medium), the spectral absorption coefficients are measured by conventional methods (absorption, optoacoustic, derivative) as well as by the pure laser method of intracavity absorption.


### 2.7.1.1. Absorption Method

The absorption method is based on measurement of the attenuation of radiation as it passes through a layer of matter, in correspondence with Bouguer's law.

The capabilities of the absorption method have been greatly enhanced by the application of tunable-frequency single-mode lasers. The high spectral power of the radiation permits the use of long paths under laboratory and atmospheric conditions and speeds the acquisition of information on the absorption coefficients of the medium [211]. The spectral resolution of the spectrometer is determined by the laser emission linewidth and the precision of adjustment of its wavelength, and it can attain values of $10^{-3}$ to $10^{-6}$ cm$^{-1}$. The accuracy of the method is maximal for attenuation of radiation by a factor of $1/1.5$ to $1/20$ [212], where the measurement error $\Delta k(\nu)/k(\nu)=1$ to 5% and the value of the absorption coefficient $k(\nu)$ that can be recorded within these error limits over a 10-km path ranges from $4\cdot10^{-7}$ to $3\cdot10^{-5}$ cm$^{-1}$. High-speed laser spectrometers attain a temporal resolution of $10^{-3}$ sec [213].

The absorption method is used extensively for the investigation of fairly strong absorption lines, $k(\nu)>10^{-6}$ cm$^{-1}$, with the use of typical atmospheric paths and multipass measurement cells. The use of lasers having a wide wavelength-tuning range, such as semiconductor and dye lasers and lasers with frequency mixing, is particularly effective. For example, semiconductor laser spectrometers with a resolution $<10^{-4}$ cm$^{-1}$ have been used successfully to resolve the structure of the $Q$ branch of the $CO_2$ band [the lines $Q(2)$ through $Q(38)$ have been recorded and their absorption coefficients measured at pressures of 1 to 50 Torr] [214] and to detect a nontrivial effect of variation of the line shape with pressure in the 5-$\mu$m region, namely collision narrowing of the spectral lines of the $H_2O$ molecule in a buffer gas (Xe, Ar, $N_2$) [215]. The spectrum of the $\nu_3$ band of $CH_4$ has been recorded with a resolution of $4 \cdot 10^{-4}$ cm$^{-1}$ in the vicinity of 3.39 $\mu$m at a pressure of 1 Torr on a laser spectrometer with frequency mixing using an argon and a dye laser [216]. The absorption method proves ineffective in the spectrum $>10,000$ cm$^{-1}$ on account of the weakness of the absorption lines (for example, practically no measurements of the absorption spectrum have been performed with a dye laser having an emission linewidth $\sim 10^{-4}$ cm$^{-1}$).

### 2.7.1.2. Derivative Method

The basic notion of the derivative method is to measure the wavelength derivative of the spectrum with modulation of the laser wavelength, i.e., to transform small signal variations $\Delta I$ occurring in a small wavelength interval $\Delta\lambda$ into a signal proportional to $(\Delta I/\Delta\lambda)\Delta\lambda$ [217]. For direct measurements of the absorption coefficient, the recording apparatus has a limited dynamic range, which is inadequate for the recording of small intensity variations $\Delta I$ against a strong background $I_0$. The derivative method has the advantage of eliminating this difficulty.

If the laser emission wavelength is modulated with a frequency $\Omega$,

$$\lambda(t) = \lambda_0 + \Delta\lambda \cos \Omega t \tag{2.140}$$

($\Delta\lambda$ is the modulation factor), the intensity of radiation transmitted through the absorbing medium is given by the expression [218]

$$I(t) = I_0 T(\lambda_0) + I_0 T^{(1)}(\lambda_0)\Delta\lambda \cos \Omega t - \tfrac{1}{4} I_0 T^{(2)}(\lambda_0)(\Delta\lambda)^2 \cos 2\Omega t + \cdots \tag{2.141}$$

in which $T(\lambda_0), T^{(1)}(\lambda_0), T^{(2)}(\lambda_0),\ldots$ are the spectral transmittance of the sample and its derivatives with respect to $\lambda$. A selective amplifier tuned to the frequency $\Omega$ or $2\Omega$ makes it possible to isolate the given component and to eliminate the large constant component of the signal $I_0 T(\lambda_0)$.

Recording of the derivative $T^{(1)}(\lambda)$ improves the sensitivity of the wavelength-modulation spectrometer to $\Delta I/I_0 = 10^{-3}$ [219], corresponding to a sensitivity $\Delta k = 10^{-9}$ cm$^{-1}$ for a cell length of 10 km. The spectral resolution of the spectrometer is determined by the wavelength modulation factor $\Delta\lambda$ and has a value of 0.02 cm$^{-1}$ for semiconductor lasers [219]. The temporal resolution is determined by the modulation frequency $\Omega$. The spectrum, exclusive of the constant component, is reconstructed by subsequent integration of the signal [217]:

$$\int \frac{d}{d\lambda}(T(\lambda))\,d\lambda = T(\lambda) + C \tag{2.142}$$

Consequently, to obtain information on the continuous absorption component, it is necessary to record both $T^{(1)}(\lambda)$ and $T(\lambda)$.

The derivative laser method is used to determine the concentration of contaminating gases in the atmosphere [219, 220] and to measure the centers of overlapping spectral lines [221]; frequency modulation of the laser radiation eliminates the influence of atmospheric turbulence on the accuracy and sensitivity of the measurements [219].

### 2.7.1.3. Optoacoustic Method

This method is based on the optoacoustic effect, which is manifested in pressure pulsations of a gas in a closed volume in conjunction with the absorption of an infrared radiation beam modulated at an acoustic frequency.

Molecules are excited when the emission frequency coincides with the frequency of an absorption line of the gas. The molecules revert to the initial state via two routes: (1) nonradiative vibration–translation relaxation with time constant $\tau_{VT}$, accompanied by heating of the gas; (2) radiative relaxation with time constant $\tau_{rad}$. The relative $\tau_{VT} \ll \tau_{rad}$ holds for the majority of molecules at pressures above 1 Torr [222], and so the absorbed energy goes mainly into heat and elicits a variation of the gas pressure, which is recorded by a sensitive diaphragm forming the sensing element of a capacitor microphone. The use of a laser as the radiation source produces orders-of-magnitude improvement of the sensitivity and resolution of this method.

The magnitude of the signal at the microphone with the use of a continuous laser is proportional to the absorption coefficient $k(\nu)$ of the gas, the gas pressure $P$, and the radiated laser power $W$:

$$U_c = \alpha_c k(\nu) P W \tag{2.143}$$

where $\alpha_c$ is the microphone sensitivity (V/cm$^{-1}$ W). The sensitivity threshold of the method is determined by the pressure fluctuations in the cell and the amplifier noise factor. The spectrophone responds to an absorbed power of the order of $10^{-10}$ W [223], so that absorption coefficients $k(\nu) = 10^{-10}$ cm$^{-1}$ can be recorded for a source power of 1 W.

It has been shown [224] that the optoacoustic method works favorably with a pulsed laser source when $\tau_p, \tau_{\rm VT} \ll \tau_{\rm diaphr} = 10^{-3}$ sec ($\tau_p$ is the pulse power, and $\tau_{\rm diaphr}$ is the response time of the diaphragm to pressure variations). In this case, the transmission of a light pulse through the measurement cell of the spectrophone induces a pressure pulse in it, and the microphone signal is proportional to the energy of the laser pulse:

$$U_p = \alpha_p k(\nu) PE \qquad\qquad (2.144)$$

where $\alpha_p$ is the microphone sensitivity (V/cm$^{-1}$ J). With the use of a spectrophone and a 30-mJ pulsed DF laser, a sensitivity of $10^{-7}$ cm$^{-1}$ is attained [225]. The sensitivity can be further increased by placing the cell in the cavity of a single-mode laser, where the radiated power is an order of magnitude greater than the output power [226]. As in the absorption method, the resolution of the spectrometer is determined by the laser emission linewidth and the smoothness of adjustment of the lasing frequency (i.e., from $10^{-3}$ to $10^{-6}$ cm$^{-1}$). Linear response over a wide range of values of $k(\nu)$, high sensitivity, and the possibility of using small volumes of the investigated gas render the optoacoustic method immensely promising for investigation of the absorption coefficients. This method was used to measure the absorption coefficients of atmospheric gases at individual emission lines of $CO_2$ [227], CO [228], and DF [219] gas lasers, as well as to investigate the profiles of absorption lines by means of tunable He–Ne lasers in the 3.39-$\mu$m region [229], ruby lasers in the 0.69-$\mu$m region [230], and liquid lasers in the 0.6-$\mu$m region [231].

### 2.7.1.4. Intracavity Absorption Methods

Intracavity absorption (ICA) methods are classified as wide band and narrow band, depending on whether the laser operates in the multimode or single-mode lasing regime.

*2.7.1.4.1. Wide-band ICA Method.* The wide-band method is based on placement of a selectively absorbing substance in the interior of the cavity of a multimode laser with a broad amplification line. Weak absorption ($10^{-4}$ to $10^{-8}$ cm$^{-1}$) causes a redistribution of the radiation intensity in different modes of the cavity. Cavity modes coinciding with the absorption lines are suppressed, i.e., selective mode suppression takes place. This effect results in the formation of sharp troughs in the laser emission spectrum, which are then recorded by means of conventional spectral instruments (spectrograph or interferometer).

Theoretical analyses of a laser using a selectively absorbing substance in the cavity and operating in the steady-state lasing regime are given in [232, 233], in which it is shown that the ratio between the depths of the spectral troughs at frequencies $\nu_1$ and $\nu_2$ for $\gamma \ll \Gamma$ ($\gamma$ is the absorption linewidth, and $\Gamma$ is the uniform amplification linewidth) is proportional to the values of the measured absorption at those frequencies:

$$\frac{\Delta I(\nu_1)}{\Delta I(\nu_2)} = \frac{k(\nu_1)}{k(\nu_2)}, \qquad \Delta I(\nu) = I_0 - I(\nu) \qquad (2.145)$$

while the sensitivity of the method depends on the loss constants ($K_n$) of the cavity and the ratio of the laser power to the spontaneous noise power.

Thus, the wide-band method in the steady-state case permits distortion-free measurements of the contours of the absorption lines, provided only that their widths are much smaller than the width of the laser spectral band. Continuous absorption is equivalent to a variation of the loss constants in the cavity; a procedure for its determination has not been developed.

In the case of pulsed laser operation, the shape of the trough in the laser spectrum does not emulate the shape of the absorption line; however, when $\gamma \ll \Gamma$ and $\tau_p \ll \tau_{\text{stead}}$ ($\tau_p$ is the laser pulse width, and $\tau_{\text{stead}}$ is the time constant for a steady-state trough), the laser intensity at frequency $\nu$ decays with the lasing time according to the law

$$I(\nu, t) = I_0(\nu, 0) \exp\left[-k(\nu)ct\right] \qquad (2.146)$$

where $c$ is the speed of light and $t$ is the time from the start of lasing [234]. The value of the absorption coefficient in this case can be obtained by recording the laser emission spectrum at two successive times $t_1$ and $t_2$:

$$k(\nu) = \frac{\ln\left[I(\nu, t_1)/I(\nu, t_2)\right]}{c(t_2 - t_1)} \qquad (2.147)$$

Several authors [213, 234] have demonstrated the feasibility of measuring the absorption coefficients from the time-integrated laser emission spectrum.

Extremely high sensitivity can be achieved in a time of $10^{-6}$ to $10^{-3}$ sec with the use of intracavity laser spectrometers having a wide, smooth spectrum. For example, in the first experiments with liquid, ruby, and neodymium lasers, the sensitivity was increased from $10^3$- to $10^5$-fold over the extracavity method, making it possible to record lines with absorption coefficients of $10^{-7}$ to $10^{-8}$ cm$^{-1}$ for a cell length of 1 m [232, 234, 235].

The resolution of the wide-band method is determined by the value of the mode spacing (which is equal to $10^{-3}$ cm$^{-1}$ for a cavity length of 5 m), but it is limited in practice by the resolution of the spectral instrument and amounts to 0.1–0.01 cm$^{-1}$.

*2.7.1.4.2. Narrow-band ICA Method.* Placement of the absorption cell in the interior of the cavity of a single-mode laser does not produce selective mode suppression as in the selective-loss method, rather it elicits a variation of the cavity $Q$ for the lasing mode, and tuning of the lasing frequency causes a variation of the laser power at frequencies corresponding to the positions of the absorption lines. Unlike the multimode lasing regime, the dependence of $\Delta I(\nu)/I_0$ on $k(\nu)$ is nonlinear in the single-mode case [233]:

$$\frac{\Delta I(\nu)}{I_0} = \frac{k(\nu)/K_n}{1+k(\nu)/K_n} \frac{1}{1-1/X_0} \tag{2.148}$$

($X_0$ is the excess of the pump level above threshold), complicating its application for measurement of the absorption coefficients.

The sensitivity of the narrow-band spectrometer exceeds that of the extracavity method only in the case of small optical thicknesses $kl \ll 1$, but even in this case it lags the sensitivity of the wide-band ICA method by three orders of magnitude due to fluctuations of the intensity [233].

A 250-fold increase in sensitivity over the extracavity method is realized in a narrow-band intracavity spectrometer using a CO laser, so that absorption coefficients of $\sim 10^{-5}$ cm$^{-1}$ can be recorded with a cell of length 30 cm [237].

The resolution of the narrow-band spectrometer is determined by the laser emission linewidth and the smoothness of adjustment of the lasing wavelength (i.e., it can attain values of from $10^{-3}$ to $10^{-6}$ cm$^{-1}$).

The advantages of ICA methods, namely the high resolution of the narrow-band version and the high sensitivity of the wide-band version, are both realized in the competing-beam method [236]. The investigated substance is placed inside a dispersive (main) cavity of a laser emitting a narrow spectral line, which can be smoothly adjusted along the spectrum. High sensitivity of the lasing process to small losses is created by the insertion of a secondary nonselective cavity into the arrangement. The secondary cavity is inserted in such a way as to provide the main and secondary cavities with a common active medium. The absorption lines are recorded photoelectrically with comparison of the output intensities of the main and secondary cavities with and without the investigated substance in the dispersive cavity of the laser.

The ICA method has been used to measure the center positions of the absorption lines of atmospheric gases in the emission regions of dye [238], ruby [234], neodymium–glass [239], and CO [237] lasers. The absorption coefficients for individual lines have been measured only in the pulsed operation of neodymium [223], ruby [234], and dye [238] lasers within 10 to 50% error limits.

## 2.7.2. Fourier Spectroscopy

Unique spectroscopic results have been obtained in recent years by means of Fourier spectroscopy (measurements of the absolute values of the center positions of the absorption lines for various gases have been measured within $\sim 10^{-4}$ cm$^{-1}$ error limits over a broad range extending from the far-infrared to the visible region of the spectrum [220]). These accomplishments are primarily attributable to the intimacy of the Fourier spectroscopy principle with the principles of computer operation, so that the vigorous growth of computer engineering has engendered a concomitant breakthrough in the development of Fourier-transform algorithms, establishing the possibility of real-time operation and the processing of $10^6$ spectral elements in a period of a few minutes [240].

In Fourier spectroscopy, the spectrum is obtained in two stages:

1. measurement of an interferogram $I(\delta)$ by recording the signal as a function of the optical path difference in a Michelson interferometer:

$$I(\delta) = \int_{\nu_1}^{\nu_2} B(\nu) \cos(2\pi\nu\delta)\, d\nu \qquad (2.149)$$

2. reconstruction of the spectrum $B(\nu)$ by Fourier transformation of the interferogram [241]:

$$B(\nu) = \mathrm{const} \int_{-\infty}^{\infty} I(\delta) \cos(2\pi\delta\nu)\, d\delta$$

For the measurement of absorption spectra, three Michelson interferometer configurations can be used, according to the placement of the cell containing the absorbing gas:

1. single-beam configuration (cell placed before or after the beam splitter);
2. dual-beam configuration (using a reference and a test beam);

3. asymmetrical configuration (cell placed in one arm of the interferometer).

In the single-beam configuration, the spectrum is measured without the
sample and with it, and the transmissivity is determined by the ratio of their
reconstructed spectra. The absorption of the sample introduces insignificant
variations in the interferogram. All information on the absorption lines is
contained in the neighborhoods of "spikes," the magnitude of which comprises a small fraction ($\sim 1\%$) of the first maximum and decreases with
increasing path difference so that the determination of the absorption
coefficients requires a large dynamic range on the part of the recording
apparatus ($> 10^4$ [242]).

The stated difficulty can be overcome in the dual-beam Fourier
spectroscopic arrangement, where only the difference between the interfero-
grams without the sample and with it is recorded. In technical implementation, however, this approach still poses an exceedingly complicated problem
and has not been sufficiently developed [243].

In the asymmetrical configuration, the spectrum is reconstructed by
complex Fourier transformation involving, rather than the intensities, the
amplitudes of the incident and transmitted waves (so-called amplitude
spectroscopy).

The absorption coefficient of the sample is expressed in terms of the
real parts $P$ and imaginary parts $Q$ of the inverse complex Fourier transform with the sample $(P, Q)$ and without it $(P_0, Q_0)$ [244]:

$$k(\nu)=\frac{1}{L}\ln\left[\frac{P_0^2(\nu)+Q_0^2(\nu)}{P^2(\nu)+Q^2(\nu)}\right]^{1/2} \tag{2.150}$$

The method is suitable for the measurement of small transmissivities, $\sim 1\%$
[243].

Measurements of absorption spectra on a Fourier spectrometer incur a
host of problems that are not met in conventional spectroscopy. First of all,
it is necessary to run a calibration of the $k(\nu)$ measurements because the
spectrum is reconstructed correct to within a constant factor, and it is also
required to be assured of a large dynamic range on the part of the recording
system. Interferogram measurement errors produce severe distortions in the
spectrum calculations.

Various types of errors of Fourier spectroscopy have been analyzed in
[241, 244] in which methods are also proposed for their elimination;

however, the problem of the precise determination of the absorption coefficients has yet to be solved.

Fourier spectrometers have a broad spectral range (up to $10^6$ spectral elements), fast response, and a high spectral resolution, which is determined by the maximum optical path difference $\Delta\nu = 1/\delta_{max}$ and at the present time attains a value of $5\times10^{-3}$ cm$^{-1}$ or even as high as $5\times10^{-4}$ cm$^{-1}$ in a recently developed interferometer with a path difference up to 20 m [240]. Cells having a path length of the order of 100 m provide a sensitivity of $10^{-5}$ cm$^{-1}$.

## 2.7.3. Comparative Highlights of the Various Methods

The foregoing analysis indicates that the method most commonly used today for measurements of the spectral absorption coefficients is the laser absorption method, by means of which the absorption spectra have been measured for a whole series of atmospheric gases ($H_2O$, $CO_2$, $CO$, $CH_4$,...) with a resolution of from $10^{-3}$ to $10^{-6}$ cm$^{-1}$ in the regions of laser emission lines. This method has the drawback of relatively low sensitivity: $10^{-6}$ cm$^{-1}$.

A higher sensitivity, $\sim 10^{-7}$ to $10^{-9}$ cm$^{-1}$, is exhibited by other laser methods currently in a state of rapid development (optoacoustic, derivative, and intracavity absorption methods), which permit spectroscopic measurements to be extended to faint absorption lines. The derivative method is the most effective for the measurement of small variations of the absorption coefficient $\Delta k$ against a strong background $k$, but are unsuitable for measurement of the continuous component of the absorption coefficient. The optoacoustic method is simpler to realize but is applicable only for molecular transitions with nonradiative relaxation of excitation. The ICA method makes it possible to record the absorption spectrum in a short time period ($\sim 10^{-3}$ sec) over a wide range, $\sim 70$ cm$^{-1}$, but so far it is applicable only in the visible region, where lasers with broad amplification lines are available.

Fourier-spectroscopic methods provide a capability for the performance of measurements in parts of the spectrum inaccessible to laser sources, with a certain sacrifice of resolution ($\sim 10^{-3}$ cm$^{-1}$) and sensitivity ($\sim 10^{-5}$ cm$^{-1}$).

We see that none of the methods discussed above for measurement of the spectral absorption coefficients is universal, so that they complement rather than duplicate one another.

## 2.8. Tables of Parameters of the Spectral Lines of Atmospheric Gases

As mentioned above, the quantitative determination of the absorption of laser radiation by atmospheric gases requires, above all, data on the absorption coefficients, which in turn can be obtained analytically if the parameters of the absorption lines contributing to the absorption at a particular frequency are known. Accordingly, the problem of determining and tabulating fundamental data on the line parameters has always been, and still is, most timely.

In this section, we briefly summarize the existing tabulated data on the basic line parameters (foremost of which are the center positions, intensities, and half-widths) for various atmospheric gases.

The most complete information on the absorption line parameters of atmospheric gases is contained in the atlas [245], which covers the water-vapor, carbon dioxide, ozone, nitric oxide, carbon monoxide, methane, and oxygen molecules. The vibration–rotation line of each gas is characterized in the tables by the center position, intensity, half-width, and energy of the lowest transition state.

The vibration–rotation bands of water vapor and carbon dioxide are most completely represented in [245] (covering the spectral range from the microwave to the visible region). The line parameters of 66 bands are calculated for water vapor, 32 of those bands corresponding to the principal isotopic modification of the molecule.

The centers of the $H_2O$ lines are determined on the basis of the empirical energy levels within error limits of $\pm 0.005$ to $\pm 0.05$ cm$^{-1}$ for the bands of the principal isotope. The error is considerably higher for the lines of the minor isotopes of water vapor. The line intensities of the vibration–rotation bands of water vapor have been determined either from experiment or according to expression (2.108).

The authors postulate $\pm 10\%$ error limits for the calculation of the line intensities of the fundamental bands of water vapor with small values of the rotational quantum numbers.

Seven isotopic modifications of the molecule are included in the calculations for gaseous carbon dioxide. The energy levels of $CO_2$ are calculated according to expression (2.132), in which the constants $B_V$ and $D_V$ and the vibrational terms are evaluated according to experimental data. As a result, the centers of the $CO_2$ lines are given within error limits of $\pm 0.01$ cm$^{-1}$. The line intensities are calculated according to (2.132), and

Coriolis interaction is taken into account by the introduction of the factor $F=(1+\xi_\nu m)^2$, in which $\xi_\nu$ is an empirical constant and $m$ is the rotational constant. In the case of bands formed by transitions with a difference of quantum numbers $\Delta l = \pm 2$, the square-law dependence of the $F$ factor on the rotational quantum numbers is used.

The atlas includes 12 vibration–rotation absorption bands of the ozone molecules, 10 of those bands referring to the principal isotopic modification of the molecule $O_3^{16}$. The tabulation covers the vibration–rotation transitions up to and including $j=60$ with regard for line intensities exceeding a value of $3.5\times10^{-23}$ cm$^{-1}$/molecules·cm$^{-2}$. The error of determination of the line centers varies from $\pm0.01$ cm$^{-1}$ (in the $O^{16}$ $\nu_1$ and $\nu_3$ bands) to 1 cm$^{-1}$ (in the $\nu_2+\nu_3-\nu_2$ band) and is not estimated at all for the series of lines of "hot" bands. The line intensities are determined according to expression (2.105) since the lack of experimental data precludes evaluation of the $F$ factor.

For $N_2O$, the atlas includes five isotopic modifications of the molecule. The line parameters for this molecule are determined according to the expressions given earlier for linear molecules with $l$ doubling. Data for CO are given for the vibration–rotation bands of four isotopes of this molecule. The error of determination of the line centers for the principal isotope is $\pm0.001$ cm$^{-1}$, and for the other isotopes it is $\pm0.01$ cm$^{-1}$. The line intensities of the fundamental band have error limits of $\pm2\%$; for the first overtone they are $\pm10\%$, and for the second overtone they are $\pm4\%$.

For methane, the tables list the line parameters for the vibration–rotation bands in the region from 3 to 8.5 $\mu$m, including five bands for the principal isotope and two bands of the isotope $^{13}CH_4$.

The parameters given in the tables for the absorption lines of atmospheric gases are undoubtedly in need of appropriate refinements, which the authors intend to do as new, more precise data are acquired. The most significant refinements, of course, are to be expected for the near-infrared region of the spectrum (0.8 to 1.5 $\mu$m), which spans the vibration–rotation absorption bands of atmospheric gases where the line parameters are most vulnerable to the effects of intra- and intermolecular interactions. This conjecture is supported by the results of appropriate measurements recently carried out by the present author's research group with the application of ultrahigh-resolution laser-spectroscopic methods.

In concluding this section, we note that, besides the data described above, spectral line parameters have also been tabulated in several other works [246–252].

The data on the absorption line parameters for molecular oxygen refer to the 1.06-, 1.26-, and 1.908-$\mu$m absorption bands, as well as to the pure rotational spectrum in the submillimeter range.

## 2.9. Absorption Functions for Laser Sources

In cases where it is impossible to ignore the wavelength dependence of the absorption coefficient within the limits of the laser emission line, the attenuation of radiation due to absorption by atmospheric gases is described by the absorption function. For the latter, in this case, it is necessary to use the most general expressions (2.7)–(2.9), which take into account the wavelength dependence of the radiation intensity from the source.

Knowing that the width of the emission spectra of lasers in the majority of cases is comparable with the half-width of the absorption lines of atmospheric gases in the lower layers of the atmosphere, we readily infer that if the emission lines overlap the absorption lines, then it is required to know the absorption functions in order to estimate the energy losses of the laser beam due to absorption.

Recent experimental studies of the absorption spectra of atmospheric gases with the use of instruments characterized by ultrahigh resolution and sensitivity have shown that not only the regions occupied by the absorption bands but also the atmospheric windows are rather densely filled with absorption lines. In particular, an enormous number of lines originating from transitions between high vibrational and rotational levels of molecules have been discovered in the visible part of the spectrum and in the transmission windows of the infrared wavelength range.

It turns out, therefore, that the concept of the absorption function must, as a rule, be recruited for quantitative assessment of the absorption of laser radiation by atmospheric gases, and only in situations where highly monochromatic laser radiation falls between absorption lines or the degree of monochromaticity is so great that the wavelength dependence of the absorption can be neglected in this part of the spectrum can the concept of spectral absorption [expression (2.5)] and, hence, Bouguer's law be used for quantitative estimation of the radiation losses due to absorption by atmospheric gases. In this latter case, the degree of monochromaticity of the laser output must be at least $10^{-3}$ cm$^{-1}$ for the lower layers of the atmosphere and at least an order of magnitude better than that for the upper layers, where the half-width of the absorption line is determined mainly by the Doppler effect.

The absorption functions of laser sources can be determined by means of an appropriate direct calculation and through direct measurements either under laboratory or under natural atmospheric conditions.

For direct calculation of the absorption functions, it is necessary to know the laser emission spectrum and the parameters of all absorption lines contributing to the absorption of laser frequencies. These parameters include the center positions, intensities, and half-widths of the lines. It may also be required to consider the coefficients of continuous absorption. It is implicit in the content of the preceding sections that the information required in order to determine the laser absorption functions is now available for the most commonly used laser sources. It is essential, however, to underscore the exceedingly high sensitivity of the values of those functions to the accuracy of the input information and, in particular, to the error of determination of the emission and absorption line centers. This problem is discussed in some detail in the present author's work [253], which indicates that the errors of determination of the absorption line centers, ranging from 0.05 to 0.1 $cm^{-1}$, are totally unacceptable for calculations of the absorption of laser radiation in the atmosphere.

In experimental studies, under controlled conditions of an artificially synthesized gaseous atmosphere or in the real atmosphere, the absorption functions can be determined with the use of specific laser prototypes as sources of emitted radiation. Examples of this kind of work may be found in papers by the author and his colleagues [254–258], which are reviewed in detail in [1]. The advantage of this mode of determining the absorption functions of laser sources lies in the fact that it does not require knowledge of the source emission spectrum, the absorption line positions, or their parameters. On the other hand, this method has a significant drawback in that the data obtained thereby are suitable only for the specific laser prototypes used in the particular measurements. It is necessary to be certain in this connection that a particular laser emits a time-invariant spectrum, otherwise it is necessary to know what those variations are, for example, as is the case of ruby lasers.

The results of field measurements of the absorption functions of laser sources are subject to the influence of aerosol scattering and signal fluctuations associated with turbulence. Both effects are always present in the atmosphere. However, this influence can be excluded with sufficient accuracy through the application of suitable innovative procedures [254, 253, 258].

## 2.10. Slant-Path Absorption of Laser Radiation in the Atmosphere

The conditions of absorption by atmospheric gas molecules vary continuously in the case of slant-path propagation of laser radiation in the atmosphere. These variations are attributable to a whole series of effects, the most significant of which are (1) the dependence of the half-widths of the absorption lines on the total and partial pressures of the gases and the temperature; (2) the pressure and temperature dependence of the center positions of the absorption lines; (3) the temperature dependence of the line intensities; (4) the dependence of the absorption coefficients in the far wings of the lines on the temperature and the total and partial pressures of the absorbing gases.

We have examined all of the foregoing dependences in detail in the preceding sections, by which we conclude that it is indeed possible to calculate directly the absorption of laser radiation propagating in the inhomogeneous atmosphere. Here we must use as the fundamental analytical equations the expressions for the spectral absorption (transmission) and the absorption (transmission) functions, written with regard for the above-indicated dependences, viz.:

$$F(\nu) = \frac{I(\nu)}{I_0(\nu)} = \exp\left[-\int_{l_1}^{l_2} \rho(l)k(\nu,l)\,dl\right] \tag{2.151}$$

$$H(\nu) = 1 - F(\nu) \tag{2.152}$$

$$F = \frac{\int_{\nu_1}^{\nu_2} I_0(\nu)F(\nu)\,d\nu}{\int_{\nu_1}^{\nu_2} I_0(\nu)\,d\nu} = \frac{\int_{\nu_1}^{\nu_2} I_0(\nu)\,d\nu \exp\left[-\int_{l_1}^{l_2} k(\nu,l)\,dl\right]}{\int_{\nu_1}^{\nu_2} I_0(\nu)\,d\nu} \tag{2.153}$$

$$H = 1 - F \tag{2.154}$$

$$k(\nu,l) = \sum \frac{S_i[T(l)]}{\pi} \frac{\gamma_i[T(l), P_a(l), P_b(l)]}{\{\nu - \nu_{0i}[T(l), P_a(l), P_b(l)]\}^2 + \gamma_i^2 T(l), P_a(l), P_b(l)]} \tag{2.155}$$

where $F(\nu)$ and $H(\nu)$ are the spectral transmittance and spectral absorptance, $F$ and $H$ are the transmission and absorption functions, $I_0(\nu)$ is the intensity of the laser radiation incident on an absorbing layer of the atmosphere of thickness $l_2 - l_1$, $\rho(l)$ is the density distribution of the absorbing gas along the beam path, and $S_i$, $\gamma_i$, $\nu_{0i}$ are the intensity, half-width, and center position of the $i$th line contributing to absorption at the frequency $\nu$. The brackets enclose the macroparameters through which $S$, $\gamma$, and $\nu_0$ depend on the coordinate $l$ associated with the path of radiation propagation.

Expressions (2.151)–(2.155) describe the absorption of radiation propagating along slant paths in the atmosphere on the assumption that the absorption lines of the atmospheric gas molecules have a dispersion contour. In the general case, where broadening of the lines due to molecular collisions and the Doppler effect must be taken into account, it is necessary to use expression (2.31), taking into account the dependence of the line parameters entering into it on the temperature and the total and partial pressures of the gases.

If the laser emission spectrum falls into a region where it is essential to consider continuous absorption associated with the far wings, the absorption coefficient in expressions (2.152)–(2.155) must include a term accounting for continuous absorption with regard for its appreciable dependence on the temperature, total pressure, and, particularly, the partial pressure of the absorbing gas.

Thus, the precise numerical calculation of the absorption of laser radiation by atmospheric gases poses a rather complex problem, particularly where one is concerned with determining the absorption functions and most especially in parts of the spectrum where it is necessary to consider both selective and continuous absorption. Nonetheless, this problem is completely accessible to solution at the present time. Accordingly, we indicate the parameters most crucial to this analysis and, on the other hand, the cases in which the corresponding dependences can be disregarded.

In calculating the component of the coefficient $k(\nu, l)$ responsible for selective absorption, we must first of all take into account the dependence of the line half-widths on the pressure and of the intensities on the temperature. It is important to consider the pressure dependence of the center positions of the lines only in situations where the laser emission line falls in the central part of an absorption line. Thus, recent measurements with ultrahigh-resolution laser spectrometers have shown that the shifts of the line centers due to pressure variations amount to tens of megahertz per Torr, so that for all atmospheric thicknesses the shifts of the line centers cannot be more than a few tenths of $1 \text{ cm}^{-1}$.

The temperature dependence of the line half-widths and center positions can be ignored for practical calculations. The same is certainly true of the dependence of $\nu_0$ on the partial pressure of the absorbing gas.

In the case of the absorption component due to the far wings, as mentioned, the dependence on the temperature and partial pressure of the absorbing gas and, so, automatically on the total pressure, is extremely significant.

It is self-evident that any calculations of the absorption of laser radiation by atmospheric gases in slant directions require knowledge of the distributions of the temperature and the total and partial gas pressures along the path of propagation of the laser beam; however, such information is not easily acquired because reliable measurement data have not been obtained to date.

The absorbtion of laser radiation along slant paths in the atmosphere can be measured indirectly, as in a homogeneous atmosphere (see the preceding section). The corresponding data are contained both in standard models of the atmosphere and in several monographs, including the author's book [1].


## 2.11. Limits of Applicability of Bouguer's Law

All preceding material in this chapter has been predicated on the assumption of applicability of Bouguer's law. It is of fundamental importance, therefore, to consider the problem of the limits of applicability of this law.

Two fundamental hypotheses underly the derivation of Bouguer's law: (1) The absorption coefficient $k(\nu)$ does not depend on the intensity of the radiation incident on the absorbing layer of the medium; (2) $k(\nu)$ does not depend on the concentration of the absorbing gas or, equivalently, all gas molecules absorb radiation independently. On the basis of these assumptions, the law in question has the following form for a homogeneous medium:

$$I(\nu)=I_0(\nu)\exp\left[-k''(\nu)lc\right] \tag{2.156}$$

where $I(\nu)$ and $I_0(\nu)$ are the intensities of the radiation transmitted through a layer $l$ of the medium and incident on it, and $c$ is the concentration of the absorbing gas.

The first hypothesis has been subjected to painstaking experimental verification by Vavilov [259], who demonstrated its validity under variation of $I_0(\nu)$ by 20 orders of magnitude for electron transitions with short lifetimes $\tau$ of atoms in the excited state. Investigations of electron transitions with large values of $\tau$ disclosed a dependence of $k(\nu)$ on $I_0(\nu)$.

The dependence of $k''(\nu)$ on $I_0(\nu)$ for vibration–rotation transitions in the absorption spectra of atmospheric gases has been tested in a number of recent experimental studies [260–266], which have disclosed a dependence of the absorption coefficient on the incident radiation intensity for values of the latter greater than $10^6$ W/cm$^2$. The details of the results obtained in those studies will be described in Chap. 5.

The hypothesis of independence of the absorption coefficient from the concentration of absorbing gas molecules has been investigated in numerous experimental papers, beginning with the earliest works of Ångström published in the period from 1889 through 1907. These studies showed that $k''(\nu)$ can be treated as independent of $c$ only for very low concentrations of the absorbing gas. An increase in the concentration of the absorbing gas and the addition of an extraneous gas have the effect of intensifying the molecular interaction processes responsible for variation of the absorption coefficient. These variations are exhibited through a dependence of the parameters of the absorption lines on the temperature and the total and partial pressures of the gases.

In application to the conditions of optical wave propagation in the atmosphere along horizontal paths, in which case the time variation of the total pressure at a given height can be neglected and the partial pressures of the absorbing gases are small in comparison with the total pressure, Bouguer's law may be regarded as valid in cases where it is permissible to neglect absorption in the far wings of the lines. The only caution here is that the absorption coefficient will have different values for different heights. If continuous absorption associated with the far wings is significant, Bouguer's law cannot be satisfied even for horizontal paths.

In addition to the above-considered true deviations from Bouguer's law, there are apparent deviations due to the limited resolving power of the spectral instruments used to measure the absorption of radiation by atmospheric gases.

It is well known that the emergent light beam from any spectrometer contains a frequency interval bounded by the resolving power of the instrument. The maximum resolution inherent in instruments with dispersive elements is at best a hundredth of 1 cm$^{-1}$ in the near- and far-infrared regions of the spectrum. It is evident from this fact that even the best models of such spectrometers cannot provide undistorted absorption spectra because the linewidths in the absorption spectra of atmospheric gases fluctuate from tenths to hundredths of 1 cm$^{-1}$ in the lower layers of the atmosphere and decrease directly with the pressure as the height is increased, i.e., decrease exponentially.

Thus, the spectral transmissivity $T(\nu)$ recorded by the spectrometer under these conditions deviates from its true value $f(\nu)$. In fact, $T(\nu)$ characterizes the spectral behavior of the absorption with distortion by the slit function of the instrument. The distorting influence of the spectrometer on the true pattern of the spectrum and the resulting apparent deviation from Bouguer's law grows increasingly pronounced with diminishing resolution of the instrument and with increasing frequency dependence of the absorption coefficient. The measured spectral absorption is equal to the true value only when $k(\nu)=$ const in the investigated spectral interval.

The measured spectral absorption $A'(\nu)$ is related to the true spectral absorption $A(\nu)$ and instrument slit function $S(\nu)$ by the expression

$$A'(\nu)=\int_{-\infty}^{\infty} S(\nu-\nu')A(\nu')\,d\nu' \tag{2.157}$$

If the slit function is specified by a Gaussian distribution, then $A'(\nu)$ assumes the form

$$A'(\nu)=\frac{(\ln 2)^{1/2}}{a^2\pi^{1/2}}\int_{-\infty}^{\infty}\exp\left[-\frac{\ln 2}{a^2}(\nu-\nu')^2\right]A(\nu')\,d\nu' \tag{2.158}$$

where $a$ is the half-width of the instrument slit-function curve.

Invoking the Fourier transform, we write

$$A(\nu)=\frac{1}{2\pi}\int_{-\infty}^{\infty}\frac{A'(\omega)}{S(\omega)}\exp(-i\omega\nu)\,d\omega \tag{2.159}$$

where $A'(\omega)$ and $S(\omega)$ are the transforms of $A(\nu)$ and $S(\nu)$.

Kostkowski and Bass [267] have carried out exhaustive calculations of $A(\nu)$ for cases in which the absorption line has a dispersion form and the instrument slit function is described by a Gaussian distribution. The influence of the spectrometer on the results of measurements of absorption spectra have been investigated in detail in many papers, a bibliography of which may be found in [1].

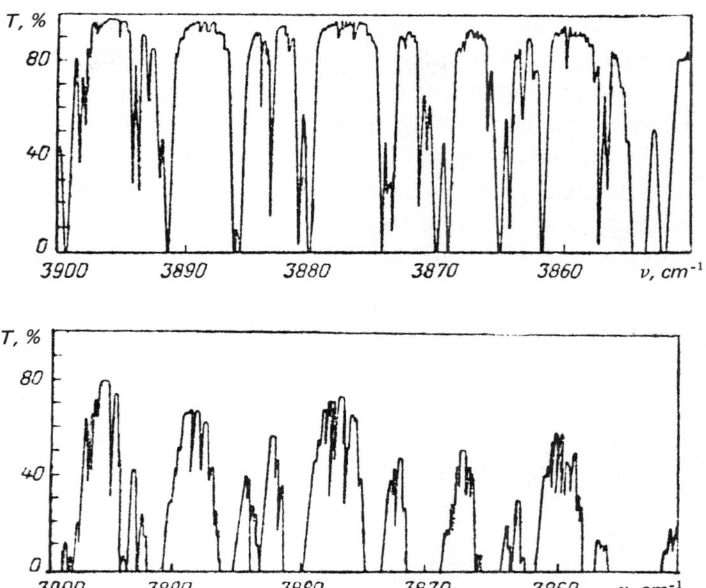

Fig. 2.11. Completely resolved absorption spectrum of water vapor in the interval 3850–3900 cm$^{-1}$ (2.56–2.6 $\mu$m) at pressure P=1.0 atm and column number densities for water $w$ =0.001 cm (upper curve) and $w$ =0.01 cm (lower curve) [268].

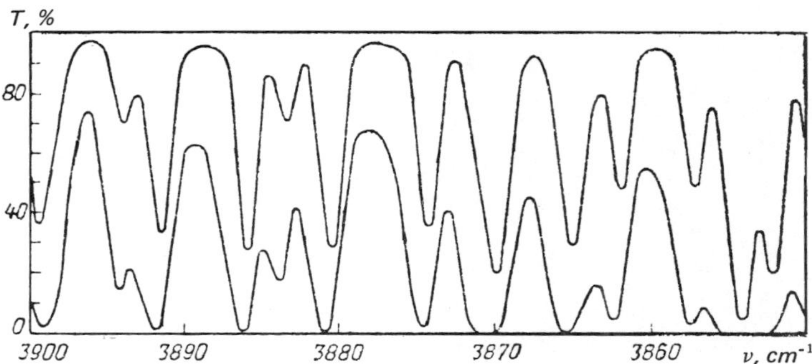

Fig. 2.12. Absorption spectrum obtained for water vapor by multiplying $T(\nu)$ (Fig. 2.11) by a slit function with width $2a$=2.0 cm$^{-1}$ [268].

We illustrate the influence of the spectrometer slit function on the form of the absorption spectrum for water vapor in the region from 3850 to 3900 $cm^{-1}$ on the basis of calculations carried out by Calfee [268]. The calculated values of the transmissivity for two layers of the atmosphere are given in Figs. 2.11 and 2.12. The first figure illustrates completely resolved spectra for the indicated layers, and the second figure gives the same spectra distorted by the spectrometer slit function with a half-width $a = 1$ $cm^{-1}$.

In conclusion, we stress the fact that only in the last few years, owing to advances in the development of laser spectroscopy and ultrahigh-resolution Fourier spectrometry, has it been possible to eliminate the distorting influence of the slit functions of spectrometers on the absorption spectra recorded by them for atmospheric gases.

# 3

# Scattering of Laser Radiation in the Atmosphere

## 3.0. Introduction

The energy of laser radiation propagating in the earth's atmosphere is lost from the directional beam as a result of various scattering effects. The main laser energy losses are attributable to aerosol and molecular scattering [1].

Molecular scattering is fairly well understood. Exhaustive tables of the scattering coefficients in the visible and infrared regions have now been compiled, providing a means for determining numerically, with reasonably good accuracy, the energy losses of waves propagating in any directions in the atmosphere. We therefore confine the description of molecular scattering for the most part to certain tabulated data on the scattering coefficients and optical thicknesses of a Rayleigh atmosphere.

In speaking of aerosol scattering, we generally think in terms not only of scattering, but also of the absorption of wave energy by particles. It would be more proper, therefore, to speak of aerosol extinction as a result of both the scattering effect and the effect of absorption of radiation flux by aerosol particles.

Despite the variety of particle-size spectra and the broad range of variation of the concentration and chemical composition of atmospheric aerosols, certain characteristic types of aerosols can be discerned, which differ significantly in their abilities to scatter electromagnetic waves in the optical range. Foremost among these types are clouds, fogs, and hazes. Also, while precipitations cannot properly be termed "aerosols," we include the extinction of radiation in transmission through them in this chapter because the nature of wave scattering by precipitation particles and by haze, cloud, and fog particles is one and the same.

Many practical problems associated with the scattering of laser radiation in the atmosphere require knowledge not only of the energy losses due to various scattering phenomena, but also of the angular (directional) distribution and polarization of the scattered radiation. Accordingly, several sections of the chapter are concerned with those problems. Especially timely today are the problems of pulsed laser radiation propagating in a scattering medium, which are treated in the section on transient scattering.

The penultimate section of the chapter summarizes the results of experimental and theoretical studies of the fluctuations of laser radiation during propagation in disperse media. Not enough importance has been attached to this phenomenon in the past, despite the fact, as will become evident in the indicated section, that it is of paramount significance in some cases.

The final section of the chapter is devoted to optical models of an aerosol atmosphere and related problems.

## 3.1. Molecular Scattering

The Cabannes–Rayleigh theory of molecular scattering of light gives the following expression for the scattering coefficient in gases:

$$\sigma_{\mathrm{Rayl}}(\lambda) = \frac{8\pi^3(n^2-1)^2}{3N\lambda^4}\frac{6+3\delta}{6-7\delta} \tag{3.1}$$

where $N$ is the number of molecules per unit volume, $n$ is the refractive index of the medium, $\lambda$ is the radiation wavelength, and $\delta$ is the depolarization factor of the scattered radiation; according to recent measurements, $\delta = 0.035$ [2].

Penndorf [3] has calculated the molecular scattering coefficient for various wavelengths in the interval from 0.2 to 20 $\mu$m according to expression (3.1). The data obtained in [3] can be used to calculate the optical thicknesses $\tau_{\mathrm{Rayl}}$ of molecular scattering for various geometrical thicknesses of the atmosphere.

Tables 3.1 and 3.2 give data on the coefficients $\sigma_{\mathrm{Rayl}}$ and $\tau_{\mathrm{Rayl}}$ for various wavelengths and geometrical thicknesses of the atmosphere. We note that the Rayleigh scattering coefficient calculated according to (3.1) has the dimensions of reciprocal length.

The values given in Table 3.1 for the molecular scattering coefficients and optical thicknesses $\tau_{\mathrm{Rayl}}$ provide a simple means for estimating the role

**Table 3.1.** Molecular Scattering Coefficients $\sigma_{\text{Rayl}}$ at Temperature $t=15°C$ and Pressure $P=1013$ mbar, and Optical Thicknesses $\tau_{\text{Rayl}}$ of a Vertical Layer of the Total Atmosphere According to Data of Penndorf [3]

| Wavelength $\lambda$, $\mu$m | $\sigma_{\text{Rayl}}$, km$^{-1}$ | $\tau_{\text{Rayl}}$ | Wavelength $\lambda$, $\mu$m | $\sigma_{\text{Rayl}}$, km$^{-1}$ | $\tau_{\text{Rayl}}$ |
|---|---|---|---|---|---|
| 0.30 | $1.446\times10^{-1}$ | 1.2237 | 0.65 | $5.893\times10^{-3}$ | 0.0499 |
| 0.32 | 1.098 | 0.9290 | 0.70 | 4.364 | 0.0369 |
| 0.34 | $8.494\times10^{-2}$ | 0.7188 | 0.80 | 2.545 | 0.0215 |
| 0.36 | 6.680 | 0.5653 | 0.90 | 1.583 | 0.0134 |
| 0.38 | 5.327 | 0.4508 | 1.06 | $8.458\times10^{-4}$ | 0.0072 |
| 0.40 | 4.303 | 0.3641 | 1.26 | 4.076 | 0.0034 |
| 0.45 | 2.644 | 0.2238 | 1.67 | 1.327 | 0.0011 |
| 0.50 | 1.716 | 0.1452 | 2.17 | $4.586\times10^{-5}$ | 0.0004 |
| 0.55 | 1.162 | 0.0984 | 3.50 | $6.830\times10^{-6}$ | 0.0001 |
| 0.60 | $8.157\times10^{-3}$ | 0.0690 | 4.00 | 4.002 | 0.0000 |

of molecular scattering in the energy losses of optical radiation propagating in the atmosphere. Thus, a quantitative measure of these losses is the transmittance $T_{\text{Rayl}}(\lambda)$ of a given layer of the atmosphere for radiation of wavelength $\lambda$. The quantity $T_{\text{Rayl}}(\lambda)$ is given by the simple expression

$$T_{\text{Rayl}}(\lambda)=\exp\left[-\tau_{\text{Rayl}}(\lambda)\right] \tag{3.2}$$

In the ground layer of the atmosphere,

$$\tau_{\text{Rayl}}(\lambda)=\sigma_{\text{Rayl}}(\lambda)l \tag{3.3}$$

where $l$ is the thickness of the layer.

**Table 3.2.** Coefficients $\sigma_{\text{Rayl}}$ for Various Heights $z$, and Optical Thicknesses $\tau_{\text{Rayl}}$ of Layers of the Atmosphere ($z-\infty$) for Wavelengths $\lambda=0.30$, 0.55, and 1.06 $\mu$ according to Data of Elterman [2]

| Height $z$, km | $\lambda=0.30\ \mu$m | | $\lambda=0.55\ \mu$m | | $\lambda=1.06\ \mu$m | |
|---|---|---|---|---|---|---|
| | $\sigma_{\text{Rayl}}$, km$^{-1}$ | $\tau_{\text{Rayl}}$ ($z-\infty$) | $\sigma_{\text{Rayl}}$, km$^{-1}$ | $\tau_{\text{Rayl}}$ ($z-\infty$) | $\sigma_{\text{Rayl}}$, km$^{-1}$ | $\tau_{\text{Rayl}}$ ($z-\infty$) |
| 0 | $1.446\times10^{-1}$ | 1.2237 | $1.162\times10^{-2}$ | 0.0984 | $8.458\times10^{-4}$ | 0.0072 |
| 5 | $8.693\times10^{-2}$ | 0.6538 | $6.988\times10^{-3}$ | 0.0526 | 5.085 | 0.0038 |
| 10 | 4.881 | 0.3212 | 3.924 | 0.0258 | 2.855 | 0.0019 |
| 15 | 2.999 | 0.1471 | 1.848 | 0.0118 | 1.345 | 0.0009 |
| 20 | 1.049 | 0.0672 | $8.436\times10^{-4}$ | 0.0054 | $6.138\times10^{-5}$ | 0.0004 |
| 30 | $2.173\times10^{-3}$ | 0.0146 | 1.747 | 0.0012 | 1.271 | 0.0001 |
| 40 | $4.716\times10^{-4}$ | 0.0035 | $3.791\times10^{-5}$ | 0.0003 | $2.758\times10^{-6}$ | 0.0000 |
| 50 | 1.212 | 0.0010 | $9.743\times10^{-6}$ | 0.0001 | $7.089\times10^{-7}$ | 0.0000 |

If we consider a vertical layer of the molecular atmosphere, its optical thickness in this case is

$$\tau_{\mathrm{Rayl}}(\lambda) = \int_0^\infty \sigma_{\mathrm{Rayl}}(\lambda, s)\, ds \qquad (3.4)$$

Here $\sigma_{\mathrm{Rayl}}(\lambda, s)$ is the molecular scattering coefficient for radiation of wavelength $\lambda$ as a function of the coordinate in the layer $s$ (or the height in the atmosphere).

Using the expressions given above and the data of Table 3.1, we readily calculate the losses of radiation with wavelengths of 0.3 $\mu$m (ultraviolet region), 0.55 $\mu$m (maximum of the solar emission spectrum and maximum sensitivity of the human eye), 0.69 $\mu$m (ruby laser emission), 0.8 $\mu$m (approximate demarcation between the visible and infrared regions of the spectrum), and 1.06 $\mu$m (neodymium glass layer emission) in the ground layer and in a vertical column of the entire atmosphere (Table 3.3).

Table 3.3 clearly exhibits the strong dependence of the radiation energy losses due to molecular scattering on the wavelength. Thus, in a vertical column running the entire thickness of the atmosphere, these losses are 70% at a wavelength of 0.3 $\mu$m, a mere 9% at 0.55 $\mu$m, and 3.9 and 0.7% for ruby and neodymium glass lasers, respectively. A similar picture emerges for the ground layer of the atmosphere.

The molecular scattering coefficients in the infrared region have values that are usually neglected in comparison with the aerosol scattering coefficients wherever any of the coefficients are used to estimate the energy losses of radiation propagating in the atmosphere.

In regard to many practical problems associated with utilization of the molecular scattering effect, it is important to know the angular distribution of the scattered radiation intensity, or the angular scattering function

**Table 3.3.** Radiation Energy Losses at Various Wavelengths due to Molecular Scattering in the Ground Layer and in a Vertical Column of the Entire Atmosphere (%)

| $\lambda$, $\mu$m | Distance | | Vertical column of entire atmosphere |
|---|---|---|---|
| | 1 km | 10 km | |
| 0.30 | 13.4 | 76.3 | 70.4 |
| 0.55 | 1.2 | 10.9 | 9.1 |
| 0.69 | 0.5 | 4.6 | 3.9 |
| 0.80 | 0.3 | 2.5 | 2.1 |
| 1.06 | 0.1 | 0.9 | 0.7 |

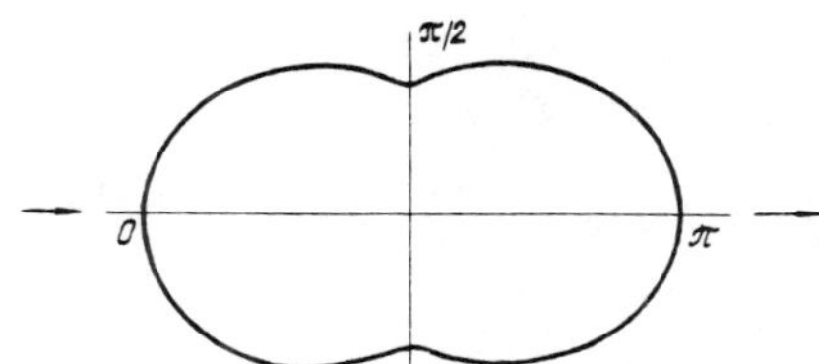

Fig. 3.1. Normalized Rayleigh scattering function.

(scattering "indicatrix"), which is defined as the ratio

$$f(\theta)=\frac{I(\theta)}{\displaystyle\int_{4\pi} I(\theta)\,d\omega} \tag{3.5}$$

in which $I(\theta)$ is the intensity of the scattered radiation in the direction of the angle $\theta$ and $d\omega$ is an element of solid angle.

The form of the Rayleigh scattering function (scattering diagram) is given in Fig. 3.1. Its single-valued character is important from the point of view of obtaining unambiguous results from investigations based on utilization of the molecular scattering effect.

## 3.2. Scattering by a Single Particle

### 3.2.1. Representation of Polarized Light

Following [4], we consider a plane monochromatic wave, whose electric field $\mathbf{E}$ is written in the complex notation

$$\mathbf{E}=\mathbf{E}_0\exp(-i\omega t+i\mathbf{k}\cdot\mathbf{r}) \tag{3.6}$$

Here $\omega$ is the frequency of the field, the direction of $\mathbf{k}$ is the same as the direction of wave propagation, $k=m_a\omega/c$, $m_a$ is the refractive index of the medium, $c$ is the velocity of light, and $\mathbf{E}_0$ is a constant vector perpendicular to $\mathbf{k}$. The magnetic field $H$ is related to $E$ by the usual equation

$$\mathbf{H}=m_a[\mathbf{n},\mathbf{E}] \tag{3.7}$$

in which

$$\mathbf{n}=\mathbf{k}/k$$

The energy flux of the electromagnetic field per unit area is given by the Poynting vector

$$\mathbf{P} = \frac{c}{4\pi}[\mathrm{Re}\,\mathbf{E}, \mathrm{Re}\,\mathbf{H}] \qquad (3.8)$$

Inasmuch as radiation detectors are sensitive to the energy characteristics of the field, the time-average components of (3.8) represent measurable variables in optics. Time averaging is dictated by the fact that the period of experimental analysis of the properties of the field is much greater than the period of the light wave.

We now consider the complete set of measurable variables. The first quantity is the total wave intensity, which is determined as the time average of $\mathbf{P}$. Next, it is also possible to measure the time-average intensity along a definite line. The corresponding oscillations can be segregated by placing an analyzer with a definite orientation in the path of the wave. The indicated characteristics form the complete set of experimentally determinable information about the light beam. This information can be quantitatively described as follows. It is necessary to substitute expressions (3.6) and (3.7) into (3.8) and to allow for the fact that the time averages of all terms with the factor $\exp(\pm i2\omega t)$ vanish. Then for the total intensity we have

$$I = \frac{c}{8\pi} m_a(\mathbf{E}_0, \mathbf{E}_0^*) \qquad (3.9)$$

We now introduce a certain Cartesian coordinate system $x, y, z$, relative to which the investigated wave propagates in the direction of the negative third axis. Then the vector $\mathbf{E}_0$ is situated in the plane formed by the unit vectors of the first two axes. The direction of the line along which it is required to measure the intensity can be specified by the angle $\eta$ relative to the first axis. If $I(\eta)$ is the intensity of the corresponding oscillations, we readily obtain from (3.9)

$$I(\eta) = \frac{c}{16\pi} m_a(S_1 + S_2\cos 2\eta + S_3\sin 2\eta) \qquad (3.10)$$

If an auxiliary device is placed in the path of the light beam, introducing a constant phase difference $\delta$ into the mutually perpendicular components of the field (for example, a quarter-wave plate), then

$$I(\eta) = \frac{c}{16\pi} m_a\left[S_1 + S_2\cos 2\eta + (S_3\cos\delta - S_4\sin\delta)\sin\eta\right] \qquad (3.11)$$

The Stokes parameters in expressions (3.10) and (3.11) are defined as follows:

$$S_1 = E_{01} E_{01}^* + E_{02} E_{02}^*$$

$$S_2 = E_{02} E_{02}^* - E_{01} E_{01}^*$$

$$S_3 = E_{02} E_{01}^* + E_{02}^* E_{01}$$

$$S_4 = i\left( E_{02} E_{01}^* - E_{02}^* E_{01} \right) \qquad (3.12)$$

Here $E_{0j}$ denotes the first and second components of the vector $\mathbf{E}_0$.

A comparison of (3.9) and (3.12) enables us to write an equation for the total intensity in the form

$$I = \frac{c}{8\pi} m_a S_1 \qquad (3.13)$$

It is easily shown that $S_1$ and $S_4$ are invariant under rotations about the third axis, while $S_2$ and $S_3$ undergo the transformations

$$S_2' = S_2 \cos 2\psi + S_3 \sin 2\psi; \qquad S_3' = -S_2 \sin 2\psi + S_3 \cos 2\psi$$

where $S_2'$ and $S_3'$ are the values of the Stokes parameters in the system rotated through an angle $\psi$ about the third axis relative to the old system.

Next, it can be shown that the end of the vector $\mathbf{E}$ for the wave (3.6) describes a certain ellipse. This type of wave is therefore said to be elliptically polarized. The polarization ellipse can be described by the angle $\varphi$ between the semimajor axis of the ellipse and the first unit vector of the adopted coordinate system and by the ellipticity $\beta$, which is defined by the relation $\tan \beta = a_2 / a_1$, in which $a_1$ and $a_2$ are the semiminor and semimajor axes, respectively; $\beta$ is positive for dextrorotation (relative to $\mathbf{k}_0$) and positive otherwise. After suitable calculations, we arrive at the relations

$$S_2 = S_1 \cos 2\beta \cos 2\varphi$$

$$S_3 = S_1 \cos 2\beta \sin 2\varphi \qquad (3.14)$$

$$S_4 = S_1 \sin 2\beta$$

Equations (3.11), (3.13), and (3.14) make it possible to calculate the characteristics of the polarization ellipse from the results of corresponding measurements.

### 3.2.2. Scattering of a Plane Monochromatic Wave

We now identify the field discussed in Section 3.2.1 with a wave incident on a particular object. Let the coordinate origin be situated at the center of the object, and let the first axis of the system coincide with the semimajor axis of the wave polarization ellipse. We denote the unit vectors of this system by $\mathbf{l}_1$, $\mathbf{l}_2$, and $\mathbf{l}_3$.

The material of the given object has a complex-valued refractive index $m_b \neq m_a$ and so comprises a certain optical inhomogeneity. Consequently, a scattered field must exist outside the object. We therefore endow all quantities characterizing the incident wave with index (0) and those for the scattered wave with index ($a$).

We consider a certain point $\mathbf{r}$, at which the scattered field is to be investigated. We denote by $Q$ the plane containing the chosen point and the direction of propagation of the incident wave (i.e., the third axis of the coordinate system).

We introduce a coordinate system $g$ with a right-handed triple of unit vectors $\mathbf{g}_1, \mathbf{g}_2, \mathbf{g}_3$, where $\mathbf{g}_3 = -\mathbf{l}_3$, $\mathbf{g}_1$ is perpendicular to the plane $Q$, and $\mathbf{g}_2$ is parallel to it. In the system $g$, the Stokes parameters $S_j^{(0)}$ for the incident wave have the form (3.14), and $\varphi$ is the azimuth angle of the point $\mathbf{r}$.

It is more practical to analyze the scattered wave in a system $j$ with the right-handed triple of unit vectors defined so that $\mathbf{j}_3 = \mathbf{r}/r$, $r = |\mathbf{r}|$, $\mathbf{j}_1$ is perpendicular to $Q$, and $\mathbf{j}_2$ is parallel to $Q$. It follows from the linearity of the Maxwell equations and the extinction condition at infinity that the scattered wave is represented in the wave zone by the expressions

$$E_1^{(a)} = \frac{e^{-i\omega t + ikr}}{ikr}\left[a_{11}(\theta,\varphi)E_1^{(0)} + a_{12}(\theta,\varphi)E_2^{(0)}\right]$$

$$E_2^{(a)} = \frac{e^{-i\omega t + ikr}}{ikr}\left[a_{21}(\theta,\varphi)E_1^{(0)} + a_{22}(\theta,\varphi)E_2^{(0)}\right]$$

$$(3.15)$$

In these expressions, $r, \theta, \varphi$ are the polar coordinates of the point $r$, $\mathbf{E}_i^{(0)}$ denotes the components of $\mathbf{E}_0^{(0)}$ in the system $g$, and $E_j^{(a)}$ denotes the components of the scattered field in the system $j$. The magnetic field $\mathbf{H}$ of the scattered wave is again calculated according to (3.7). The functions $a_{ij}(\theta,\varphi)$ are determined by the size, shape, and material properties of the particle.

The wave (3.15) has the form analyzed in Section 3.2.1 since its characteristics are constant at all points of a sphere of fixed radius; $E_3^{(a)} = 0$

in the wave zone, and the factors $\exp(-i\omega t + i\mathbf{k}\cdot\mathbf{r})$ and $\exp(-i\omega t + ik\cdot r)$ are essentially the same. In the system $j$, therefore, we can introduce the Stokes parameters $S_j^{(a)}$ for the scattered light and again determine relations (3.12). If the Stokes parameters are written in the single-column matrix form $\{S\}$, we readily infer that

$$\{S^{(a)}\} = \frac{1}{k^2 r^2}\{M\}\{S^{(0)}\} \tag{3.16}$$

Relation (3.16) describes the scattering matrix $\{M\}$, which, as the significance of the Stokes parameters implies, contains essentially all information about the scattered light. We now write components of the scattering matrix in explicit form:

$$M_{ij} = \frac{1}{2}\sum_{\alpha,\beta=1}^{2}|a_{\alpha\beta}|^2\varepsilon_{\alpha\beta ij}, \qquad i,j=1,2$$

$$\varepsilon_{\alpha\beta ij} = \begin{pmatrix} 1 & 1 & 1 & 1 \\ -1 & 1 & -1 & 1 \\ -1 & -1 & 1 & 1 \\ 1 & -1 & -1 & 1 \end{pmatrix}$$

$$M_{13} = \mathrm{Re}(a_{12}a_{11}^* + a_{21}a_{22}^*); \qquad M_{41} = -\mathrm{Im}(a_{12}a_{22}^* + a_{21}a_{11}^*)$$

$$M_{23} = \mathrm{Re}(a_{21}a_{22}^* - a_{12}a_{11}^*); \qquad M_{43} = -\mathrm{Im}(a_{11}a_{22}^* + a_{12}a_{21}^*)$$

$$M_{31} = \mathrm{Re}(a_{12}a_{22}^* + a_{21}a_{11}^*); \qquad M_{44} = \mathrm{Re}(a_{11}a_{22}^* - a_{12}a_{21}^*)$$

$$M_{32} = \mathrm{Re}(a_{12}a_{22}^* - a_{21}a_{11}^*); \qquad M_{24} = \mathrm{Im}(a_{21}a_{22}^* - a_{12}a_{11}^*)$$

$$M_{33} = \mathrm{Re}(a_{11}a_{22}^* - a_{12}a_{21}^*); \qquad M_{42} = -\mathrm{Im}(a_{12}a_{22}^* - a_{21}a_{11}^*)$$

$$M_{14} = \mathrm{Im}(a_{12}a_{11}^* + a_{21}a_{22}^*); \qquad M_{34} = -\mathrm{Im}(a_{11}a_{22}^* - a_{12}a_{21}^*)$$

The explicit form of the coefficients $a_{ij}$ is determined once the corresponding electrodynamical boundary-value problem has been solved, which entails solution of the Maxwell equations subject to the condition that the tangential component of the field is continuous at the interface between media with different electromagnetic characteristics. This problem is very complex, and so its solutions have been found only in certain special cases.

In the case of spherical particles, $a_{12}=a_{21}=0$, the coefficients $a_{11}$ and $a_{22}$ depend only on $\theta$, and for $\theta=\pi$, i.e., when the direction of propagation of the scattered wave coincides with the direction of the incident wave, $a_{11}=a_{22}$. We also note that $M_{11}$ has the same significance as the angular scattering function.

### 3.2.3. Scattering, Absorption, and Extinction Coefficients

It follows from relations (3.13) and (3.16) that the scattered light intensity is determined from the expression

$$I^{(a)} = \frac{m_a c}{16\pi k^2 r^2} \left( S_1^{(0)}M_{11} + S_2^{(0)}M_{12} + S_3^{(0)}2M_{13} + S_4^{(0)}M_{14} \right) \quad (3.17)$$

Also, the direction of the Poynting vector, according to expressions (3.7), (3.8), and (3.15), coincides with the direction of $\mathbf{j}_3$. Consequently, the energy flux of the scattered field $P^{(a)}$ through a sphere of sufficiently large radius is equal to $\int I^{(a)} r^2 \sin\theta\, d\theta\, d\varphi$. The ratio of the latter quantity to the incident light intensity determines the scattering coefficient $\sigma_s$.

Substituting (3.17) into the definition of the flux and making use of expression (3.13) for calculation of the incident light intensity, along with relations (3.14), we find

$$\sigma_s = \frac{1}{2k^2} \int ( M_{11} + M_{12}\cos 2\beta \cos 2\varphi + 2M_{13}\cos 2\beta \sin 2\varphi$$

$$+ 2M_{14}\sin 2\beta)\sin\theta\, d\theta\, d\varphi \qquad (3.18)$$

From (3.18) we readily deduce expressions for $\sigma_s$ in the case of scattering of linearly polarized light ($\beta=0$) and circularly polarized light ($\beta=\pm\pi/4$, depending on the direction of polarization). If the particle is spherical, then, using the properties of $a_{ij}$, we obtain in this case

$$\sigma_s = \frac{\pi}{k^2} \int_0^\pi M_{11}\sin\theta\, d\theta \qquad (3.19)$$

independently of the polarization state of the incident light.

The absorption coefficient $\sigma_a$ is defined as minus the ratio of the Poynting vector for the total field through a sphere of radius $r$ to the intensity of the incident light. It is seen at once that the absolute value of the flux defined above is equal to the field energy absorbed in the investigated volume. A minus sign represents an energy sink.

The Poynting vector **P** for the total field can be written as follows on the basis of the field superposition principle and expressions (3.8):

$$\mathbf{P}=\mathbf{P}^{(0)}+\mathbf{P}^{(a)}+\mathbf{P}'$$

where

$$\mathbf{P}'=\frac{c}{8\pi}\,\mathrm{Re}\left\{[\mathbf{E}^{(a)},\mathbf{H}^{(0)}*]+[\mathbf{E}^{(0)},\mathbf{H}^{(a)}*]\right\} \tag{3.20}$$

The vector **P'** is time averaged in (3.20).

By the definition of the absorption coefficient,

$$\sigma_a=-\frac{1}{I^{(0)}}\int(\mathbf{P},\mathbf{j}_3)\,ds \tag{3.21}$$

where, as usual, $ds=r^2\sin\theta\,d\theta\,d\varphi$.

We define the sum of the scattering and absorption coefficients as the extinction coefficient:

$$\sigma=\sigma_a+\sigma_s \tag{3.22}$$

If the expression for **P** is substituted into (3.21) and allowance is made for the fact that the integral with the first term vanishes and the integral with the second term yields the scattering coefficient, we obtain from (3.22)

$$\sigma=-\frac{1}{I_0}\int(\mathbf{P}',\mathbf{j}_3)\,ds \tag{3.23}$$

Upon substitution of (3.20) into (3.23), we can write the integrand in explicit form, making use of (3.6) and (3.15) for the components of the electric field and (3.7) for the components of the magnetic field.

We then arrive at integrals of the type $\int F(\theta,\varphi)\exp[ikr(1+\cos\theta)]\sin\theta\,d\theta$. Inasmuch as $kr\gg 1$ in the wave zone, the indicated integrals can be computed by the stationary-phase principle. After suitable calculations, we obtain the following expression for $\sigma$ [5]:

$$\sigma=-\frac{1}{k^2}\,\mathrm{Re}\int_0^{2\pi}\Big[(a_{11}-a_{22})+\cos^2\beta\cos 2\varphi(a_{22}-a_{11})$$

$$+(a_{12}+a_{21})\cos 2\beta\sin 2\varphi+i(a_{21}-a_{12})\sin 2\beta\Big]\,d\varphi \tag{3.24}$$

All the functions $a_{ij}$ in (3.24) have the argument $\theta=\pi$.

The results (3.24) essentially represent a well-known optical theorem generalized to the case of elliptically polarized light and a scattering particle of arbitrary geometry.

For spherical particles, on the basis of the corresponding properties of $a_{ij}$ and (3.24), we write

$$\sigma = -\frac{4\pi}{k^2}\,\mathrm{Re}\,a(\pi) \qquad\qquad (3.25)$$

independently of the polarization state of the incident wave. Here $a(\pi) = a_{11}(\pi) = a_{22}(\pi)$ represents the forward-scattered wave amplitude.

It is evident from (3.24) that in order to calculate the extinction coefficient it is necessary to know the amplitude of the wave scattered at a small angle relative to the direction of propagation of the incident wave. The reasons for this need are fairly simple, considering that any experimental scheme for the determination of $\sigma$ essentially involves investigation of the interference of the incident wave with a small-angle scattered wave. Since integrals of the form given above are independent of the upper limit when computed by the stationary-phase principle, it can be shown that $\sigma$ defined by (3.22) coincides with the screening number $\eta$. The latter is a specific property of the experimental scheme: $\eta = I_0^{-1}(\Pi_0 - \Pi)$, where $\Pi$ and $\Pi_0$ are the energies recorded by the radiation detector when, respectively, the particle is situated in the radiation flux and is far removed from it. From the purely computational point of view, expression (3.24) is useful in the sense that it permits any approximate information about the small-angle scattered light amplitudes to be used for the determination of $\sigma$.

### 3.2.4. Extinction, Scattering, and Absorption Efficiency Factors

The concepts of the efficiency factors of extinction $K$, scattering $K_s$, and absorption $K_a$ are introduced in the investigation of electromagnetic wave scattering by a spherical particle:

$$K = \frac{\sigma}{\pi a^2}; \qquad K_s = \frac{\sigma_s}{\pi a^2}; \qquad K_a = \frac{\sigma_a}{\pi a^2} \qquad\qquad (3.26)$$

The functions $K$, $K_s$, and $K_a$, as is evident from (3.26) and the definitions of the coefficients $\sigma$, $\sigma_s$, and $\sigma_a$ given in Section 3.2.3, are numerically equal to the ratio of the energy attenuated, scattered, and absorbed by the particle, respectively, to the energy entrained within its geometrical cross section $\pi a^2$.

#### 3.2.4.1. Analytical Expressions for the Functions $K$, $K_s$, and $K_a$

General expressions for $K$, $K_s$, and $K_a$ are given by Mie theory, which is described schematically and in detail in the books [6, 7]. The expressions for $K$, $K_s$, and $K_a$ comprise infinite series; $K$, $K_s$, and $K_a$ depend on two arguments characterizing the relative radius $\rho$ and relative refractive index $m$ of the particle:

$$\rho = \frac{2\pi a}{\lambda} \tag{3.27}$$

$$m = \frac{m_1}{m_2} \tag{3.28}$$

where $\lambda$ is the wavelength of the scattered radiation and $m_1$ and $m_2$ are the complex-valued refractive indices of the particle and the medium.

In application to radiation scattering conditions in the atmosphere, the relative complex refractive index may be assumed to be equal to the particle refractive index, i.e., we can put $m = m_1 = n - i\kappa$, where $n$ is the ordinary refractive index and $\kappa$ is the refractive index of the particle material.

Expressions for the function $K$, $K_s$, and $K_a$ have been obtained in finite form for a number of asymptotic situations. Some of the asymptotic expressions that will be needed later on are given below.

**3.2.4.1.1. Small Particles.** Particles are considered to be small when $\rho \ll 1$. In this case, asymptotic expressions are obtained for $K$ and $K_s$ by expanding the Bessel and Hankel functions occurring in the expressions for $K$ and $K_s$ into powers of $\rho$. Different expressions are obtained for different $|m|$. We are interested in the case where $|m|$ is small, for which the following expressions have been obtained [6, 8]:

$$K(\rho, m) = \sum_{n=1}^{5} P_n \rho^n, \qquad P_1 = 4\,\mathrm{Im}\left(\frac{1-m^2}{m^2+2}\right), \qquad P_2 = 0$$

$$P_3 = 2\,\mathrm{Im}\left[\frac{-2(m^2-1)(m^2-2)}{(m^2+2)^2} + \frac{m^2-1}{15} - \frac{m^2-1}{3(2m^2+3)}\right]$$

$$P_4 = \frac{8}{3}\,\mathrm{Re}\left(\frac{m^2-1}{m^2+2}\right)^2 \tag{3.29}$$

$$P_5 = 2\,\mathrm{Im}\left[\frac{3}{175}\frac{m^2-1}{m^2+2}\frac{m^6+20m^4-200m^2+200}{m^3-2}\right.$$

$$\left. -\frac{1}{56}\cdot\frac{m^2-1}{3m^2+4} - \frac{(m^2-1)(2m^2-3)}{315}\right]$$

For transparent particles, putting $\kappa=0$ in (3.29), we obtain

$$K(\rho,m)=K_s(\rho,m)=\frac{8}{3}\rho^4\left(\frac{m^2-1}{m^2+2}\right)^2 \qquad (3.30)$$

It is evident from (3.30) that the single-particle scattering coefficient in this special case, if its real refractive index is assumed to be constant, is inversely proportional to the fourth power of the wavelength, as in the case of molecular (Rayleigh) scattering. In other cases, the dependence turns out to be extremely complex and is not similar to the implication of the well-known Rayleigh law.

Expressions for $K(\rho,m)$ and $K_s(\rho,m)$ in the case of large values of $m$ and $m=\infty$ are given in [6, 7].

**3.2.4.1.2. Large Particles.** Large particles are considered to be those for which $\rho\gg1$. An analysis of the problem with the direct application of the Mie equations is exceedingly difficult in this case because it is necessary to retain in the sums, as shown by Debye, all terms containing $n$ with values from 1 to $\rho$. For example, in the case of raindrops, it is necessary to retain several thousand terms. Shifrin [9] has analyzed this case for a transparent particle with the scattered field treated as comprising geometrical-optics rays and rays diffracted by the contours of the drop. Following arguments similar to those in [9] in application to the case of an absorbing particle, we obtain for $K(\rho,m)$

$$K(\rho,m)=2-\frac{8(n^2-\kappa^2)^{1/2}}{(n+1)^2+\kappa^2}\frac{n}{n-1}\frac{\exp(-2\rho\kappa)}{\rho}$$

$$\times\sin\left[2\rho(n-1)-2\tan^{-1}\frac{(n^2+\kappa^2)^{1/2}}{(n^2+\kappa^2)^{1/2}+1}\frac{\kappa}{(n^2+\kappa^2)^{1/2}+n}\right]$$

$$(3.31)$$

For transparent particles, we obtain from (3.31)

$$K_s(\rho,m)=2-\frac{8n^2}{\rho(n+1)^2(n-1)}\sin\left[2\rho(n-1)\right] \qquad (3.32)$$

It follows from (3.31) and (3.32) that the functions $K$ and $K_s$ tend to 2 in the case $\rho\to\infty$, regardless of the value of $m$. This means that extremely large particles scatter twice as much radiation as impinges on their geometrical cross section.

*3.2.4.1.3. Particles with $|m-1|\to 0$ ("Soft" Particles).* This case has been analyzed in detail in Van de Hulst's book [7]. We note that water and water–aerosol particles can be regarded as "soft" with sufficient practical accuracy.

A reasonably simple and practical expression has been obtained [7] for large "soft" particles ($\rho\gg 1$):

$$K(\rho,m)=2-4\exp\left(-\rho'\tan\beta\frac{\cos\beta}{\rho'}\right)\sin(\rho'-\beta)$$

$$-4\exp\left[-\rho'\tan\beta\left(\frac{\cos\beta}{\rho'}\right)^2\right]\cos(\rho'-2\beta)+4\left(\frac{\cos\beta}{\rho'}\right)^2\cos^2\beta$$

$$(3.33)$$

where

$$\rho'=2\rho(n-1),\qquad \tan\beta=\frac{\kappa}{n-1} \tag{3.34}$$

and for a transparent particle

$$K_s(\rho,m)=2-\frac{4}{\rho'}\sin\rho'+\frac{4}{\rho'^2}(1-\cos\rho') \tag{3.35}$$

Expressions (3.33)–(3.35) adequately conform to the behavior of the $K$ and $K_s$ curves (including those for small values of $\rho$) plotted on the basis of a tabulation of the exact Mie equations.

### 3.2.4.2. Results of Tabulation of the Functions $K$, $K_s$, and $K_a$

In the situation where none of the foregoing conditions is satisfied, the functions $K$, $K_s$, and $K_a$ can only be obtained by calculations based on the exact Mie equations. The number of terms retained in the series expansions in order to obtain acceptable computational accuracy must be of the order of $\rho$. The calculations are exceedingly cumbersome and, so, prior to the advent of high-speed electronic computing equipment, had been carried out only for selected values of the parameters $m$ and $\rho$.

Quite a few calculations for various values of $m$ and $\rho$ have now been carried out in view of the considerable need for data on the functions $K$, $K_s$, and $K_a$ on the part of specialists in many branches of scientists, primarily

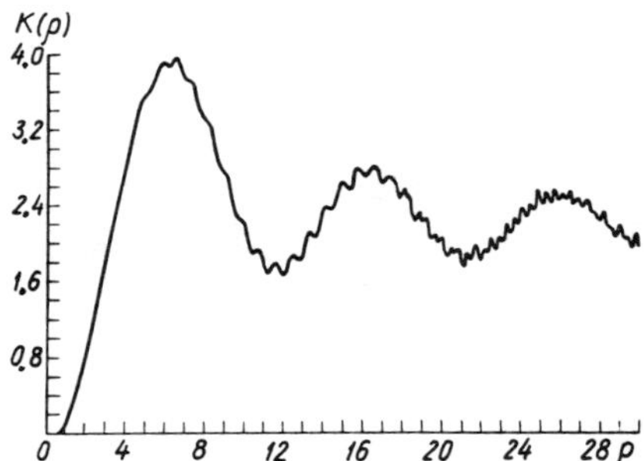

Fig. 3.2. Extinction efficiency factor, $|m| = 1.33$.

chemists, geophysicists, and meteorologists. By far, the most calculations have been carried out for real-valued refractive indices: $0.60 \leqslant m \leqslant 2.105$ and $m = \infty$.

With reference to atmospheric aerosol particles, the most complete data have been obtained in [10–18]. The present author has published detailed illustrations of the results of pertinent computations in a recent book [4]. We restrict the present discussion to one such illustration, Fig. 3.2, which gives the dependence of the efficiency factor $K_0 \simeq K_s$ as a function of the parameter $\rho$ for water spheres with refractive index $n = 1.33$ (visible spectrum).

### 3.2.4.3. Approximation Relations for K

A number of authors have obtained approximation relations for the dependence of the function $K$ on $\rho$ for various values of $m$. Levin [19] has derived a corresponding relation for $K(\rho)$ in the case of arbitrary $\rho$ and $m = 1.33$ (water spheres in the visible region of the spectrum).

The same author has also [20] adopted an approximation relation for $K(\rho, m)$ that is valid for any values of $\rho$ and complex values of $m$ satisfying the condition $|m| < 2$. In that work, $K$ is written in the form

$$K = (1 + D)K_1 \tag{3.36}$$

where $K_1$ is the function specified by expressions (3.33) and (3.35) and $(1 + D)$ is an approximation factor.

The function $D(\rho, m)$ is given by the expressions

$$D_1 = \frac{n-1}{2n} \frac{5(n-1)}{4.08}[d(\beta)+1] - \frac{5(n-1)-\rho'}{5(n-1)d(\beta)}$$

$$\rho' \leqslant 5(n-1) \leqslant \frac{4.08}{1+3\tan\beta}$$

$$D_2 = \frac{n-1}{2n}\left[d(\beta)+1\right]\frac{\rho'}{4.08}, \qquad 5(n-1)\leqslant\rho'\leqslant\frac{4.08}{1+3\tan\beta} \quad (3.37)$$

$$D_3 = \frac{n-1}{2n}\frac{d(\beta)+1}{1+3\tan\beta}, \qquad \frac{4.08}{1+3\tan\beta}\leqslant\rho'\leqslant\frac{4.08}{1+\tan\beta}$$

$$D_4 = \frac{n-1}{2n}\frac{d(\beta)+1}{d(\beta)}\frac{4.08}{\rho'}, \qquad \rho'>\frac{4.08}{1+\tan\beta}$$

$$d(\beta)=(1+\tan\beta)(1+3\tan\beta)$$

The values of $\rho'$ and $\beta$ are given by expressions (3.35).

It is shown in [20] that the functions $K(\rho, m)$ obtained by means of (3.36) and (3.37) approximate the results of calculations [21] according to the exact Mie equations within 4% error limits. We note that calculations of $K(\rho, m)$ in [20] are carried out up to $\rho=17.5$. Our own comparison of the results obtained according to (3.36) and (3.37) and according to the asymptotic relation (3.31) shows that the above-indicated approximation error is applicable for $\rho>17.5$.

### 3.2.5. Angular Scattering Functions

Calculations of the angular scattering function, or scattering indicatrix, have been undertaken in many papers, bibliographies of which may be found in several books [4, 6, 7]. The most comprehensive data have been obtained in [10, 11]. Shifrin and Zel'manovich [10] have tabulated the scattering functions for angles of 0° (0.1°) 5° (1°) 90° (all angles from 0 to 5° in steps of 0.1°, etc.) and in the angular interval of the primary bow for water droplets, 135–140° in steps of 0.2°. The values of all components of the scattering matrix and the components of the scattered-wave field are given in [11] for water droplets in the wavelength range from 0.4 to 12 $\mu$m. The wavelengths are chosen to span the entire range of values of the components of the complex refractive index of water with a definite approximation.

All the characteristics of the scattered field are calculated for 51 values of the parameter $\rho=0.5$ (0.5) 6 (1) 20 (2) 50 (5) 100 and 43 values of the scattering angle $\theta=0, 0.05, 0.1, 0.2, 0.5, 1, 2, 5, 10$ (10) 130, 135 (0.5) 140 (10) 170, 175, 178, 179, 179.5, 179.8, 179.9, 179.95, 180°. Thus, very detailed data have been obtained for small-angle forward and back scattering.

Penndorf [22] has analyzed the behavior of the function $i_1+i_2$ in the expressions for the particulate extinction coefficient and scattering function for angles $\theta=0, 90, 180°$ and for $m=1.33$; this function exhibits strong oscillations with variation of $\rho$. The frequency and amplitude of the oscillations increase with the value of the angle $\theta$. Thus, if the oscillation amplitude at $\theta=0$ is taken as equal to 0.1, it increases to 5 and 500 at angles of 90 and 180°, respectively.

An analysis of the results obtained in calculations of the scattering functions for spherical particles enables us to sketch the following qualitative picture of how their general behavior is affected by the particle size and the components of the complex-valued refractive index of the particle. Small particles with $m \sim 1$ and $\rho \to 0$ have a symmetrical Rayleigh scattering function, and small particles with $m = \infty$ reflect radiation backward more strongly than forward. We note that different authors adopt values of $m$ in the interval from 1.33 to 1.5 for atmospheric aerosols in the visible spectrum [4].

As $\rho$ increases from 0 to $\infty$, the scattering diagram for atmospheric aerosol particles changes its shape continuously, becoming increasingly asymmetrical and protracted in the forward direction (Mie effect). Volz [23] gives the following numerical example, illustrating this process. For particles with $m = 1.5$ and radii $a = 0.5$, 1.5, 5.0, and 12.5 $\mu$m the ratios between the radiant energy fluxes at a wavelength of 0.5 $\mu$m ($\rho = 6.28$, 18.84, 62.8, and 157) for forward and back scattering are equal to 17, 74, 823, and 16,000, respectively. This ratio is often called the asymmetry factor of the angular scattering function (or diagram).

The foregoing pattern of variation of the scattering function with the size of atmospheric aerosol particles is significantly affected by the complex-valuedness of the refractive index and the intensity oscillations of radiation scattered at various angles, those oscillations depending on $\rho$, $\theta$, and $m$.


### 3.2.6. Scattering by Nonspherical Particles

Despite the observation by many researchers that the shape of the great majority of aerosol particles can be approximated by spheres, this particle nonetheless deserves special consideration insofar as dust particles, minute ice crystals, and crystalline cloud particles actually have rather arbitrary configurations. It is important to know how the shapes of the particles influence their optical properties. A great many results pertaining to this problem have been gathered and compiled in Van de Hulst's book [7] (for ellipsoids, circular cylinders, and particles having other geometries with various values of $\rho$ and $m$ and different orientations relative to the incident radiation). Shifrin [6] has investigated the optical characteristics of rod- and disk-shaped particles approximated by ellipsoids.

An analysis of the existing results shows that the optical characteristics of particles of various geometries depend strongly on the ratio between the maximum and minimum particle radii, their orientations relative to the incident radiation, the degree of polarization of the latter, and the values of the complex refractive index. For example, in the case of a greatly elongated transparent rod, all linear dimensions of which are much smaller than the wavelength, the ratio of the scattering coefficients for orientation parallel and antiparallel to the field is equal to 6.25 for $m=2$ and 1.64 for $m=1.64$ [7]. Naturally, the ratio will differ for the same absorbing rod. A variation of the dimensions of the rod incurs a corresponding variation of the given ratio.

The optical characteristics of particles of different geometries can differ markedly from those of the spherical particle having the same volume. The results of Mie theory must therefore be applied to nonspherical particles with utmost caution. On the other hand, if the particle shape does not depart too radically from spherical (as in the cases of ellipsoids with ratios of the semiaxes up to 1.5–2, cubes, cylinders with a length-to-diameter ratio close to unity, etc.), then such characteristics of the particle as the angular scattering function and the extinction, scattering, and absorption coefficients will differ only slightly from the corresponding characteristics of a spherical particle of the same volume.

We now indicate an important practical way in which the results of Mie theory can be applied to nonspherical particles. If we average a particular optical characteristic of a particle over all its possible orientations in space, we can then express the volume of the particle analytically in terms of the volume of a spherical particle having the same optical characteristic. Shifrin [6] has derived such a relation for the angular scattering function of ellipsoidal particles:

$$v^* = \left[\varphi(t)\right]^{1/2} v$$

where $v^*$ and $v$ are the volumes of the sphere and the ellipsoid with identical scattering functions, $t=a/b$ is the ratio of the semiaxes of the ellipsoid, and $\varphi(t)$ is a function taking values from 1 to 0.23 as $t$ varies from 1 to 10. In particular, $\varphi(t)=0.93$ and 0.71 for $t=2$ and 3.

Relations of a similar type can be obtained for different scattering characteristics and for particles of other geometries.

## 3.3. Scattering by a System of Particles

The rigorous electrodynamical formulation of the problem of wave scattering by a system of particles, methods for its solution, and certain results obtained to date have been discussed quite extensively in the literature (see, e.g., [24–29]). The fundamental methodological aspect of the solution of the stated problem is as follows. It is postulated that the solution of the single-particle light-scattering problem is known, and all required physical variables can be obtained by suitable statistical averaging processes over the particle positions.

In a medium filled with particles there exists a certain field, which is made up of the fields of the incident wave entering the system of particles and the waves scattered by the individual particles. The latter fields are formulated on the basis of the known solution, where each particle is acted upon by its own so-called effective field. We can therefore write

$$\psi(\mathbf{r}) = \psi_0(\mathbf{r}) + \sum_{j=1}^{N} T(\mathbf{r}, \mathbf{r}_j) \tilde{\psi}(\mathbf{r}_j)$$

$$\tilde{\psi}(\mathbf{r}_j) = \psi_0(\mathbf{r}) + \sum_{j' \neq j} T(\mathbf{r}_j, \mathbf{r}_{j'}) \tilde{\psi}(\mathbf{r}_{j'}) \tag{3.38}$$

where $\psi$ is a certain component of the field, $\mathbf{r}_j$ denotes the coordinates of the $j$th particle, $\psi_0$ is the corresponding component of the incident wave, $\mathbf{r}$ is the radius vector of an arbitrary point, $T$ is the scattering operator, and $\tilde{\psi}$ is the effective field. The first eq. (3.38) gives the value of the field in the medium, and the second essentially represents a system of equations for determining the values of the effective field acting on each particle. The sum in (3.38) determines a fixed configuration of scattering particles.

The next step is to average Eqs. (3.38) over all configurations. This is accomplished formally by multiplying both sides of the equations by the configuration distribution function and integrating with respect to the appropriate variables. The distribution function of the configurations depends significantly, in the general case, on the nature of the interaction between particles. The pertinent calculations can be carried out to completion in general form if the particles are assumed to be noninteracting (as in a model of the ideal-gas type) or if the analysis is limited to the first few terms of the expansion in virial coefficients. It is also necessary to assume that the distances between particles are significantly greater than the light wavelength in order to be able to use the asymptotic form of the scattering operator in the wave zone. We note, in addition, that the effective field is normally taken to be equal to the average field at the particle site since the two fields differ by order of magnitude $1/N$, where $N$ is the number of particles. This assumption means that only one equation for the average field has to be considered.

The same scheme is applicable to the light-intensity problem. The expressions obtained by multiplying both sides of Eqs. (3.38) by the corresponding complex-conjugate terms are again averaged over all configurations for a definite distribution function.

If we consider noninteracting particles, we obtain the usual transport equation for the radiation intensity in the medium; if particle interaction is included in the customary way, we obtain certain corrections to the indicated equation.

In this kind of analysis, a relation automatically emerges for the extinction coefficient $\alpha(\lambda)$ per unit path length of the ray:

$$\alpha(\lambda) = N \int_0^\infty \sigma(a, \lambda) f(a)\, da \tag{3.39}$$

where $N$ is the number of particles per unit volume, $\sigma(a, \lambda)$ is the coefficient of extinction of radiation with wavelength $\lambda$ by a particle of radius $a$ (here, as elsewhere, the scattering particles assumed to be spherical), and $f(a)$ is the particle-size distribution function, the significance of which is defined by the relation $N_a\, da = N f(a)\, da$, in which $N_a$ is the number of particles having radii in the interval from $a$ to $a + da$.

The origin of expression (3.39) is easily traced by means of the optical theorem (see Section 3.2.2). The extinction coefficient of a certain volume can be determined according to the scheme described in 3.2.3 for evaluating the screening parameter. This procedure yields the relation $\alpha = 4\pi/k^2 \mathrm{Im}\, A$, in which $A$ is the amplitude of the field scattered forward by all particles. By the superposition principle, $A = \Sigma A_j$, where $A_j$ is amplitude of the wave scattered forward by the $j$th particle. The last two relations in combination with (3.25) shows that $\alpha = \Sigma\sigma_j$, where $\sigma_j$ is the coefficient of extinction by the $j$th particle. After introduction of the distribution function $f(a)$, the latter sum can be written in the form (3.39).

From relation (3.39) and the equation $\sigma(\lambda, a) = \sigma_s(\lambda, a) + \sigma_a(\lambda, a)$, in which $\sigma_s$ and $\sigma_a$ are the coefficients of scattering and absorption of radiation of wavelength $\lambda$ by a particle of radius $a$, we automatically arrive at expressions for the polydisperse coefficients of scattering $\alpha_s(\lambda)$ and $\alpha_a(\lambda)$:

$$\alpha_s(\lambda) = N \int_0^\infty \sigma_s(\lambda, a) f(a)\, da \qquad (3.40)$$

$$\alpha_a(\lambda) = N \int_0^\infty \sigma_a(\lambda, a) f(a)\, da \qquad (3.41)$$

Using the coefficient $\alpha(\lambda)$, we can write the customary expression for the variation of the intensity $I$ of radiation propagating along a particular path:

$$dI(\lambda) = -I(\lambda)\alpha(\lambda)\, dl \qquad (3.42)$$

The integration of (3.42) yields the well-known relation for the aerosol component of the transmittance of the atmosphere:

$$T(\lambda) = I/I_0$$

where $I_0$ is the radiation intensity at the start of the path and

$$T(\lambda) = \exp\left[-\int_{(l)} \alpha(\lambda, l)\, dl\right] \qquad (3.43)$$

The integration in (3.43) is carried out over points of the path, and $\alpha(\lambda)$ varies along the path in general. This variation is associated with the corresponding variation of the particle-size spectrum and particle concentration.

Relation (3.43) describes the intensity variation of the direct radiation carrying particular information. We note that it is impossible to record the direct radiation experimentally in isolation because to do so would require receivers with zero angular aperture. The angular aperture of the receiving system can be indefinitely small, generally speaking, but not equal to zero. Consequently, in addition to the direct radiation attenuated according to the law (3.43), the receiving systems always record light that is singly and multiply scattered by aerosol particles, which must be treated as one kind of background noise. This fact accounts for the dependence of the measured quantities [scattering coefficient, transmittance $T(\lambda)$, etc.] on the experimental conditions.

## 3.4. The Scattering Matrix

As already mentioned in Section 3.2.2, the scattering matrix $M$ contains complete information on the particle-scattered light field. Knowledge of this matrix suffices for the quantitative solution of any problem related to particulate scattering.

The matrix $M$ has the simplest form in the case of molecular scattering:

$$M(\theta) = \frac{3}{4+3d} \begin{pmatrix} 1+\cos^2\theta+d & -\sin\theta & 0 & 0 \\ -\sin^2\theta & 1+\cos^2\theta & 0 & 0 \\ 0 & 0 & 2\cos\theta & 0 \\ 0 & 0 & 0 & 2\cos\theta \end{pmatrix} \quad (3.44)$$

For radiation scattering by atmospheric aerosol particles, in general, the matrix $M$ can have all 16 components different. However, the symmetry of the particles and their orientation in space diminishes the number of independent components of the matrix and causes others to be equal to zero. Thus, the matrix $M$ for essentially spherical particles has the form [30]

$$M(\theta) = \begin{pmatrix} M_{11} & M_{12} & 0 & 0 \\ M_{21} & M_{22} & 0 & 0 \\ 0 & 0 & M_{33} & M_{34} \\ 0 & 0 & M_{43} & M_{44} \end{pmatrix} \quad (3.45)$$

where $M_{11}=M_{22}$, $M_{12}=M_{21}$, $M_{33}=M_{44}$, and $M_{34}=M_{43}$. For spherical particles, therefore, we have a total of four independent components, which can be calculated on the basis of the appropriate Mie equations.

Malkova [31] has calculated all four components of $M(\theta)$ for spherical water particles. The values of the complex refractive index are chosen so as to be representative of the wavelength interval from 2 to 12 $\mu$m, the parameter $\rho$ takes values from 0.1 to 1.0, and the angle $\theta$ is assigned values ranging from 0 to 180° in 5° steps. Shifrin and Zel'manovich have published comprehensive tables of the angular dependences of all components of the scattering matrix for water spheres in the infrared region of the spectrum. Detailed calculations of the scattering components $M_{43}(\theta)$ [32] indicate a high sensitivity of the given characteristic to the particle-size spectrum and the complex-valued refractive index of particles of polydisperse scattering media.

The results of Deirmendjian's [33] calculations of the components of the scattering matrix for a number of typical models of polydisperse aerosols have been used extensively in practice. Interesting analytical results have been obtained by Prishivalko [34] in a study of the variation of the components of the scattering matrix with variation of an aerosol model constructed on the basis of experimental results [35]. A power-law distribution function is adopted as the initial particle-size distribution. The calculations show that the relative humidity and inhomogeneous composition of the particles has a significant influence on the light-scattering properties of aerosols. The results of the calculations exhibit satisfactory agreement with the existing experimental data.

The most complete set of experimental data on the components of the scattering matrix have been obtained from systematic investigations conducted over a period of many years at the Zvenigorod base of the Institute of Physics of the Atmosphere of the Academy of Sciences of the USSR [36–41]. These measurements show that the scattering matrix for sufficient atmospheric turbidities has a form consistent with scattering by spherical particles, i.e., $M_{11} = M_{22}$, $M_{33} = M_{44}$, $M_{34} = -M_{43}$, $M_{12} = M_{21}$, while all other components are vanishingly small. This result justifies the assumptions made by Pritchard and Elliott [42] in their interpretation of the corresponding experimental data.

A statistical analysis of the results of measurements of the scattering components has made it possible to develop a classification of aerosol formations corresponding to various states of the disperse phase of the atmospheric aerosol. It has been found that individual types of scattering matrices can be discerned, along with the corresponding types of optical weather: (dry) haze, damp haze or mist, wet mist, fog, and drizzling mist. The components of the scattering matrix $M_{11}$, $M_{21}$, $M_{33}$, and $M_{43}$ exhibit definite types of behavior for each of these conditions.

Mist is typified by the absence of any vestiges of bows, aureoles, halos, or glories in the angular dependence of the scattering components, smoothness of the dependence on the optical parameters, and a high correlation between the values of all the optical parameters of the mist.

Wet mist is characterized by the appearance of comparatively faint bows and aureoles originating from the fractions of particles that occur in the course of the condensation process.

In fogs there are distinct bows and an aureole part of the angular scattering function, which projects far forward in the region of small scattering angles.

The optical properties of drizzling mist are determined mainly by the finely disperse fraction, and only in the vicinity of aureoles and bows are precipitating rain droplets observed.

It is important to emphasize, however, that the results described here were obtained in a definite geographical region and can scarcely be extended to other regions, at least not without appropriate statistically supported investigations.

In future experimental studies of the components of the scattering matrix under natural conditions, it will be essential to pay special attention to the particular locale of the investigation and, in particular, the nature of the atmospheric aerosol particles, including their geometry, chemical composition, size spectrum, concentration, and manner of transformation under the action of variable meteorological conditions.

## 3.5. Scattering by Clouds and Fogs

A quantitative measure of the attenuation of radiation by clouds and fogs, as in the case of other aerosol systems, is the volume extinction coefficient $\alpha(\lambda)$, or coefficient of extinction per unit radiation pathlength in the medium, defined by expression (3.39). It is evident from the latter that $\alpha(\lambda)$ is determined by the particle concentration per unit volume, the particle-size distribution function, and the single-particle extinction coefficient. We now give a brief description of these characteristics and the results of calculations of the coefficients $\alpha(\lambda)$.

### 3.5.1. Microphysical Parameters of Clouds and Fogs

Cloud and fog formation processes involve a multivariety of factors, which vary between wide limits and govern the growth of droplets (dependence of the growth rate on the concentration, size distribution, and nature of the condensation nuclei, on the air temperature and cooling rate, and on the turbulence scales and intensities). All of these considerations have so far prevented a theoretical solution of the particle-size distribution problem.

The existing analytical expressions have been derived as approximations in the processing of pertinent experimental histograms. The vast majority of experimental data obtained by various researchers indicate that the particle-size distribution function for clouds and fogs represent an asymmetrical single-peak curve similar to that shown in Fig. 3.3 [4].

Here we give the most common approximation relations used for the particle-size distribution functions in liquid-droplet clouds and fogs, includ-

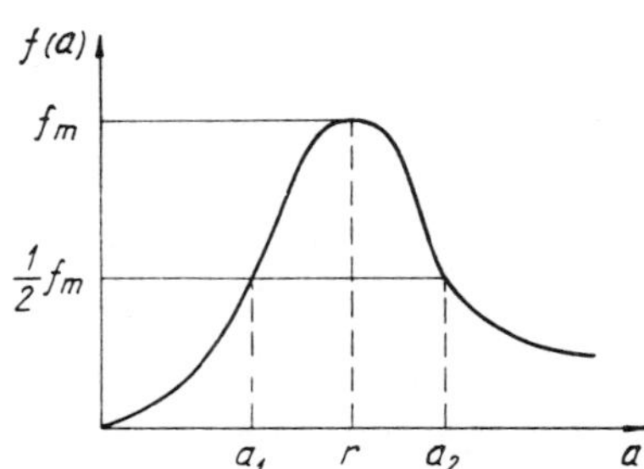

Fig. 3.3. Typical particle-size distribution curve for water clouds and fogs.

ing the gamma distribution:

$$f(a) = \frac{1}{\Gamma(\mu+1)} \mu^{\mu+1} \frac{a^{\mu}}{r^{\mu+1}} \exp(-\mu a/r) \tag{3.46}$$

and the log–normal distribution

$$f(a) = \frac{1}{(\pi t)^{1/2}} \frac{1}{r} \exp\left[ -\frac{1}{4} - \frac{1}{t}(\ln \tau)^2 \right] \tag{3.47}$$

In expression (3.46), $\Gamma(\mu+1)$ is the gamma function, which is equal to $\mu!$ for integral-valued $\mu$, and $r, \mu$ are parameters characterizing the most probable particle radius and half-width of the distribution. In (3.47), $\tau = a/r$, and $r, t$ have the same significance as $r, \mu$ in the distribution (3.46).

The average values of the most probable particle radius for various types of clouds fall roughly in the interval from 3 to 10 $\mu$m, and the parameter $\mu$ fluctuates from a few tenths (wide distributions) to 10–12 (narrow distributions). The most frequent values of $r$ and $\mu$ are approximately equal to 5 and $2\mu$m, respectively.

To characterize completely the microstructure of a cloud or fog, it is necessary to know, besides the particle-size distribution function, the concentration of particles per unit volume $N$. This parameter can be determined if the function $f(a)$ is known, along with the water content $q$, which is interpreted as the quantity of liquid water contained in droplets per unit volume, usually expressed in grams per cubic meter.

The average water contents of various types of clouds, with the exception of cumulus congestus, fall in the interval from 0.1 to 0.3 g/m³.

The solution of many problems of laser propagation in clouds and fogs requires knowledge of the relations between the water content or particle concentrations, meteorological range of visibility, and geometrical cross section of the particles per unit volume. For spherical particles with a gamma distribution of sizes, these relations have the form

$$N = \frac{3.912\mu^2}{S_M F(0.5)\pi r^2(\mu+2)(\mu+1)} \tag{3.48}$$

$$q = \frac{3.912 \times 4r(\mu+3)d}{3S_M F(0.5)\mu} \tag{3.49}$$

$$Q = N \int_0^{\infty} \pi a^2 f(a)\, da \tag{3.50}$$

Table 3.4. Water Content $q$ and Particle Concentration $N$ of
Certain Water Clouds and Fogs [4]

| Type of cloud | Values of microstructural parameters | | $S_M$, km | $Q$, g/m³ | $N$, cm⁻³ |
| | $r, \mu$m | $\mu$ | | | |
|---|---|---|---|---|---|
| Fine droplet | 1 | 2 | 0.2 | 0.031 | 971 |
| | 1 | 10 | | 0.015 | 2050 |
| Medium droplet | 6 | 2 | 0.2 | 0.194 | 28 |
| | 6 | 10 | | 0.101 | 65 |
| Large droplet | 10 | 2 | 0.2 | 0.324 | 10 |
| | 10 | 10 | | 0.168 | 2.3 |

where $N$ is the particle concentration per unit volume, $q$ is the water
content, $Q$ is the geometrical cross section of the particles per unit volume, $r$
and $\mu$ are the parameters of the gamma distribution function, $d$ is the
density, $S_M$ is the meteorological range of visibility, given by the equation

$$S_M = \frac{3.912}{\alpha(0.5)} \tag{3.51}$$

$F(0.5) = \alpha(0.5)/Q$ is the average extinction efficiency factor at a wavelength
of 0.5 $\mu$m, and $\alpha(0.5)$ is the volume extinction coefficient at a wavelength of
0.5 $\mu$m.

Values of $q$ and $N$ calculated according to (3.48)–(3.50) for characteristic sets of parameters of the microstructure of clouds and fogs are given in
Table 3.4 for a meteorological range of visibility $S_M = 0.2$ km.

It is evident from the table that the water content and, in particular, the
concentration of clouds and fogs for one given value of the meteorological
visibility $S_M = 0.2$ km, which happens to correspond to its most probable
value, vary between wide limits.

### 3.5.2. Volume Extinction Coefficients

Fairly complete theoretical and experimental data on the volume
extinction coefficients of clouds and fogs have been obtained at the Institute
of Optics of the Atmosphere of the Siberian Branch of the Academy of
Sciences of the USSR [4].

Figure 3.4 gives some results of calculations of the volume extinction
coefficients for water clouds and fogs in the wavelength range from 0.3 to
25.0 $\mu$m for various values of the parameters of the particle-size distribution
function.

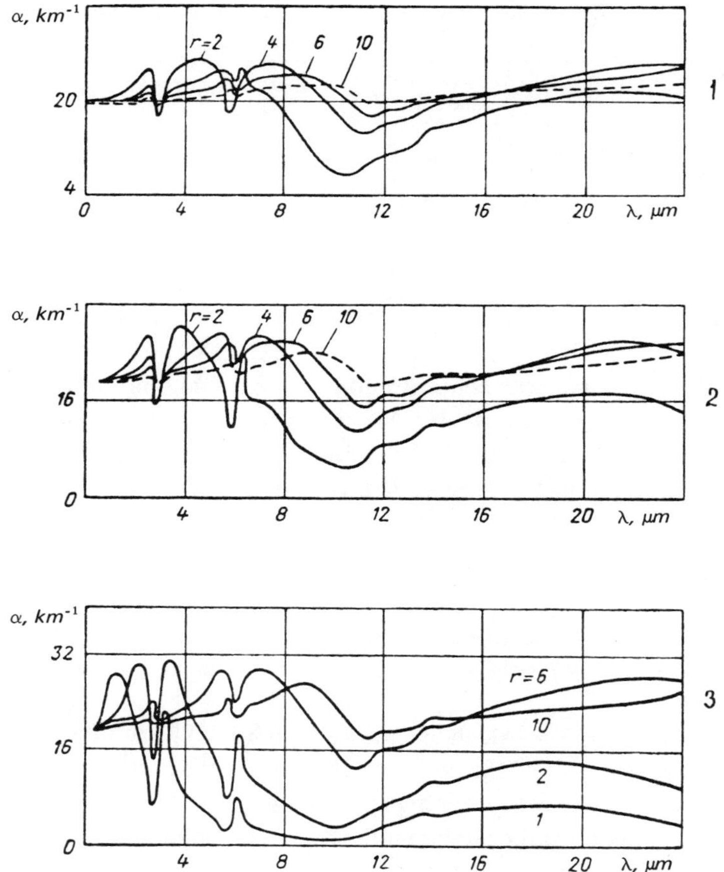



Fig. 3.4. Extinction coefficients of water clouds and fogs in the wavelength range 0.5–25 $\mu$m for various values of $\mu$ and $r$. (1) $\mu=2$; (2) $\mu=4$; (3) $\mu=10$; the values of $r$ are indicated in the parts of the figure.

Figure 3.4 clearly reveals the dependence of both the absolute values and the spectral behavior of the spatial absorption coefficients of water clouds and fogs on their microstructural parameters. We note that these data on the volume extinction coefficients have been obtained with regard for the absorption of radiation by the actual cloud and fog particles and exhibit satisfactory agreement with the results of our experiments. Absorption is taken into account in the calculations on the basis of our data on the complex-valued refractive index for water.

It follows from the data in Fig. 3.4 that clouds and fogs present a very serious obstacle to laser radiation propagating in them. The only exception is found in very infrequently encountered fine-droplet formations with a most probable particle radius of the order of 1 $\mu$m or smaller and a small distribution half-width.

## 3.6. Scattering by Hazes

### 3.6.1. Microphysical Parameters of Hazes

By a haze we mean a turbid state of the atmosphere due to the presence of relatively small-size particles with a visibility in the ground layer greater than 1 or 2 km. Haze restricts the visibility range in comparison with its approximate value of 340 km for a molecular atmosphere.

Atmospheric haze particles together with condensation nuclei are conditionally divided into three parts according to size: (1) Aitken nuclei (0.001 to 0.1 $\mu$m); (2) large particles (0.1 to 1.0 $\mu$m); (3) giant particles (radii greater than 1.0 $\mu$m). The majority of investigations indicate that particles with linear dimensions greater than 0.01 $\mu$m usually exhibit single-peak curves for the function $f(a)$ with a maximum in the vicinity of a few hundredths or tenths of a micrometer. Young has proposed the following simple power-law function for the size distribution of particles of radius greater than 0.1 $\mu$m:

$$f(a) = Aa^{-\beta} \tag{3.52}$$

where $A$ is a scale factor, $a$ is the particle radius, and $\beta$ is an empirical constant. The constant $\beta$ can take values from 2 to 5, depending on the time and place. Young's equation, of course, gives a very approximate description of the actual pattern of the particle-size distribution.

Specific individual-size distributions of the number of particles can depart considerably from expression (3.52). In particular, multiple-peak distributions are found in the literature. It is important to bear in mind, in this connection, that if the maxima of single- or multiple-peak distribution functions occur at particle radii smaller than 0.1 $\mu$m, Young's equation is fully applicable because particles of radius smaller than 0.1 $\mu$m are optically inactive due to their small dimensions and the small value of the extinction efficiency factor.

The concentration of particles with radii greater than 0.1 $\mu$m varies between very wide limits as a function of the time and place. Despite this fact, it is possible to indicate certain common laws in the variation of the particle concentration with height. A rapid exponential decay of this parameter is normally observed in the lower troposphere. A strong dependence of the concentration on the height is not observed in the upper troposphere, while in the stratosphere it begins to increase with the height, attains a maximum at height of 15 to 23 km, and then decreases.

The existing data of particle-concentration measurements at heights above 30 km are inadequate so that it is impossible at the present time to draw any definite conclusions as to its absolute values or height dependence. However, the fact that there are aerosol particles in the atmosphere up to heights of the order of 500 km is undisputed.

Fine structure in the stratification of the aerosol layers of the troposphere and stratosphere has been discerned in a number of studies. Highly promising results in this vein are anticipated through application of the method of laser probing of aerosols with its fantastically high potential spatial resolving power.

In addition to the variation of the particle-size spectrum and particle concentration of the atmospheric aerosol, it is also important to consider the chemical composition of the particles, which determine the components of their complex refractive index. The variation of these components can exert a significant influence on the corresponding optical characteristics of the aerosol (scattering coefficients, angular scattering functions, etc). It is to be expected that these characteristics will differ not only between overwater and overland aerosols, but also between different categories of either of those, depending on their origin.

Of no small significance either are the shape and homogeneity of the aerosol particles. According to published data, haze particles often comprise conglomerates of small particles, all differing in their shape and chemical composition. The size of these conglomerates depends strongly on the relative humidity.

In summary, we stress the fact that all the experimental studies to date of the microphysical parameters of the atmosphere have disclosed only the extreme diversity of the concrete realizations of sets of these parameters, but in no case can they be used to synthesize statistically supported models of atmospheric hazes. The successful solution of this problem will require enormous efforts on the part of all working groups engaged in the detailed investigation of the space and time distributions of the concentration, size spectra, chemical composition, and geometry of atmospheric haze particles.


### 3.6.2 Volume Extinction Coefficients

Figure 3.5 presents some of the results of calculations of the volume scattering coefficients of hazes by the author and others [4]. Young's

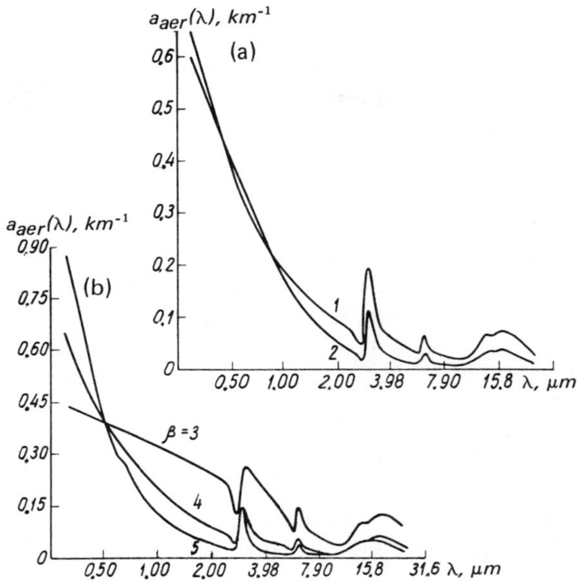



Fig. 3.5. Volume scattering coefficients of hazes in the wavelength range 0.3–25 $\mu$m for a visibility of 10 km. (a) $\beta=4$, $a_{min}=0.1$ $\mu$m, $a_{max}=1.0$ $\mu$m (curve 1); $\beta=4$, $a_1=0.01$ $\mu$m, $a_2=10$ $\mu$m (curve 2); (b) $a_{min}=0.05$ $\mu$m, $a_{max}=5.0$ $\mu$m, $\beta=3,4,5$.

distribution function with a power exponent $\beta=3$, 4, 5 is adopted in the calculations as the size distribution of the particles (water spheres). The particles are assumed to have minimum radii of 0.01, 0.05, and 0.1 $\mu$m and maximum radii of 1.0, 5.0, and 10.0 $\mu$m.

Figure 3.5 rather clearly delineates the role of the microstructural parameters of haze in both the spectral composition and the absolute values of the scattering coefficients. The steepest decay of the scattering coefficient with increasing wavelength in the spectral region from 0.3 to 2.7 $\mu$m is attributable to the corresponding steep decline of the function $K(\rho)$ in the visible and near-infrared regions for small particles (cf. Fig. 3.2). The majority of the haze particles have values of the parameter $\rho$ corresponding to the left wing of the function $K(\rho)$. Also, since $\rho$ decreases inversely as the wavelength, $K(\rho)$ decreases simultaneously, as does the scattering coefficient, the latter even more rapidly, inasmuch as it represents the product of $K(\rho)$ and the geometrical cross section of the particles, which decreases in proportion to the particle radius squared.

The maxima in the spectral dependence of the scattering coefficients around wavelengths of 2.9, 6.0, and 17 $\mu$m coincide with the maxima of the absorption bands for liquid water.

Table 3.5. Volume Scattering Coefficients of Haze for
Laser Radiation of Various Wavelengths

| $\lambda, \mu m$ | 0.5 | 0.53 | 0.63 | 0.69 | 0.84 | 1.06 | 1.15 | 2.36 | 3.39 | 10.6 |
|---|---|---|---|---|---|---|---|---|---|---|
| $\alpha, km^{-1}$ | 0.40 | 0.38 | 0.32 | 0.29 | 0.24 | 0.18 | 0.17 | 0.07 | 0.08 | 0.01 |

The values of the volume scattering coefficient of hazes for the most common lasers with a visibility range of 10 km and the most probable microstructural parameters ($\beta = 4$, $a_{min} = 0.05$ $\mu$m, $a_{max} = 5.0$ $\mu$m) according to the indicated calculations are summarized in Table 3.5.

The scattering coefficients for other values of the visibility range are easily obtained directly from Table 3.4 since they are inversely proportional to the visibility range.

Systematic experimental studies of the spectral transmittance of hazes over a wide range of wavelengths are currently in progress at the Zvenigorod Test Site of the Institute of Physics of the Atmosphere of the Academy of Sciences of the USSR, at the Tomsk Test Site of the Institute of Physics of the Atmosphere of the Siberian Branch of the Academy of Sciences of the USSR, and in the coastal region of the Black Sea.

Measurements performed at the Zvenigorod site [43, 44] have made it possible to obtain an approximate expression for the volume extinction coefficient of hazes in the spectral interval from 0.59 to 10 $\mu$m:

$$\alpha(\lambda) = \alpha(0.59)\left(n_0 + n_1\lambda^{-k}\right) \tag{3.53}$$

where $n_0$, $n_1$, and $k$ are empirical parameters, which have been tabulated for 10 types of climatic conditions: summer and winter hazes, spring and autumn hazes, wet haze, drizzling mist, postdrizzle mist, mist with rain, mist with snow, and "ice fog."

It is important to note that expression (3.53) describes the spectral behavior of the volume extinction coefficient of overland hazes typical of the region around Moscow, and its application for other geographical regions requires additional substantiation. Moreover, it may be stated with certainty that this expression is unsuitable, for example, for overwater hazes, as evinced by our measurements conducted the last few years in the Black Sea coastal region [45, 46], which indicate a much slower decrease of the coefficients $\alpha(\lambda)$ with increasing wavelength than according to (3.53). The processing of measurement data obtained during the summer period yields the following expression for the coefficients $\alpha(\lambda)$, which is valid up to a wavelength $\lambda = 12$ $\mu$m:

$$\alpha(\lambda) = \left\{\left[\alpha(0.59) - C\right]K\right\}^n \tag{3.54}$$

where $C$, $K$, and $n$ are empirical parameters, which differ for different spectral intervals.

Equation (3.54) mirrors the high correlation that exists between the coefficients $\alpha(\lambda)$ in the infrared region and the coefficient $\alpha(0.59)$. It describes all measurement situations without the need for classifying hazes by separate types.

A comparison of the results of calculations of the coefficients $\alpha(\lambda)$ according to expressions (3.53) and (3.54) indicates a substantial disparity between them, as high as an order of magnitude, in the vicinity of the long-wave atmospheric window centered near 10 $\mu$m. This fact is attributed to the marked difference between the microphysical parameters of over-water and overland hazes.

The experimental studies conducted at the Tomsk site of the Institute of Optics of the Atmosphere of the Siberian Branch of the Academy of Sciences of the USSR in collaboration with Leningrad University on the spectral dependence of the volume extinction coefficients of overland hazes [47, 48] have disclosed a very complex dependence of the coefficients $\alpha(\lambda)$ on various aerosol fractions. This discovery has been made possible by simultaneous measurements of the coefficients $\alpha(\lambda)$, the particle-size spectra, and the chemical composition of the haze particles. It was found, for example, that short-wave ($\lambda < 2.0$ $\mu$m) and long-wave ($\lambda > 2$ $\mu$m) radiations are attenuated predominantly by different species of particles. One very intriguing fact is the reliable detection of maxima in the spectral behavior of the coefficients $\alpha(\lambda)$ in the vicinity of 10–12 $\mu$m due to the large imaginary part of the complex refractive index of the smoke particles. We note in Fig. 3.5 that the deepest and broadest minimum in the values of the coefficients $\alpha(\lambda)$ for polydisperse wet haze is observed in this spectral region. This result constitutes further evidence of the multivariety of physical parameters of overland haze particles.

The next interesting result of the given comprehensive investigations is the dependence of the volume aerosol extinction coefficient on the relative humidity in the visible region of the spectrum. As the relative humidity varies from 40 to 100%, the volume extinction coefficient increases at first; then at roughly 70% humidity begins to decrease with increasing humidity up to 85%, and thereafter it is observed to increase again. This behavior pattern was observed in identical seasons for two years under conditions such that significant replacement of the air mass did not take place. Statistical processing of the data characterizing the above-described relative humidity dependence of the aerosol extinction coefficient indicates a correlation coefficient equal to 0.6.

The set of microphysical parameters of hazes in the ground layer of the atmosphere should be manifested to some degree or other in the boundary layer and at different heights. However, altogether insufficient data have been gathered to date to permit any definite conclusions to be drawn. Considerable hopes for the acquisition of such data can only be invested in the application of methods for laser probing of the atmosphere, which are discussed in Chapter 7.

## 3.7. Scattering by Precipitations

All precipitations are typified by their content of large particles, for which the parameter $\rho$ is much greater than unity. The existing data on the particle-size distributions of rainfall indicate that they have a form similar to the distribution functions in clouds and fogs. The values of the microstructural parameters of rains vary with their intensity and the distance from the clouds generating them and, as such, lie within the following intervals: particle concentration, 100 to 20,000 $m^{-3}$; particle radii, from hundredths of a millimeter to several millimeters; water content, from hundredths of grams per cubic meter to units of grams per cubic meter; intensity, from tenths to tens of millimeters per hour.

Since the condition $\rho \gg 1$ holds over the entire range of laser wavelengths for all rain particles, we have for the spatial attenuation coefficient

$$\alpha(\lambda) = N \int_0^\infty \pi a^2 K(\rho, m) f(a)\, da = 2Q \tag{3.55}$$

where $Q$ is the geometrical cross section of the particles per unit volume, as given by expression (3.50).

Thus, the volume extinction coefficient for precipitations in the ultraviolet, visible, near-IR, and middle-IR ranges of the electromagnetic spectrum does not depend on the wavelength and is quantitatively determined by the geometrical cross section of the particles per unit volume.

The dependence of the coefficient $\alpha(\lambda)$ on the variations of the microstructural parameters is inconsequential in comparison with the correlation between $\alpha(\lambda)$ and the rainfall intensity $I$ (see [4]):

$$\alpha(\lambda) = 0.21 \cdot I^{0.74}$$

where $I$ is given in mm/h and $\alpha$ in $km^{-1}$. The correlation coefficient between $\log \alpha$ and $\log I$ is equal to $0.95 \pm 0.01$. Still higher correlation obtains between $\log \alpha$ and $\log q$, where $q$ is the moisture content of the rain in $g/m^3$. The correlation coefficient in this case is equal to $0.97 \pm 0.01$.

The behavior of the coefficient $\alpha(\lambda)$ is similar to that described in the case of snowfalls.

The numerical value of the extinction coefficient for rains with an average intensity of 10 mm/h is approximately equal to 1 $km^{-1}$. Rain of such intensity in the path of a laser beam at a distance of 1 km extracts roughly 60% of the energy from it.

The theoretically predicted neutral spectral variation of the volume extinction coefficients of precipitations is not corroborated by experimental investigations. The discrepancy between theory and experiment grows with the difference between the wavelengths at which the extinction coefficients are determined. The reason for these discrepancies lies in the fact that in optical measurements using a measurement setup with specific geometrical and optical parameters it is necessary to make allowance for the fact that large particles are characterized by concentration of their scattered light in a very narrow forward cone. The angular aperture of the cone depends significantly on the parameter $\rho$ and, hence, on the radiation wavelength. As a result, not only transmitted and attenuated radiation but also a large part of the forward-scattered radiation is recorded in precipitation measurements, and the measured spectral transmittance can differ appreciably from the calculated nonselective value [49, 50].

The wavelength dependence of the measured extinction coefficients in precipitations has been studied experimentally in several papers [51–55]; Kabanov and Pkhalagov [55] also give an interpretation of the observed spectral behavior of the transmittance of precipitations.

The experiments on the wavelength dependence of the extinction coefficient in [55] were carried out in the range from 1 to 10 $\mu$m over a path of length equal to 3.5 km in rains and snowfalls of various intensities. The spectral intervals near wavelengths of 1 and 10 $\mu$m were adopted as the basis of the experiments. The errors incurred in the determination of the signals at the two wavelengths by fluctuations of the precipitation intensity did not exceed 10%. The results of the measurements indicate that with increasing rainfall intensity the transmittance in the spectral region around 10 $\mu$m decreases more rapidly than around 1 $\mu$m. Inasmuch as the measurements were performed in the regions of atmospheric "windows," the signal attenuated in the precipitations can be represented by the equation

$$I(\lambda) = I^0(\lambda) e^{-\tau(\lambda)}$$

in which $I^0(\lambda)$ is the initial signal and $\tau(\lambda)$ is the measured optical thickness for a 3.5-km layer, which in the case of large scatterers is related to the true (theoretical) optical thickness $\tau_0$ by the relation $\tau(\lambda)=K(z,z_0)\tau_0$ [49], where the function $K(z,z_0)$ obtained in [49] characterizes the dependence of the measured volume extinction coefficient for large particles on the parameters of the scattering medium and the geometrical properties of the radiation detector:

$$K(z,z_0)=R(z_0)\frac{z}{z_0}+z\int_z^{z_0}\frac{\varphi(z)}{z^2}dz$$

$$\varphi(z)=\begin{cases} R(z_0) & \text{for } z\geqslant z_0 \\ R(z) & \text{for } z<z_0 \end{cases} \tag{3.56}$$

Here $z_0=\rho\Psi$, $z=\rho D_{in}/2L$, $R(z)=1+J_0^2(z)+J_1^2(z)$, $J_0(z)$ and $J_1(z)$ are the zeroth- and first-order Bessel functions, $L$ is the photometrically measured thickness of the scattering layer, and $D_{in}$ is the diameter of the receiving aperture.

The results of calculations of $K(z,z_0)$ are given in Fig. 3.6, in which the upper curve corresponds to $z_0\to 0$, i.e., the case of a very small receiver field of view (f.o.v.) $\Psi\leqslant D_{in}/2L$, and the lower curve ($z_0\to\infty$) refers to the case in which the angle of reception of the scattered radiation is determined only by the ratio $D_{in}/2L<\Psi$. The intermediate dashed curves correspond to specific values of $z_0$ realized in the experiment (which are indicated above the curves). The dashed curves for large values of $z$ coincide with the upper curve after intersection with it.

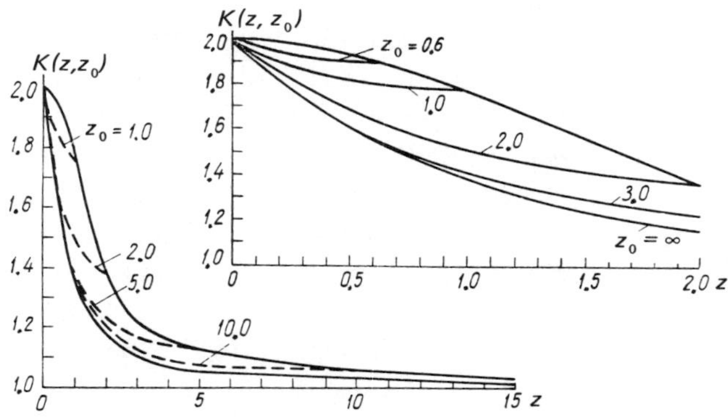


Fig. 3.6. Function $K(z,z_0)$ versus $z$ for various values of $z_0$ (indicated in the figure).

Processing of the measurement results shows that the measured extinction coefficients for precipitations turn out in every case to be greater for a wavelength of 10 than for 1 $\mu$m, unless corrections are introduced by means of the function $K(z, z_0)$. The observed difference between the extinction coefficients at wavelengths of 10 and 1 $\mu$m is readily explained in the qualitative sense by the considerable elongation of the angular scattering diagram at 1 $\mu$m relative to 10 $\mu$m. Accordingly, the detection device senses not only the direct radiation, attenuated according to Bouguer's law, but also the forward-scattered radiation. The latter part is greater for $\lambda = 1$ $\mu$m. The values obtained with correction by the function $K(z, z_0)$ for the extinction coefficients coincide within the experimental error limits. With this fact in mind, Fig. 3.7 gives the calculated values of $\tau_{\lambda_1}/\tau_{\lambda_{10}}$ as a function of $D_{\text{in}}$ for an angle $\Psi = 30'$ and various distances $L$. The scattering particles are assumed to have a radius of 3 mm in the calculations in order to be able to estimate the maximum possible effect created by the influence of forward-scattered radiation on the measured scattering coefficient.

It is evident from Fig. 3.7 that for sufficiently large entrance apertures the calculated value of $\tau_{\lambda_1}/\tau_{\lambda_{10}}$ increases in a regular manner with decreasing path length, tending to unity in the limit. This means that for small values of $L$ the influence of scattered light on the measured extinction coefficients is the same for both wavelengths and the measured transmittance of the precipitations becomes nonselective.

By systematic examination of one of the curves in Fig. 3.7 (say, for $L = 500$ m) it is possible to obtain a complete picture of the physics of the effect. As $D_{\text{in}} \to 0$, the ratio $\tau_{\lambda_1}/\tau_{\lambda_{10}}$ tends to unity (theoretical case of nonselective extinction); then at $D_{\text{in}} = 7.5$ cm the ratio $\tau_{\lambda_1}/\tau_{\lambda_{10}}$ drops

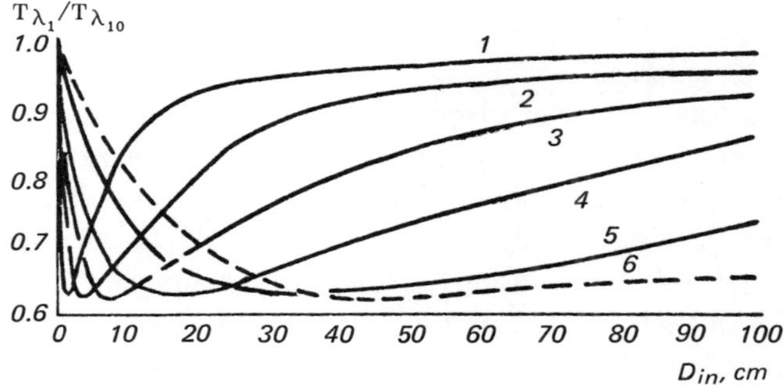


Fig. 3.7. Ratio of optical thicknesses at two wavelengths, 1 and 10 $\mu$m, versus aperture diameter of receiving system with 30' f.o.v., at various distances: (1) 0.1 km; (2) 0.25 km; (3) 0.5 km; (4) 1 km; (5) 2 km; (6) 3.5 km.

abruptly, assuming a value of 0.625. This means that a sizable portion of the scattered radiation is recorded by a receiving system with this diameter at a wavelength of 1 $\mu$m, so that the value of $\tau_{\lambda_1}$ is too low in comparison with $\tau_{\lambda_{10}}$. With a further increase in $D_{in}$, the fraction of the scattered radiation recorded at a wavelength of 10 $\mu$m increases steadily, but such growth does not occur for short-wave radiation because practically all the scattered radiation has been recorded already for $D_{in} = 7.5$ cm. As a result, with an increase in the diameter of the receiving system (beginning with a certain value thereof), the ratio $\tau_{\lambda_1}/\tau_{\lambda_{10}}$ increases, tending to unity in the limit. Consequently, the measured transmittance of precipitations becomes non-selective for any path length and sufficiently large diameters (and f.o.v.) of the receiving system.

## 3.8. Angular Scattering Functions of Polydisperse Aerosols

The volume extinction coefficient of aerosols, being a quantitative measure of the directional radiation extracted by the scattering medium, in effect sums the energy losses due to scattering in all directions. In this regard, we have no interest whatsoever in the angular distribution of that energy.

In many problems related to the propagation of laser radiation in aerosol media, it is very important to know not only the energy losses, but also the nature of the angular distribution of such losses. This knowledge is essential, for example, in interpreting the results of laser probing of the atmosphere, as well as in lidar (light detection and ranging) and many other problems.

The calculation of the polydisperse angular scattering functions of ensembles of spherical particles does not present any major difficulty at the present time and has been carried out for a large set of wavelengths and microstructural parameters of water clouds, fogs, and hazes.

Some typical results of calculations of the scattering functions of clouds, fogs, and hazes are given in Figs. 3.8–3.11 for the most common laser sources: gas lasers using mixtures of helium and neon (emission wavelengths $\lambda = 0.63$, 1.15, 3.39 $\mu$m), helium and xenon ($\lambda = 3.51$ $\mu$m), and carbon dioxide and nitrogen ($\lambda = 10.6$ $\mu$m); solid-state lasers using ruby ($\lambda = 0.69$ $\mu$m) and neodymium glass ($\lambda = 1.06$ $\mu$m); gallium arsenide semi-conductor lasers ($\lambda = 0.84$ $\mu$m).

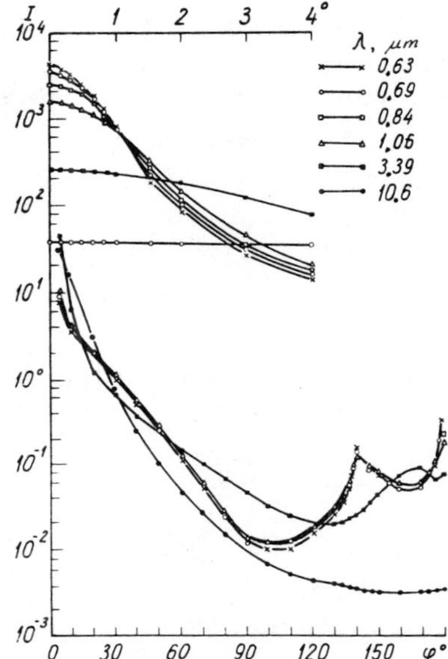



Fig. 3.8. Angular scattering functions of water clouds and fogs for gamma-distribution parameters $r = 5$ $\mu$m and $\mu = 2$ at various laser wavelengths.

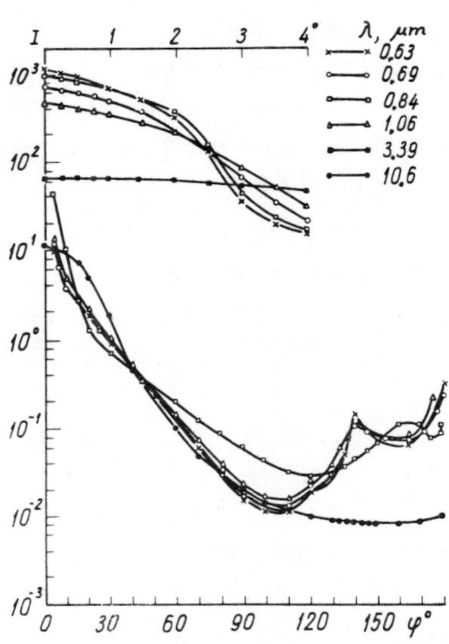



Fig. 3.9. Angular scattering functions of water clouds and fogs for gamma-distribution parameters $r = 5$ $\mu$m and $\mu = 8$ at various laser wavelengths.

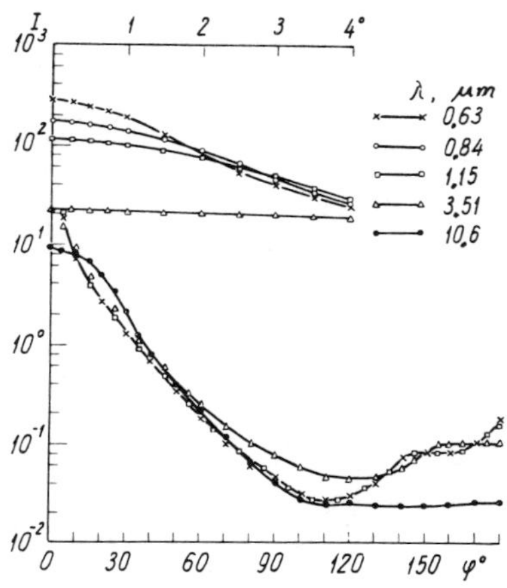

Fig. 3.10. Angular scattering functions of water haze with Young particle-size distribution function ($\beta = 3$, $a_{min} = 0.05$ $\mu$m, $a_{max} = 5.00$ $\mu$m) at various laser wavelengths.

Figures 3.8 and 3.9 refer to water clouds and fogs, whose particle-size spectra are described by a gamma distribution function with values of the parameters $r = 5$ $\mu$m, $\mu = 2$ and 8, respectively. We recall that the most probable radius $r = 5$ $\mu$m occurs most often in real clouds and fogs, while the values $\mu = 2$ and $\mu = 8$ characterize wide and narrow particle-size distributions.

Figures 3.10 and 3.11 refer to atmospheric hazes consisting of spherical water particles with a particle-size spectrum described by Young's equation with power exponents $\beta = 3$ and 4 and values of the minimum and maximum radii equal to 0.05 and 5 $\mu$m.

It is evident from the figures that the scattering diagrams of water clouds, fogs, and hazes at the given laser emission wavelengths have a rather smooth configuration. In the case of clouds and fogs, radiation is scattered

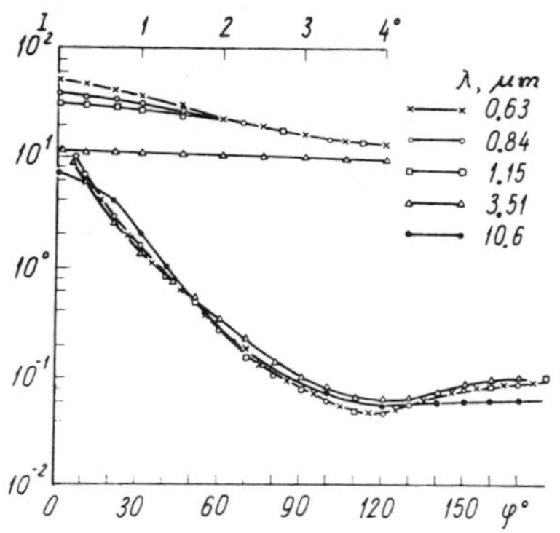

Fig. 3.11. Angular scattering functions of water haze with Young particle-size distribution function ($\beta = 4$, $a_{min} = 0.05$ $\mu$m, $a_{max} = 5.00$ $\mu$m) at various laser wavelengths.

in directions close to 0° (forward direction) approximately 2 to 4 orders of magnitude more than in directions close to 180° (backward direction). The quantity of light scattered in directions close to 0 and 180° in the case of hazes differs by 2 or 3 orders.

The results of a considerable number of experimental studies on the angular scattering functions of atmospheric aerosols are described in detail in the present author's book [4]. They qualitatively confirm the results of calculations. As far as quantitative comparison is concerned, it is impossible in the majority of cases because measurements of the scattering functions have not been accompanied by measurements of the microphysical parameters of the scattering aerosols. It is also important to note that the overwhelming majority of measurements of the scattering functions have been carried out at wavelengths in the visible region of the spectrum. An important objective of future experimental investigations of the angular scattering functions of atmospheric aerosols will be to expand the range of emission wavelengths used, and it will be imperative that these investigations be supported by appropriate measurements of the microphysical parameters of the aerosols. Special emphasis must be given to the investigation of the scattering functions at various heights, bearing in mind that variations of the scattering function mirror corresponding variations in the microphysical parameters.

## 3.9. Luminance of Forward- and Backscattered Radiation

When spatially confined light beams propagate in an aerosol atmosphere, the radiation is attenuated and particulate scattering of the light field takes place. Upon superposition of the direct and scattered radiation, the luminance distribution of the radiation in the beam cross section depends in a complex way on the optical thickness of the layer, the geometrical dimensions of the beam, the properties of the scattering medium, and the polarization state of the incident radiation. This pattern can be distorted by the instruments used in experimental work.

The objective of this section is to examine the indicated laws of propagation of laser beams in various atmospheric aerosols. Our primary attention is focused on analyzing the structure of the light field in the direction of small scattering angles (forward scattering) and at scattering angles close to 180° (backscattering) because it is most essential in connection with the use of lasers in communications, data transmission, lidar, and other systems to have data on forward- and backscattering.

### 3.9.1. Luminance of Forward-Scattered Radiation

#### 3.9.1.1. Theoretical

The light field produced by scattering of radiation by aerosol particles is described by a transport equation, the solution of which involves sizable mathematical difficulties in the general case [56]. In the case of small-angle scattering, the luminance of forward-scattered radiation can be calculated by the method of small-angle approximation of the transport equation. This method, however, has significant limitations insofar as it does not allow for polarization effects and is suitable only for beams of unbounded width and large particles (highly elongated scattering diagrams).

The theoretical determination of the luminance of forward-scattered radiation poses an exceedingly complex problem in the case of narrow collimated light beams. So far, the problem has been solved only for certain special cases.

Kabanov [57] gives expressions for calculating the luminance of singly scattered light for various geometrical parameters of a narrow beam, the divergence of which is equal to the f.o.v. of the receiving system:

$$V = V_0 e^{-\tau}\left[1 + \frac{\tau}{2}\int_0^\Theta \int_0^\Psi f(m,\rho,\psi+\vartheta)\,d\psi\,d\vartheta\right] = V_0 e^{-\tau}[1+\tau D] \quad (3.57)$$

where $V_0$ is the magnitude of the signal without attenuation in the medium, $\tau$ is the optical thickness of the layer, $\Theta$ and $\Psi$ are the f.o.v. of the radiation source and detection system, $f(m,\rho,\psi+\vartheta)$ is the normalized angular scattering function, which depends on the scattering angle $\varphi=\psi+\vartheta$, the parameter $\rho$, and the complex-valued refractive index of the scatterers, and $D$ characterizes singly scattered radiation for various parameters $\Psi$ and $\Theta$ in different scattering media.

If the distance between the source and detector of radiation satisfies the condition $l \gg d/\Theta$, where $d$ is the diameter of the receiving objective, expression (3.57) can be used to describe the extinction of a narrow collimated beam.

Kabanov [57] has derived an expression for the function $D$ in the case where $\Theta$ and $\Psi$ are small quantities, equal to one another, and the angular scattering function is expressed in terms of Legendre polynomials:

$$D = \frac{1}{2}\left\{\Psi\Theta + \sum_{n=1}^\infty a_n \int_0^\Psi \int_0^\Theta P_n[\cos(\psi+\vartheta)]\,d\psi\,d\vartheta\right\}$$

$$\cong \frac{1}{2}\varphi^2 \sum_{n=0}^\infty a_n = \frac{1}{2}\varphi^2 A_n \quad (3.58)$$

where $\varphi=\Psi=\Theta$ and the coefficients $a_n$ of the Legendre polynomials depend on the optical properties of the scattering medium.

Equation (3.58) is inapplicable for very large values of $\rho$ since it was derived without regard for the angular dependence of the Lengendre polynomials in the case of small $\varphi$. Accordingly, Kabanov [57] had derived an expression for $D$ with the angular scattering function expressed in terms of Bessel functions:

$$D=\frac{1}{2}\int_0^{\varphi}\int_0^{\varphi}f(\psi+\vartheta)d\psi d\vartheta=\frac{1}{2}\int_{\rho\varphi}^{2\rho\varphi}\left[2\frac{J_1(z)}{z}\right]^2 dz$$

$$+2\left[1-J_0^2(\rho\varphi)-J_1^2(\rho\varphi)\right]-\left[1-J_0^2(2\rho\varphi)-J_1^2(2\rho\varphi)\right] \quad (3.59)$$

where $J_0$ and $J_1$ are Bessel functions.

We note that the representation of the scattering function in terms of Bessel functions describes the angular intensity distribution of the scattered light in the interval of scattering angles $\varphi$ of several degrees within 3% error limits for particles with $\rho\geqslant60$.

The results of calculations of $D$ according to (3.59) are given in Fig. 3.12. The results indicate that in situations where the f.o.v. of the detection system and source coincide for narrow collimated radiation beams with a spread of a few thousandths of a radian it is permissible to neglect single forward scattering in comparison with the direct beam, up to optical thicknesses of a few tenths in fogs and, even more so, in hazes. In the case of rains, the value of $D$ is close to unity under the same conditions, so that even for $\tau=1$ singly scattered light in the zone of the beam will have the same luminance as the direct beam.

The Monte Carlo method is a powerful tool for the solution of radiation transport problems for spatially confined light beams in scattering and absorbing media. The Monte Carlo method is extremely effective in the solution of multidimensional radiation transport problems in media having

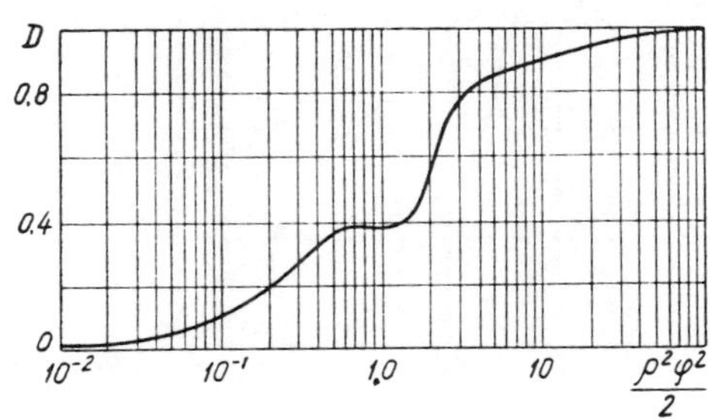

Fig. 3.12. Parameter $D$ versus $\rho^2\varphi^2$ for a collimated beam.

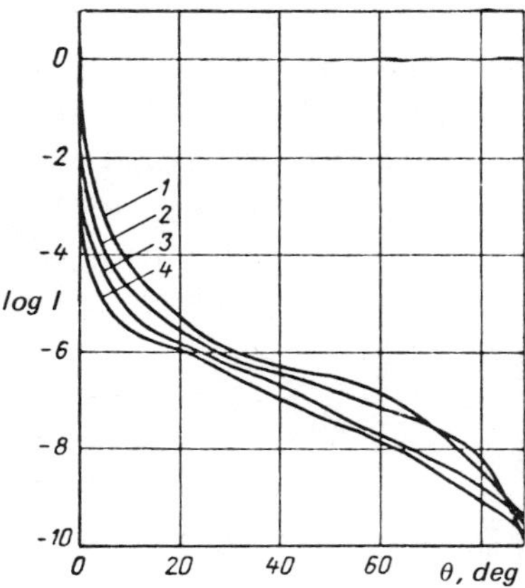

Fig. 3.13. Results of calculations of the angular distribution of intensity of multiple-forward-scattered radiation ($\lambda=0.45$ $\mu$m) in a water cloud with optical thickness $\tau=5.0$ for various beam spreads of source: (1) $\theta=6'$; (2) $1°$; (3) $5°$; (4) $10°$ (source and receiver diameters: 4 and 150 mm, respectively).

diverse optical characteristics in conjunction with a finite geometry on the part of the radiation sources and detectors. The relatively slow convergence of the method depends only on the number of statistical tests and the quality of the modeling. The development of various modifications of the method and the use of advanced electronic computers have made it possible to solve many problems in atmospheric optics. The application of the method to the solution of atmospheric-optical problems is discussed in a paper by Marchuk and Mikhailov [58].

Improved algorithms for implementation of the method and the results of calculations of forward-scattered radiation fields are given in several papers [59–67] (see Figs. 3.13 and 3.14).

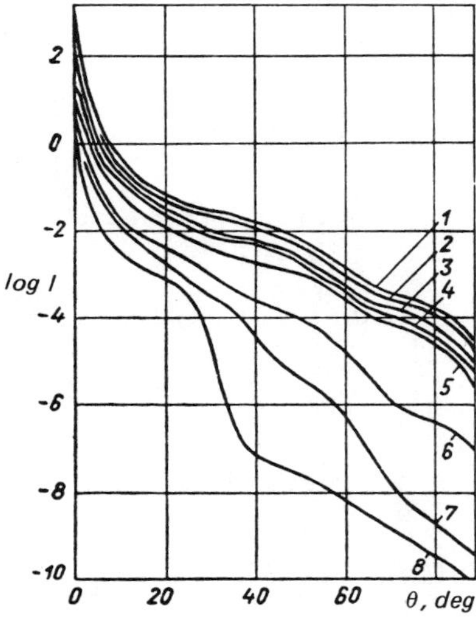

Fig. 3.14. Results of calculations of the angular distribution of intensity of multiple-forward-scattered radiation ($\lambda=0.45$ $\mu$m) in a water cloud with optical thickness $\tau=4.0$ for various receiver diameters: (1) $D(r)=4.0$ m; (2) 3.0 m; (3) 1.5 m; (4) 1.0 m; (5) 0.5 m; (6) 0.2 m; (7) 0.15 m; (8) 0.1 m (source diameter and beam spread: 4 mm and $30'$, respectively).

### 3.9.1.2. Experimental

Detailed experimental studies of the luminance of forward-scattered laser radiation in various media have been carried out by the present author and co-workers [4]. The radiation sources were a helium–neon laser with a wavelength of 6328 Å, beam diameter of 4 mm, and divergence of 6′ and a ruby laser with a wavelength of 6943 Å, beam diameter of 20 to 100 mm, and divergence of 30″ to 40″.

The measurements were performed in a chamber, in which wood smoke (particle diameter 0.8 to 1.0 $\mu$m) and artificial water fogs (rms droplet diameter 8 to 15 $\mu$m) were created. The choice of scattering media was dictated by the hope of obtaining suitable data for analysis of the laws of propagation of narrow collimated beans in the earth's atmosphere. The luminances of the direct and scattered radiation were measured by means of two measurement arrangements. In one, the source and receiving system were set up on the same straight line (direct-beam scheme). In the second version, the light beam from the source was returned by a plane mirror to the receiver which was set up next to the source (reflected-beam scheme).

The results of measurements of the luminance of forward-scattered radiation in artificial water fogs and smokes according to the reflected-beam scheme with the use of a gas laser are given in Fig. 3.15. All the measurement data were processed relative to the initial luminance of the source $B = 1$.

It is evident from Fig. 3.15 that a nonzero background luminance exists at an optical thickness $\tau = 0$. To determine the background luminance

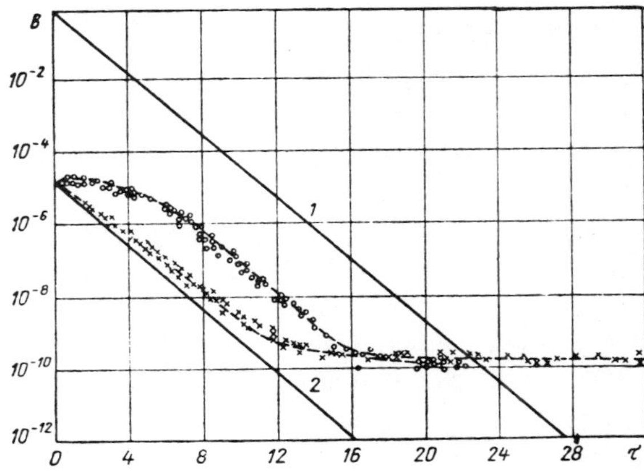

Fig. 3.15. Total luminance of forward- and backscattered radiation versus optical thickness $\tau$ in fogs (circles) and smokes (crosses). (1,2) Reduction in luminance of direct beam and initial source background with decreasing $\tau$ according to Bouguer's law.

associated only with light scattering, it is necessary to extract the luminance of the initial source background from the measured total background luminance. It may be assumed that the extinction of the initial source background is described by Bouguer's law (line 2). The contribution of the latter to the total background proves significant for fogs with $\tau < 4$ and for smokes with $\tau < 14$. It may be asserted in light of these remarks that the background luminance becomes equal to the luminance of the direct radiation for optical thicknesses $\tau \cong 22\text{--}24$ for both fogs and smokes, even though the media differ sharply in the sizes of the scattering particles. In the range of optical thicknesses roughly from 2 to 13, the background luminance is approximately 1 to 1.5 orders of magnitude greater in fogs than in smokes. Beginning with a certain value of the optical thickness in smokes and fogs, the background brightness curves acquire a bend. It sets in at a smaller value of $\tau$ for smokes than for fogs. For optical thicknesses greater than 20, the background luminance curves practically coincide for both smokes and fogs and do not depend on $\tau$.

The results of the background luminance measurements for fogs and smokes in Fig. 3.15 were obtained by the reflected-beam scheme. This means that not only the background due to small-angle forward scattering, but also the background due to small-angle backscattering in propagation of the beam from the source to the return mirror was recorded in the measurements. It is important to determine the luminance values for both background components. For this purpose, the return mirror was covered, and the background luminance associated with backscattering only was measured. These measurements showed that the background luminance for large $\tau$ is determined mainly by backscattered radiation.

Figure 3.16 gives the results of measurements of the luminance of forward-scattered radiation in fogs and smokes by the direct-beam scheme. It is seen that the background luminance is considerably less than the luminance of the direct radiation over the entire investigated range of $\tau$. The behavior of the background luminance is satisfactorily described by results of calculations according to the single-scattering expression.

Along with the above-described measurements in the artificial fog chamber, we also investigated the luminance of forward-scattered radiation im model media (a slightly cloudy solution of milk in water with an rms particle diameter of $3.5 \pm 1.5$ $\mu$m, and a suspension of lycopodium powder in an alcohol–water mixture with a particle radius of $15 \pm 0.5$ $\mu$m). The beam width was characterized by the optical diameter

$$\Delta = \alpha d$$

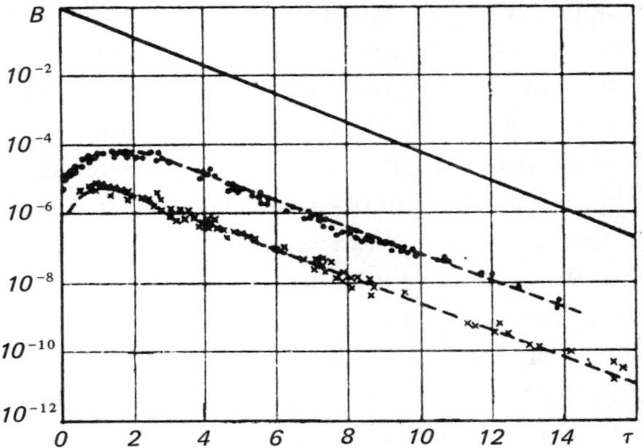

Fig. 3.16. Luminance of forward-scattered radiation versus optical thickness in fogs (dots) and smokes (crosses), plotted on the basis of calculations according to single-scattering theory (dashed curves) and Bouguer's extinction law for the direct radiation (solid line).

where $\alpha$ is the extinction coefficient and $d$ is the geometrical diameter of the beam. The quality $\Delta$ was equal to 0.34 in our measurements. The angular aperture of the detector was equal to the angle of divergence of the source beam.

Figure 3.17 gives the results of the measurements for a slightly cloudy milk solution. The optical thickness of the medium is plotted along the horizontal axis in these figures, and the measured luminances of the direct and scattered light are plotted on the vertical axis. The luminance of the direct laser radiation in the absence of the scattering medium was taken as unity. The curves in the figures are drawn through the experimental points, which have a maximum 5% spread relative to the luminance values. Curve 1 characterizes the luminance variation of the direct and scattered (in the zone

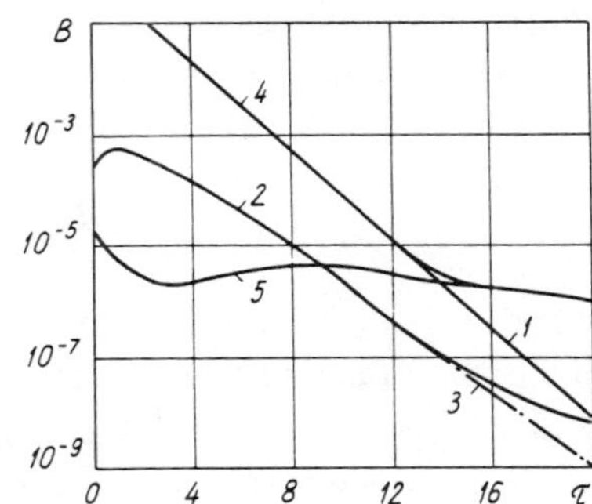

Fig. 3.17. Luminance of direct radiation and radiation scattered in the beam zone versus optical thickness in a slightly cloudy milk solution.

of the beam) radiation for an optical diameter of the receiving objective $\Delta = 0.5$; curve 2 was obtained under the same conditions and describes the luminance variation of the scattered radiation only; curve 3, which coincides with curve 2 for values of $\tau < 15$, is plotted according to the results of luminance calculations for singly scattered radiation under the same measurement conditions as in the determination of curve 2; curve 4 is similar to curve 1, except that the optical diameter of the receiving objective is $\Delta = 9$; curve 5 describes the luminance variation of multiple scattering only for an optical diameter of the receiving objective $\Delta = 9$.

It is evident from Fig. 3.17 that in the zone of a light beam characterized by a divergence of 6' and an optical diameter $\Delta = 0.34$ and for a receiving objective with an optical diameter of 0.50 the luminance of the scattered light is described by the single-scattering expressions [68] up to values of the optical thickness $\tau = 15$, and its absolute value is at least an order of magnitude smaller than the luminance of the direct radiation, attenuated according to Bouguer's law, in the interval of values $\tau = 0$ to 18. An increase in the optical diameter of the receiving objective, being equivalent in our experiments to a corresponding increase in its geometrical diameter since the beam width and density of the scatterers were constant, significantly enhanced the role of multiple scattering in the formation of the forward-scattered field for various optical thicknesses. Thus, for values of $\tau > 15$ (optical diameter of the receiving objective equal to 9.0), the multiple-scattering luminance turns out to be greater than the luminance of the direct radiation. The absolute value of the multiple-scattering luminance is greater than the single-scattering luminance for $\tau > 9$, depending slightly on the value of $\tau$ in this case.

Simultaneously with the investigations of the luminance of multiple-forward-scattered radiation, it was deemed important to ascertain the limiting optical thicknesses for which the dominant role in forward scattering in various scattering media is taken by single scattering, which is fairly simple to calculate.

The intensity of singly forward-scattered radiation is written [68] in the form

$$I_s = I_0 \tau e^{-\tau} \frac{\omega}{4\pi} f(0) \tag{3.60}$$

where $I_0$ is the intensity of the radiation incident on the scattering layer, $\tau$ is the optical thickness of the layer, $\omega$ is the solid aperture angle of the beam, and $f(0)$ is the value of the angular scattering function at the scattering angle $\Theta = 0$ (forward scattering). For small collimation angles, we can put

$\omega = \pi \alpha^2$, where $\alpha$ is the aperture angle of the beam. If Penndorf's approximation formula is used [69]:

$$\frac{\omega}{4\pi} f(\Theta) = \frac{\alpha^2 \rho^2}{4} K(\rho, m) \tag{3.61}$$

we obtain from (3.60)

$$I_s = I_0 \tau e^{-\tau} \frac{\alpha^2 \rho^2 K(\rho, m)}{16} \tag{3.62}$$

where $K(\rho, m)$ is the extinction efficiency factor of a particle of radius $a$, $\rho = 2\pi a / \lambda$, and $\lambda$ is the wavelength.

Equation (3.62) can be rewritten in the form

$$I_s = I_0 \eta \tau e^{-\tau} \tag{3.63}$$

where

$$\eta = \frac{\alpha^2 \rho^2 K(\rho, m)}{16} \tag{3.64}$$

is a parameter characterizing the fraction of light scattered by the particle in the forward direction. The values of this parameter can be determined from the experimentally measured value of $I_s$.

The experimentally determined extreme values of $\eta$ provide a means for determining the limiting optical thicknesses for which multiple-scattering effects can be neglected in determining the forward-scattered radiation. It is found that for a beam divergence in the interval $\alpha = 30'$ to $10''$ the equations describing the intensity of forward-scattered light due to single scattering alone are valid up to values of the optical thickness $\tau < 18$ for particles with a value of the parameter $\rho$ ranging from 1 to 3000. This range of $\rho$ covers practically all sizes of atmospheric aerosol particles for the visible and infrared regions of the spectrum (hazes, clouds, fogs, drizzle, smoke, dust).

Experimental studies of the luminance of forward-scattered light propagating in various model media for optical thicknesses $\tau \leqslant 20$ have been carried out by Ivanov and Khairullina [70, 71]. The parameters characterizing the radiation source, receiver, and scattering medium were varied between wide limits (angle of divergence of the source from $7'$ to $1°44'$; angular aperture of the detector from $16''$ to $7°$; optical diameter of the radiation beam from 0 to 0.30; optical diameter of the radiation detector from 0 to 0.40). The results enabled the authors to make a quantitative estimation of the systematic error of measurements of the extinction coefficient of the scattering medium due to the recording of forward-scattered radiation by the detector. This error is determined uniquely if the optical characteristics of the scattering medium and the geometrical parameters of the source and receiver are known.

### 3.9.2. Luminance of Backscattered Radiation

Detailed results of theoretical and experimental investigations of the luminance of backscattered radiation in various scattering media have been obtained by the present author's group [4]. Numerical experiments were conducted with the use of the Monte Carlo method. Measurements were performed under laboratory and natural conditions.

We discuss the results of the numerical experiments later in section 3.12 in connection with transient scattering and in Chap. 7 in connection with methods for laser probing of the atmosphere. At this point, we give some of the most representative experimental data pertaining to the controlled conditions of an artificial fog and smoke chamber and affording a clear quantitative idea of the magnitude of the luminance of backscattered laser radiation for various optical thicknesses of these media.

The results of measurements of the luminance of radiation emitted by a gas laser ($\lambda = 0.63$ $\mu$m, beam diameter 1 cm, beam spread 6$'$) and scattered at an angle of 171°30$'$ in artificial fogs with various optical thicknesses are plotted in Fig. 3.18 (crosses). Also given in this figure are data from measurements of the total luminance of forward- and backscattered radiation (circles) as obtained in the scheme: source–rotatable mirror–detector (angle of beam rotation 8°30$'$). In measuring the luminance of radiation scattered at 171°30$'$, the rotatable mirror was covered.

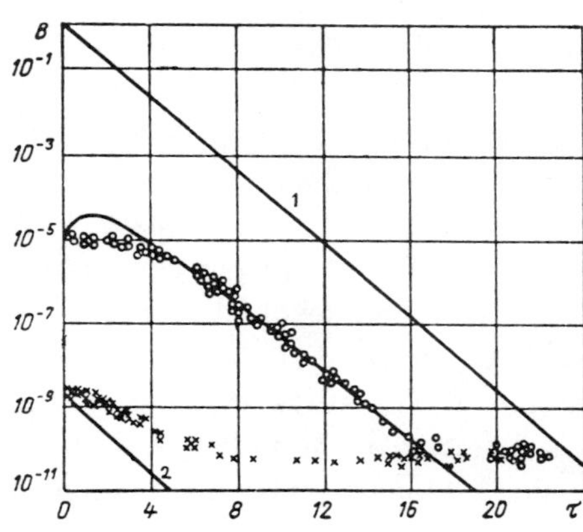

Fig. 3.18. Total luminance of forward- and backscattered radiation (circles) and luminance of backscattered radiation (crosses) versus optical thickness of fogs. (1,2) Reduction in luminance of direct beam and initial source background according to Bouguer's law.

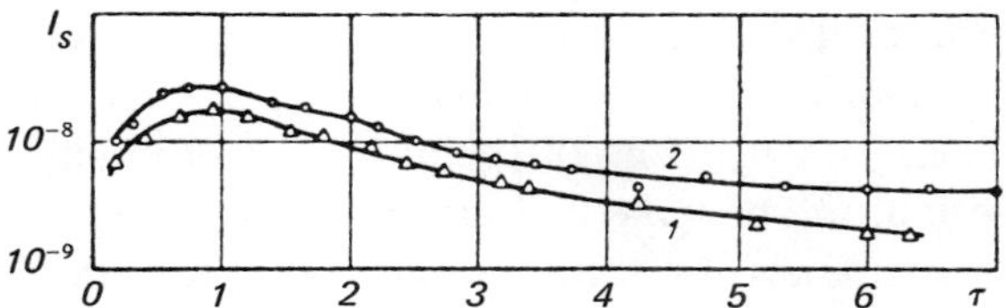

Fig. 3.19. Variation of intensity of laser radiation ($\lambda = 0.63$ $\mu$m) scattered at 172° by fogs (1) and wood smokes (2).

If the initial source background is eliminated from the measurement results, it is seen that as the optical thickness is increased from 0 to 1 the luminance of backscattered light increases, attaining a maximum, and then decreases with increasing $\tau$, comparatively rapidly at first and then more slowly. For $\tau > 8$, it remains practically constant, attaining a value equal to the brightness of the direct beam for $\tau \cong 23$.

Measurements of the luminance of radiation emitted by a gas laser and scattered at an angle of 171°30′ by wood smoke have shown that its values coincide with those obtained in fogs for $\tau > 20$. For smaller values of $\tau$, the luminance of the backscattered light in fogs is smaller than in smokes.

Figure 3.19 gives the results of measurements of the luminance of radiation emitted by a 0.63-$\mu$m laser and scattered at an angle of 172° by fogs and smokes. The measurements were conducted without the use of a rotatable mirror, with a beam having a diameter of 0.4 cm and a 6′ spread. The optic axes of the detector and source intersected at an 8° angle. The optical thicknesses plotted in the figure refer to the scattering layer from the source to the receiver. The luminance values are referred to the initial luminance of the direct beam. Each point of the figure represents the average of five to ten measurements.

It is evident from Fig. 3.19 that the absolute values of the luminance of light scattered at 172° in fogs and smokes in the investigated interval of optical thicknesses have an order of magnitude of $10^{-8}$ to $10^{-9}$ times the initial luminance of the direct beam.

Numerous measurements of the volume coefficients of back scattering by aerosols with the application of methods of laser probing of aerosols will be analyzed in Chap. 7.

## 3.10. Limits of Applicability of Bouguer's Law

The direct monochromatic radiation of a collimated beam propagating in a scattering medium without self-radiation is attenuated according to

Bouguer's law, provided that the particles of the medium scatter independently of one another. The direct radiation usually carries certain useful information. Consequently, from the point of view of practical applications it is very important to know the limiting conditions under which the direct radiation can be separated from the background of forward-scattered radiation. It is clear that this can be done under conditions such that the luminance of the direct radiation is greater than the background radiation. But if the luminance of the background is greater than that of the direct radiation, insurmountable difficulties can stand in the way of extracting the useful information carried by the beam, in connection with the fact that the forward-scattered radiation is, in the final analysis, created by the beam itself. In this case, in order to select the direct-radiation signal against the scattered-radiation background, it is necessary that the luminance of the signal be greater than the luminance of forward-scattered light. It is readily perceived that the most favorable conditions for measurement of the useful signal are those wherein the angular aperture of the receiver and the angle of divergence of the source are identical. In this event, the detection system will capture the entire beam and a minimum-scattered radiation background since the background noise signal will be greater for larger values of the entrance pupil, given the same useful signal.

In the case where the useful signal is considerably stronger than the signal from forward-scattered light, it is reasonable to postulate the applicability of Bouguer's law for description of the measured attenuation of a narrow collimated beam propagating in a scattering medium and completely captured by the detection system. Thus, the analysis of the limits of applicability of Bouguer's law for the description of the measured attenuation in the medium will eventually provide an answer to the question of the range of a particular system utilizing narrow collimated light beams for the transmission of useful information through various scattering media.

A detailed investigation of the limits of applicability of Bouguer's law for various specific measurement arrangements in different scattering media has been carried out in the work of the author and others, cited in the preceding section, where the luminance of the direct beam was determined concurrently with measurement of the luminance of the forward-scattered radiation. Here we summarize the highlights of these investigations from the standpoint of the limits of applicability of Bouguer's law. We stress once again the fact that the discussion pertains to the limits of applicability of Bouguer's law for the description of the experimentally measured attenuation of a light beam propagating through a scattering medium. It is clear that these limits will depend not only on the optical properties of the scattering medium, but also on the geometrical parameters of the beam and the detection system. We examine the case in which the angle of divergence of the beam and the angular aperture of the detector are equal.

Figure 3.20 presents the results of measurements of the luminance $B$ of a laser beam as a function of the optical thickness of water-diluted milk. A gas laser with a 6′ beam spread and beam diameter $d=0.4$ cm was used in the measurements. Each curve in the figure refers to a definite value of the optical beam diameter $\Delta=\alpha d$. The value of $\Delta$ was varied over the range from 0.09 to 12.0 by increasing the scatterer density. All the measurement results are reduced to unit luminance of the beam incident on the scattering layer.

The critierion of applicability of Bouguer's law for the description of the measured luminance attenuation of a beam with variation of $\tau$ is the presence of a linear relationship between $\log B$ and $\tau$. It is evident from Fig. 3.20, in which $B$ is plotted on logarithmic scale, that the linear segments of the curves depend strongly on the optical diameter of the beam. An especially sharp variation of the limiting values of $\tau$ occurs for small values of $\Delta(\Delta<0.74)$. As $\Delta$ is increased, the limiting values of $\tau$ decrease more and more slowly, and for $\Delta>1.48$ they are practically independent of $\Delta$, being approximately equal to $\tau=12$.

The resulting dependence of the limits of applicability of Bouguer's law on the optical diameter of the beam in regard to the description of the

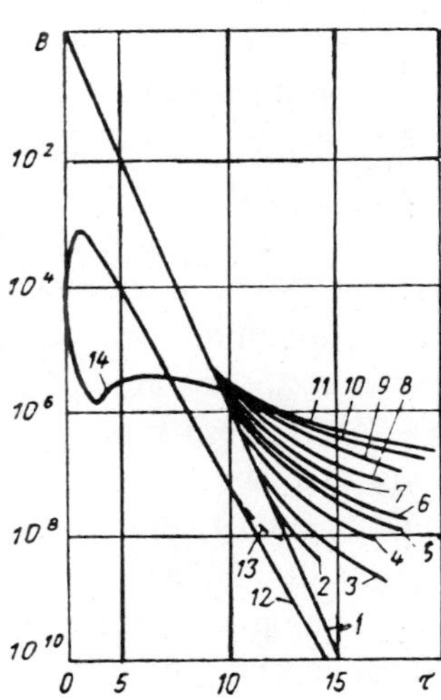


Fig. 3.20. Dependence of limits of applicability of Bouguer's law for description of the measured extinction of a narrow collimated light beam in a scattering medium on the optical diameter of the beam $\Delta$. (1) $\Delta=0.09$; (2) 0.34; (3) 0.74; (4) 1.11; (5) 1.48; (6) 2.22; (7) 2.96; (8) 3.56; (9) 7.12; (10) 9.0; (11) 12.0; (12) calculated intensity of single scattered radiation; (13) measured intensity of single scattered radiation; (14) measured intensity of multiple scattered radiation..

variation of the measured luminance of the beam with $\tau$ can be explained by the diversified role of multiple light scattering in the zone of the beam for different values of $\Delta$. When $\Delta$ is increased by a variation of the particle concentration at a constant geometrical diameter of the beam or by an increase in the latter with a constant scatterer concentration, the role of multiple scattering in the formation of light scattered in the zone of the beam relative to singly scattered radiation becomes stronger. For sufficiently large values of $\Delta$, "saturation" of the multiple-scattering contribution sets in. For small values of $\Delta$, single scattering yields a more significant contribution to the forward-scattered field. This fact tends to shift the limits of applicability of Bouguer's law for describing the measured attenuation of the beam toward larger values of $\tau$.

It is inferred from the preceding section that similar variations of the limits of applicability of Bouguer's law take place with an increase in the optical diameter of the objective of the receiving collimator for a constant optical diameter of the light beam.

The results of measurements in a model medium in Fig. 3.20 bring us to a number of conclusions about the applicability of Bouguer's law for describing the attenuation of narrow collimated light beams in various atmospheric aerosols. The optical diameters of these beams in the aerosols of greatest optical density—clouds and fogs, with a meterological range $S_M = 50$ m—do not exceed the lowest of the investigated values of $\Delta$ in Fig. 3.20 in the visible part of the spectrum for a geometrical beam diameter $d = 0.4$ cm. Thus, the extinction coefficient in the given case is approximately equal to $8 \times 10^{-4}$ cm$^{-1}$, so that $\Delta = 0.0003$ for $d = 0.4$ cm. In terms of their microphysical and optical properties, clouds and fogs do not differ very significantly from a dilute solution of milk in distilled water. Therefore, the results given in Fig. 3.20 can be used for an approximate analysis of the limits of applicability of Bouguer's law for the description of the attenuation of a collimated beam in clouds and fogs. Bearing in mind that the value of $\Delta$ for $d = 0.4$ cm in a dense cloud or fog ($S_M = 50$ m) is considerably smaller than its minimum value in Fig. 3.17, we can state with certainty that the limits of applicability of Bouguer's law in this case fall outside the limits of $\tau = 25$. This assertion is completely consistent with our own experimental data obtained in measurements in the artificial water fogs. It is expected that the indicated limit will apply even when the geometrical beam diameter is equal to 100 cm since $\Delta = 0.08$ in this case.

The optical diameters of beams propagating through hazes, precipitations, and dry aerosols have, as a rule, a smaller value than in clouds and fogs. Bouguer's law should therefore describe the measured attenuation of collimated light beams when the spread and diameter of the beam are less than or equal to 6′ and 100 cm, respectively, and the angular aperture of the detector is equal to the beam spread in all atmospheric aerosols for an optical thickness $\tau$ not less than 25 in the visible region of the spectrum. We note that the most sensitive radiation detectors in the visible spectrum record radiation transmitted through a layer of the medium with $\tau = 30$–$35$ if the energy density input to the layer is equal to $10^3$ W. This conclusion can also be extended to the infrared part of the spectrum, which differs from the visible part in its relatively smaller values of the parameter $\rho$ and larger values of the absorption coefficient of the medium. Both factors merely increase the limiting values of $\tau$ for which Bouguer's law remains applicable for describing the measured attenuation of the beam in the scattering medium.

Our discovery of the preservation of the brightness contrast of direct laser radiation against the background associated with multiple scattering of that radiation in the forward direction up to large optical depths affords remarkable potentials for the application of lasers in various navigational systems in aerosol scattering media, including clouds, fogs, hazes, and precipitations.

## 3.11. Polarization Characteristics of Scattered Laser Radiation

The polarization state of radiation scattered at various angles is important in the solution of many practical problems associated with information transmission by means of a narrow beam of radiation. Thus, if a scattering layer of a medium is irradiated with a linearly polarized beam, the particles of the layer can depolarize the incident radiation in scattering. Polarizing devices can be used in the detection of direct and scattered radiation to diminish the contribution of the scattered field to the signal relative to the contribution of the direct beam. This possibility can be utilized to increase the range of the appropriate technical system. For example, it has been shown [72] that the use of polaroids in detection systems enhances underwater visibility at least twofold. An analogous effect should be anticipated in the atmosphere.

The depolarization of radiation scattered by aerosol particles follows qualitatively from simple considerations since only in the forward and backward directions does the degree of polarization of singly scattered radiation coincide with the degree of polarization of the incident radiation in the case of homogeneous spherical particles [6, 7]. Hence, it is clear that in the case of multiple scattering, radiation is incident on the particles of the scattering volume with different polarizations. The superposition of secondary scattered waves results in depolarization of the scattered radiation. If the scattering particles are irregularly shaped, as in the cases of dust particles, minute crystals of ice clouds, etc., then depolarization of the scattered radiation takes place for all angles even in single scattering.

Of special interest is the investigation and application of polarization effects of scattered radiation in the case of small optically inactive particles, i.e., particles that have scarcely any influence on the attenuation of a laser beam.

The primary information about the polarization state of aerosol-scattered laser radiation is still obtained from appropriate experimental investigations. Here we give a few illustrations of the results of such investigations [73, 74]. We shall return to this problem in Chap. 7 in a discussion of the methods of laser probing of aerosols.

As a source of linearly polarized radiation, lasers afford an excellent tool for investigating the polarization characteristics of a light field scattered by aerosol particles. From the practical standpoint, we are interested mainly in the investigation of scattering in the forward and backward directions.

The results given below are taken from measurements carried out in an artificial aerosol chamber with water fogs and wood smokes at scattering angles of $1°30'$ and $172°$. The measured variables were the intensity $I_1$ of light with the vector $\mathbf{E}$ situated in the scattering plane, along with the intensity $I_2$ of light with the vector $\mathbf{E}$ perpendicular to that plane. The ratio $\Delta = I_1/I_2$ characterizes the depolarization of the radiation. Knowledge of the value of $\Delta$ makes it possible to determine the degree of polarization of the scattered light:

$$p = \frac{1-\Delta}{1+\Delta} \tag{3.65}$$

Figures 3.21 and 3.22 give the results of measurements of $I_1$ and $I_2$ and the degree of polarization $p$ of the backscattered radiation in fogs and wood smokes, calculated on the basis of those intensities. The values of $I_1$ and $I_2$ are reduced to the initial intensity of the direct-beam incident on the scattering layer. It is evident from the figures that the dependence of the degree of polarization of the backscattered radiation on the optical thickness of the layer $\tau$ can be approximated in the investigated range of $\tau$ values by the straight line

$$p(\tau) = p_0 - k\tau \tag{3.66}$$

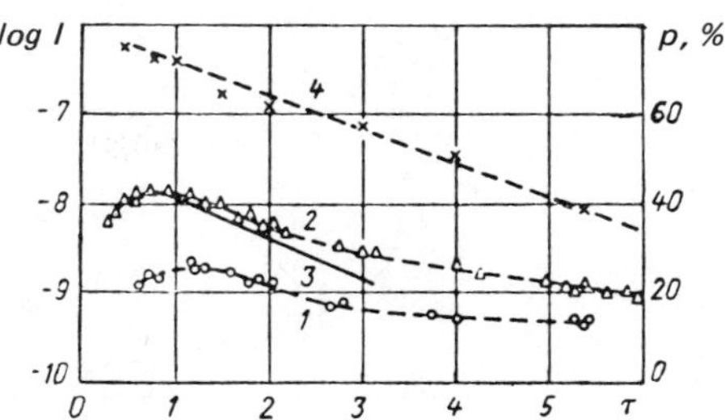

Fig. 3.21. Intensity of backscattered light with vector **E** in the scattering plane (1), intensity of backscattered light with vector **E** in a plane perpendicular to the scattering plane (2), intensity of backscattered radiation, calculated according to single-scattering theory (3), and degree of polarization of backscattered radiation (4) versus optical thickness of fog.

where $p_0$ and $k$ are empirical parameters, the values of which depend on the properties of the scattering medium and, as investigations have shown, vary only slightly with the angle of divergence of the source between the limits from 40″ to 6′.

The degree of polarization of backscattered radiation differs from the value of $p$ for the source even for the smallest of the investigated values of $\tau \cong 0.5$. Extrapolation of the linear relation (3.66) to $\tau = 0$ yields a value of $p$ smaller than for the source (the degree of polarization of the source, according to measurements, is greater than 0.99). This means that the dependence of $p$ on $\tau$ cannot be linear in the interval of small $\tau$.

The results of measurements of the polarization characteristics of reflected radiation from artificial fogs of various densities with separation of the total radiation flux and of the multiply scattered radiation flux alone [74] are given in Fig. 3.23. The indicated separation can be realized by a scheme in which the optic axes of the source and detector coincide. Representing the total flux by the sum $I_\Sigma = I_0 + I_m$, we write the following

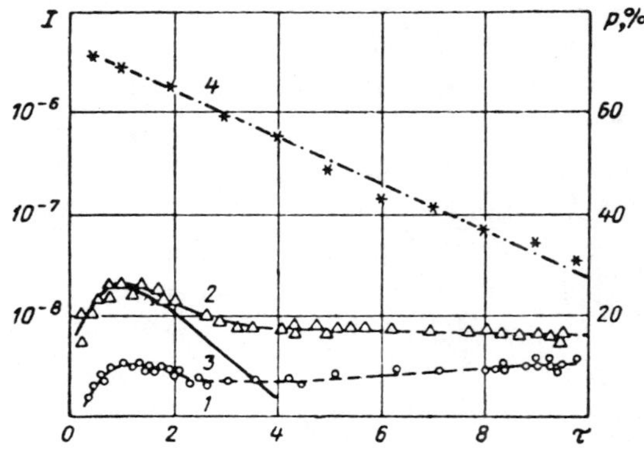

Fig. 3.22. Intensity of backscattered light with vector **E** in the scattering plane (1), intensity of backscattered light with vector **E** in a plane perpendicular to the scattering plane (2), intensity of backscattered radiation, calculated according to single-scattering theory (3), and degree of polarization of backscattered radiation (4) versus optical thickness of wood smoke.

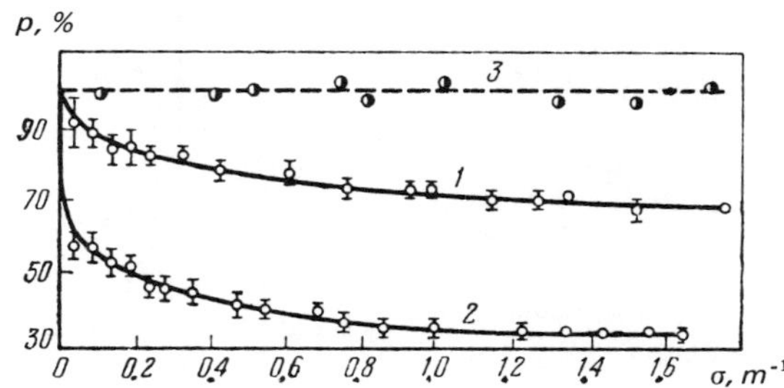

Fig. 3.23. Degree of polarization of backscattered radiation in fogs versus scattering coefficient. (1) For total flux; (2) for multiple-scattered radiation alone; (3) calculated in single-scattering approximation.

expression for the degree of polarization:

$$p_\Sigma = \frac{I_{\Sigma_1} - I_{\Sigma_2}}{I_{\Sigma_1} + I_{\Sigma_2}} = \frac{p_0 + p_m \delta(\alpha)}{1 + \delta(\alpha)} \tag{3.67}$$

where $I_0$ and $p_0$ are the intensity and degree of polarization of singly scattered radiation, $I_m$ and $p_m$ are the same quantities for multiply scattered radiation, and $\delta(\alpha) = (I_{m_1} + I_{m_2})/(I_{01} + I_{02})$ is the ratio of intensities of multiply and singly scattered radiation.

The foregoing data show that the cause of the reduction in the degree of polarization for backscattered radiation with increasing density of the medium is the increasing role of multiple-scattering effects, where the degree of polarization varies only slightly for large extinction coefficients ($\sigma \sim 1.5$ m$^{-1}$) and is close to 70% for the total flux and approximately equal to 35% for multiple scattering of radiation.

It follows from a comparison of Figs. 3.21 and 3.23 that the degree of polarization of the recorded reflected radiation decreases with increasing distance between the source and detector but remains larger than for multiply scattered radiation. This result is a consequence of the relatively greater role of multiple-scattering effects in zones farther from the beam axis. Similar results have been obtained for water media [75].

Figure 3.24 gives the results of measurements of the intensities $I_1$ and $I_2$ of forward-scattered (at 1°30′) radiation in fogs and smokes for various optical thicknesses. As expected, the sum $I_1 + I_2$ for the fog measurements is the same as the value of $I_1$ within the measurement error limits, indicating that the forward-scattered radiation is not depolarized. The value of $I_1$ in wood smokes, as the figures discloses, is greater than $I_2$ by 2.5 orders of

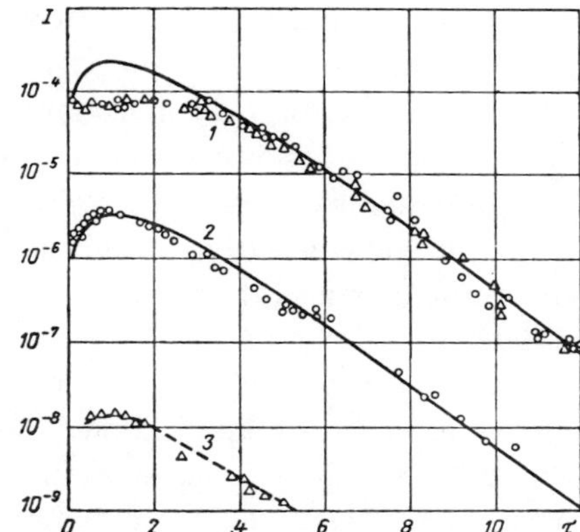

Fig. 3.24. Total intensity $I_1 + I_2$ (triangles) and intensity $I_1$ of forward-scattered radiation (circles) versus optical thickness $\tau$. Intensities versus $\tau$, calculated according to theoretical single-scattering formula: (1) $I_1 + I_2$ and $I_1$ in fogs; (2) $I_1$ in wood smokes; (3) $I_2$ in wood smokes.

magnitude. Thus, the depolarization of radiation in small-angle forward scattering is also practically nonexistent in the case of wood smokes. The solid and dashed curves in the figure have been obtained by calculations according to the single-scattering expression. An analysis of the measurement results shows that the forward-scattered radiation signal is formed in the given experimental arrangement predominantly as a result of single-scattering events up to values of the optical thickness $\tau = 12$. This is what accounts for the absence of depolarization of the indicated radiation. Considering the fact that the contribution of multiple-scattering effects in the forward direction depends significantly on the geometrical parameters of the source (diameter and beam spread) and the detector, the distance from the source to the investigated volume of the aerosol medium, and the angular scattering function of the latter, we infer that the values of the limiting thicknesses for which multiple-scattering effects and, hence, the depolarization of forward-scattered radiation can be neglected vary between rather wide limits. The details of this problem will be discussed in Chap. 7.

## 3.12. Transient Scattering

The use of pulsed laser radiation in lidar systems and many other devices operating under atmospheric conditions requires knowledge of the laws of transient scattering of spatially confined light beams in various scattering media characterized by, for example, the photon survival probability. The latter can vary considerably in atmospheric aerosols as a function of the pulsed radiation wavelength.

One of the most timely transient scattering problems has to do with the distortion of a pulse as it propagates to various depths in absorbing and scattering media. In this connection, it is of paramount importance to know how the shape of an infinitesimally short pulse varies because any pulse can be represented by a set of delta ($\delta$) pulses.

In the general setting, the given problem requires a rigorous solution of the transient transport equation, and such a solution has not been obtained to date.

Approximate methods for the solution of the transport equation have limited domains of application [76–79]. Of the numerical methods, the Monte Carlo method has definite advantages, and its possibilities are persuasively illustrated in a paper by Krekov [80]. One of the results obtained in [80] is shown in Fig. 3.25, which gives the angular distribution of the photon flux in the plane of a detector with a diameter of 150 mm for a propagating $\delta$ pulse with a diameter of 8 mm, spread angle of 30′, and a wavelength of 0.7 $\mu$m in a water cloud with an optical thickness $\tau = 5$. The sequence of curves 1–4 corresponds to time differences of roughly 10 nsec and illustrates the spreading of the $\delta$ pulse with time. Similar results have been obtained for other optical thicknesses, aerosol models, and radiation pulse wavelengths. Also, the distributions of photons of various scattering multiplicities with respect to transit time across the entrance area of the detector have been obtained in the same paper. We emphasize the fact that the computational algorithms developed in that work permit the sorting of photons emitted by the $\delta$ pulse according to transit angles of the scattering multiplicity and transit times across the entrance area of a detector situated

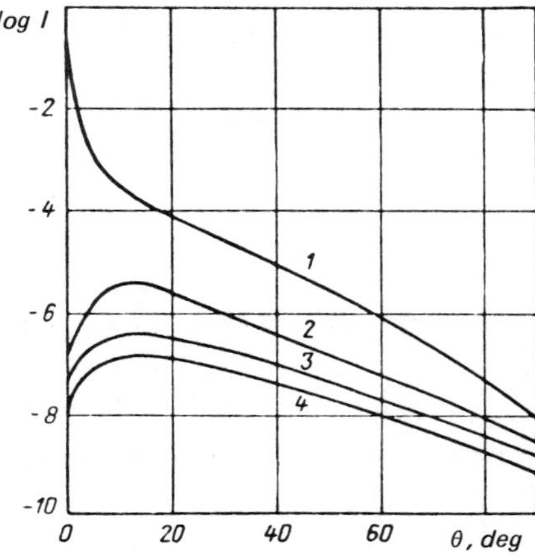


Fig. 3.25. Results of calculations of the angular distribution of photon flux in the plane of a receiver with diameter of 150 mm for propagation of a light beam of diameter 8 mm with 30′ spread and wavelength of 0.7 $\mu$m in a water cloud with optical thickness $\tau = 5.0$. (1–4) Values of parameter $t$ with successive increments $\Delta t = 0.05 \approx 10$ nsec.

at an arbitrary point of the scattering medium relative to the radiation source.

The Monte Carlo method makes it possible to form a complete pattern of the distortion of a pulse having a given shape during propagation in various scattering media. The corresponding results have direct bearing on the methods of laser probing of aerosols, and for this reason their discussion is deferred to Chap. 7.

In situations where the radiation pulse propagates in a scattering medium of small optical density, the theoretical treatment of the problem is simplified because the applicability of the simple expressions for single scattering can be counted on. Ivanov and others [81, 82] have derived single-scattering expressions for the typical experimental setup comprising a point source of pulses with a radiation cone of vertex angle $\Theta$ plus a detection system with a circular aperture of diameter $d_{\text{det}}$ and f.o.v. $\Psi$. When the medium is nonabsorbing and homogeneous along the path, we obtain the following equation for the recorded reflected signal $v(t)$ in the case of a source-detector distance $z \gg d_{\text{det}}/2$:

$$v(t) = \frac{\sigma f(\pi) d_{\text{det}}^2}{\sigma c \Theta t^2} e^{-\sigma ct} \varphi(t) \tag{3.68}$$

$$\varphi(t) = \begin{cases} 0, & 0 < \dfrac{2z}{c(\gamma - \Psi - \Theta)} \leqslant t \leqslant \dfrac{2z}{c(\gamma + \Psi + \Theta)} \\[2ex] \gamma + \Psi + \Theta - \dfrac{2z}{ct}, & \dfrac{2z}{c(\gamma + \Psi - \Theta)} \leqslant t \leqslant \dfrac{2z}{c(\gamma + \Psi - \Theta)} \\[2ex] 2\Theta, & \dfrac{2z}{c(\gamma + \Psi - \Theta)} \leqslant t \leqslant \dfrac{2z}{c(\gamma - \Psi + \Theta)} \\[2ex] \dfrac{2z}{ct} + \Psi + \Theta - \gamma, & \dfrac{2z}{c(\gamma - \Psi + \Theta)} \leqslant t \leqslant \dfrac{2z}{c(\gamma - \Psi - \Theta)} \end{cases} \tag{3.69}$$

Here $\sigma$ is the volume scattering coefficient, $f(\pi)$ is the value of the angular scattering function in the backward direction, $c$ is the speed of light, $t$ is the time reckoned from the instant of pulse transmission, and $\gamma$ is the scattering angle. The angles $\Psi$, $\gamma$, and $\Theta$ are assumed to be small. It is evident from expressions (3.68) and (3.69) that the shape of the reflected pulse in single scattering represents a single-peaked asymmetrical curve in every case and is determined by the relationship between the angles $\gamma$, $\Psi$, and $\Theta$. The position of the maximum of the curve depends on the scattering coefficient $\sigma$ only for large values of the latter, as specified by the condition $\sigma \geqslant (\gamma + \Psi - 5\Theta)(\gamma + \Psi - \Theta)/4z\Theta$. An experimental verification of expressions (3.68) and (3.69) [82] for atmospheric hazes has demonstrated good agreement between the experimental and calculated data for scattering coefficients smaller than 5 km$^{-1}$ and values of $t$ up to 20 $\mu$sec. It was shown on the basis of the measurements that the temporal structure of the reflected pulse signal under conditions of high atmospheric transmissivity ($\sigma \leqslant 0.3$ km$^{-1}$) is determined mainly by the geometry of the experiment rather than by the optical properties of the atmosphere. In a highly turbid atmosphere ($\sigma > 10$ km$^{-1}$), on the other hand, the geometrical parameters of the experiment are observed to have only a slight influence on the temporal structure of the reflected pulse. The properties of the medium are decisive here.

A significant dependence of the pulse duration and delay time on the extinction coefficient in natural fogs has been observed experimentally in earlier studies [83, 84]. In particular, as the extinction coefficient increases from 1 to 10 km$^{-1}$, the duration of the reflected pulse is observed to vary from 2–3 to 0.5 $\mu$sec. But the dependence of the characteristics of the reflected pulse on the experimental geometry, as has been demonstrated for water media with an extinction coefficient of 0.8 m$^{-1}$ [85], causes at most a twofold broadening relative to the width of the pulse transmitted into the medium. Thus, the factor of primary concern for dense scattering media is the dependence of the characteristics of the reflected pulse on the optical properties of the medium.

Kabanov and Samokhvalov [86] have conducted a detailed experimental investigation of the reflection of light pulses for dense fogs and smokes. The measurements were carried out with the use of a semiconductor laser having a wavelength of 0.84 $\mu$m and a pulse duration of 8 nsec at the 0.5 level in an artificial fog chamber. The extinction coefficients of the medium were varied from 0.02 to 1.0 m$^{-1}$. The radiation detector and source were situated in such a way that their optic axes intersected in the investigated medium at an angle of 1° at a distance of 7 m from the leading edge.

An analysis of the results shows that with a decrease in the optical density of the medium the duration of the leading edge of the reflected pulse increases, while its slope decreases. At the same time, the duration of the trailing edge of the reflected pulse also increases.

Figure 3.26 gives the duration $\Delta t$ of pulses reflected from fogs (upper curve) and smokes (lower curve) as a function of the extinction coefficient. It is evident from the figure that the duration of the reflected pulses in both cases decreases with increasing extinction coefficient, tending to be pulse

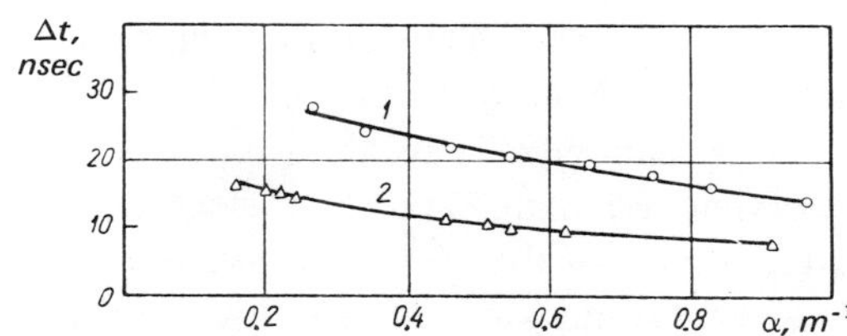

Fig. 3.26. Durations of pulses reflected from fogs (1) and smokes (2) versus extinction coefficient.

duration for the source. This result is attributable to the fact that the reflected signal is formed primarily in the layer immediately adjacent to the source. The extent of these layers decreases with increasing density of the medium. The different durations of pulses reflected from fogs and smokes for identical values of $\alpha$ are clearly associated with the concomitant difference in the angular scattering functions of these media.

Figure 3.27 gives the dependence of the delay times $t_m$ of pulses reflected by fogs (curve 1) and smokes (curve 2) on the values of the extinction coefficient. We note that the pulse delay time is interpreted as the time interval between transmission of the pulse and the maximum value of the received signal. It is apparent from the figure that the value of $t_m$ for fogs decays more rapidly with increasing $\alpha$ than for smokes. For values of $\alpha > 0.5$ m$^{-1}$, the difference between the values of $t_m$ for fogs and smokes practically disappears. The following qualitative explanation is offered for the different behavior of the dependence of $t_m$ on $\alpha$ in fogs and smokes for small values of $\alpha$. For small optical densities of the medium, the principal role in the formation of the reflected signal is taken by small scattering multiplicities, in which case the difference between the scattering functions of the media significantly affects the result of formation of that signal. The reflected pulse in fogs is formed from more distant layers than in smokes.

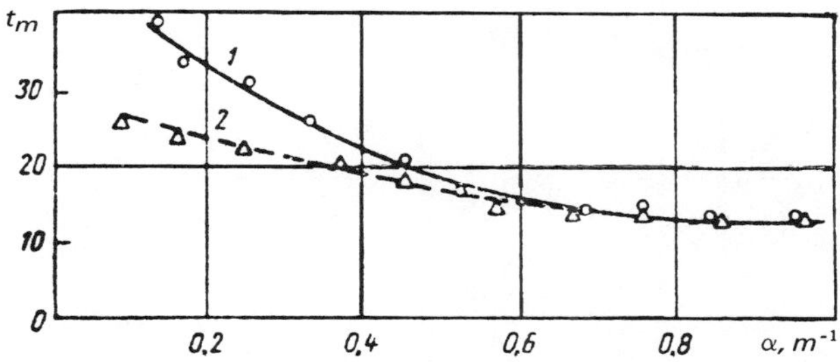

Fig. 3.27. Delay times of pulses reflected from fogs (1) and smokes (2) versus extinction coefficient.

We note in conclusion that the results described here from experimental studies of the distortion of a reflected pulse from fogs have also been obtained analytically by the Monte Carlo method [87]. The analytical and experimental data exhibit satisfactory agreement, further supporting the effectiveness of the Monte Carlo method when used for investigation of the laws of propagation of spatially confined light beams in scattering and absorbing media.

We conclude with some quantitative data obtained on the basis of calculations of the characteristics of a reflected pulse by Monte Carlo algorithms for a number of typical conditions of lidar applications in the atmosphere [88, 89]. Figure 3.28 gives the results of calculations of the intensity of cloud-reflected radiation for the case of aligned optic axes of the transmitter and detection system (and a monostatic monitoring scheme). The lidar conditions are as follows: distance to cloud 1000 m; optical thickness of cloud 5; cloud droplet-size spectrum described by a "broad" gamma distribution function $n(r) = ar^{-2}\exp(-0.4r)$, where $a$ is a normalizing factor; the optical properties of the aerosol atmosphere beneath the cloud are determined by a standard atmosphere [90] with meteorological range $S_M = 10$ km; width of Gaussian pulse at half-power points 0.06 $\mu$sec; optical wavelength 0.69 $\mu$m; angular spread of laser beam 12′. The solid curves in the figure represent the variation of the shape of the reflected pulse as a function of the cloud density, and the dashed curves together with curve 3 indicate the influence of the f.o.v. $\Psi$ of the detection system. As is apparent from Fig. 3.28, a decrease in the density of the cloud or a constant density and an increase in the f.o.v. of the detection system results in broadening of the reflected pulse almost entirely due to delay of the trailing edge. This analytical result is a natural consequence of the major role of multiple-scattering effects for large detector f.o.v. The broadening of the reflected pulse with decreasing cloud density is a result of the increase in the dimensions of the scattering volume.

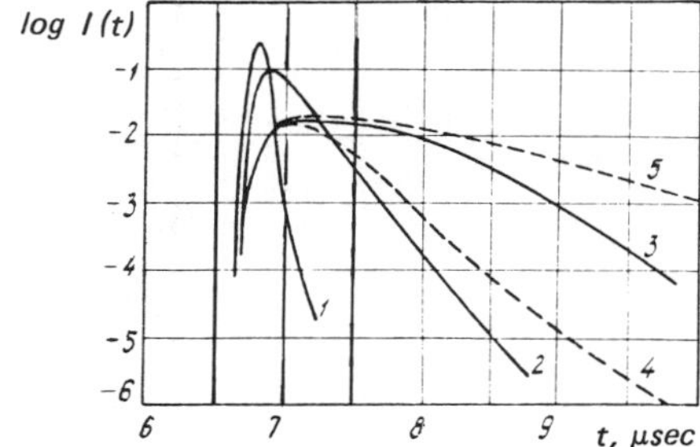


Fig. 3.28. Variation of reflected-signal shape with volume extinction coefficient of a cloud with constant optical thickness, $\Psi = 10°$: (1) $\sigma = 0.5$ m$^{-1}$ (cloud thickness $L = 10$ m); (2) $\sigma = 0.1$ m$^{-1}$ ($L = 50$ m); (3) $\sigma = 0.02$ m$^{-1}$ ($L = 300$ m); (4) $\Psi = 1°$, $\sigma = 0.02$ m$^{-1}$ ($L = 300$ m); (5) $\Psi = 180°$, $\sigma = 0.02$ m$^{-1}$ ($L = 300$ m).

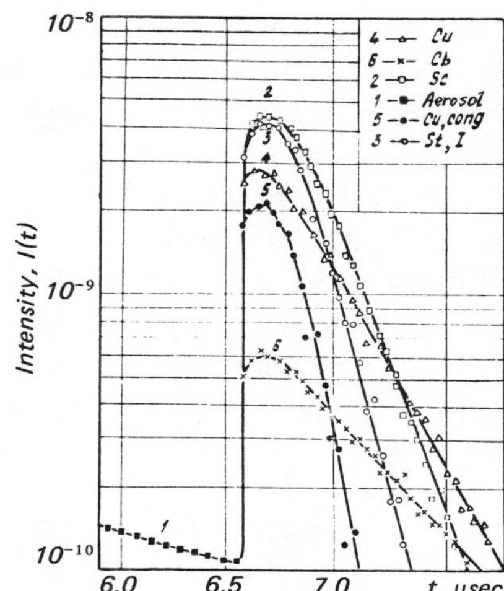


Fig. 3.29. Combined influence of the extinction coefficient and angular scattering function of clouds on the shape of the reflected signal (10.6 µm).

Figure 3.29 presents analytical data [89] for the intensity of radiation reflected by cloud formations with various densities and microphysical characteristics. The cloud parameters taken from the data of Carrier and others [91] for $\lambda = 10.6$ µm and used in the calculations are summarized in Table 3.6. The initial duration of the lidar pulse is assumed to be 30 nsec, and the optical thickness of the cloud $\tau = 3$. Absorption by atmospheric gases is disregarded. The data of Fig. 3.29 imply considerable sensitivity of the shape and amplitude of the reflected pulse at a wavelength of 10.6 µm to the microphysical parameters of the cloud formations. Similar results have been obtained [89] for the intensity of reflected pulses with wavelengths of 0.69 and 2.36 µm.

Several researchers [74, 92–96] have analyzed the role of various scattering multiplicities, the geometrical parameters of the source and

Table 3.6.

| Parameters | Type of cloud | | | | |
|---|---|---|---|---|---|
| | Sc | St, I | Cu | Cu, cong | Cb |
| Extinction coefficient $\varepsilon$, km$^{-1}$ | 27.62 | 32.37 | 13.21 | 44.48 | 21.30 |
| Scattering coefficient $\sigma$, km$^{-1}$ | 16.85 | 19.24 | 7.83 | 26.59 | 12.11 |
| Backscattering coefficient $\sigma\pi$, km$^{-1}$ | 0.386 | 0.391 | 0.187 | 0.194 | 0.0721 |
| Droplet concentration $N$, cm$^{-3}$ | 358 | 446 | 168 | 211 | 69 |

detector, the angular scattering function, and the volume scattering coefficient on the deformation of a laser pulse propagating in media with different photon survival probabilities. The fundamental results obtained in these studies may be summarized as follows.

With the application of sources having an angular spread of the order of 10′ to 20′, detectors with a f.o.v. of the same order, and a baseline (distance between source and detector) less than 3 m, the single-scattering expressions satisfactorily describe the shape and intensity of pulses reflected from scattering media up to optical thickness values $\tau \leqslant 1$–2. The particular value of $\tau$ in this case depends on the scattering function. For example, $\tau \leqslant 2$ in the case of wood smokes ($\rho = 6 \pm 3$), and $\tau \leqslant 1.5$ for water fogs ($\rho = 60 \pm 20$).

Under conditions of high transmissivity of the atmosphere (with volume extinction coefficient $\alpha \leqslant 0.15$ km$^{-1}$), the temporal structure of a radiation pulse reflected from a scattering medium is determined mainly by the geometrical parameters of the experiment rather than by the optical parameters of the medium. In dense media ($\alpha \geqslant 15$ km$^{-1}$), the role of the geometrical parameters diminishes, but in the case of parallel axes of the source and detection system the dependence on the baseline becomes very strong. A decrease in the diameter of the detector induces only a slight increase in the slope of the leading edge of the pulse.

The expressions describing double-scattering effects permit advancement into the range of optical thickness with values up to 2 or 3, beyond which it is necessary to take higher scattering multiplicities into account.

In very dense media ($\alpha > 100$ to 200 km$^{-1}$), the form of the luminance distribution of backscattered radiation depends mainly on the angular scattering function and only slightly on $\alpha$. The zone of significance of double-scattering events is concentrated to a greater degree around the beam axis for fogs than for smokes. The corresponding difference due to the influence of the scattering function is of the same order. It is inferred from this result that the range of variations of the radiation pulse shape due to variations in the geometrical parameters of the experiment should be correspondingly greater in fogs.

We note in conclusion that the complete solution of the transient scattering problem will require additional theoretical as well as experimental investigation of the propagation of pulsed radiation in media with different photon survival probabilities in order to acquire data on the space–time distortions of pulses in the regions of linear interactions of the radiation with the medium. The problem of the durations of radiation pulses commensurate with the corresponding relaxation times of the indicated interaction processes, where nonlinear effects become possible, will be discussed in Chap. 7.

## 3.13. Intensity Fluctuations of Spatially Confined Beams in Scattering Media

Investigations of the aerosol component of the transmittance of highly turbid atmospheres [50, 97] show that the slow variations of this quantity with changing meteorological conditions are accompanied by small-scale fluctuations of the transmittance. Such high-frequency transmittance fluctuations have also been observed in the case of a system of coarsely dispersed scatterers under laboratory conditions [98]. The cause of these fluctuations for invariant optical properties of the medium as a whole should logically be sought in the temporal variations of the optical cross section of the system of scatterers in the zone of the beam due to spatial displacement of the total system or of individual scatterers in it. Accordingly, it is necessary to include among the principal factors affecting the fluctuation characteristics of the transmittance, together with the optical properties of the scatterers, their translational velocity and the geometrical parameters of the optical beam. We now give the results of theoretical and experimental studies of the statistical characteristics and nature of the transmittance fluctuations of disperse media.

### 3.13.1 Experiments in Model Media

For fixed optical properties of the disperse media serving as model media, we are mainly concerned with the dependence of the fluctuation characteristics on the diameter of the optical beam and on the geometrical or optical thickness of the scattering layer that this beam must penetrate.

The results of measurements of the fluctuation characteristics for various diameters of the light beam have been described in detail by Denchik and others [98]. The scattering medium is represented by a suspension of spherical paraffin particles in an alcohol–water solution. The rms particle radius is $215 \pm 5$ $\mu$m, the relative refractive index is 1.20, and the scatterer concentration is $250 \pm 15$ cm$^{-3}$. The nature of the fluctuations of the recorded signal is given in Fig. 3.30 in the form of segments of time traces of the signal for several values of the optical thickness of the scattering layer. Processing of the experimental data has shown that the distribution of the fluctuations for optical thicknesses greater than 5 is well described by a log-normal function, and the spectrum of the signal fluctuations depends significantly on the diameter of the optical beam as well as on the velocity of the scatterers.

The results of calculations of the variance of the fluctuations on the basis of traces of a random signal for three light beam diameters are given

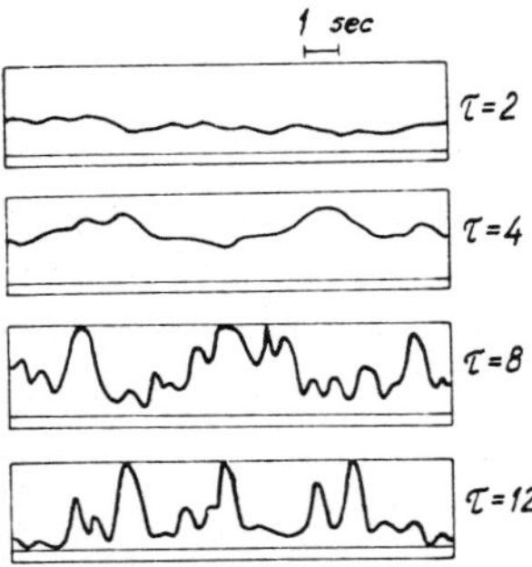

Fig. 3.30. Sample time traces of incoming radiation intensity for various optical thicknesses of the scattering layer.

in Fig. 3.31, in which the optical thickness of the medium $\tau$ is plotted along the horizontal axis and the standard deviation (square root of the variance) along the vertical axis. It is seen in the figure that monotonic growth of the variance with increasing $\tau$ is observed over the entire investigated range of optical thicknesses.

Goryachev and others [99] have carried out corresponding measurements for spherical polystyrene latexes in water with a relative refractive index of 1.2, an rms particle radius of 0.285 mm, and a scatterer concentration of 193 $cm^{-3}$. The beam diameter in the measurements was 4 mm, and the angular spread of the beam and f.o.v. of the detector were both 4′.

Processing of the measurements results shows that the values of the standard deviation increase with the optical thickness, attaining a maximum of $\sigma \cong 1.3$ at $\tau = 20$–$24$, and then dropping rapidly to a value of $\sigma \cong 0.1$ at $\tau = 30$. The latter result is explained by the rapid spreading of the beam at large depths due to multiple-scattering effects. The distribution of the fluctuations in this case changes from a normal distribution for $\tau < 4$ to a log-normal function for larger values of $\tau$.

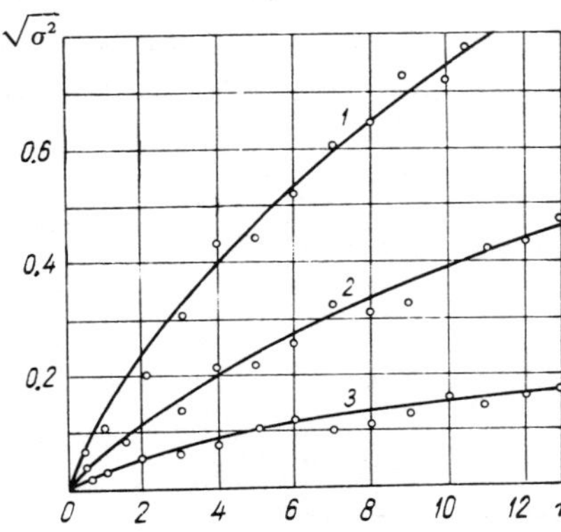

Fig. 3.31. Standard deviation of incoming radiation intensity versus optical thickness. (1) Optical beam of diameter 2 mm; (2) 5 mm; (3) 20 mm.

## 3.13.2. Transmittance Fluctuations of Precipitations

The results of experimental studies of low-frequency transmittance fluctuations of a turbid atmosphere (samples were taken every 6 min) have been obtained [97] by means of a transmittance recorder with a time constant of 20 sec. Table 3.7 gives the results of measurements of the mean visibility range $S$ and variance of the visibility $\sigma^2$ for various meteorological conditions.

More detailed investigations of fluctuation phenomena in the transmittance of the atmosphere have been conducted by Kabanov and others [100, 101] with the use of fast-response equipment. These investigations disclosed both low- and high-frequency fluctuations of the transmittance. The experimental arrangement used for the measurements ensured the possibility of varying the diameter of the optical beam between the limits of 10 and 75 mm. The measurements were carried out in a part of the spectrum including the wavelength of 1.03 $\mu$m, which was segregated from the mercury-arc radiation by means of an interference-type light filter. The receiving and recording system was suitable for the investigation of random processes in the frequency range from 0 to 600 Hz.

An analysis of the probability distribution functions of the intensity fluctuations shows that in the majority of cases in rains and light snowfalls a normal law prevails, while in heavy snowfalls the distribution is skewed in the sense of increasing small values. The skewness is diminished by increasing the diameter of the detection system.

The results of a correlation analysis of the transmittance fluctuations of precipitations indicate a strong dependence of the correlation time on the microstructure of the precipitations. Figure 3.32 gives the spectral density functions $G(\omega)$ for snowfalls of various microstructures. It is evident from the figure that the high-frequency contribution in the spectrum of observable intensity fluctuations increases with the maximum size of the snowflakes. In the case of large flocculent snowflakes, the fluctuation spectrum is close to a white-noise spectrum over the entire range of investigated frequencies.

A total of 57 records was processed to determine the variance of the transmittance fluctuations of the atmosphere in the presence of snowfalls,

Table 3.7.

| Parameter | Fog | Drizzle | Rain | Snowstorm | Snowfall | Mist | Haze |
|---|---|---|---|---|---|---|---|
| Variance $\sigma^2$ | 0.082 | 0.45 | 0.61 | 0.56 | 0.75 | 0.49 | 0.99 |
| $S$, km | 0.71 | 2.55 | 6.19 | 2.27 | 3.28 | 3.03 | 3.18 |

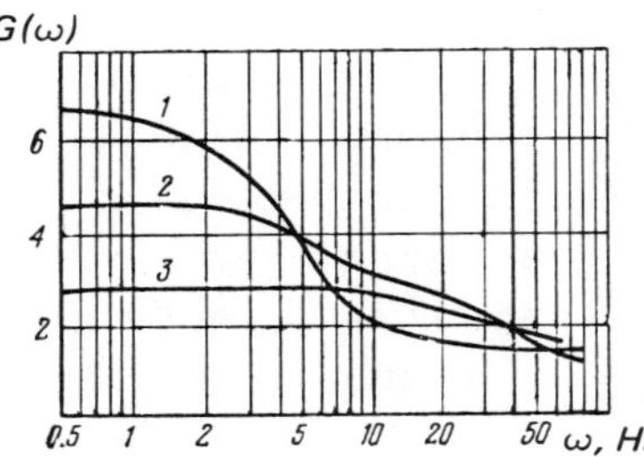

Fig. 3.32. Frequency spectra of transmittance fluctuations of precipitations. (1) Small snowflakes (2 mm or less); (2) snowflakes 5–10 mm in diameter; (3) large flocculent flakes (20–30 mm).

hail, rain, and clear weather. The results of processing of experimental data obtained under diverse meteorological conditions with various beam diameters (from 10 to 75 mm) over a 200-m path are given in Table 3.8.

We see in the table that the variance of the observed transmittance fluctuations depends significantly on the sizes of the scatterers, the intensity of the precipitations, and the geometrical parameters of the experiment; specifically, the variance increases with increasing precipitation intensity and with decreasing detector aperture or diameter of the optical beam. The indicated properties of the variance and other statistical characteristics of the transmittance of precipitations lead to the conclusion that the scattering of optical radiation by hydrometers exerts a strong influence of the properties of the observed fluctuations. Gurvich and Pokasov [102] arrive at the same conclusion in measurements of the spectra of atmospheric transmittance fluctuations before a rain and during light drizzle.

### 3.13.3. Calculation of Fluctuation Characteristics

It follows from the results of an analysis of the mean luminance values for transmitted and scattered radiations in scattering media that the fraction of recorded scattered radiation (relative to the direct radiation) for narrow optical beams and comparatively small optical thicknesses is relatively small. Consequently, the principal effect responsible for fluctuations of the transmitted signal must be optical screening of the direct radiation by the

Table 3.8.

| Meteorological conditions | Normalized variance | Meteorological significance | Normalized variance |
|---|---|---|---|
| Heavy snowfall (flocs) | 0.14 | Heavy rain | 0.09–0.25 |
| Moderate snowfall | 0.03–0.06 | Moderate rain | 0.01 |
| Hail (to 1 cm) | 0.02 | Cloudless | 0.01–0.20 |

system of scatterers. This effect is such that attenuation by a system of scatterers distributed randomly along the path and in the beam cross section in the case of independent scattering is equivalent to attenuation by a system of overlapping screens in a plane layer with a certain effective transverse attenuation. The effect can be quantitatively described on the basis of the results of the mathematical statistics of random tossing of pennies onto a square [103] or the model of granular structure in the photographic recording of an image [104]. With this approach, the effect of statistical screening of transmitted radiation takes into account both the fluctuations of the number of scatterers in the visual volume and the statistical variation of their relative spatial positions. We carry out a calculation of the statistical characteristics, following Kabanov and Krutikov [105].

We denote by $I(\mathbf{r}_1)$ the illuminance created at the point $\mathbf{r}_1$ (with coordinates $x_1$, $y_1$) by the transmitted optical beam in the plane of the receiving aperture. If the dimensions of the latter are greater than the correlation radius of the illuminance fluctuations, then the fluctuations of the recorded signal will be averaged. To describe the averaging effect of the receiving aperture, we introduce the function $S(\mathbf{r})$, which is equal to zero outside the aperture surface and to unity on it and which has the significance of the pulse response of the receiving aperture. Then the optical radiation signal recorded by a detection system with a finite aperture at a point $\mathbf{r}$ is given by the expression [104, 106]

$$I(\mathbf{r}) = \int_{-\infty}^{\infty} S(\mathbf{r} - \mathbf{r}_1) I(\mathbf{r}_1) d\mathbf{r}_1 \tag{3.70}$$

and the corresponding fluctuation component of the signal is

$$I'(\mathbf{r}) = \int_{-\infty}^{\infty} S(\mathbf{r} - \mathbf{r}_1) I'(\mathbf{r}_1) d\mathbf{r}_1 \tag{3.71}$$

where $I' = I - \langle I \rangle$. The autocorrelation function of the signal fluctuations is written in the form

$$B_{I'}(\rho) = \langle I'(\mathbf{r}) I'(\mathbf{r} + \rho) \rangle = \int_{-\infty}^{\infty} B_{I'}(\mathbf{r}) d\mathbf{r} \int_{-\infty}^{\infty} S(\mathbf{r} + \rho - \xi) S(\xi) d\xi \tag{3.72}$$

The inner integral in (3.72) is readily evaluated for a typical circular receiving aperture of radius $R$ used in optical measurements [104]:

$$\int_{-\infty}^{\infty} S(\mathbf{r} + \rho - \xi) S(\xi) d\xi = \pi R^2 F\left(\frac{|\mathbf{r} + \rho|}{2R}\right) \tag{3.73}$$

where

$$F(x) = \begin{cases} \dfrac{2}{\pi}\left[\cos^{-1}x - x(1-x^2)^{1/2}\right] & \text{for } x \leqslant 1 \\ 0 & \text{for } x > 1. \end{cases}$$

For the determination of the function $B_{I'}(\mathbf{r})$, we make use of the fact that the measured optical scattering diameter of the system of particles is described by the expression [49]

$$\sigma_{\text{meas}} = \sigma k(z, z_0) \tag{3.74}$$

where $k(z, z_0) = K(z, z_0)/2$, $K(z, z_0)$ is described by expression (3.56) and is plotted in Fig. 3.6, $\sigma$ is the optical scattering diameter (volume scattering coefficient), $z = \rho R/L$, $z_0 = \rho \Psi$, $L$ is the geometrical thickness of the scattering layer, $\Psi$ is the f.o.v. of the detection system, $\rho = 2\pi a/\lambda$, and $a$ is the particle radius. A system of particles with scattering diameter $\sigma_{\text{meas}}$ is equivalent to a system of overlapping circular grains of radius $a$ and transmittance $h = 1 - k(z, z_0)$. The autocorrelation function $B_{I'}(\mathbf{r})$ for such a system with a Poisson distribution of grain centers (i.e., the limit of the binomial distribution for a constant average number of grains) is given by the expression [107]

$$B_{I'}(\mathbf{r}) = \langle I \rangle^2 \left\{ \exp\left[\tau(1-h)^2 F(r/2a)\right] - 1 \right\} \tag{3.75}$$

where $\langle I \rangle = I_0 e^{-\tau(1-h)}$, $\tau = (a/R)^2 \langle n \rangle$, and $\langle n \rangle$ is the average number of grains on the photometrically measured area (in our case, the number of scatterers in the photometrically measured volume of the medium $\langle n \rangle = L\pi R^2 N_0$, where $N_0$ is the scatterer concentration).

Finally, for the autocorrelation function of the recorded optical signal transmitted through the scattering layer we obtain the following upon substitution of (3.73) and (3.75) into (3.72):

$$B_{I'}(|\boldsymbol{\rho}|) = 2\pi(\pi R^2)\langle I \rangle^2 \int_0^{2R} \left\{ \exp\left[\tau(1-h)^2 F\frac{r}{2a}\right] - 1 \right\} F\left( \frac{|\mathbf{r}+\boldsymbol{\rho}|}{2R} \right) r\,dr$$

$$\tag{3.76}$$

From (3.76) we readily obtain two asymptotic cases for the autocorrelation function and variance $B_{I'}(0)$. For radii of the receiving aperture (or beam radii) $R \gg a$, the function $F(r/2R)$ in the integrand of (3.76) can be expanded into a series in $r/2R$ and restricted to the first term. Then the variance is written in the form

$$\sigma_{I'}^2 = B_{I'}(0) = \frac{8\tau}{\langle n \rangle} \langle I \rangle^2 \int_0^1 \left\{ \exp\left[\tau k^2 F(x)\right] - 1 \right\} x\, dx \qquad R \gg a \qquad (3.77)$$

which is analogous to the expression obtained by Shifrin and others [103] under the same assumptions for a rectangular aperture.

In the other limiting case, where $R \ll a$ (very narrow optical beams), the function $F(r/2a)$ in (3.76) can be expanded into a series in $r/2a$. Restricting the expansion to the first term, we obtain

$$\sigma_{I'}^2 = B_{I'}(0) = (\pi R^2)^2 I_0^2 \exp(-2\tau k)\left[\exp(\tau k^2) - 1\right], \qquad R \ll a \qquad (3.78)$$

which coincides with the analogous result obtained in [104].

The results of calculations according to the expressions derived above are compared with the available experimental data for fluctuations of transmitted radiation in disperse media in Fig. 3.33. The solid curves represent the results of measurements of the standard deviation of the signal as a function of the optical thickness of the scattering layer according to the results of Denchik and others [98] (curve 1, $\rho = 2.2 \times 10^3$) and [99] (curve 2, $\rho = 2.8 \times 10^3$), and the dashed curves characterize the results of calculations using the approximate expression (3.77), which is justified for the given experimental conditions. It is evident from Fig. 3.33 that the analytical data for curve 1 agree satisfactorily with the experimental over the entire range of measured variances. In the case of curve 2, systematic discrepancies set in at optical thicknesses $\tau = 16$. Such discrepancies in large thicknesses are naturally attributed to the influence of multiple scattering of radiation, which is ignored in the calculations. If we assume that the influence of a very weakly

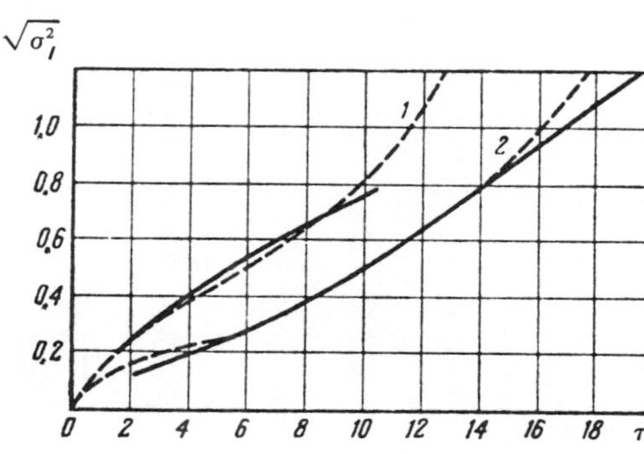

Fig. 3.33. Comparison of calculated (dashed curves) and measured (solid curves) variances of fluctuations of transmitted radiation intensity.

fluctuating multiple-scattering background is felt at large optical thicknesses, then for the total normalized standard deviation we have the relation

$$\sigma_{I_{\text{tot}}} = \sigma_I \frac{\langle I \rangle}{\langle I_{\text{tot}} \rangle} = \sigma_I \frac{\langle I \rangle}{\langle I \rangle + \langle I_{\text{av}} \rangle} \tag{3.79}$$

Here $\langle I \rangle$ is the average intensity of the transmitted radiation, whose attenuation is described by the equation

$$\langle I \rangle = I_0 \exp(-\tau_{\text{meas}}) = I_0 \exp(-\tau k) \tag{3.80}$$

in which $I_0$ is the initial average intensity of the beam and $\langle I_{\text{av}} \rangle$ is the average intensity of the multiple forward-scattering background. According to the measurement results, the dependence of $\langle I_{\text{av}} \rangle$ on $\tau$ can be neglected in comparison with the same dependence for $\langle I \rangle$. Thus, we finally obtain

$$\sigma_{I_{\text{tot}}} = \sigma_I / [1 + e^{k(\tau - b)}] \tag{3.81}$$

where $b$ characterizes the average intensity level of multiple-scattered radiation. Figure 3.34 gives a comparison of the results of calculations of $(\sigma_{I_{\text{tot}}}^2)^{1/2}$ according to expression (3.81) (curve 2) for a value of $b = 24$ corresponding to the results of measurements of the average intensities, with the experimental data of Goryachev and others [99] (solid curve), indicating good agreement over the entire investigated range of optical thicknesses.

Thus, it follows from a comparison of the calculated and experimental data for the variances of the fluctuations of transmitted radiation that statistical screening is a definite cause of the fluctuations of transverse radiation in disperse media. The limits of applicability of the statistical screening expressions are determined by the optical thicknesses at which the total luminance of the direct and singly forward-scattered radiation is less than the luminance of multiply forward-scattered radiation. For large

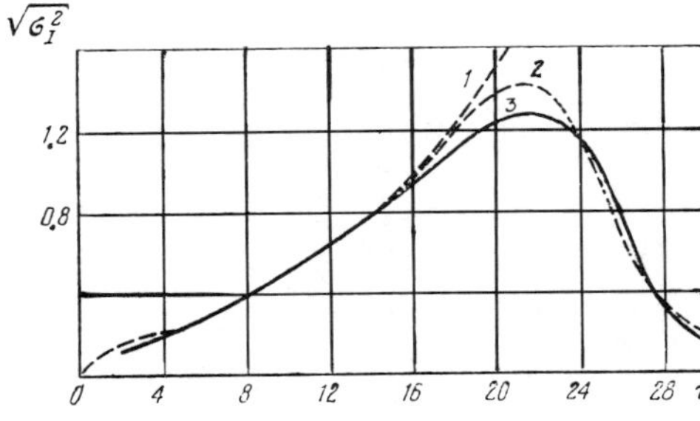


Fig. 3.34. Variance of fluctuations of transmitted radiation intensity versus optical thickness. (1) Calculated according to screening formulas; (2) calculated according to (3.81) (dashed curves); (3) experimental (solid curve)

optical depths, the variances can be approximately calculated with sufficient accuracy for practical purposes according to expression (3.81).

## 3.14 Optical Models of Atmospheric Aerosols

The enormous variety of microphysical and, accordingly, optical properties of atmospheric aerosols in real situations can, despite its size, be classified according to specific criteria based on statistical processing of the existing experimental data. The end result of such a classification comprises optical models of an aerosol atmosphere, which has an important bearing on quantitative calculations of the many and diverse laws of propagation of optical waves and, in particular, laser radiation in the atmosphere.

The most commonly used constructs in practice are the cloud, precipitation, and haze models proposed by Deirmendjian [90] on the basis of an analysis of vast experimental material. A modified gamma distribution is postulated as the general particle-size distribution function:

$$n(r) = ar^{\alpha}\exp(-br^{\gamma}), \qquad 0 \leqslant r \leqslant \infty \qquad (3.82)$$

where $r$ is the particle radius and $a$, $b$, $\alpha$, $\gamma$ are empirical parameters of the distribution. The parameter $b$ is related to the model radius $r_M$ [the function $n(r)$ has a maximum at this value of the radius] by the equation $b = \alpha/\gamma r_M^{\gamma}$. The value of the distribution parameters for the proposed models are given in Table 3.9, along with the number of particles per unit volume $N$ and the values of the maximum particle radii $r_{\max}$ (at the level below $10^{-3}$ times the peak value of the distribution function). The given tables clearly illustrate the broad range of variation of the microphysical and, accordingly, the optical parameters of atmospheric aerosols.

Models of the microstructure of aerosols in water hazes and the results of calculations of the extinction coefficients have been proposed and described in detail [4, 108]. Refinements of these models on the basis of direct microphysical measurements of the microstructure of atmospheric hazes in the ground layer and at various heights are obtained through statistical data and their analysis [48, 109].

A consequence of the generalization of the experimental optical and microphysical characteristics is the set of optical models of noctilucent clouds proposed by Zuev and others [110]. The optical parameters of these models are calculated on the assumption that the scattering particles of noctilucent clouds are either ice particles or particles that behave as such in the optical sense.

Table 3.9.

| Model | $N$ | $a$ | $r_M$ | $r_{max}$ | $\alpha$ | $\gamma$ | Type of distribution |
|---|---|---|---|---|---|---|---|
| Haze M | $100\ \mathrm{cm}^{-3}$ | $5.3333\times10^4$ | $0.05\ \mu\mathrm{m}$ | $3\ \mu\mathrm{m}$ | 1 | $\frac{1}{2}$ | Overwater or coastal aerosol |
| Haze L | $100\ \mathrm{cm}^{-3}$ | $4.9757\times10^6$ | $0.07\ \mu\mathrm{m}$ | $2\ \mu\mathrm{m}$ | 2 | $\frac{1}{2}$ | Overland aerosol |
| Haze H | $100\ \mathrm{cm}^{-3}$ | $4.0000\times10^5$ | $0.10\ \mu\mathrm{m}$ | $0.6\ \mu\mathrm{m}$ | 2 | 1 | High and stratospheric aerosols |
| Rain M | $100\ \mathrm{m}^{-3}$ | $5.3333\times10^5$ | $0.05\ \mathrm{mm}$ | $3\ \mathrm{mm}$ | 1 | $\frac{1}{2}$ | Light to moderate rainfall |
| Rain L | $1000\ \mathrm{m}^{-3}$ | $4.9757\times10^7$ | $0.07\ \mathrm{mm}$ | $2\ \mathrm{mm}$ | 2 | $\frac{1}{2}$ | Heavy rainfall |
| Hail H | $10\ \mathrm{m}^{-3}$ | $4.0000\times10^4$ | $1.00\ \mathrm{mm}$ | $6\ \mathrm{mm}$ | 2 | 1 | Hail with large content of small particles |
| Cumulus cloud C.1 | $100\ \mathrm{cm}^{-3}$ | $2.3730$ | $4.00\ \mu\mathrm{m}$ | $15\ \mu\mathrm{m}$ | 6 | 1 | Cumulus and stratiform clouds, fogs |
| Cloud C.2 | $100\ \mathrm{cm}^{-3}$ | $1.0851\times10^{-2}$ | $4.00\ \mu\mathrm{m}$ | $7\ \mu\mathrm{m}$ | 8 | 3 | Clouds exhibiting colored rings (halos) |
| Cloud C.3 | $100\ \mathrm{cm}^{-3}$ | $5.5556$ | $2.00\ \mu\mathrm{m}$ | $3.5\ \mu\mathrm{m}$ | 8 | 3 | Nacreous clouds |
| Cloud C.4 | $100\ \mathrm{cm}^{-3}$ | $5.5556$ | $4.00\ \mu\mathrm{m}$ | $5.5\ \mu\mathrm{m}$ | 8 | 3 | Clouds exhibiting double or triple rings around sun |

The results of calculations of various optical characteristics of aerosols, primarily the volume aerosol extinction coefficients, on the basis of the models discussed above are given in the relevant sections of this chapter.

The next important problem related to optical models of the aerosol atmosphere is the distribution of the optical characteristics with height. This problem mainly concerns the profiles of the volume aerosol extinction coefficients because data on the other characteristics are available only in very limited quantity. The most common model of the height distribution of the volume aerosol extinction coefficient to date is Elterman's model [111], in the construction of which it is postulated that the aerosol extinction coefficient up to heights $H=5$ km can be related one to one with meteorological range $S_M$ on the earth's surface by the expression $\varepsilon_a(H;\lambda)=\varepsilon_a(0;\lambda)\exp(-H/H_a)$, in which $\varepsilon_a(0;0.5)=3.9/S_M$ and the empirical constant $H_a$ is made different for different values of $S_M$ in such a way that the aerosol extinction coefficient will be constant ($5\times10^{-3}$ km$^{-1}$ at a wavelength of 0.55 $\mu$m) at a height $H=5$ km. At heights greater than 5 km, the decay of the extinction coefficient is assumed to be independent of $S_M$. The spectral dependence of the extinction coefficient is chosen in correspondence with the results of measurements [112] over a ground-level path. The extinction coefficients are calculated at heights of 0 to 50 km and for wavelengths of 0.27, 0.28 (0.02) 0.40 (0.28 to 0.40 in steps of 0.02), 0.40

(0.05) 0.70, 0.80, 0.90, 1.06, 1.26, 1.67, and 2.17 $\mu$m. Besides the aerosol extinction and Rayleigh scattering coefficients, the model incorporates data for the absorption coefficient of ozone and the total extinction coefficient.

McClatchey and others [113] have proposed a model of the stratification of the atmosphere for the aerosol extinction coefficient over a broader spectral interval. The particle-size distribution is presumed to be characterized by a function describing an "overland" haze according to Diermendjian [90] with the difference that the function is cut off at a particle radius of 10 rather than 5 $\mu$m. The height distribution of the particle concentration is chosen as in Elterman's model. Two kinds of turbidity are considered in this connection: (1) a "clear" atmosphere ($S_M =$ 23 km at ground level); (2) a "hazy" atmosphere ($S_M = 5$ km). The refractive index of the particles is specified by the real part for $\lambda = 0.6$ $\mu$m. In the interval $\lambda > 0.6$ $\mu$m, the imaginary part of the refractive index is assumed to be linearly growing to 0.1 for $\lambda \geqslant 2$ $\mu$m. The wavelength dependence of the scattering and extinction coefficients for the given model remains the same at different heights and for both types of turbidity, i.e., $\varepsilon_a(H, \lambda) = k(\lambda)\varepsilon_a(0; 0.5745)$. The individual laser wavelengths at which the calculations are carried out, the working media of the lasers, and the values of $k(\lambda)$ are listed in Table 3.10.

The above-described models of the vertical profiles of the volume aerosol extinction coefficients disregard the multilayered character of aerosols due to vertical stratification, which has been observed repeatedly in related studies. In this connection, a model has been proposed [114] on the basis of statistical processing of data on the microphysical parameters of an overland aerosol according to the results of numerous measurements by members of Leningrad University in various regions of the Soviet Union

Table 3.10.

| Wavelength $\lambda, \mu$m | $k(\lambda)$ | Laser medium |
|---|---|---|
| 0.3371 | 1.40 | Nitrogen |
| 0.4880 | 1.05 | Argon |
| 0.5145 | 1.00 | Argon |
| 0.6328 | 0.827 | Helium–neon |
| 0.6943 | 0.756 | Ruby |
| 0.86 | 0.625 | Gallium arsenide |
| 1.06 | 0.522 | Neodymium glass |
| 1.536 | 0.382 | Erbium glass |
| 3.392 | 0.192 | Helium–neon |
| 10.591 | 0.0601 | Carbon dioxide |

Table 3.11. Complex Refractive Indices of Aerosol-Particle
Substance as a Function of Relative Humidity

| $\lambda, \mu$m | $\theta = 10\%$ | | $\theta = 40\%$ | | $\theta = 70\%$ | |
|---|---|---|---|---|---|---|
| | Re | Im | Re | Im | Re | Im |
| 0.6943 | 1.54 | $0.5 \times 10^{-2}$ | 1.38 | $1 \times 10^{-3}$ | 1.34 | $1 \times 10^{-4}$ |
| 1.06 | 1.53 | $0.5 \times 10^{-2}$ | 1.37 | $1 \times 10^{-3}$ | 1.33 | $1 \times 10^{-4}$ |
| 2.36 | 1.50 | $1.3 \times 10^{-2}$ | 1.34 | $1 \times 10^{-3}$ | 1.27 | $1 \times 10^{-3}$ |
| 10.6 | 1.91 | $1.4 \times 10^{-1}$ | 1.47 | $9 \times 10^{-2}$ | 1.26 | $7 \times 10^{-2}$ |

Table 3.12. Vertical Profiles of Aerosol Extinction and
Scattering Coefficients at Wavelengths of 0.6943 and 1.06 $\mu$ (Model of [114])[a]

| $H$, km | $\lambda = 0.6943\ \mu$m | | $\lambda = 1.06\ \mu$m | |
|---|---|---|---|---|
| | $\sigma$, km$^{-1}$ | $\varepsilon_a$, km$^{-1}$ | $\sigma$, km$^{-1}$ | $\varepsilon_a$, km$^{-1}$ |
| 5 | 1.450 − 03 | 1.639 − 03 | 1.427 − 03 | 1.572 − 03 |
| 6 | 2.485 − 03 | 2.809 − 03 | 2.447 − 03 | 2.694 − 03 |
| 7 | 1.450 − 03 | 1.639 − 03 | 1.427 − 03 | 1.572 − 03 |
| 8 | 1.036 − 03 | 1.171 − 03 | 1.020 − 03 | 1.122 − 03 |
| 9 | 6.213 − 04 | 7.023 − 04 | 6.117 − 04 | 6.735 − 04 |
| 10 | 2.628 − 03 | 2.871 − 03 | 2.325 − 03 | 2.508 − 03 |
| 11 | 1.752 − 03 | 1.914 − 03 | 1.550 − 03 | 1.672 − 03 |
| 12 | 8.760 − 04 | 9.57  − 04 | 7.750 − 04 | 8.360 − 04 |
| 13 | 3.540 − 04 | 3.828 − 04 | 3.100 − 04 | 3.344 − 04 |
| 14 | 3.330 − 04 | 3.598 − 04 | 2.926 − 04 | 3.128 − 04 |
| 15 | 4.995 − 04 | 5.397 − 04 | 4.389 − 04 | 4.692 − 04 |
| 16 | 6.660 − 04 | 7.196 − 04 | 5.852 − 04 | 6.256 − 04 |
| 17 | 1.665 − 03 | 1.799 − 03 | 1.463 − 03 | 1.564 − 03 |
| 18 | 2.498 − 03 | 2.698 − 03 | 2.194 − 03 | 2.346 − 03 |
| 19 | 1.665 − 03 | 1.799 − 03 | 1.463 − 03 | 1.564 − 03 |
| 20 | 1.166 − 03 | 1.259 − 03 | 1.024 − 03 | 1.095 − 03 |
| 25 | 1.702 − 04 | 1.801 − 04 | 1.461 − 04 | 1.541 − 04 |
| 30 | 3.574 − 04 | 3.782 − 04 | 3.068 − 04 | 3.236 − 04 |
| 35 | 3.759 − 05 | 3.903 − 05 | 2.768 − 05 | 2.856 − 05 |
| 40 | 1.253 − 05 | 1.301 − 05 | 9.225 − 06 | 9.520 − 06 |
| 50 | 1.002 − 05 | 1.041 − 05 | 7.380 − 06 | 7.616 − 06 |
| 60 | 2.506 − 06 | 2.602 − 06 | 1.845 − 06 | 1.904 − 06 |
| 70 | 6.265 − 07 | 6.505 − 07 | 4.612 − 07 | 4.760 − 07 |
| 80 | 2.506 − 07 | 2.602 − 07 | 1.845 − 07 | 1.904 − 07 |
| 90 | 8.771 − 08 | 9.107 − 08 | 6.458 − 08 | 6.664 − 08 |
| 100 | 3.76  − 08 | 3.903 − 08 | 2.768 − 08 | 2.856 − 08 |

[a] The numbers $-03, -04, \ldots, -08$, to the right of each entry gives the power of ten by which the
entry is to be multiplied.

during the period 1967–71. Calculations of the optical characteristics (volume aerosol extinction and scattering coefficients) have been carried out according to the exact Mie equations with allowance for the complex-valued refractive index. The value of the latter was determined on the basis of investigations of the chemical composition of the particulate substance under the assumption that all the compounds are mixed uniformly in the proportions obtained from chemical analysis. Finally, the magnitudes of the complex refractive indices used in the calculations are summarized in Table 3.11.

The height profile of the calculated particle concentration at heights above 5 km were representative of many measurements at middle latitudes (45 to 60°).

Table 3.13. Vertical Profiles of Aerosol Extinction and Scattering Coefficients at Wavelengths of 2.36 and 10.6 $\mu$m (Model of [114])[a]

| $H$, km | $\lambda = 2.36\ \mu$m | | $\lambda = 10.6\ \mu$m | |
| --- | --- | --- | --- | --- |
| | $\sigma$, km$^{-1}$ | $\varepsilon_a$, km$^{-1}$ | $\sigma$, km$^{-1}$ | $\varepsilon_a$, km$^{-1}$ |
| 5 | 1.226 −03 | 1.390 −03 | 3.652 −04 | 6.307 −04 |
| 6 | 2.102 −03 | 2.383 −03 | 6.262 −04 | 1.081 −03 |
| 7 | 1.280 −03 | 1.422 −03 | 3.804 −04 | 6.514 −04 |
| 8 | 8.761 −04 | 9.932 −04 | 2.609 −04 | 4.505 −04 |
| 9 | 5.256 −04 | 5.958 −04 | 1.565 −04 | 2.703 −04 |
| 10 | 1.954 −03 | 2.151 −03 | 4.440 −04 | 7.804 −04 |
| 11 | 1.303 −03 | 1.434 −03 | 2.960 −04 | 5.203 −04 |
| 12 | 6.515 −04 | 7.171 −04 | 1.481 −04 | 2.601 −04 |
| 13 | 2.606 −04 | 2.868 −04 | 5.921 −05 | 1.042 −04 |
| 14 | 1.992 −04 | 2.212 −04 | 6.151 −05 | 1.020 −04 |
| 15 | 2.988 −04 | 3.318 −04 | 9.225 −05 | 1.530 −04 |
| 16 | 3.984 −04 | 4.424 −04 | 1.230 −04 | 2.041 −04 |
| 17 | 9.961 −04 | 1.106 −03 | 3.075 −04 | 5.102 −04 |
| 18 | 1.494 −03 | 1.659 −03 | 4.612 −04 | 7.653 −04 |
| 19 | 9.961 −04 | 1.106 −03 | 3.075 −04 | 5.102 −04 |
| 20 | 6.972 −04 | 7.742 −04 | 2.152 −04 | 3.571 −04 |
| 25 | 9.481 −05 | 1.021 −04 | 7.459 −06 | 1.248 −05 |
| 30 | 1.991 −04 | 2.144 −04 | 1.566 −05 | 2.620 −05 |
| 35 | 9.726 −06 | 1.053 −05 | 2.960 −07 | 8.007 −07 |
| 40 | 3.242 −06 | 3.511 −06 | 9.868 −08 | 2.669 −07 |
| 50 | 2.593 −06 | 2.808 −06 | 7.894 −08 | 2.135 −07 |
| 60 | 6.484 −07 | 7.022 −07 | 1.973 −08 | 5.338 −08 |
| 70 | 1.621 −07 | 1.755 −07 | 4.934 −09 | 1.334 −08 |
| 80 | 6.501 −08 | 7.051 −08 | 1.992 −09 | 5.342 −09 |
| 90 | 2.269 −08 | 2.457 −08 | 6.907 −10 | 1.868 −09 |
| 100 | 9.726 −09 | 1.053 −08 | 2.960 −10 | 8.001 −10 |

[a]See footnote to Table 3.12.

The results of the calculations of the aerosol scattering ($\sigma_a$) and extinction ($\varepsilon_a$) coefficients are given in Tables 3.12 and 3.13. At heights below 5 km, the calculations were carried out with regard for the exponential decay of the aerosol concentration with height, as in Elterman's model. The computational procedure was as follows: The quantity $\sigma_a(0)$ was determined at the earth's surface either experimentally or analytically; the empirical coefficient $H_a$ in the relation $\sigma_a(H) = \sigma_a(0)\exp(-H/H_a)$ is calculated, where $\sigma_a(H)$ is evaluated at $H = 5$ km according to Tables 3.12 and 3.13; the scattering (or attenuation) coefficient at any height $H \leqslant 5$ km is calculated for the known quantities $\sigma_a(0)$ and $H_a$.

Further details on the optical models of the aerosol atmosphere, including the results of detailed experimental studies of the optical and microphysical characteristics of various aerosols may be found in Zuev and Kabanov [115].

# 4

# Propagation of Laser Radiation in a Turbulent Atmosphere

## 4.0. Introduction

In addition to energy losses associated with absorption and scattering effects and refraction-induced variations of the trajectory, a laser beam propagating in the atmosphere also experiences amplitude and phase fluctuations due to the random space–time distribution of the refractive index of the medium. Turbulent fluctuations of the refractive index are caused by disordered turbulent air mixing and, accordingly, temperature variations.

Estimates show that a 1°C variation of the air temperature is accompanied by an order of $10^{-6}$ variation of the refractive index. The amplitude of the observed air-temperature fluctuations at a given point attains tenths of a degree Celsius. The period of the fluctuations varies from a few milliseconds to several seconds. The amplitude of the temperature fluctuations along horizontal paths in the atmosphere can attain several degrees for points situated at distances of the order of $10^2$ to $10^3$ m [1].

Inasmuch as the atmosphere is always turbulent, it is particularly important to study the laws by which turbulence affects the parameters of laser radiation, both from the standpoint of purely scientific interests and more specifically in connection with the extraordinary possibilities afforded by the application of lasers in communications systems, data-transmission systems, linear and angular distance-measuring facilities, etc.

The turbulent state of the atmosphere disrupts the coherence of laser radiation and can, therefore, limit the capabilities of lasers in devices that utilize the coherence property. Wave front distortions induced by turbulent fluctuations of the refractive index elicit broadening of laser beams, random variations of the position of the beam "centroid," redistribution of the beam energy within the cross section, and related intensity fluctuations.

It is quite clear at this time that the entire set of phenomena involving the interaction of laser radiation with a turbulent atmosphere must be understood and taken into account in designing the sundry laser systems intended for operation in the atmosphere in order to be able to articulate the technical specifications for a particular system. On the other hand, knowledge of the indicated laws is essential to the solution of the corresponding inverse problems in laser monitoring of the characteristics of atmospheric turbulence. Finally, it is important in connection with the development of means for compensating the influence of turbulence on laser parameters, i.e., so-called adaptive systems.

The intention of this chapter is to delineate the present state of the problem of the propagation of laser radiation in a turbulent atmosphere on the basis of all available fundamental results of theoretical and experimental research conducted in the last few years, including those discussed in earlier surveys [2, 3] and the author's previous book [1].

## 4.1 General

Air movements are characterized by disordered variations of both the magnitude and the direction of the velocity at any point. The result is vigorous mixing. Such motion is called turbulent, as distinct from laminar motion in which mixing does not occur and the velocity at a given point is either constant or varies in a regular fashion.

The transition from laminar to turbulent motion takes place at a definite critical value of the Reynolds number [4]:

$$\mathrm{Re} = uL/\nu_m$$

where $u$ is a characteristic velocity, $L$ is a characteristic space scale of the flow process, and $\nu_m$ is the kinematic viscosity.

In the ground layer of the atmosphere, for a height $L = 2$ m, characteristic velocities $u = 1$–$5$ m/sec, and $\nu_m = 0.15$ cm$^2$/sec, the Reynolds numbers have values $\mathrm{Re} = (2.5$–$7) \times 10^5$, i.e., are very large, and so the motion is highly turbulent.

Turbulent air motion represents a set of vortices of various diameters, from extremely large with a characteristic scale $L_0$ to extremely small with a scale $l_0$. The value of $L_0$ is determined by the space scale of the flow on the whole and is called the outer turbulence scale. Under the influence of inertial forces, large vortices break up into smaller ones. This cascade process of the breakup of vortices continues until the Reynolds numbers attain values of unit order and viscous forces begin to play a decisive role in comparison with the inertial forces. The scale $l_0$ is customarily referred to as the inner turbulence scale. The interval of scales between $L_0$ and $l_0$ is called inertial in connection with the fact that vortices falling within this interval of scales behave mainly in accordance with the action of the inertial forces. Vortices with scales $r \leqslant l_0$ belong to the viscous dissipation interval.

The cascade mechanism of transfer of kinetic energy from larger vortices to smaller ones is constantly maintained in the atmosphere through external sources of energy, which feed the overall flow of moving air. The dissipation of kinetic energy is realized in the smallest vortices.

The scale $L_0$, as mentioned, is determined by the total flux. Thus, the value of $L_0$ in the ground layer is of the order of the height of the point of observation, and even though larger vortices may be present in the flow, they are perceived in this case merely as variations of the total flux. The scale $l_0$ is of the order of 1 to 10 mm near the earth's surface.

The field of fluctuations of the refractive index $n_1(\mathbf{r})$ of a medium containing random inhomogeneities is normally characterized by the structure function, which in the case of real random functions is written in the form [4]

$$D_n(\mathbf{r}) = \left\langle \left[ n_1(\mathbf{r}_1 + \mathbf{r}) - n_1(\mathbf{r}_1) \right]^2 \right\rangle \tag{4.1}$$

where the angle brackets signify statistical averaging. The quantity $D_n(\mathbf{r})$ represents the mean-square increment of the refractive index between the points $\mathbf{r}_1 + \mathbf{r}$ and $\mathbf{r}_1$.

Index fluctuations in the optical wavelength range, at least within the atmospheric windows, are generated mainly by temperature microfluctuations, which, in turn, occur as a result of turbulent mixing of atmospheric air layers having different temperatures on the average. The temperature fluctuations are also characterized by a structure function

$$D_T(\mathbf{r}) = \left\langle \left[ T(\mathbf{r}_1 + \mathbf{r}) - T(\mathbf{r}_1) \right]^2 \right\rangle \tag{4.2}$$

The functions $D_n(\mathbf{r})$ and $D_T(\mathbf{r})$ for locally homogeneous and isotropic turbulence, according to hypotheses advanced by Kolmogorov and Obukhov [5, 6], are described in the inertial interval by the Kolmogorov–

Obukhov two-thirds law:

$$D_n(\mathbf{r}) = C_n^2 r^{2/3}, \qquad l_0 \ll r \ll L_0 \qquad\qquad (4.3)$$

$$D_T(\mathbf{r}) = C_T^2 r^{2/3}, \qquad l_0 \ll r \ll L_0 \qquad\qquad (4.4)$$

The quantities $C_n^2$ and $C_T^2$ are called the structural characteristics of the index and temperature fields, respectively. The characteristic $C_T^2$ is given by the expression [4]

$$C_T^2 = C_\nu^2 \varepsilon_T \varepsilon_k^{-1/3} \qquad\qquad (4.5)$$

in which $C_\nu$ is a number determined from the experimental data, $\varepsilon_T$ is the rate of equalization of the temperature inhomogeneities per unit mass measured in $({}^\circ K)^2 sec^{-1}$, and $\varepsilon_k$ is the rate of dissipation of kinetic energy per unit mass measured in $cm^2 sec^{-3}$.

For dry air, $C_n^2$ is related to $C_T^2$ as follows:

$$C_n = \frac{10^{-6}}{T}\left(\frac{77.6P}{T} + \frac{0.584P}{T\lambda^2}\right) C_T = 10^{-6} N_{0,\infty} \frac{288}{T} \frac{P}{1013} k(\lambda) C_T$$

$$(4.6)$$

where $P$ and $T$ are the pressure and temperature, $\lambda$ is the wavelength, $N_{0,\infty} = 273$ is the refractivity of dry air in the radio range under standard conditions $P = 1013$ mbar and $T = 288^\circ K$, $k(\lambda) = N_\lambda / N_\infty$, $N_\lambda$ is the refractivity at wavelength $\lambda$: $N_\lambda = (n_\lambda - 1) \cdot 10^6$, and $n_\lambda$ is the refractive index.

The data of Table 4.1, obtained at a height of 2.5 m in the July–August period of 1964–69 in Tsimlyansk [7], provide a clear notion of the nature of $C_n^2$ in the ground layer over an open level territory. The table gives the percentage repeatability of the values of $C_n^2$ at different times of day.

The values of $C_T^2$ and $C_n^2$ vary both with height and in horizontal directions, thereby mirroring the presence of inhomogeneities of the wind-velocity and temperature gradients in space and time.

**Table 4.1.** Distribution of Values of $C_n^2$ by Time of Day [7]

| Time of day (clock time) | $C_n^2$, $cm^{-2/3}$ | | | | |
|---|---|---|---|---|---|
| | $0.2 \times 10^{-16}$ | $(0.25\text{--}2.5)$ $\times 10^{-16}$ | $(0.25\text{--}2.5)$ $\times 10^{-15}$ | $(0.25\text{--}2.5)$ $\times 10^{-14}$ | $2.5 \times 10^{-14}$ |
| Midday (1115–1515) | 0.2 | 0.8 | 12.2 | 83.5 | 3.4 |
| Evening (1615–1845) | 8.4 | 16.8 | 48.8 | 26.0 | — |
| Night (1915–2345) | 1.0 | 10.5 | 69.6 | 19.0 | — |

The most complete data of measurements of $C_T^2$ at various heights from 50 m to 5 km have been obtained in aircraft measurements [8–10]. All the $C_T^2$ profiles are divided [10] into three groups: The first group includes situations in which $C_T^2$ is practically invariant with the height, the third group is characterized by a very abrupt variation of $C_T^2$ with height, and, finally, the second group comprises intermediate cases.

An analysis of the data shows that the behavior of the vertical $C_T^2$ profiles are most substantially influenced by the value of $P$ at a height of 50 m. Thus, the ground layer exerts a significant influence on the shape of the vertical $C_T^2$ profiles up to heights of several kilometers.

Byzova and Vyal'tseva [11] have published statistically supported data on the height profiles of $C_T^2$ obtained by means of a meteorological tower, indicating that in the atmospheric layer up to a height of 50 m, even in the presence of unstable temperature stratification, the height profile of $C_n^2(z)$ is close to the law $C_n^2(z) \sim z^{-2/3}$, whereas heights greater than 50 m are characterized by the law $C_n^2(z) \sim z^{-4/3}$.

A more comprehensive compilation of data on the vertical profiles of $C_n^2(z)$ and $C_T^2(z)$ is presented in the author's book [4], in which an analysis of the data leads to the conclusion that the values of $C_n^2$, as a rule, diminish with height, the most rapid decay taking place in the bottom kilometer layer of the atmosphere.

For a complete description of the propagation of laser radiation in a turbulent atmosphere it is necessary to know the probability distribution function of the radiation field. The probability density function of a random function yields a complete description of that function, but its determination usually presents an extremely complicated problem. It is customary, therefore, to describe the random functions in terms of the moments of the distribution, which in the case of a univariate random function are given by the relation

$$M_t^{(n)}(f) = \left\langle [f(t)]^n \right\rangle = \int_{-\infty}^{\infty} f_1^n P_t(f_1)\, df_1 \qquad (4.7)$$

in which $f(t)$ is a random function of the argument $t$, $n$ is the order of its moment, and $P_t(f_1)$ is the density function, which depends on the arguments $t$ and $f_1$ and satisfies the normalization condition $\int_{-\infty}^{\infty} P_t(f)\, df = 1$ as well as the positivity condition $P_t(f_1) \geqslant 0$ for all $t$.

It follows from expression (4.7) that the first moment of the random function is its mean value. The variance $\sigma_f^2$ is expressed in terms of the first and second moments:

$$\sigma_f^2 = \left\langle (f - \langle f \rangle)^2 \right\rangle = M_t^{(2)}(f) - \left[ M_t^{(1)}(f) \right]^2 \qquad (4.8)$$

If the random function is the field $U(\mathbf{r})$ of a laser beam, then the first moment, or $\langle U(\mathbf{r})\rangle$, characterizes the coherent component of the wave field in a turbulent medium. The second moment, or second-order cross-correlation function $\Gamma_2 = \langle U(\mathbf{r}_1)U^*(\mathbf{r}_2)\rangle$, for identical observation points characterizes the directional intensity distribution of the radiation scattered in a randomly inhomogeneous medium. The fourth moment, or fourth-order coherence function $\Gamma_4 = \langle U(\mathbf{r}_1)U^*(\mathbf{r}_2)U(\mathbf{r}_3)U^*(\mathbf{r}_4)\rangle$ describes the intensity fluctuations of the laser radiation.

We now give several other definitions pertinent to the given problem and necessary in the ensuing discussion. The random spatial modulation of the intensity in the beam cross section is characterized by the relative variance $\sigma_I^2$, which is given by the equation

$$\sigma_I^2(\mathbf{R}) = \langle I^2(\mathbf{R})\rangle / \langle I(\mathbf{R})\rangle^2 - 1 \tag{4.9}$$

in which $I(\mathbf{R}) = U(\mathbf{R})U^*(\mathbf{R})$ is the random value of the intensity at a point $\mathbf{R}$ of the observation plane.

The degree of statistical coupling between the random values of the intensity in the beam cross section is described by the correlation coefficient $b_I$:

$$b_I = \frac{\langle I(\mathbf{R}_1)I(\mathbf{R}_2)\rangle - \langle I(\mathbf{R}_1)\rangle\langle I(\mathbf{R}_2)\rangle}{\left[\left(\langle I^2(\mathbf{R}_1)\rangle - \langle I(\mathbf{R}_1)\rangle^2\right)\left(\langle I^2(\mathbf{R}_2)\rangle - \langle I(\mathbf{R}_2)\rangle^2\right)\right]^{1/2}} \tag{4.10}$$

where $\mathbf{R}_1$ and $\mathbf{R}_2$ are the radius vectors of points in the observation plane. The distance at which the correlation coefficient decreases to the $1/e$ level is called the correlation radius.

For homogeneous isotropic fields, the correlation function $B_{ff}(r)$ depends only on the distance between observation points and can be written in Fourier integral form [4]:

$$B_{ff}(r) = 2\int_0^\infty V_{ff}(\kappa)\cos\kappa r\, d\kappa \tag{4.11}$$

where $V_{ff}$ is the one-dimensional spectrum of the random field $f(\mathbf{r})$.

The interrelationship between the correlation function and the three-dimensional spectrum in the case of homogeneous isotropic fields is expressed by the equations

$$B_{ff}(r) = 4\pi\int_0^\infty \Phi_{ff}(\kappa)\frac{\sin\kappa r}{\kappa r}\kappa^2\, d\kappa \tag{4.12}$$

$$\Phi_{ff}(\kappa) = \frac{1}{2\pi^2}\int_0^\infty \frac{\sin\kappa r}{\kappa r}B_{ff}(r)r^2\, dr \tag{4.13}$$

Using expressions (4.11) and (4.12), we can show that the three-dimensional and one-dimensional spectra are related by the expression

$$\Phi_{ff}(\kappa) = -\frac{1}{2\pi\kappa} \cdot \frac{dV(\kappa)}{d\kappa} \tag{4.14}$$

The one-dimensional spectrum can be calculated with the use of the structure function $D(r)$ according to the expressions

$$V_{ff}(\kappa) = \frac{1}{2\pi\kappa} \int_0^\infty D'(r)\sin\kappa r\, dr$$

$$V_{ff}(\kappa) = \frac{1}{2\pi\kappa^2} \int_0^\infty D''(r)\cos\kappa r\, dr \tag{4.15}$$

in which $\kappa$ is the spatial frequency. The expression in which the integral converges is the one used in the calculations.

If the expression $D(r) = Cr^\alpha$ $(0 < \alpha < 2)$ is used as the structure function, then on the basis of Eqs. (4.15) we obtain

$$V_{ff}(\kappa) = \frac{C\alpha}{2\pi\kappa^{\alpha+1}} \int_0^\infty x^{\alpha-1}\sin x\, dx, \qquad 0 < \alpha < 1$$

$$V_{ff}(\kappa) = \frac{C\alpha(\alpha-1)}{2\pi\kappa^{\alpha+1}} \int_0^\infty x^{\alpha-2}\cos x\, dx, \qquad 1 < \alpha < 2$$

whence it is clear that the power-law structure function $D(r) = Cr^\alpha$, $0 < \alpha < 2$, corresponds to a power-law spectrum $V_{ff}(\kappa) = A\kappa^{-\alpha-1}$, $A = (C/2\pi)\Gamma(1+\alpha)\sin(\pi\alpha/2)$. We note that power-law structure functions play a major role in the description of atmospheric turbulence.

An important characteristic of the fluctuations is the temporal spectrum

$$W_{ff}(\omega) = \frac{1}{\pi} \int_0^\infty \cos(\omega\tau)R_{ff}(\tau)\, d\tau \tag{4.16}$$

in which $R_{ff}(\tau)$ is the temporal autocorrelation function and $\omega$ is the cyclic frequency.

When the "frozen turbulence" hypothesis holds, implying that the random field is transported with a constant velocity $v$, thereby remaining stationary in a moving coordinate system:

$$f(r, t + t_1) = f(r - vt_1, t)$$

both the one-dimensional and the three-dimensional spatial spectra can be expressed in terms of the temporal spectrum in the form

$$V_{ff}(\omega/v) = vW(\omega) \tag{4.17}$$

$$\Phi_{ff}(\kappa) = -\frac{v^3}{2\pi\omega} \frac{dW_{ff}(\omega)}{d\omega} \tag{4.18}$$

These relations play an important role because it is considerably easier in practice to measure the frequency spectra than the spatial spectra.


## 4.2. Turbulence Broadening of a Laser Beam in the Atmosphere

A laser beam propagating in a turbulent atmosphere is broadened as a result of losses of spatial coherence of the wave field. As a consequence of this effect, the average or effective width of a beam in a turbulent atmosphere is greater than its width in vacuum.

Let us suppose that a radiation source is situated in the plane $x' = 0$, and let the effective width of the beam in the turbulent atmosphere be denoted by $\rho_e(x)$. The value of $\rho_e(x)$ can be determined from the decay of the average radiation intensity $\langle I(x, \rho) \rangle$ at, say, the $1/e$ level. The distribution function $I(x, \rho)$ coincides with the second-order coherence function $\Gamma_2(x, \rho, \rho) = \langle U(x, \rho)U^*(x, \rho) \rangle$ for identical observation points, where $U(x, \rho)$ is the field of the beam in the plane $x' = x = \text{const}$.

The coherence function $\Gamma_2(x, \rho_1, \rho_2)$ satisfies the second-order partial differential equation [2–4]

$$2ik\frac{\partial\Gamma_2(x, \rho_1, \rho_2)}{\partial x} + (\Delta_1 - \Delta_2)\Gamma_2 + \frac{i\pi k^3}{2}H(x, \rho_1 - \rho_2)\Gamma_2 = 0 \tag{4.19}$$

in which

$$H(x, \rho) = 8\int d^2\kappa \; \Phi_n(x, \kappa)(1 - \cos\kappa\rho)$$

is expressed in terms of the spectrum of index fluctuations in the atmosphere.

The following solution has been obtained [12–14] for Eq. (4.19):

$$\Gamma_2\left(x,\mathbf{R}+\frac{\boldsymbol{\rho}}{2},\mathbf{R}-\frac{\boldsymbol{\rho}}{2}\right)=\frac{k^2}{4\pi^2x^2}\int d^2R'\int d^2\rho'\Gamma_2^0\left(\mathbf{R}'+\frac{\boldsymbol{\rho}'}{2},\mathbf{R}'-\frac{\boldsymbol{\rho}'}{2}\right)$$

$$\times\exp\left\{\frac{ik}{x}(\mathbf{R}-\mathbf{R}')(\boldsymbol{\rho}-\boldsymbol{\rho}')-\frac{\pi k^2x}{4}\int_0^1 d\xi H\right.$$

$$\left.\times\left[\frac{\boldsymbol{\xi}}{x},\left|\frac{\xi}{x}\boldsymbol{\rho}+\left(1-\frac{\xi}{x}\right)\boldsymbol{\rho}'\right|\right]\right\} \tag{4.20}$$

In expression (4.20), $\Gamma_2^0(\mathbf{R}+\boldsymbol{\rho}/2,\mathbf{R}-\boldsymbol{\rho}/2)=\langle U_0(\mathbf{R}+\boldsymbol{\rho}/2)U_0(\mathbf{R}-\boldsymbol{\rho}/2)\rangle$ is the initial value of the coherence function.

Normally the statistical characteristics of laser radiation in a turbulent atmosphere are analyzed [4] for the model of a single-mode Gaussian beam, the complex amplitude of whose field in the plane of the emitting aperture is written in the form

$$U_0(\boldsymbol{\rho})=U_0\exp\left(-\frac{\rho^2}{2a^2}-\frac{ik\rho^2}{2F}\right) \tag{4.21}$$

where $U_0$ is the source amplitude, $a$ is the effective beam radius, $F$ is the radius of curvature of the phase front of the beam at the center of the aperture, $k=2\pi/\lambda$ is the wave number, and $\lambda$ is the radiation wavelength. In the case of the beam (4.21), the expression for the average intensity $\langle I(x,\mathbf{R})\rangle=\Gamma_2(x,\mathbf{R},\mathbf{R})$ given by (4.20) is reducible to a single integral, which can then be analyzed [12–14] by numerical and asymptotic methods for any set of turbulent conditions of propagation and any beam parameters $a$ and $F$. In later papers [15, 16], a Gaussian approximation has been proposed for the average intensity:

$$\langle I(x,\boldsymbol{\rho})\rangle=|U_0^2|\frac{a^2}{\rho_e^2}\exp\left(-\frac{\rho^2}{\rho_e^2}\right) \tag{4.22}$$

where

$$\rho_e(x)=a\left[\left(1-\frac{x}{F}\right)^2+\Omega^{-2}\left(1+\frac{4}{3}\frac{a^2}{\rho_0^2}\right)\right]^{1/2} \tag{4.23}$$

$\Omega=ka^2/x$ is the Fresnel parameter of the emitting aperture and $\rho_0=$

$(1.45C_n^2k^2x)^{-3/5}$ is the coherence radius of a plane wave in the turbulent atmosphere (see Section 4.3 below).

Within 4% error limits, expression (4.22) coincides in the domain $\rho \lesssim \rho_e$ with the results of numerical calculations [12–14].

In the event of focusing of radiation, i.e., for $x/F=1$, Eq. (4.23) assumes the form

$$\rho_e(x) = \frac{x}{k}\left(\frac{1}{a^2} + \frac{4}{3\rho_0^2}\right)^{1/2} \tag{4.24}$$

whence we infer that the effect of saturation of focusing of the beam takes place [13] in the turbulent atmosphere. Thus, in the propagation of radiation in vacuum, the quantity $\rho_e(x)=x/ka$ for $x/F=1$, and so the size of the focal spot can be made as small as desired by an appropriate increase of the radius $a$. In a turbulent atmosphere with $a \gg \rho_0$, the quantity $\rho_e(x)$ no longer depends on the size of the emitting aperture and becomes saturated at the value

$$\rho_e(x) = \frac{2}{\sqrt{3}}\,\frac{x}{k\rho_0} \tag{4.25}$$

It is readily perceived that the broadening of a laser beam in a turbulent atmosphere leads to a corresponding reduction in the intensity and, hence, with the use of highly directional detection systems, in which case the whole beam cannot be captured, to a reduction in the received signal level, which can be interpreted as an apparent reduction in the transmittance of the atmosphere in connection with its turbulence.

The results of calculations of $\rho_e(x)$ according to expressions (4.22) and (4.23) are in satisfactory agreement with the corresponding experimental data obtained in measurements [17–21] of the effective widths of laser beams and average intensities under various conditions of propagation in the atmosphere (different values of the parameter $\rho_0$), as well as for various values of $a$ and $F$.

Mironov and Khmelevtsov [22] have investigated the broadening of laser beams due to atmospheric turbulence in connection with the propagation of radiation along slant paths. The results of this work indicate that expressions (4.22) and (4.23) can be used to determine the beam broadening in the case of slant paths, except that the actual path length in the expression for $\rho_0$ must be replaced by the equivalent distance

$$X(x,\Theta)=\frac{x}{C_n^2(h_0)}\int_0^1 C_n^2\left(\frac{\xi}{x},\Theta\right)\left(1-\frac{\xi}{x}\right)^{5/3}d\xi$$

which is governed by the height profile of the structural characteristic $C_n^2(\xi/x,\Theta)/C_n^2(h_0)$ and the zenith angle of the path $\Theta$, and $C_n^2$ must be replaced by the expression $C_n^2(h_0)$, which is equal to the value of the structural characteristic at the point of the emitting aperture. The values of the equivalent distances for certain profiles are given in [22].

An ideal Gaussian distribution of the beam field at the exit aperture cannot always be realized, either because of certain technical constraints on the construction of the optical emitting system, or because of the multiple-mode nature of the laser radiation, or finally, in the application of higher transverse laser modes. Aspects of the calculation of the average intensity of a laser beam emitted in a turbulent atmosphere by an aperture of the Cassegrainian type and of the transformation of the average intensity distribution in asymmetrical transverse modes due to atmospheric turbulence have been investigated in [23, 24], respectively. The multimode emission of laser sources is taken into consideration in [25].

Turbulent broadening of laser beams is primarily attributable, as we infer from expressions (4.22) and (4.23), to deterioration of the coherence of the laser field in the atmosphere (decrease of the parameter $\rho_0$). In the next section, we discuss the problems of distortion of the coherence of the laser field in greater detail.

## 4.3. Distortion of Coherence of the Field of a Laser Beam in a Turbulent Atmosphere

The spatial coherence of the field of an optical wave is characterized [26] by the degree of coherence

$$\gamma\left(x,\mathbf{R}+\frac{\rho}{2},\mathbf{R}-\frac{\rho}{2}\right)=\frac{\left|\Gamma_2\left(x,\mathbf{R}+\frac{\rho}{2},\mathbf{R}-\frac{\rho}{2}\right)\right|}{\Gamma_2^{1/2}\left(x,\mathbf{R}+\frac{\rho}{2},\mathbf{R}+\frac{\rho}{2}\right)\Gamma_2^{1/2}\left(x,\mathbf{R}-\frac{\rho}{2},\mathbf{R}-\frac{\rho}{2}\right)}$$

$$(4.26)$$

The space scale of decay of the degree of coherence $\gamma(x,\mathbf{R}+\boldsymbol{\rho}/2,\mathbf{R}-\boldsymbol{\rho}/2)$ with respect to the difference coordinate $\boldsymbol{\rho}=\boldsymbol{\rho}_1-\boldsymbol{\rho}_2$, say by a factor $1/e$, is called the spatial coherence radius. The coherence radius characterizes the distance at which the random difference in the phase angles of wave front approaches the value $\pi$, so that with any further separation of the observation points the wave front loses its cophasality.

In the simplest case of an unbounded plane ($a\to\infty$) or spherical ($a\to0$) wave, the degree of coherence is deduced from (4.20) and (4.26) in the form

$$\gamma(x,\rho)=\exp\left[-\left(\frac{\rho}{\rho_c}\right)^{5/3}\right] \tag{4.27}$$

where

$$\rho_c=\rho_0=\left(1.45C_n^2k^2x^2\right)^{-3/5} \tag{4.28}$$

$$\rho_c=\rho_s=\left(0.55C_n^2k^2x^2\right)^{-3/5} \tag{4.29}$$

for a plane wave and a spherical wave, respectively. The coherence radius decreases with an increase in the path length and the intensity of turbulent microfluctuations as well as in transition to shorter wavelengths.

Equation (4.27) has been tested experimentally [27] by measuring the distribution of the average intensity in the focal plane of a receiving lens illuminated through the atmosphere by a broad collimated laser beam. The distribution measured in this way coincides well with the Fourier spectrum of the function (4.27).

The degree of coherence in a spatially confined laser beam under arbitrary conditions of propagation with focusing and spreading of the beam has been investigated in several papers [15, 28–32]. Belen'kii and Mironov [32] discovered that if the radius of the emitting aperture of the collimated beam satisfies the condition

$$\rho_0\ll a\ll\frac{x}{k\rho_0} \tag{4.30}$$

then, given the same turbulent conditions of propagation, the coherence radius of the field of the beam is greater than the corresponding values in unconfined plane and spherical waves. This effect is attributable to diffraction at the emitting aperture and is observed when the radius of the first Fresnel zone is much greater than the coherence radius of the field ($k\rho_0^2/x \ll 1$). The Gaussian approximation obtained in [32] for the degree of coherence of the field of the laser beam (4.21) has the form

$$\gamma(x, R, \rho) = \exp\left(-\frac{\rho^2}{\rho_c^2}\right) \tag{4.31}$$

where

$$\frac{\rho_c^2}{\rho_0^2} = \frac{[1-(x/F)]^2 + \Omega^{-2} + \frac{4}{3}(a^2/\rho_0^2)\Omega^{-2}}{1-(x/F) + \frac{1}{3}(x/F)^2 + \frac{1}{3}\Omega^{-2} + \frac{1}{3}(a^2/\rho_0^2)\Omega^{-2}} \tag{4.32}$$

Expressions (4.31) and (4.32) give values of the coherence radius $\rho_c$ that agree, within a maximum 5% error limits, with expressions (4.28) and (4.29) and with the results obtained for the case of confined beam [29, 30] by numerical calculations. We note that certain expressions analogous to (4.31) in other papers [15, 28] contain errors, which, in particular, lead to an incorrect value of the coherence radius in transition to a spherical wave as $\Omega \to 0$ and $x/F \to \infty$ in [15] and as $x/F \to \infty$ in [28].

It follows from (4.32) that the ratio of the coherence radius of the field of a collimated beam to the same quantity for a plane wave has the form

$$\frac{\rho_c^2}{\rho_0^2} = \frac{3(1+\Omega^{-2}) + 4(\Omega\Omega_0)^{-1}}{3 + \Omega^{-2} + (\Omega\Omega_0)^{-1}} \tag{4.33}$$

where $\Omega_0 = k\rho_0^2/x$.

It is readily verified on the basis of this result that if the coherence radius $\rho_0$ is greater than the radius of the first Fresnel zone ($\Omega_0 = k\rho_0^2/x \gg 1$), the value of the coherence radius $\rho_c$ will almost always fall between the values corresponding to plane and spherical waves, $\rho_0 \leqslant \rho_c \leqslant \rho_s$. An exception is the point $\Omega \simeq 1/12\Omega_0^2$, in the neighborhood of which the coherence radius slightly exceeds the spherical-wave value

$$\rho_c = 3^{1/2}\rho_0\left(1 + \Omega_0^2/72\right)^{1/2} \tag{4.34}$$

But if the coherence radius becomes smaller than the radius of the first Fresnel zone (and the inequality $k\rho_0^2/x \ll 1$ holds), then for values of the beam radius satisfying condition (4.30) the coherence radius acquires a maximum at the point $\Omega \simeq \frac{1}{3}(1-2\Omega_0)$, and the value of the coherence radius at the point of the maximum is approximately equal to $\rho_c = 2\rho_0(1 - \frac{3}{2}\Omega_0)^{1/2}$. In this case, therefore, we observe an appreciable excess of the coherence radius for the field of a spatially confined beam even in comparison with the

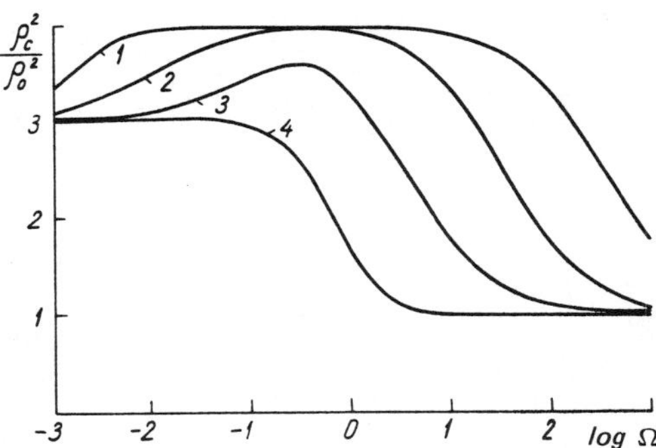

Fig. 4.1. Coherence radius of the field of a collimated beam in a turbulent atmosphere. (1) $\beta_0 = 16.5$; (2) 6.3; (3) 2.4; (4) 0.34.

coherence radius for a spherical wave. The correlation between the coherence radii for unconfined plane and spherical waves and a collimated laser beam propagating in a turbulent atmosphere under various atmospheric conditions (characterized by the parameter $\beta_0$) and various diameters of the emitting aperture, is illustrated in Fig. 4.1. It is evident from Fig. 4.1 that the increase in the coherence radius of the laser beam in comparison with unconfined waves as the parameter $\beta_0$ is decreased takes in an ever-increasing range of values of the aperture diameter in the interval specified by condition (4.30). The behavior of the coherence radius of the field of a partially coherent (multimode) laser beam propagating in a turbulent atmosphere has also been investigated in [32].

Experimental confirmation of the increase in the coherence radius in a spatially confined beam, quantitatively consistent with the values obtained from expression (4.33), has been obtained in [33]. The effects discussed above, i.e., violation of the spatial coherence of the laser field in a turbulent atmosphere and a concomitant increase in the angular spread of the beam, are mainly due to small-scale phase fluctuations of the wave front of the beam, where the scale of the fluctuations is much smaller than the transverse dimension of the beam. Large-scale phase fluctuations commensurate with the beam diameter or greater induce gross transverse displacements of the beam as a whole in space, i.e., random beam wander. This phenomenon will be discussed in the next section.

## 4.4. Random Wander of Laser Beams in a Turbulent Atmosphere

The displacement of spatially confined beams in a turbulent atmosphere was first observed long before the advent of lasers. The quivering of the image of an astronomical object at the focus of a telescope is typical, where the light beam is confined by focusing.

The intense interest in the study of fluctuations of the direction of propagation of laser beams in a turbulent atmosphere is stimulated by the need for appropriate data in support of the design of communications, information-transmission, geodesic, ranging, telemetry, and other laser-operated systems functioning in the atmosphere.

The theory of fluctuations of the centroid of a spatially confined beam in a turbulent atmosphere is essentially similar to the theory of displacements of the centroid of an image in the focal plane of a telescope [34]. The random displacements of a laser beam in the atmosphere have been studied theoretically in various approximations [14, 16, 35–43].

Using a Markov approximation and the parabolic equation approximation [2, 4], Tatarskii [14] and Klyatskin and Kon [36] have derived an expression for the centroid vector of a random distribution of the intensity in the plane transverse to the direction of propagation at a distance $x$ from the source:

$$\rho_c(x) = \frac{\int_0^x (x-\xi)\, d\xi \int d^2\rho\, I(\xi,\rho)\, \nabla_\rho n_1(\xi,\rho)}{\int d^2\rho\, I(\xi,\rho)} \tag{4.35}$$

where $n_1(\xi,\rho)$ is the fluctuation component of the refractive index. It is apparent from expression (4.35) that the centroid vector is determined by the transverse (to the direction of propagation) index gradient summed along the path over a scale of the order of the beam width. The same expression also implies that the main contribution to the value of $\rho_c(x)$ comes from inhomogeneities located near the emitting aperture ($\xi = 0$).

Inasmuch as the random intensity distribution $I(\xi,\rho)$ serves in (4.35) merely as a scale of summation of the index inhomogeneities, Klyatskin and Kon [36] postulate that this function can be replaced by its average value, $I(\xi,\rho) \cong \langle I(\xi,\rho) \rangle$, without incurring appreciable errors in the statistical characteristics of the centroid fluctuations. Qualitative estimates [16] have shown that this substitution is acceptable in the case of weak intensity fluctuations and is valid for strong fluctuations to the extent that the beam width exceeds the space scale of correlation of the intensity fluctuations. Quantitative estimates of the error of using the phase approximation of the Huygens–Kirchhoff method [44] for $I(\xi,\rho)$ were obtained in later papers [42, 43]. Expression (4.35) yields the following expression [4] for the variance

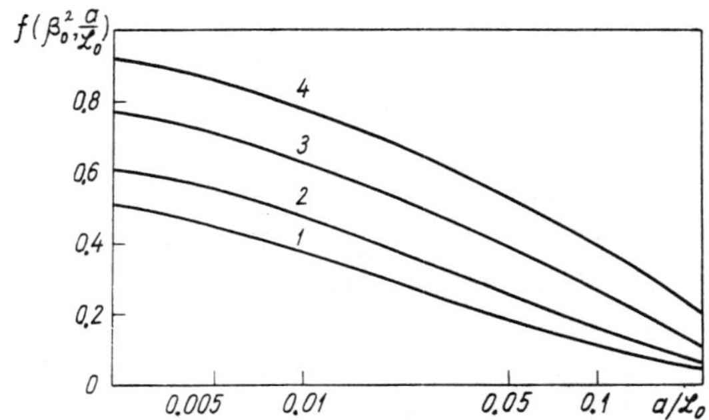

Fig. 4.2. Function $f(\beta_0^2, a/L_0)$, $x/F = 1$, $\Omega = 100$. 1) $\beta_0 = 108$; 2) 60; 3) 20; 4) 0.

of the centroid in the Fresnel zone of a collimated light beam of radius $a$:

$$\sigma_{c,0}^2 = 1.08 C_n^2 x^2 a^{1/2} \tag{4.36a}$$

Equation (4.36a) does not allow for the spreading of the beam due to diffraction and turbulent broadening. The influence of these factors has been investigated in detail in several papers [16, 36, 43] in which it is shown that they tend to decrease the variance of the displacements. When the size of the emitting aperture approaches the outer turbulence scale ($a/L_0 \sim 1$), an appreciable reduction of the variance of the centroid fluctuations is also observed [16]. The influence of the outer scale is particularly noticeable in beam propagation along ground-layer paths. Figure 4.2 gives the function $f(\beta_0^2, a/L_0)$ [16], which characterizes the reduction in the variance $\sigma_c^2 = \sigma_{c,0}^2 f_c$ with an increase in the effective turbulent thickness of the atmosphere as characterized by the parameter $\beta_0^2 = 1.23 C_n^2 k^{7/6} x^{11/6}$, and with an increase in the outer turbulence scale. If this factor is taken into account, deviations are observed from the linear relationship, characteristic of (4.36a), between the angular displacement of the beam axis $\sigma_c/x$ and the distance $x$.

As an example, Fig. 4.3 gives a comparison of the results of calculations according to expression (4.36a) and an experiment [45] for the variance of the displacements of the centroid of a laser beam along a ground-layer path. The data are fairly consistent with each other and indicate that turbulence-induced wandering of the beam axis in the real atmosphere can attain 8 to 10 angular seconds. On the whole, experimental data obtained over short paths by Gel'fer and others [46] are also consistent with expression (4.36a).

As mentioned, diffraction and turbulent spreading as well as the influence of the outer turbulence scale can cause the experimental data for

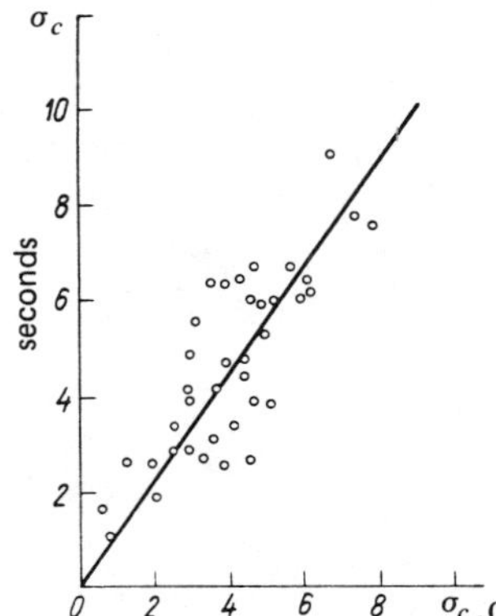



Fig. 4.3. Comparison of theory with experiment [9], $\Omega=86$, $x/F=1$, $\lambda=0.63\ \mu$m, $x=250$ m.

the variance to deviate from the values given by (4.36a). Such a deviation has been observed by V. Ya. S″edin over a long path ($x=18.5$ km) and has been noted in [3]. Mironov and Nosov [43] have taken the influence of the state factors into account and obtained the asymptotic expression

$$\sigma_c^2 = 1.77 \frac{a^2 D_s^{5/8}(2a)}{x^2 \Omega^{11/18}}\left[(1+\beta)^{7/48}-1\right]$$

$$+\frac{a^2 D_s^{1/2}(2a)}{x^2 \Omega^{3/2}}$$

$$\times\left\{0.5\beta^{-1/6}\left[(1+\beta)^{1/12}-1\right]+\kappa(\beta)\right\}+O\left(\frac{a^2 D_s^{2/5}(2a)}{x^2 \Omega^{4/3}}\right),$$

$$D_s(2a)\gg\Omega^{5/3}\max\left\{2^{11/15}\left(\Omega^{-2}+\frac{x^2}{F^2}\right)^{4/3},\right.$$

$$\left.\times 2^{47/15}\left|\frac{x}{F}\right|^{8/3},2^{5/6}(1+\beta)^{5/6},\beta^{-5/6}\Omega^{-5/3}2^{5/6}\right\}, \quad (4.36b)$$

$$\Omega\gtrsim 1,\qquad 0<\frac{x}{F}\leqslant 1$$

where $D_s(2a)=1.1C_n^2 k^2 x(2a)^{5/3}$ is the structure function of the phase fluctuations of a spherical wave, referred to the diameter of the emitting aperture:

$$\kappa(\beta)\simeq 1.86(1-1.22\beta^{-1/12}),\qquad \beta=L_0^2/2\pi^2 a\gg 1$$

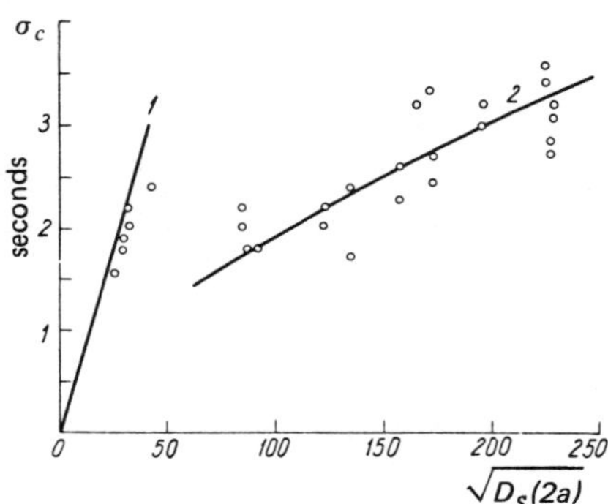

Fig. 4.4. Comparison of theory with experimental data of V. Ya. S″edin in [3], $\Omega = 18.4$, $x/F = 1$, $\lambda = 0.63$ $\mu$m, $x = 18.5$ km, $\beta = 0.73$. (1) According to (4.36a); (2) (4.36b).

Figure 4.4 gives the results of calculations according to expressions (4.36a) and (4.36b) and the experimental data of V. Ya. S″edin. It is evident from the data that allowances for turbulent spreading and a finite outer turbulence scale make it possible to obtain satisfactory agreement between theory and experiment in this case as well.

The spatial cross correlation of random displacements of laser beams propagating along parallel paths has been investigated theoretically [16, 37–39]. It is shown in this work that the correlation of the displacements of focused and collimated beams in the diffraction near zone $(ka^2/x \gg 1)$ decreases considerably when the centers of the emitting apertures are separated by a distance of the order of the aperture diameter $(r \sim 2a)$, while in the far zone $(ka^2/x \ll 1)$ the separation should be of the order of the diffraction width of the beam: $r \sim a_d = a[(1 - x/F)^2 + x^2/k^2a^4]^2$. If the spacing of the beams is greater than these scales, the form of the correlation function is determined [16, 38, 39] by the behavior of the spectrum of fluctuations of the refractive index in the region of the outer turbulence scale. The influence of the latter on the spatial correlation [16] is illustrated in Fig. 4.5. Experimental data for the spatial correlation of the beam displacements have been obtained along ground-layer paths [38, 47]. They agree satisfactorily, as shown in [38, 39], with the analytical results for an appropriate choice of outer turbulence scale.

A characteristic attribute of the frequency spectra [40] is their exponential decay in the frequency interval $f \gg f_0$, where $f_0 = v/\pi\sqrt{2}\,a$ is the fundamental frequency of the beam displacements and $v$ is the transverse component of the wind velocity. This fact indicates that frequencies $f > f_0$ scarcely contribute at all to the displacement spectrum. Beam focusing is significant in the diffraction near zone. The spectra of focused beams have an extended interval of power-law decay for $f > f_0$. A variation of the outer

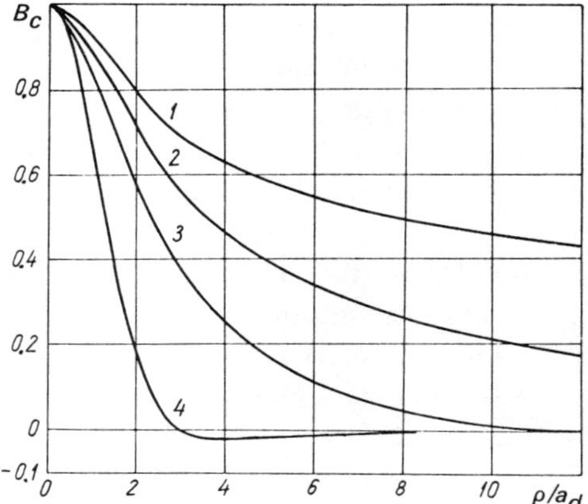

Fig. 4.5. Correlation coefficient of random displacements of parallel collimated laser beams for various outer space scales, $\Omega = 100$. (1) $\beta = L_0^2/2\pi^2 a^2 = \infty$; (2) $\beta = 10^3$; (3) 50; (4) 1.

scale dimensions is strongly felt in the beam displacement spectra. An increase in $L_0$ causes the beam displacements to acquire lower frequencies (Fig. 4.6). These conclusions have been corroborated by recent experimental work [48] over a horizontal ground-layer path.

The results of [16, 35–41] form the basis for calculating the random wander of a laser beam in a turbulent atmosphere as a whole as well as the correlation functions and spectra of the displacements for various propagation conditions. The approximation used in these studies, $I(x, \rho) \simeq \langle I(x, \rho) \rangle$, as we infer from [42, 43], is applicable to, for example, the case of a collimated beam if the size of the source aperture is much greater than the

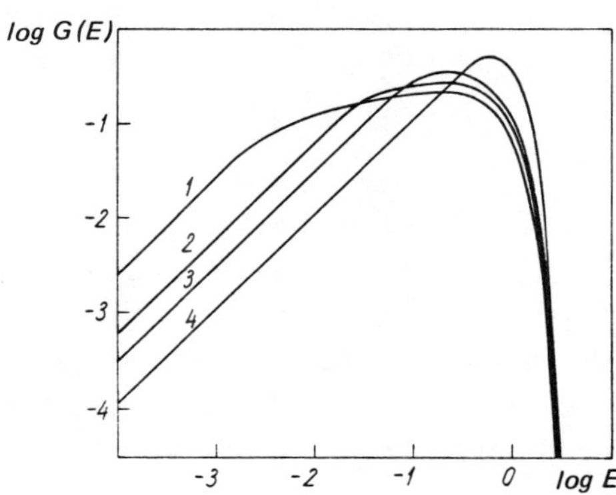

Fig. 4.6. Normalized temporal spectrum of the displacements of a collimated laser beam $G(E) = f W_c(f)/\sigma_c^2$, $E = f/f_0$, $\Omega = 100$. (1) $\beta = 10^5$; (2) $10^3$; (3) $10^2$; (4) 1.

diffraction scale at the coherence radius of the field $(a \gg x/k\rho_0)$ or, conversely, if it is much less than that quantity $(a \ll x/k\rho_0)$. Only in a certain intermediate range does this approximation give underestimated results for the variance of the deviations of the beam centroid, whereas the error for the correlation functions and normalized frequency spectra is clearly much smaller.

Besides beam wander in the plane transverse to the direction of propagation, the instantaneous pattern of illumination in its cross section is also a disordered product of interference between different parts of the wave front. The intensity fluctuations elicited by this kind of interference will be discussed in the next section.

## 4.5. Intensity Fluctuations of Laser Radiation in a Turbulent Atmosphere

The pattern of fluctuations of the intensity of a laser beam in a turbulent atmosphere depends essentially on the distance traveled by the beam for a fixed value of the turbulence strength and, conversely, on the turbulence strength for a fixed distance between source and receiver.

In the case of weak atmospheric turbulence or over the span of short paths, the relative intensity fluctuations are small. An increase in the path length or the turbulence strength is accompanied by an increase in the relative intensity fluctuations.

The conditions of propagation of a laser beam in a turbulent atmosphere are customarily [4] characterized by the parameter $\beta_0^2 = 1.23 C_n^2 k^{7/6} x^{11/6}$. This parameter is related to the ratio of the radius of the first Fresnel zone to the coherence radius (4.23) of the wave field in the turbulent medium according to the expression $\beta_0^2 \sim (x/k\rho_0^2)^{5/6}$. If $\beta_0^2$ is not greater than unity, the relative variance of the intensity fluctuations

$$\sigma_I^2 = \langle I^2 \rangle / \langle I \rangle^2 - 1$$

also turns out to be less than unity. Such conditions of optical wave propagation are usually referred to as the weak fluctuation region. When the parameter $\beta_0^2$ attains values of the order of unity and increases beyond that, the variance of the intensity fluctuations, accordingly, attains a maximum and then decreases slightly, tending to a finite limit. These propagation conditions refer to the strong fluctuation region.

According to the physical significance of the coherence radius (see Section 4.3), it is clear that the strong fluctuation region begins when the random phase difference over a distance equal to the first Fresnel zone attains a value of the order of $\pi$. This condition leads to strong random interference between different parts of the wave front during propagation in the turbulent medium and, hence, to strong intensity fluctuations. An exception is a focused beam in the atmosphere, where the parameter characterizing the corresponding fluctuation region is specified in terms of the ratio of the diameter of the focusing mirror to the coherence scale, $D_s(2a) \sim (2a/\rho_s)^{5/3}$. Inasmuch as focusing entails summation of the field from all points of the focusing aperture, rather than just from an area of the order of the first Fresnel zone, the replacement of the parameter $\beta_0^2$ by $D_s(2a)$ in this case is physically meaningful.

It is readily verified on the basis of the data in Table 4.1 that the boundary between weak and strong fluctuations of the dependence of the intensity of microfluctuations of the refractive index in the optical wavelength range for ground-layer paths in the atmosphere varies from a few tenths to several hundred meters in the case of collimated or divergent beams and can be decreased to a few meters in the focusing of radiation in the atmosphere by large apertures.

The smooth perturbation method (SPM) developed by Rytov is fully valid for the description of weak fluctuations. The results of application of this method are discussed in detail in books [4, 34, 49] and surveys [50, 51], from which we learn that is is applicable for describing the behavior of laser radiation over short paths or in the presence of weak turbulence. However, the greatest practical importance attaches primarily to long paths, where effects of multiple wave scattering by index fluctuations prevail. The magnitude of the relative intensity fluctuations in this case is of unit order and becomes saturated with any further increase in the path length and turbulence strength.

In this section, we consider the fundamental theoretical results and experimental data on the characteristics of the intensity fluctuations of laser radiation for various propagation conditions, resting mainly on the results of pertinent studies carried out in recent times.

## 4.5.1. Approximate Calculations of Strong Fluctuations

The calculations of strong fluctuations of the intensity of laser radiation propagating in the atmosphere are based on the equation for the fourth moment of the field [52–56] or the fourth-order cross-coherence function

$$\Gamma_4(x,\boldsymbol{\rho}_1,\boldsymbol{\rho}_2,\boldsymbol{\rho}_3,\boldsymbol{\rho}_4)=\langle U(x,\boldsymbol{\rho}_1)U^*(x,\boldsymbol{\rho}_2)U(x,\boldsymbol{\rho}_3)U^*(x,\boldsymbol{\rho}_4)\rangle$$

$$\frac{\partial}{\partial x}\Gamma_4(x,\boldsymbol{\rho}_1,\boldsymbol{\rho}_2,\boldsymbol{\rho}_3,\boldsymbol{\rho}_4)-\frac{i}{2k}(\Delta_1-\Delta_2+\Delta_3-\Delta_4)\Gamma_4+V\Gamma_4=0 \qquad (4.37)$$

where

$$V=\frac{\pi}{4}k^2\big[H(\boldsymbol{\rho}_1-\boldsymbol{\rho}_2)+H(\boldsymbol{\rho}_1-\boldsymbol{\rho}_4)+H(\boldsymbol{\rho}_2-\boldsymbol{\rho}_3)$$

$$+H(\boldsymbol{\rho}_3-\boldsymbol{\rho}_4)-H(\boldsymbol{\rho}_1-\boldsymbol{\rho}_3)-H(\boldsymbol{\rho}_2-\boldsymbol{\rho}_4)\big]$$

An exact solution of the equation for $\Gamma_4$ can be written in explicit form only in terms of continuous integrals [56, 57], the analysis of which, either numerical or analytical, is rather complicated. The first asymptotic solutions of the equation for the fourth moment were published by Shishov [58–60]. The method of solution proposed by him has been further elaborated in later papers [61–65]. In these studies, a description is given for the variance and spatial correlation of strong intensity fluctuations for a turbulent atmosphere in the region of saturation of the variance for the case in which the initial mode of radiation is a plane and a spherical wave. For a beam focused in the atmosphere, an approximate solution of the fourth-moment equation has been formulated by Gochelashvili [66–68]. This solution describes the saturated intensity fluctuations of a focused beam due to focusing by large apertures under conditions such that the intensity fluctuations of a plane or spherical wave are small, $\beta_0^2\lesssim1$. The results of [58–68] are generalized in a recent survey paper [3].

In later papers [69–73], simpler methods have been proposed for solving the equation for the fourth moment of the field in the case of a plane wave in the region of strong intensity fluctuations, yielding results identical to those given in [3]. Finally, Zavorotnyi and others [74] have very recently succeeded in obtaining asymptotic estimates of the continuous integrals and, in the case of a plane wave, arriving at results consistent with [3].

Along with the attempts to obtain an asymptotic ($\beta_0^2\gg1$) solution of Eq. (4.37), a different approach has been developed for solving the problem of intensity fluctuations of a laser beam [75–78]. As an approximate solution of the wave equation (in the parabolic approximation)

$$2ik\frac{\partial U(x',\boldsymbol{\rho}')}{\partial x'}+\Delta\rho'U(x',\boldsymbol{\rho}')+\frac{k^2}{2}n_1(x',\boldsymbol{\rho}')U(x',\boldsymbol{\rho}')=0 \qquad (4.38)$$

it is proposed that the representation for the complex amplitude in Huygens–Kirchhoff form [79, 80] be used:

$$U(x, \boldsymbol{\rho}) = \int d^2\rho' U_0(\boldsymbol{\rho}') G(x, x_0; \boldsymbol{\rho}, \boldsymbol{\rho}') \tag{4.39}$$

where $U_0(\boldsymbol{\rho}')$ is the initial distribution of the field in the plane of the emitting aperture $x' = x_0$, $G(x, x_0; \boldsymbol{\rho}, \boldsymbol{\rho}')$ is the field of a spherical wave propagating from the point $(x, \boldsymbol{\rho})$ to the point $(x_0, \boldsymbol{\rho}')$. The Green's function $G(x, x'; \boldsymbol{\rho}, \boldsymbol{\rho}')$ in this case is interpreted as the phase approximation

$$G(x, x'; \boldsymbol{\rho}, \boldsymbol{\rho}') \simeq G^0(x, x'; \boldsymbol{\rho}, \boldsymbol{\rho}') = G_0(x, x'; \boldsymbol{\rho}, \boldsymbol{\rho}') \exp\left[iS(x, x'; \boldsymbol{\rho}, \boldsymbol{\rho}')\right]$$

$$\tag{4.40}$$

where

$$G_0(x, x'; \boldsymbol{\rho}, \boldsymbol{\rho}') = k\left[2\pi i(x - x')\right]^{-1} \exp\left[\frac{ik}{2}(\boldsymbol{\rho} - \boldsymbol{\rho}')^2(x - x')^{-1}\right]$$

satisfies Eq. (4.38) in a homogeneous $[n_1(x', \boldsymbol{\rho}') \equiv 0]$ medium and the function

$$S(x, x'; \boldsymbol{\rho}, \boldsymbol{\rho}') = ik \int_{x'}^{x} d\xi\, n_1\left(\xi, \boldsymbol{\rho}\frac{\xi - x'}{x - x'} + \boldsymbol{\rho}'\frac{x - \xi}{x - x'}\right) \tag{4.41}$$

is equal to the random phase of a spherical wave, calculated in the first geometrical-optics approximation [34].

Banakh and Mironov [44] have found an integral equation, equivalent to (4.38), for the complex field amplitude:

$$U(x, \boldsymbol{\rho}) = \int d^2\rho' U_0(\boldsymbol{\rho}') G^0(x, x_0; \boldsymbol{\rho}, \boldsymbol{\rho}')$$

$$+ \frac{i}{2k} \int_{x_0}^{x} dx' \int d^2\rho' U(x', \boldsymbol{\rho}') G_0(x, x'; \boldsymbol{\rho}, \boldsymbol{\rho}') \Delta'$$

$$\times \Delta' \exp\left[iS(x, x'; \boldsymbol{\rho}, \boldsymbol{\rho}')\right] \tag{4.42}$$

in which the Huygens–Kirchhoff phase approximation (HKPA) is assigned to the role of the free term. Averaging of this equation shows that the average-field equation in the case of a homogeneous isotropic field of index fluctuations, subject to the condition that the path length is much greater than the outer scale of the field $n_1(x', \boldsymbol{\rho}')$, viz.,

$$\langle U(x, \boldsymbol{\rho}) \rangle = \int d^2\rho' U_0''(\boldsymbol{\rho}') \langle G^0(x, x_0; \boldsymbol{\rho}, \boldsymbol{\rho}') \rangle \tag{4.43}$$

strictly satisfies the equation obtained in the local small-perturbation approximation [3, 49] or in the Markov process approximation [2, 57].

The equation obtained by the same approach for the coherence function of order $2n$

$$\Gamma_{2n}(x, \boldsymbol{\rho}_1, \boldsymbol{\rho}_2, \ldots, \boldsymbol{\rho}_{2n-1}, \boldsymbol{\rho}_{2n})$$

$$= \langle U(x, \boldsymbol{\rho}_1) U^*(x, \boldsymbol{\rho}_2) \cdots U(x, \boldsymbol{\rho}_{2n-1}) U^*(x, \boldsymbol{\rho}_{2n}) \rangle$$

has the form

$$\Gamma_{2n}(x, \boldsymbol{\rho}_1, \ldots, \boldsymbol{\rho}_{2n}) = \Gamma_{2n}^0(x, \boldsymbol{\rho}_1, \ldots, \boldsymbol{\rho}_{2n}) + \frac{i}{2k} \int_0^x dx' \int d^2\rho_1' \cdots d^2\rho_{2n}'$$

$$\times \Gamma_{2n}(x', \boldsymbol{\rho}_1', \ldots, \boldsymbol{\rho}_{2n}') G_{2n,0}(x, x'; \boldsymbol{\rho}_1, \ldots, \boldsymbol{\rho}_{2n}, \boldsymbol{\rho}_1', \ldots, \boldsymbol{\rho}_{2n}')$$

$$\times \sum_{j=1}^{2n} (-1)^{j+1} \Delta j \left\langle \exp\left[ i \sum_{\nu=1}^{2n} (-1)^{\nu+1} S(x, x'; \boldsymbol{\rho}_\nu, \boldsymbol{\rho}_\nu') \right] \right\rangle$$

$$\tag{4.44}$$

where

$$\Gamma_{2n}^0(x, \boldsymbol{\rho}_1, \ldots, \boldsymbol{\rho}_{2n}) = \int d^2\rho_1' \cdots d^2\rho_{2n}' G_{2n,0}(x, x'; \boldsymbol{\rho}_1, \ldots, \boldsymbol{\rho}_{2n}, \boldsymbol{\rho}_1', \ldots, \boldsymbol{\rho}_{2n}')$$

$$\times \left\langle \exp\left[ i \sum_{j=1}^{2n} (-1)^{j+1} S(x, x_0; \boldsymbol{\rho}_j, \boldsymbol{\rho}_j') \right] \right\rangle$$

and

$$G_{2n,0}(x, x_0; \boldsymbol{\rho}_1, \ldots, \boldsymbol{\rho}_{2n}) = G_0(x, x_0; \boldsymbol{\rho}_1, \boldsymbol{\rho}_1') G_0^*(x, x_0; \boldsymbol{\rho}_2, \boldsymbol{\rho}_2')$$

$$\cdots G_{2n-1}(x, x_0; \boldsymbol{\rho}_{2n-1}, \boldsymbol{\rho}_{2n-1}')$$

$$G_{2n}^*(x, x_0; \boldsymbol{\rho}_{2n}, \boldsymbol{\rho}_{2n}')$$

is the phase approximation of the coherence function of order $2n$. In solving

Eq. (4.44) for $\Gamma_2(x, \boldsymbol{\rho}_1, \boldsymbol{\rho}_2)$ for the case of homogeneous isotropic turbulence for $x \gg L_0$ by the iterative method, the Neumann series is truncated at the first term. The resulting coherence function $\Gamma_2(x, \boldsymbol{\rho}_1, \boldsymbol{\rho}_2) = \Gamma_2^0(x, \boldsymbol{\rho}_1, \boldsymbol{\rho}_2)$ coincides with expression (4.20) and therefore obeys the equation (4.19) obtained in the local small-perturbation or Markov process approximation.

In the case of the fourth moment, the iterative series for Eq. (4.44) contains infinitely many terms. For the variance of the relative intensity fluctuations, the first term of the series, which coincides with the phase approximation, yields a uniform approximation to the solution in the case of a collimated laser beam under the condition $ka/x \gtrsim 1$, both in the weak ($\beta_0 < 1$) and in the strong ($\beta_0 \gtrsim 1$) intensity fluctuation region. Another advantage of the HKPA is the fact that it gives an explicit expression not only for the average field and average moments, but also for the complex amplitude and its statistical moments. These expressions represent simple quadratures and are useful for the solution of various practical problems such as occur, for example, in theoretical studies of the correlation·for turbulent distortions of the field of laser beams.

The characteristics of the intensity fluctuations of spatially confined beams has been investigated by numerical and asymptotic methods [62–64, 75–78] for weak and strong fluctuations as well as in the intermediate region of turbulent beam-propagation conditions. It is also important to cite a very recent study [81] in which the method of solution developed in [73] is used to obtain certain results for the variance of the intensity fluctuations in the saturation region for a collimated beam with an emitting aperture of arbitrary diameter.

We note that definite progress has been realized in the development of numerical algorithms for the solution of Eq. (4.37) on the basis of the Monte Carlo method. For example, Marchuk and others have published [82] numerical data on the variance of the relative fluctuations of a plane wave according to this method. We now describe some specific physical results obtained in theory for the relative variance, spatial correlation, and frequency spectra of the intensity fluctuations of laser radiation in a turbulent atmosphere.

The most important practical characteristic of the intensity fluctuations in the cross section of a laser beam is the relative variance, defined as follows:

$$\sigma_I^2(x, \mathbf{R}) = \frac{\Gamma_4(x, \mathbf{R}) - \Gamma_2^2(x, \mathbf{R})}{\Gamma_2^2(x, \mathbf{R})}$$

In the case of weak intensity fluctuations, it follows from the solution [3,4,14] of Eq. (4.37) that the relative variance of intensity fluctuations for plane and spherical waves is written in the form

$$\sigma_{I,p}^2 = \beta_0^2$$

$$\sigma_{I,s}^2 = 0.41\beta_0^2 \tag{4.45}$$

respectively. The value of the variance grows with the path length and turbulence strength. These results are completely consistent with those obtained in the solution of the stochastic equation (4.38) by the smooth-perturbation method [34]. It is shown on the basis of the SPM that the form (4.21) of the variance in the case of an arbitrary Gaussian beam can be determined from the expression

$$\sigma_I^2 = f_\sigma(\Omega, x/F, R)\beta_0^2 \tag{4.46}$$

in which the factor $f_\sigma$ is determined by the relative size of the emitting aperture $\Omega$, the curvature of the phase front at the aperture $x/F$, and the position of the observation point relative to the axis of the laser beam. Curves of the function $f_\sigma(\Omega, x/F, R)$ are given in [4]. The variance can vary more than fourfold as a result of the function $f_\sigma(\Omega, x/F, R)$. The domain of applicability of Eq. (4.46), according to experiments [4], is limited to values $\sigma_I \lesssim 0.8$.

There is an important exception, which arises in the case of a focused beam, where calculation of the function $f_\sigma(\Omega, 1, \beta_0^2)$ by the SPM [83] yields results in the region $\beta_0^2 \lesssim 1$ that are an order of magnitude too low in comparison with the experimental data [84, 85]. In the region of strong intensity fluctuations, the variances for a plane wave $\sigma_{I,p}^2$ and a spherical wave $\sigma_{I,s}^2$ can be estimated from the asymptotic expressions [3]

$$\sigma_{I,p}^2 = 1 + 0.86\beta_0^{-4/5} \tag{4.47}$$

$$\sigma_{I,s}^2 = 1 + 2.8\beta_0^{-4/5}, \qquad \beta_0^2 \gg 1 \tag{4.48}$$

These expressions have been derived for the case of a pure power-law spectrum of the index fluctuations. The variance for a collimated laser beam has been calculated [77, 86] with regard for the behavior of the spectrum $\Phi_n(\kappa)$ in the internal scale region. It has been shown [86] that expressions (4.47) and (4.48) are applicable only for certain intermediate conditions where the ratio of the inner scale to the coherence radius is small ($l_0/\rho_0 \ll 1$).

Otherwise ($l_0/\rho_0 \gtrsim 1$), the relative variance is observed to depend significantly on the inner turbulence scale. Thus, the following asymptotic relations are valid for a collimated beam [86]:

$$\sigma_{I,b}^2 = 1 + 2.7\Omega^{-1/3}\beta_0^{-4/5}, \qquad \text{for} \begin{cases} \beta_0^2 \gg 1 \\ \beta_0^{-12/5} \ll \Omega \ll \beta_0^{12/5} \\ l_0/\rho_0 = 0 \end{cases} \tag{4.49}$$

$$\sigma_{I,b}^2 = 1 + 2\Omega^{-1/3}l_f^{2/3} + 3\Omega^{-2/3}l_f^{4/3} + 2\beta_0^{-2}\left[\Omega^{-1/3}l_f^{-1} + 3.8\Omega^{-2/3}l_f^{-1/3}\right]$$

$$\text{for} \begin{cases} \beta_0^2 \gg 1 \\ \beta^{12/5} \ll \Omega \ll \beta_0^{12/5} \\ l_0/a \ll 1 \end{cases} \tag{4.50}$$

In expression (4.50), the quantity $l_f$ is equal to the inner scale normalized to the radius of the first Fresnel zone:

$$l_f = l_0(k/x)^{1/2}$$

It follows from expressions (4.49) and (4.50), in particular, that the level of saturation of the variance of the intensity fluctuations of a collimated laser beam for $l_0 \neq 0$ turns out to be greater than unity, and its value is determined by the ratio of the inner turbulence scale to the radius of the source aperture, $\Omega^{-1/3}l_f^{2/3} = (l_0/a)^{2/3}$. Banakh and others [77] give the results of a numerical calculation of the dependence of the variance $\sigma_I^2$ on the parameters $\beta_0^2$ and $l_f$ with the inclusion of weak fluctuations $\beta_0^2 \ll 1$ and in the intermediate region $\beta_0^2 \sim 1$ for the case $\Omega = 1$. It follows from the asymptotic relations (4.49) and (4.50) and from the numerical calculations [77] that allowance for the inner scale, given a fixed value of the parameter $\beta_0^2$, produces an increase in the variance of strong intensity fluctuations of the laser field.

Expressions (4.49) and (4.50) break down as $\Omega \to 0$. The behavior of the variance of saturated fluctuations ($\beta_0^2 \gg 1$) of a collimated beam for arbitrary values of the parameter $\Omega$ and $l_0 = 0$ is described in [81]. It has the form

$$\sigma_I^2 = 1 + f_b(\Omega, \beta_0^2)\beta_0^{-4/5} \tag{4.51}$$

where $f_b(\Omega, \beta_0^2)$ is a special function, the values of which are given for $\beta_0 = 2.4$ in [81].

                                                          

The values of the variance calculated according to (4.47) have been compared [3, 4] with measurements [87, 88] over a ground-layer path of length $x = 1750$ m in the case of a collimated beam for which the relative radius of the source aperture is $a(k/x)^{1/2} = 11.4$. The experimental data for $\sigma_I$ in the interval $1 \leqslant \beta_0 \leqslant 7$ differ, on the large side, from the calculations according to (4.47) at most by 10 to 15%. The results of calculations according to (4.48) are consistent with the experimental data [87–89], within the same limits, for a divergent beam (1-mrad spread) propagating along a ground-layer path over a distance $x = 1750$ m. A comparison of the results of an experiment [90] conducted over a path $x = 16.5$ km for a collimated beam with apertures $0.1 \leqslant \Omega \leqslant 2$ and in the interval of values $4 \leqslant \beta_0 \leqslant 7$ has shown [81] that the experimental data are more than $1\frac{1}{2}$ times greater than the calculated results (4.51), although the analytical curve is qualitatively consistent with the dependence of $\sigma_I$ on the parameter $\Omega$ (see Fig. 4.7).

Allowance for the finiteness of the inner turbulence scale according to Eq. (4.50) yields values for the variance for $\Omega \gtrsim 1$ with better agreement with experiment than the data of Yakushkin [81]. The dependence of the variance of strong intensity fluctuations on the inner scale has been demonstrated experimentally [91] in measurements performed over a 30-km path with a collimated ($\Omega \simeq 1$) laser beam.

We note that the results presented above for the variance refer to an observation point on the beam axis. It has been shown [75] that if the detector is displaced from the axis, the variance increases. This effect is

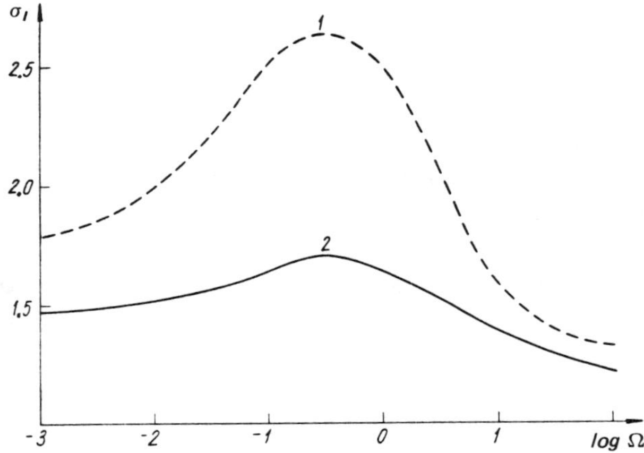

Fig. 4.7. Relative variance of strong intensity fluctuations of a collimated laser beam versus source diameter. (1) Experimental [90], $4 \leqslant \beta_0 \leqslant 7$; (2) theoretical [81], $\beta_0 = 2.4$.

most conspicuous in the region of weak fluctuations [92] and in transition from weak to strong fluctuations. If the detector is displaced by a distance the order of the effective beam radius (see Section 4.2), the variance can increase severalfold. This result has been corroborated experimentally [93–95].

The asymptotic expression for the variance in the case of a focused laser beam [3] coincides with (4.49):

$$\sigma_{I,b}^2 = 1 + 4.1\, D_s^{-2/5}(2a), \qquad D_s(2a) \gg 1 \tag{4.52}$$

A numerical calculation of the variance for arbitrary values of the parameter $D_s(2a)$ has been carried out in [75,76]. The analytical data [4] are given in Fig. 4.8 and compared with the results of experiments [85,96] conducted over ground-layer paths. It is evident from the figure that for $D_s(2a) \sim 50$ the variance of the intensity fluctuations acquires a maximum. It may be assumed that a "focal plane" for the random effective lenses formed in the atmosphere by refractive index fluctuations is created at a definite distance from the source under fixed propagation conditions. The results of calculations according to (4.52) are somewhat below the numerical results, but certain ones agree satisfactorily with experiment, the quantitative agreement of the data improving with allowance for the finiteness of the inner scale.

The scatter of the experimental data in Fig. 4.8 is typical of such experiments conducted in the real atmosphere and is clearly a result of the nonstationarity of the measured intensity-fluctuation process.

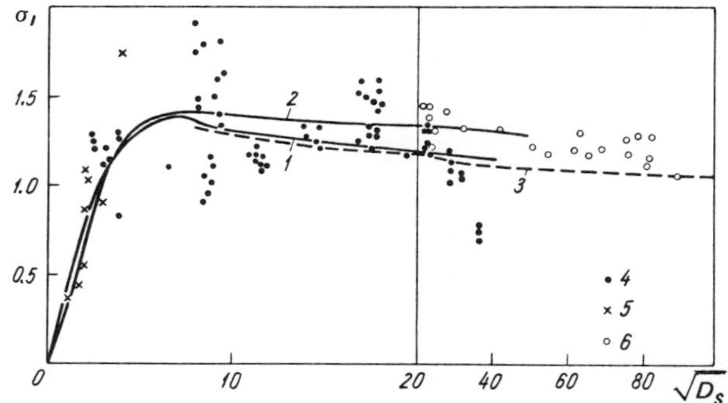


Fig. 4.8. Relative variance of intensity fluctuations at the focus of a laser beam versus parameter $D_s$. (1, 2) Numerical calculation according to expressions in [77]: (1) $l_f = 0$; (2) $l_f = 0.5$; (3) calculated according to asymptotic expression (4.52); (4) experimental data of [96]; (5) experimental data of [85]; experimental data of I. A. Starobinets in [75].

Besides the variance, another important characteristic of the intensity fluctuations of a laser beam in a turbulent atmosphere is the correlation coefficient, which characterizes the statistical coupling between the random values of the intensity in the beam cross section $b_I$ (see Section 4.1). The distance at which the correlation coefficient decreases to the $1/e$ level is called the radius of correlation $\rho_c$.

Under weak fluctuation conditions, $\beta_0^2 \ll 1$, it has been verified [34, 4] by the SPM that the correlation radius $\rho_c$ is determined by the radius of the first Fresnel zone $(\lambda x)^{1/2}$ independently of the initial field distribution. Narrow (in the diffraction sense) collimated beams are characterized by a much stronger negative correlation than in the cases of plane and spherical waves.

In the case of propagation of laser radiation over atmospheric paths, such that the condition $\beta_0^2 \ll 1$ is violated, there is an appreciable redistribution of the intensity in the beam cross section. The characteristic diffraction pattern in the reception plane ultimately fades out, and the beam represents a set of bright spots, which contain the bulk of the radiant energy, against a general gray background.

An analysis of relevant analytical and experimental data shows that this pattern of the intensity distribution in the beam cross section in the strong fluctuation region is explained by the presence of two correlation scales [3, 4]. The first scale is determined by the correlation radius $\rho_c$, which is considerably smaller than $(\lambda x)^{1/2}$, while the second (decay of the correlation coefficient to zero) is much greater than the radius of the first Fresnel zone.

The expressions obtained in [3] for the spatial correlation coefficient of strong intensity fluctuations in the case of plane and spherical waves have the form

$$b_{I,p} = \frac{\exp\left[-2.37\beta_0^2(k/x)^{5/6}\rho^{5/3}\right] + 0.86\beta_0^{-4/5}h_p(q_p)}{1 + 0.86\beta_0^{-4/5}}$$

$$b_{I,s} = \frac{\exp\left[-0.89\beta_0^2(k/x)^{5/6}\rho^{5/3}\right] + 2.8\beta_0^{-4/5}h_s(q_s)}{1 + 2.8\beta_0^{-4/5}} \tag{4.53}$$

where $q_p = 0.6\rho\beta_0^{-6/5}(k/x)^{1/2}$, $q_s = 1.07\rho\beta_0^{-6/5}(k/x)^{1/2}$, and $\rho$ is the spacing of the observation points. To simplify expressions (4.53), the term of order $\beta^{-4/5}$ is dropped from the numerators in the interval $\rho \lesssim (x/k)^{1/2}\beta_0^{-4/5}$. The functions $h_p(q_p)$ and $h_s(q_s)$ are special functions, which are tabulated in [3] and are summarized here in Tables 4.2 and 4.3.

### Table 4.2.

| $q_p$ | 0 | 0.25 | 0.5 | 0.75 | 1 | 1.25 |
|---|---|---|---|---|---|---|
| $h_p$ | 1 | 0.68 | 0.45 | 0.27 | 0.14 | 0.06 |

In complete correspondence with the foregoing, it follows from (4.53) that the first scale of the intensity fluctuations $\rho_{c,1} \sim (x/k)^{1/2}\beta_0^{-6/5} \sim \rho_0$ is determined by the coherence radius of the plane or spherical wave field, respectively, while the second scale is of the order of the diffraction scale at the coherence radius $\rho_{c,2} \sim x/k\rho_{c,1} \sim (x/k)^{1/2}\beta^{6/5}$. Under strong fluctuation conditions, the ratio of these scales is large: $\rho_{c,2}/\rho_{c,1} \sim \beta_0^{12/5} \gg 1$.

Experimental confirmation of the two-scale nature of the spatial correlation of strong fluctuations under conditions close to plane and spherical wave propagation is given in [87–89]. It has been shown [72] that the experimental results of Gracheva and others [87] agree with the calculated results for the plane wave case, within the experimental error limits. In the case of a focused beam, the asymptotic expression [3] for the correlation coefficient has the form

$$b_{I,f} = \frac{\exp\left[-(k\Omega/2x)\rho^2\right] + 0.87\Omega^{-1/3}\beta_0^{-4/5}\left[1.58h_{f,1}(q_1) + 1.43h_{f,2}(q_2)\right]}{1 + 2.7\Omega^{-1/3}\beta_0^{-4/5}}$$

$$(4.54)$$

where $q_1 = (2k\Omega/x)^{1/2}\rho$, $q_2 = 1.62(k/x)^{1/2}\rho\beta^{-6/5}$, and the values of the special functions $h_{f,1}$ and $h_{f,2}$ are given in Tables 4.4 and 4.5.

Equation (4.54) is valid for $D_s(2a) \gg 1$. It follows from expression (4.54) that the first correlation scale is of the order of the radius of the Airy disk corresponding to the focusing aperture $(\rho_{c,1} \sim x/ka)$, while the second scale is determined by the diffraction scale at the coherence radius $\rho_{c,2} \sim (x/k)^{1/2}\beta_0^{6/5} \sim x/k\rho_0$. It can be shown by means of the Huygens–Kirchhoff phase approximation [75, 76] that the first scale is equal to $(2x/k\Omega)^{1/2}$ only under the condition $\Omega \gg \beta_0^{12/5}$, in which case the average width of the beam (4.23) in the focusing plane does not exceed the diameter of the emitting aperture. With a further increase in the parameter $\beta_0^2$, the scale $\rho_{c,1}$ approaches the coherence radius of the field $\rho_0$.

### Table 4.3.

| $q_s$ | 0 | 0.2 | 0.4 | 0.6 | 0.8 | 1 | 1.2 |
|---|---|---|---|---|---|---|---|
| $h_s$ | 1 | 0.63 | 0.37 | 0.23 | 0.12 | 0.05 | 0.02 |

Table 4.4.

| $q_1$ | 0 | 0.25 | 0.5 | 0.75 | 1 | 1.25 | 1.5 | 1.75 | 2 | 2.25 | 2.75 |
|---|---|---|---|---|---|---|---|---|---|---|---|
| $h_{f,1}$ | 1 | 0.96 | 0.83 | 0.68 | 0.44 | 0.27 | 0.11 | 0 | $-0.06$ | $-0.07$ | $-0.05$ |

In certain instances, it is sufficient to know the first correlation scale of the intensity fluctuations. For a source aperture of arbitrary diameter and under the conditions of focusing in the strong fluctuation region, it has been shown [81] that this scale coincides with the coherence radius given by (4.31) and (4.32). We note that, according to (4.31) and (4.32), the correlation radius in a collimated beam, judging from the analysis carried out in Section 4.3, is greater than the corresponding values for plane and spherical waves under identical propagation conditions ($\beta_0^2 = \mathrm{const}$).

A numerical analysis [75] of the representations obtained for the correlation coefficient in the Huygens–Kirchhoff phase approximation makes it possible to trace the variations of the correlation scales and the form of the correlation function continuously with respect to the parameter $\beta_0^2$, even for values of $\beta_0^2$ of the order of unity. Figure 4.9 gives the results of calculations of the correlation coefficient of focused and collimated laser beams for various values of the parameter $D_s(2a) = 2.84\beta_0^2\Omega^{5/6}$, which characterizes turbulent conditions of beam propagation and is chosen in such a way as to take in weak intensity fluctuations, the interval of maximum variance (see Fig. 4.8) (interval of focusing of intensity fluctuations), and finally the variance saturation interval (decay of $\sigma_I^2$ according to the $D_s^{-2/5}$ law). The spacing of the observation points is plotted along the horizontal axis in fractions of the diffraction width of the beam in a homogeneous medium.

It is evident from the curves in Fig. 4.9 that the spatial correlation scale for weak intensity fluctuations is of the order of the diffraction width of the beam in a homogeneous medium. A characteristic attribute of the correlation coefficient in this region is a strong negative correlation of the intensities observed at a distance of the order of the actual beam width [for $D_s(2a) \sim 1$ the effective beam width $\rho_e$ practically coincides with its diffraction width]. This strong autocorrelation has been observed even in calculations of the spatial correlation coefficient by the smooth-perturbation

Table 4.5.

| $q_2$ | 0 | 1 | 2 | 3 | 4 | 5 | 7 | 9 |
|---|---|---|---|---|---|---|---|---|
| $h_{f,2}$ | 1 | 0.88 | 0.57 | 0.32 | 0.18 | 0.12 | 0.07 | 0.06 |

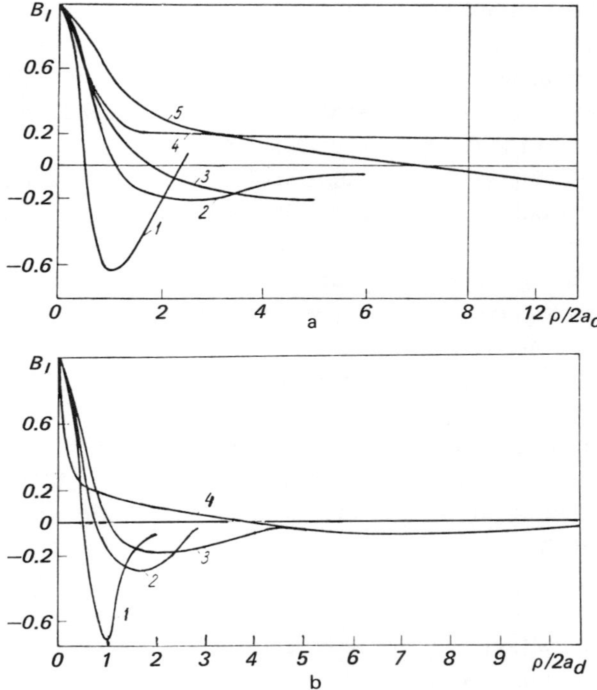

Fig. 4.9. Spatial correlation coefficient of intensity fluctuations of a focused and a collimated laser beam for various values of $D_s(2a)$. (a) focused beam, $x/F=1$, $\Omega=25$: (1) $D_s=2$; (2) $D_s=10$; (3) $D_s=50$; (4) $D_s=1400$; (5) $D_s=400$. (b) Collimated beam, $x/F=0$, $\Omega=1$: (1)$D_s=3$; $D_s=16$; (3) $D_s=32$; (4) $D_s=158$.

method [92] and has been experimentally confirmed [93,94]. It occurs, clearly, as a consequence of beam wander relative to two detectors so that an increase in the intensity in one detector situated at a given time on the beam axis is accompanied by a decrease of the intensity in the second detector, which as a result of physical spacing is located at that same time at the edge of the beam. With an increase in the parameter $D_s(2a)$, the correlation function acquires a two-scale character. In the case of a focused beam, the diffraction width in vacuum remains as the first scale, while for a collimated beam this scale approaches the coherence radius and turns out to be much smaller than the diffraction width of the beam. Measurements of the spatial correlation functions of the intensity fluctuations in a focused beam [96–100] under strong fluctuation conditions indicate the diffraction width of the beam in vacuum as the correlation radius.

It follows from certain experiments [90, 101] that the first correlation scale in the case of a narrow collimated beam, $\beta_0^{-12/5} \ll \Omega \ll \beta_0^{12/5}$, given identical turbulence conditions of propagation, is greater than the corresponding values obtained for broad collimated and divergent beams, in full agreement with the theoretical conclusions.

The next important characteristic of the intensity fluctuations of a laser beam in a turbulent atmosphere is the frequency spectrum, the knowledge of which is always important in regard to the selection of techniques for the encoding and reception of optical signals traveling through the atmosphere and carrying a particular kind of useful information.

Under weak fluctuation conditions, the frequency spectra have been well studied by the smooth-perturbation method [34, 102–105]. It follows from these studies that the main contribution to the frequency spectrum of the intensity fluctuations for $\beta_0^2 < 1$ occurs at a frequency $f_0 \sim \tau_f^{-1}$, where $\tau_f = (\lambda x)^{1/2}/v$ is the transfer time of inhomogeneities of the refractive index over a distance equal to the radius of the first Fresnel zone with the average wind velocity $v$.

Banakh and Mironov [78] have carried out a theoretical investigation of the frequency spectra of strong intensity fluctuations using the Huygens–Kirchoff phase approximation to carry out relevant calculations under various conditions of propagation and for various values of the source parameters. The results of calculations of the temporal correlation function have shown that the temporal correlation radius for strong fluctuation conditions is determined by the radiation wavelength, the path length, and the turbulence conditions. The dependence on the diffraction radius of the emitting aperture and focusing, on the other hand, practically disappears.

Figure 4.10 gives the spectral densities of the intensity fluctuations $U_I(f) = fW_I(f)/B_I(0)$ for various values of the parameter $D_s(2a)$. The frequency spectrum $W_I(f)$ is calculated by means of the well-known expression relating $W_I(f)$ to the temporal correlation function $B_I(\tau)$:

$$W_I(f) = 4\int_0^\infty B_I(\tau)\cos 2\pi f\tau\, d\tau \qquad (4.55)$$

It is evident from the figure that for small values of $D_s$ the function $U_I(f)$ has a distinct maximum at a frequency of order $f_0$, as is entirely consistent with the results obtained by the smooth-perturbation method. With an increase in the parameter $D_s$, the maximum of the function $U_I(f)$ shifts toward higher frequencies, and for very large $D_s$ the main contribution to the spectral density occurs at a frequency $f_c \sim \tau_c^{-1}$, where $\tau_c \sim \rho_0/v$ is the

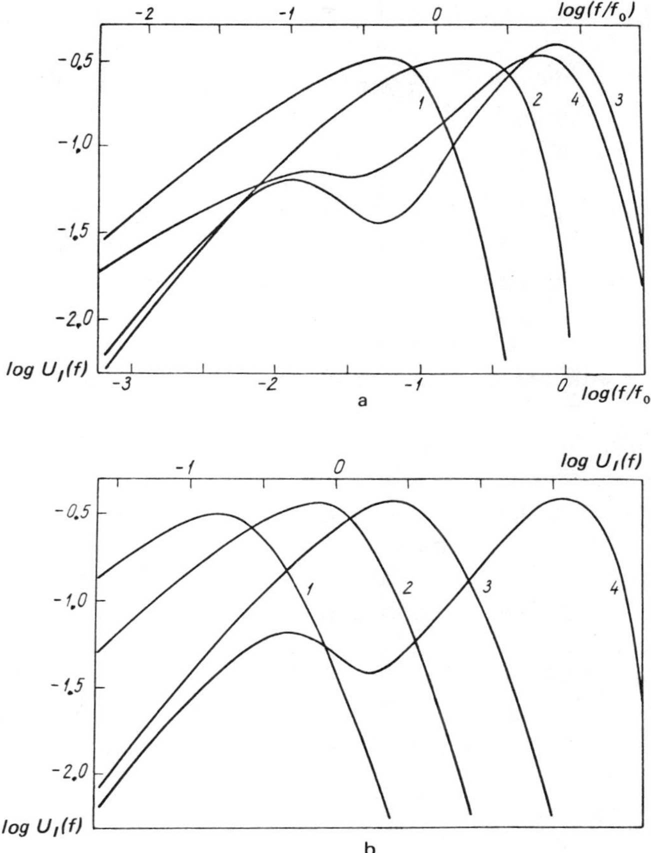

Fig. 4.10. Normalized spectral density of intensity fluctuations of collimated and focused laser beams. (a) Collimated beam, $f_0 = v/2a$, $f_c = v/5\pi p_s$, $x/F = 0$, $\Omega = 1$: (1) $D_s = 3$; (2) $D_s = 160$; (3) $D_s = 1400$, $\beta_0^2 = 493$; (4) experimental curve from [87] ($x/F = 0$, $\Omega = 26$, $v = 1.5$–$8$ m/sec, $\beta_0^2 = 625 \ldots 900$). (b) Focused beam, $x/F = 1$, $\Omega = 25$: (1) $D_s = 2$; (2) $D_s = 50$; (3) $D_s = 400$; (4) $D_s = 1400$.

transfer time of spatial inhomogeneities of the intensity over a distance of the order of the coherence radius of the radiation field $\rho_0$ with the average wind velocity. The appearance of a second maximum in the low-frequency interval is associated with the presence of a second correlation scale in the temporal correlation function, analogous to the corresponding effect in the case of spatial fluctuations.

A comparison [78] of the results of calculations of the intensity fluctuation spectra with experimental data obtained for a collimated beam along a ground-layer path [87–89] exhibits satisfactory agreement between the two.

In concluding this section, we stress the fact that the main problems of quantitative estimation of the various characteristics of laser beam fluctuations due to atmospheric turbulence may be regarded as solved, provided, of course, that statistically supported data are available on turbulent atmosphere models. Unfortunately, the latter circumstance is still a long way from realization and, accordingly, remains a timely problem.

Among the newer problems associated with the investigation of intensity fluctuations of laser radiation in a turbulent atmosphere, it is essential to mention the study of intensity fluctuations of a laser beam reflected from various objects. These problems are of considerable practical significance in connection with the development of more sophisticated lidar and laser telemetry devices. The first steps have already been taken in this direction. For example, Vinogradov and others [106, 107] have solved the problem of the scattering of a spherical wave by a point scatterer in a randomly inhomogeneous medium containing large-scale inhomogeneities. They have shown, in the case of strict backward reflection, that the effect of amplifying intensity fluctuations, and a residual correlation of intensity fluctuations in the reflected wave, have their place in this situation.

To calculate the variance and correlation functions of the intensity fluctuations of laser radiation reflected from a circular plane mirror of finite diameter, Aksenov and others [108] use the Huygens–Kirchhoff phase approximation, which enables them to obtain a number of interesting results.

Numerical calculations of the relative variance and spatial correlation coefficient of the reflected-wave intensity [108] show that the variance of strong intensity fluctuations of a wave from a mirror whose diameter is commensurate with the radius of the first Fresnel zone is more than twice the variance of the intensity fluctuations of the direct wave. The spatial correlation scales of the intensity fluctuations in the region of weak and strong intensity fluctuations are of the same order of magnitude as in a beam traversing the path once. The quantitative values of the correlation radius, which now depend on, *inter alia*, the diffraction parameters of the reflecting mirror, differ from the corresponding quantities in the direct beam under the same turbulent propagation conditions.

Attempts have also been made [109] to calculate the intensity fluctuations of laser radiation reflected under turbulent atmospheric conditions from diffusely scattering objects. The first results of such calculations indicate a significant dependence of the spatial correlation radius of strong intensity fluctuations of the reflected wave primarily on the size of the reflecting body. In this same vein, studies have also been carried out on the reflected-wave coherence [110, 111]. It has been shown that under certain conditions the coherence radius of the reflected-wave field can (under identical propagation conditions in the atmosphere) exceed the largest attainable value of this quantity for the field of a wave traversing the path one time.

Next we examine in closer detail the experimental work carried out on intensity fluctuations in laser beams.

## 4.5.2. Experimental Research

The results of experimental investigations of the intensity fluctuations of spatially confined light beams in a turbulent atmosphere are surveyed in detail in the author's earlier book [4]. Inasmuch as we have discussed in the preceding section the results of calculations that exhibit satisfactory agreement with the data of corresponding experimental studies, we limit this section mainly to a summary of the principal experimental work, devoting special attention only to those situations in which the results are intractable by theoretical methods.

Measurements of the variance of the intensity fluctuations of broad collimated and divergent beams are described in [112–122]. Khmelevtsov and Tsvyk [121, 122] have investigated the relative variance in the Fresnel diffraction zone of a beam over measurement paths of 0.2, 0.5, 1.36, and 18.5 km. Gracheva and others [116] have measured the statistical parameters of fluctuations of the logarithm of the amplitude for broad collimated beams over 0.25- and 1.75-km paths. Others [112, 113] have investigated the variance over a 1.75-km path in the case of divergent laser beams with angular spreads of 60″ and 2 mrad. Several authors [114, 117, 120] have performed simultaneous measurements of the variance of intensity fluctuations for lasers with wavelengths $\lambda_1 = 0.488$, $\lambda_2 = 1.15$, $\lambda_3 = 10.6$ $\mu$m [120]; $\lambda_1 = 0.6328$, $\lambda_2 = 1.084$ $\mu$m [117]; and $\lambda_1 = 0.6328$, $\lambda_2 = 10.6$ $\mu$m [114], showing that a universal relation $\sigma_I^2 = \sigma_I^2(\beta^2)$ holds with variation of the optical wavelength.

Measurements have been performed with multimode lasers [115, 118, 119]. Corresponding theoretical investigations have not been published to date. The fundamental result of this work is essentially that the variance of saturated intensity fluctuations in the case of multimode divergent beams is smaller than in the single-mode case.

Khmelevtsov and others [121–124] have carried out experimental studies of the variance of intensity fluctuations of narrow collimated beams. An investigation of the influence of the size of the collimated beam at the exit aperture on the variance of the intensity fluctuations on the beam axis is described in [123]. The dependence of weak intensity fluctuations on the curvature of the phase front at the exit aperture has also been investigated [121]. The increase in the relative variance with displacement of the observation point from the beam axis toward the edge under weak fluctuation conditions has been studied [124].

Detailed studies of the spatial correlation of intensity fluctuations of laser radiation in a turbulent atmosphere are described in [125–129]. Data on the correlation coefficient of the intensity fluctuations have been obtained for broad collimated and divergent beams [126, 127]. The spatial correlation functions of the intensity of a focused laser beam has also been measured [128]. Data on the spatial correlation of the intensity of a collimated laser beam have been obtained on the basis of measurements of averaging functions derived with the use of a variable-diameter receiving aperture [129]. D'yachenko and others [128] have photographed the illumination created on a screen irradiated by a pulsed ruby laser to determine the correlation coefficients in a focused laser beam.

For an investigation of the spatial correlation of the intensity of divergent and focused laser beams, Andreev and others [126] have relied on a photographic determination of the second moment with the use of an optical correlometer.

The frequency spectra of the intensity fluctuations of laser beams in a turbulent atmosphere have been investigated in a number of papers [21, 85, 87, 103, 112, 130–132]. The most detailed studies for a quasiplane wave are reported by Gurvich and others [87, 131, 132]. Their complex measurement technique yielded data on the spectrum in the frequency range from 2 Hz to 6.3 kHz. The spectra disclose a strong dependence on the parameter $\beta_0^2$, the behavior of which we have already discussed in the preceding section in relation to the results of a calculation of the frequency spectra on the basis of the Huygens–Kirchhoff phase approximation.

The processing of results of measurements with lasers at wavelengths of 0.63 and 10.6 $\mu$m over 0.25- and 16.3-km paths has shown that the frequency spectra span a very broad frequency range. The positions of their maxima differ by more than 3 orders of magnitude.

Gurvich [103] and Time [130] have measured the spectra of fluctuations of the logarithm of the intensity over short paths (50 m for a quasiplane wave [130] and 50 and 100 m for a divergent laser beam). The spectra of a focused beam have been investigated over a 1.75-km path [4, 21, 85]. The intensity fluctuation spectrum obtained in the latter case contains a dominant high-frequency part. However, with an increase in the diameter of the receiving aperture, the small-scale fluctuations are averaged, and, accordingly, the high-frequency contribution to the variance of the recorded light flux decreases.

## 4.6. Distribution Function of Intensity Fluctuations

Knowledge of the probability distribution function of intensity fluctuations of laser beams propagating in the atmosphere is essential to the design and operational analysis of communications, lidar, telemetry, and other atmospheric laser systems.

Theoretical studies using the smooth-perturbation method have shown that a log–normal distribution and normal distribution hold for the intensity and phase fluctuations, respectively, in the weak fluctuation region.

In the case of strong intensity fluctuations, it has been shown very recently [74, 133] by asymptotic solution of the equations for the coherence functions

$$\Gamma_{2n}(x, \boldsymbol{\rho}_1, \ldots, \boldsymbol{\rho}_n, \boldsymbol{\rho}_1', \ldots, \boldsymbol{\rho}_n') = \langle U(x, \boldsymbol{\rho}_1) U^*(x, \boldsymbol{\rho}_1') \cdots U(x, \boldsymbol{\rho}_n) U^*(x, \boldsymbol{\rho}_n') \rangle$$

in the case of an unconfined plane wave that, as the parameter $\beta_0^2$ increases, the normalization of the field of a light wave with respect to the higher moments $\langle I^n \rangle$ slows down and so the distribution function of the intensity for arbitrarily large values of $\beta_0^2$ deviates from exponential, while the probabilities of the field amplitude deviate from a Rayleigh distribution.

The experimental studies performed to date along real atmospheric paths under various conditions yield, in the majority of cases, distribution functions close to a log–normal.

Gracheva and others [87, 134] have performed pertinent measurements with a helium–neon laser ($\lambda = 0.63$ $\mu$m) operating in axial modes over ground-layer paths of 0.65, 1.75, and 8.5 km.

The collimator used in this work ensured an essentially plane phase front at an aperture 50 cm in diameter with a Gaussian beamwidth $2a = 30$ cm, so that the beam could be regarded approximately as a quasiplane wave. In the weak fluctuation region ($\beta_0 < 1$), the measured distribution is well approximated by a log–normal function. In the interval of values of $\beta_0^2$ extending roughly from 25 to 100 we find the greatest deviations from this function. Deviations from a log–normal distribution in the interval $\beta_0^2 \sim 1$ have also been observed in [113, 135].

The nature of the distribution of the intensity fluctuations can be affected by the size of the source and receiving apertures, the divergence or focusing of the laser beam, and the multimodality of the emitters, which determines the degree of coherence at the exit aperture. The influence of these factors has been investigated to some extent experimentally.

The distribution functions of the intensity fluctuations in a focused laser beam have been investigated [85, 128]. It was found that the empirical distributions obtained in the strong fluctuation region differ significantly from a log–normal function in connection with deep fading. The amplitude distributions in this case also deviate from the Rayleigh and generalized Rayleigh functions.

Series of measurements in the ground layer of the atmosphere have been performed with the use of divergent laser beams [113, 125, 135], a continuous semiconductor laser with a large number of transverse modes ($\lambda = 0.905$ $\mu$m) [124], and pulsed lasers ($\lambda = 1.06$, 0.53, 0.69 $\mu$m) [126]. Measurements along an earth–space path have been carried out [136]. The results of these studies support the presence of a log–normal distribution of the intensity fluctuations. Other investigations [137, 138] have shown that increasing the dimensions of the receiving aperture has a natural averaging effect on the intensity fluctuations and decreases the variance accordingly but does not distort the log–normal distribution, which persists even when the radius of the receiving aperture is considerably greater than the correlation radius of the intensity fluctuations.

## 4.7. Random Spatial Intensity Peaks

The random redistribution of intensity in the cross section of a laser beam is characterized by spatial peaks; it is important in practice to understand the laws governing their occurrence in relation to the development of laser systems operating in the atmosphere. This consideration is particularly significant in situations where the linear dimensions of the receiving aperture are of the same order of magnitude as the linear dimensions of the random intensity peaks.

A number of theoretical studies of random intensity peaks have been published [139–143]. Bunkin and Gochelashvili [139, 140], postulating a normal joint distribution of the logarithm of the intensity and its derivative and an isotropic random field, have derived expressions for the average area

$\langle S(I_1)\rangle$ of a peak above a specified intensity level $I_1$, the average number $\langle N(I_1)\rangle$ of such peaks per unit area, and the average distance ($\langle l(I_1)\rangle$ between peaks:

$$\langle S(I_1)\rangle = -\frac{\pi^2}{b_x''(0)}\left[1-\Phi(\xi)\right]^2\exp(\xi^2)$$

$$\langle N(I_1)\rangle = -\frac{b_x''(0)}{2\pi^2}\left[1-\Phi(\xi)\right]^{-1}\exp(-\xi^2)$$

$$\langle l(I_1)\rangle = -\frac{\pi}{\left[2b_x''(0)\right]^{1/2}}\left[1-\Phi(\xi)\right]^{1/2}\exp(\tfrac{1}{2}\xi^2)$$

where $\xi = (1/2\sigma_x)[2\sigma_x^2 + \ln(I_1/\langle I\rangle)]$, $\sigma_x^2$ is the variance of the intensity level, $\langle I\rangle$ is the average intensity, $\Phi(\xi) = (2/\pi)^{1/2}\int_0^\xi\exp(-x^2/2)dx$, and $b_x''(0)$ is the second derivative of the correlation coefficient of the logarithm of the amplitude, evaluated at zero.

In order to calculate $\langle S(I_1)\rangle$, $\langle N(I_1)\rangle$, and $\langle l(I_1)\rangle$ according to the expressions given above, it is necessary to know the variance of the fluctuations of the logarithm of the amplitude and the second derivative of the spatial correlation function for those fluctuations. Specific approximative calculations of the characteristics of the peaks in both the weak and the strong intensity fluctuation regions are given in [141, 142].

For strong fluctuations in the region of saturation of the variance, it is postulated that the field of the laser beam has an asymptotically normal distribution; Aksenov and others [143] have obtained both analytical and numerical results for $\langle S(I_1)\rangle$, $\langle N(I_1)\rangle$, and $\langle l(I_1)\rangle$.

Gel'fer and others [144] have derived an approximate expression describing the random intensity peaks in terms of experimentally measurable quantities, namely the effective radius $a_e = (\langle S(I > I_1)\rangle/\pi^{1/2}$, where $S(I > I_1)$ is the area of the focal plane in which the intensity is greater than the given level $I_1$ and the structural characteristic $C_n^2$ of the field of the refractive index. The effective radius $a_e$ has been measured [144] in the ground layer of the atmosphere over 180- and 650-m paths at heights of 1.5 to 2 m above a uniform level steppe area. Figure 4.11, which is taken from [4], gives the results of measurements performed in the experiment described above, along with calculated curves. The ratio of the specified level to the intensity at the focus of the beam in vacuum $\alpha = I_1/I_0$ is plotted on the vertical axis. A comparison of these results shows that the expression obtained in [144] is suitable for approximate calculations of the fraction of the beam area wherein the intensity, on the average, exceeds a certain specified level.

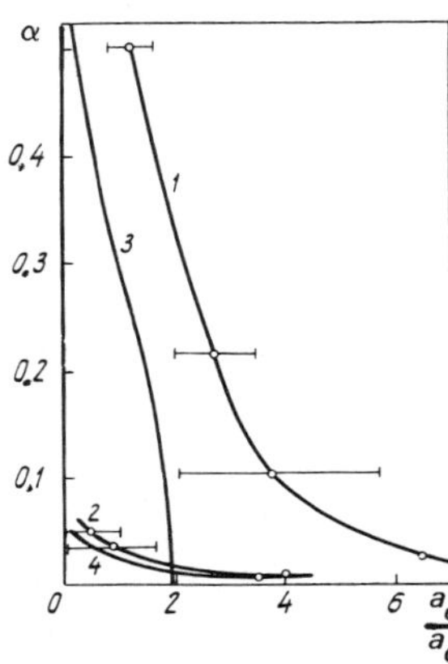

Fig. 4.11. Analytical curves and experimental values of effective radius of a focused beam corresponding to $\alpha$ peak level. Experimental: (1) $D_s = 5$; (2) $D_s = 5 \ldots 20$. Analytical: (3) $D_s = 2$; (4) $D_s = 10$.

## 4.8. Averaging Effect of the Receiving Aperture

Inasmuch as the intensity fluctuations in a light wave incident on a detector have a finite spatial correlation radius, it is quite clear that the experimental data on the power fluctuations of the flux transmitted through an aperture of finite size will necessarily depend on the diameter of the receiving mirror. Without knowledge of this dependence, it is virtually impossible to interpret and analyze the large set of results of related experimental investigations. On the other hand, this knowledge is important in relation to the development of various laser systems designed to operate in the atmosphere.

A quantitative measure of the averaging effect of a receiving aperture of finite dimensions is the function $G(R)$ introduced by Tatarskii [34], which indicates the factor by which the magnitude of the relative fluctuations of the total light flux recorded by an objective of radius $R$ is smaller than in the case of a point objective

$$G(R) = \frac{4}{\pi R^2} \int_0^{2R} b_I(\rho) \left[ \cos^{-1} \frac{\rho}{2R} - \frac{\rho}{2R} \left( 1 - \frac{\rho^2}{4R^2} \right)^{1/2} \right] \rho \, d\rho$$

where $b_I(\rho) = B_I(\rho)/B_I(0)$ is the correlation coefficient of the intensity fluctuations in the incident wave on the detector.

Theoretical studies of the function $G(R)$ have been carried out for the case of weak intensity fluctuations when a plane [34] and a spherical [145] wave is incident on a circular aperture, as well as in the reception of the field of a plane wave by a circular aperture of the Cassegrainian type [146].

Fante [72] has calculated the function $G(R)$ numerically for the field of a plane incident wave in the case of strong intensity fluctuations. Measurements of the averaging effect of the receiving aperture have been repeated many times [16, 122, 129, 135, 137, 138, 147–149]. Before discussing the fundamental results of these investigations we stress the fact, which is evident from the expression for $G(R)$, that it depends significantly on the spatial correlation function of the intensity fluctuations, which, in turn, depends on the equivalent thickness of the turbulent atmosphere, as characterized either by the parameter $\beta_0^2 = 1.23 C_n^2 k^{7/6} x^{11/6}$ in the case of a plane wave or by the parameter $D_s(2a) = 1.1 C_n^2 k^2 x (2a)^{5/3}$ when the radiation is focused by a source aperture of diameter $2a$. It is therefore essential to know $C_n^2$ for the appropriate interpretation of the measurement data. Earlier studies [17, 135, 137] failed to monitor $C_n^2$ to the extent that it warranted.

The most complete experimental data on the averaging effect of the receiving aperture over long measurements paths have been obtained in [122, 129, 138, 147–149]. Figure 4.12, which is taken from [4], gives typical representation of these data. Kazaryan and others [138] performed measurements over a 25-km path in a mountainous locale. Curve 1 in the figure has been obtained as the average of five curves with close values of $C_n^2 = (3.1, 3.5, 3.6, 3.8, 4.4) \times 10^{-16}$ cm$^{-2/3}$. Curves 2 and 4 are taken from [122] and [148] in which the measurements were also performed under the

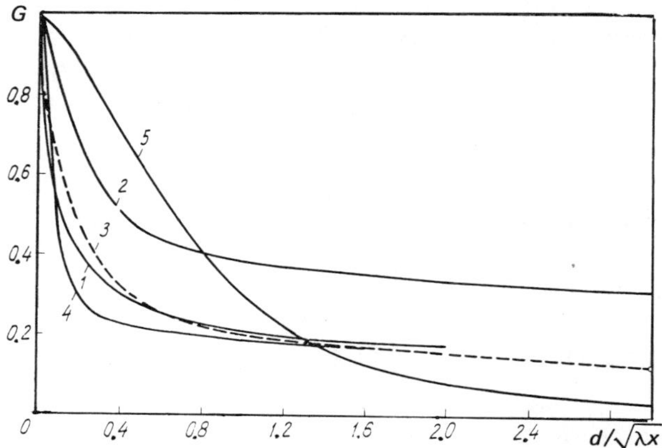


Fig. 4.12. Empirical receiving-aperture averaging function. (1) Data of [138], $x = 25$ km; (2) data of [148], $x = 30$ km; (3) renormalized curve 2; (4) data of [122], $x = 24$ km; (5) calculated weak-fluctuation curve [34].

conditions of a mining region over 30- and 24-km paths. Curves 1, 2, and 4 were obtained with the use of a continuous helium–neon laser having an emission wavelength of 0.63 $\mu$m. Curve 2 is the result of averaging of 13 measurement series performed over a period of two summer months.

On the basis of the fact that the minimum size of the receiving aperture in [148] was smaller than the size of the entrance slit in [138], curve 2 is renormalized accordingly, and curve 3, representing the result of this operation, exhibits good agreement with curve 1, thus evincing the fact that the meteorological conditions of the measurements in [138] and [140] were similar.

Curve 5 in Fig. 4.12 has been obtained theoretically for the case of weak fluctuations. Comparison with the experimental curves 1–4 indicates the presence of two spatial correlation scales for strong intensity fluctuations. ·

Belen'kii and others [129] have obtained results from which it is possible to systematize the measurement data as a function of the meteorological conditions. The measurements were carried out over an 11.8-km path at a height of 42 m above a sea surface. The quantity $C_n^2$, measured by an optical method, varied from $1.58 \times 10^{-16}$ to $7 \times 10^{-16}$ cm$^{-2/3}$. Simultaneous measurements by the gradient method at a height of 10 m above an arid plain yielded larger values, from $1.7 \times 10^{-15}$ to $1.4 \times 10^{-14}$ cm$^{-2/3}$, the increase being fully attributable to the differences in heights at which the measurements were performed. The general behavior of the function $G(R)$ for different values of $C_n^2$ is similar to that shown in Fig. 4.12.

Experimental investigations of the averaging effect of the receiving aperture in the case of a focused beam are described in [97]. The averaged experimental curves indicate that the greater the aperture diameter of the aperture focusing the radiation, the steeper will be the curve of $G(R)$. An analysis of the results leads to the conclusion that the correlation radius of the intensity fluctuations is proportional to the diffraction width of the beam.


## 4.9. Phase Fluctuations in Laser Beams

Fluctuations of the refractive index in a turbulent atmosphere induce random phase shifts. This effect is extremely important in application to laser radiation because it destroys its coherence. In this section, we briefly characterize the present status of the problem.

The phase fluctuations of spatially confined beams in a turbulent atmosphere have been studied theoretically [150–152]. Kon and Tatarskii [150] and Schmeltzer [151] have derived expressions for the structure functions of the amplitude and phase for a Gaussian beam and an arbitrary spectrum of index fluctuations. Ishimaru [152] has carried out related calculations for a turbulent spectrum $\Phi_n(\kappa)$, obtaining the following relation for the structure function of the phase fluctuations in the case of a collimated Gaussian beam [92]:

$$D_s(\boldsymbol{\rho}_1,\boldsymbol{\rho}_2)=1.77\beta_0^2\int_0^1\left\{2A^{5/6}\left[\mathrm{Re}_1F_1\left(-\tfrac{5}{6},1;-\frac{P}{A}\right)-{}_1F_1\left(-\tfrac{5}{6},1;\frac{\gamma_2^2r_1^2}{A}\right)\right.\right.$$
$$\left.\left.-{}_1F_1\left(-\tfrac{5}{6},1;\frac{\gamma_2^2r_2^2}{A}\right)\right]-2\mathrm{Re}C^{5/6}\left[1-{}_1F_1\left(-\tfrac{5}{6},1;-\frac{Q}{C}\right)\right]\right\}dx'$$

$$(4.56)$$

where ${}_1F_1(-\tfrac{5}{6},1;z)$ is the confluent hypergeometric function,

$$C=s^2+i\gamma(1-x'),\qquad A=s^2+\gamma_2(1-x')$$

$$P=n^2\gamma_1^2-\gamma_2^2t^2-2i\gamma_1\gamma_2nt\cos\Psi,\qquad Q=\gamma^2n^2$$

$$\gamma=\gamma_1-i\gamma_2=\frac{1+ix'/\Omega-x/Fx'}{1+il/\Omega-x/F},\qquad s=\frac{kl_0^2}{(5.91)^2x}$$

$$r_1^2=t^2+n^2+2nt\cos\Psi,\qquad r_2^2=t^2+n^2-2nt\cos\Psi$$

The quantities $t=|\boldsymbol{t}|=(k/x)^{1/2}|(\boldsymbol{\rho}_1+\boldsymbol{\rho}_2)/2|$ and $n=|\boldsymbol{n}|=(k/x)^{1/2}|(\boldsymbol{\rho}_1-\boldsymbol{\rho}_2)/2|$ represent the distance of the centroid of observation points from the center of the beam and half the distance between observation points, respectively, both normalized to the radius of the first Fresnel zone, and $\Psi$ is the angle between the vectors $\boldsymbol{t}$ and $\boldsymbol{n}$.

Mironov and Patrushev [92] have carried out a numerical analysis of expression (4.56) making it possible to trace the behavior of the structure function of the phase fluctuations, normalized to the variance of the intensity fluctuations in a plane wave as a function of the dimensionless spacing of the observation points $n$ for various diameters of the transmitting aperture and radii of curvature of the phase front at the exit aperture (see Fig. 4.13).

Lukin and others [153] give the following asymptotic expressions for the phase structure function in a collimated beam for two observation-point

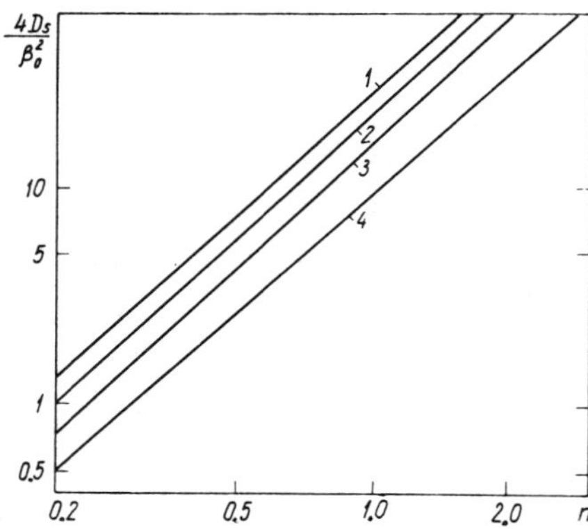

Fig. 4.13. Normalized structure function for phase fluctuations in a collimated laser beam (central dispersion of observation points, $t = 0$), $s^2 = 0.237 \cdot 10^{-3}$. (1) Plane wave; (2) $\Omega = 2$; (3) $\Omega = 1$; (4) spherical wave.

configurations:

$$D_s(\rho, 0) = 2.91 b_1 C_n^2 k^2 x \rho^{5/3}; \qquad \rho_1 = \rho, \qquad \rho_2 = 0 \qquad (4.57)$$

$$D_s(\rho, -\rho) = 2.91 b_2 C_n^2 k^2 x (2\rho)^{5/3}; \qquad \rho_1 = \rho, \qquad \rho_2 = -\rho \qquad (4.58)$$

where $b_1$ and $b_2$ are constants, the values of which are given for various $\Omega$ in Table 4.6.

A comparison of the results of calculations according to (4.57) and (4.58) with exact calculations of the function $D_s$ for $\Omega = 1$ yields good agreement between the data so that the simple expressions (4.57) and (4.58) can be recommended for practical calculations.

The behavior of the structure function $D_s(\rho)$ in the range of large values of $\rho$ has been investigated [154–156] with the use of a Kármán spectrum of index fluctuations $\Phi_n(\kappa) = 0.033 C_n^2 (\kappa^2 + \kappa_0^2)^{-11/6}$, and the variance and correlation function of the phase fluctuations have been estimated in the same work.

The smooth perturbation method has been used in conjunction with a modified Kármán fluctuation spectrum [the original spectrum multiplied by $\exp(-\kappa^2/\kappa_m^2)$] to deduce the following expression [156] for the normalized

Table 4.6.

| $\Omega$ | $\infty$ | 10 | 2 | 1 | 0 |
|---|---|---|---|---|---|
| $b_1$ | 1.0 | 0.96 | 0.78 | 0.45 | 0.375 |
| $b_2$ | 1.0 | 0.95 | 0.84 | 0.63 | 0.375 |

phase fluctuation spectrum of a collimated beam $\overline{W}_S(f) = W(f)/W_S(0)$:

$$\overline{W}_S(f) = \frac{\Gamma(11/6)}{2\Gamma(4/3)} \left( \int_0^x d\xi \frac{C_n^2}{v_\perp} \kappa^{-8/3} \right)^{-1} \int_0^x d\xi \frac{C_n^2}{v_\perp} \left( b^2 + \kappa_0^2 \right)^{-4/3}$$

$$\times \left\{ \exp\left( -\beta_1 b^2 \right) \Psi\left[ \tfrac{1}{2}, -\tfrac{1}{3}; \beta_1\left( b^2 + \kappa_0^2 \right) \right] \right.$$

$$+ \tfrac{1}{2} \exp\left( -\beta_2 b^2 \right) \Psi\left[ \tfrac{1}{2}, -\tfrac{1}{3}; \beta_2\left( b^2 + \kappa_0^2 \right) \right]$$

$$\left. + \tfrac{1}{2} \exp\left( -\beta_2^* b^2 \right) \Psi\left[ \tfrac{1}{2}, -\tfrac{1}{3}; \beta_2^*\left( b^2 + \kappa_0^2 \right) \right] \right\} \tag{4.59}$$

where $b = 2\pi f/v$, $v_\perp$ is the component of the wind velocity normal to the beam axis, $\Psi(\alpha, \beta, z)$ is the confluent hypergeometric function,

$$\beta_1 = \frac{(1-s)^2}{\Omega/2 + 2/\Omega} \cdot \frac{x}{k} + \frac{1}{\kappa_m^2}, \qquad \beta_2 = \beta_1 - i(1-s)\frac{\Omega/2 - 2s/\Omega}{\Omega/2 + 2/\Omega} \qquad s = \frac{\xi}{x}$$

The spectrum (4.59) was obtained for the case in which $C_n^2$, $v_\perp$, and $\kappa_0$ can depend on the variable of integration along the measurement path. Expression (4.59) is somewhat simplified in the case of a homogeneous path.

For comparison with the results of measurements, it is more practical, than the function $\overline{W}_S(f)$, to work with the expression $u_S(f) = W_S(f)/\sigma_S^2$, where $\sigma_S^2$ is the variance of the phase fluctuations:

$$\sigma_S^2 = 8\pi^2 k^2 \int_0^x d\xi \int_0^\infty d\kappa\, \Phi_n(\kappa) \exp\left( \frac{\kappa^2}{k} \Omega \frac{x - \xi}{(1 - x/F)^2 + \Omega^{-2}} \right)$$

$$\times \left[ 1 + \cos\left( \frac{\kappa^2}{k}(x - \xi) \frac{x/F(x/F - 1) + \Omega^{-2}}{(1 - x/F)^2 + \Omega^{-2}} \right) \right] \tag{4.60}$$

Figure 4.14 gives the spectrum $q u_S(f)/f$ as a function of the dimensionless frequency $q = 2\pi f/\kappa_0 v_\perp$ for a plane wave ($\Omega = 2 \times 10^3$), a confined beam ($\Omega = 2$), and a spherical wave ($\Omega = 2 \times 10^{-5}$) for $\kappa_0^2 x/k = 10^4$, $\kappa_m/\kappa_0 = 10^3$. It is evident from the figure that all three curves coincide in the low-frequency range, and the function increases linearly with the dimensionless frequency $q$. After attaining a maximum, the function $u_S(f)$ decreases inversely as the frequency to the $-\tfrac{5}{3}$ power. In the high-frequency range, the phase fluctuation spectrum for a confined beam decreases more rapidly than the corresponding spectra for unconfined waves.

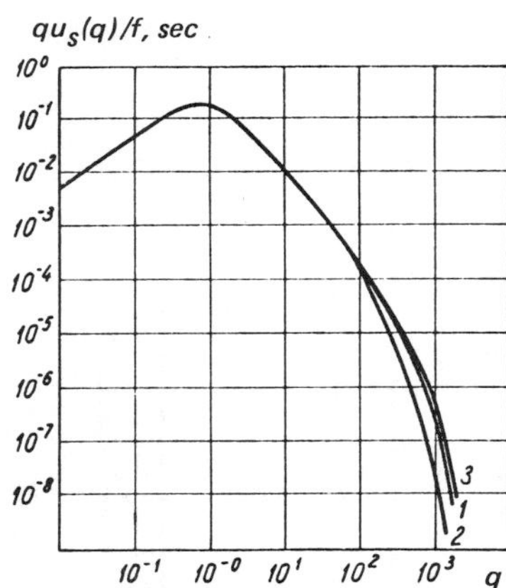



Fig. 4.14. Spectrum of phase fluctuations, $\kappa_0^2 x/k = 10^4$, $\kappa_m^2 \kappa_0^2 = 10^3$. (1) Plane wave, $\Omega = 2 \cdot 10^3$; (2) confined beam, $x/F = 0$, $\Omega = 2$; (3) spherical wave, $\Omega = 2 \cdot 10^{-5}$.

Experimental investigations of the phase fluctuations in laser beams in a turbulent atmosphere have been carried out [157–162] either with the application of a photometric procedure for determining the contrast of the interference fringes or by an optical-range heterodyning technique with the subsequent application of a digital phase meter. Pokasov and Khmelevtsov [157] and Bertolotti and others [158] have investigated the dependence of the structure function of the phase fluctuations on the spacing of the observation points and observed a tendency toward saturation of the function. Arsen'yan and others [159] measured the phase fluctuation correlation functions.

The experimental results given in [158–160] for the function $D_s(\rho)$ indicate that this function reaches saturation in the ground layer of the atmosphere along measurement paths at heights of 1.5 to 2 m, and models of the spectrum of atmospheric turbulence with an outer scale $L_0$ must be used to obtain correct estimates of the function.

Lukin and others [161] have measured the probability density functions and temporal statistical characteristics of the phase fluctuations. An analysis of these measurements shows that the phase fluctuation density function is well approximated by a normal law. The statistical characteristics of the phase-difference fluctuations were measured by a two-beam configuration; specifically, the temporal realization of the phase difference was determined at the centers of two Gaussian beams separated by a distance $\rho$, which was varied from 2 cm to 1.5 m. It was found that a decrease in the baseline substantially decreases the temporal autocorrelation radius of the phase difference, while an increase in the spacing of the beam increases that radius and simultaneously increases the negative autocorrelation depth.

A comparison of the experimental data on the structure and correlation functions of the phase fluctuations and the phase fluctuation spectra in laser beams in a turbulent atmosphere with the results of corresponding theoretical calculations indicate satisfactory agreement between those results, confirming the applicability of the expressions given above for quantitative estimates of the phase fluctuation characteristics.

## 4.10. Correction for Turbulent Distortions of Laser Beams

The fluctuations of the parameters of laser beams due to atmospheric turbulence limit the possibilities for the practical utilization of lasers for communications, information transmission, lidar, telemetry, and other applications. Consequently, the development of methods and means for the correction or compensation of the turbulent distortions of laser beams is of paramount practical importance. We emphasize the fact that the problem here is not one of minimizing the influence of the turbulent atmosphere on laser beams by an appropriate selection of spectral and geometrical parameters for the radiation sources and detectors, although certainly this consideration is also important for the development of atmospheric laser systems. Corrective or adaptive systems are designed, if not for complete eradication of the influence of turbulence on the operation of the corresponding laser systems, then at least for the partial compensation of that influence.

Adaptive systems can incorporate the following: (1) a transmitter station housing the radiation source, a transmitted-information encoding system, a controllable optical system, and instrumentation; (2) a turbulent medium with unknown, but measurable characteristics; (3) a reception station with a reference source (beacon) and instrumentation generating the signals for the controllable optics.

The following systems are realizable according to their functional criteria: (1) The source and reception stations are accessible, the measurement system (instrumentation) can be placed at the reception station, fluctuation data are transmitted by means of feedback to the controllable optics located at the transmitter station, corresponding distortions are introduced into the primary signal, and either an undistorted or a partially distorted signal is obtained at the reception station; (2) the reference point source (beacon) is placed at the reception station, where it is used for the performance of measurements at the transmitter station to obtain input information for the compensation of turbulent distortions of the laser beam; (3) only the transmitter station is accessible, as is the case in the majority of lidar systems; indirect information about the fluctuations of the optical wave at the receiver is used for compensation purposes.

In any adaptive system configuration, a necessary condition for its successful operation is the availability of reliable data on the fluctuations of the laser beam parameters for the particular source–receiver systems and conditions of atmospheric turbulence. Information about the fluctuations of the optical wave in the turbulent atmosphere can be obtained on the basis of appropriate monitoring data as well as by measurements of lidar signals reflected from various objects (reflectors, topographical features, aerosols) [163, 164].

We now consider a phase compensation system using a reference point source (beacon) situated at the reception station [165]. For an arbitrary field at the transmitter, the field in the reception plane is

$$U(x,\boldsymbol{\rho})=\frac{k}{2\pi ix}\int d^2\rho_1 U_0(\boldsymbol{\rho}_1)\exp\left[\frac{ik}{2x}(\boldsymbol{\rho}-\boldsymbol{\rho}_1)+\chi(x,\boldsymbol{\rho},\boldsymbol{\rho}_1)+iS(x,\boldsymbol{\rho},\boldsymbol{\rho}_1)\right]$$

$$(4.61)$$

where $\chi(x,\boldsymbol{\rho},\boldsymbol{\rho}_1)+iS(x,\boldsymbol{\rho},\boldsymbol{\rho}_1)$ is the additional complex phase induced by atmospheric turbulence for a spherical wave propagating from the point $(0,\boldsymbol{\rho}_1)$ to the point $(x,\boldsymbol{\rho})$ and $\boldsymbol{\rho}=\boldsymbol{\rho}(x,y)$ is the position vector in the plane transverse to the direction of propagation.

The phase distribution of the field from a beacon situated at the point $\rho=0$ in the plane $x'=x$ is characterized by the factor

$$U_b(0,\boldsymbol{\rho}_1)=\exp\left[-i\frac{k}{2x}\rho_1^2-iS(0,\boldsymbol{\rho}_1)\right] \qquad (4.62)$$

We consider only values of $\boldsymbol{\rho}$ for which $|\boldsymbol{\rho}|\lesssim\rho_S$, where $\rho_S$ is the coherence radius for a spherical wave. We can then use the approximate relation $S(\boldsymbol{\rho},\boldsymbol{\rho}_1)\simeq S(0,\boldsymbol{\rho}_1)$, and if the measured phase (4.62) from the beacon is used for correction, then the field at the receiver is written for the case of total phase correction:

$$U_c(x,\boldsymbol{\rho})=\frac{k}{2\pi ix}\int d^2\rho_1 U_0(\boldsymbol{\rho}_1)\exp\left[i\frac{k}{x}\boldsymbol{\rho}\boldsymbol{\rho}_1+i\frac{k}{2x}\rho^2+\chi(\boldsymbol{\rho},\boldsymbol{\rho}_1)\right] \quad (4.63)$$

where the symbol $c$ indicates that a phase-correction system is involved. To estimate the efficiency of this kind of system it is necessary to calculate the relative variance of the intensity fluctuations of the received radiation

$$\sigma_{I,c}^2 = \langle I_c^2 \rangle / \langle I_c \rangle^2 - 1 \tag{4.64}$$

where $I_c$ is the field intensity at the receiver.

It can be shown that for large transmitting apertures ($\Omega = ka^2/x \gg 1$, transmitter with large Fresnel number), correct to within terms of order $\Omega^{-1}$,

$$\langle I_c \rangle \simeq \exp\left(-\sigma_\chi^2\right) I_0(\rho), \qquad \langle I_c^2 \rangle \simeq \exp\left(-2\sigma_\chi^2\right) I_0^2(\rho) \tag{4.65}$$

where $\sigma_\chi^2 = \langle (\chi - \langle \chi \rangle)^2 \rangle$ and $I_0(\rho)$ is the intensity of the field of the beam in a homogeneous medium.

Thus, substituting Eq. (4.65) into Eq. (4.64), we see that if phase fluctuations are completely compensated in the system, then for large apertures the quivering of the source is almost entirely eliminated ($\sigma_{I,c}^2 \simeq 0$).

For small receiving apertures, $\Omega \ll 1$, it turns out that phase correction is ineffectual. It is necessary in this case to introduce control of the source power.

Phase correction is realizable whenever the wavelength of the reference source differs from the wavelength of the transmitter because atmospheric turbulence is weakly selective with respect to wavelength variations [166]. A detailed study of the effectiveness of such a system [167] has resulted in the recommendation of performance criteria for the cases of weak and strong fluctuations and of large and small Fresnel numbers. As in the preceding case, the system turns out to be effective for large values of $\Omega$. For complete phase correction in this case, it suffices to measure the instantaneous distribution of the random phase from a point source.

To obtain information about the instantaneous random phase distribution at the receiving aperture and make appropriate phase corrections at the transmitting aperture, various dynamic aperture configurations have been proposed [168–171]. Typical of such proposals are either multielement (segmented) apertures whose elements have independent servos for longitudinal translations and rotations or a special system comprising a deformable mirror, membrane mirrors, or a dynamic array of focusing elements. If the system consists of a large number of small elements, the phase distortions can be compensated only by translational movements of the elements [170, 172]. All of these systems are highly complex from the standpoint of technical implementation.

A much simpler system for the correction of distortions of the phase front of a laser beam transmitted through a layer of a turbulent atmosphere is a system for compensation of the fluctuations of the angle of arrival associated with the inclination of the phase front. This kind of correction reduces the angular spread of the beam and, hence, increases the intensity of the field incident on the receiving aperture. This system is effective, for example, when it is required to eliminate the influence of effects ranging from beam wander in the large to low-frequency random refraction [163, 173]. We now estimate the effectiveness of the given correction mode.

Let the instantaneous random phase at the receiver be $S(\boldsymbol{\rho}, t)$, and let the phase of the wave at this same point after compensation for the inclined aperture be

$$S_c(\boldsymbol{\rho}, t) = S(\boldsymbol{\rho}, t) - \boldsymbol{a}\boldsymbol{\rho} \tag{4.66}$$

where $2\pi a / \lambda$ is the angle formed by the plane of the wave front with the plane of the aperture. The algorithm for selecting the vector $\boldsymbol{a}$ must be such that $\boldsymbol{a}\boldsymbol{\rho}$ will best approximate the phase $S(\boldsymbol{\rho}, t)$ at the receiver. It has been proposed [173] that $\boldsymbol{a}$ be chosen so as to yield the best approximation to the phase of the field in the sense of the mean square with respect to the aperture. The following equations are obtained for an aperture with weighting function $W(\boldsymbol{\rho})$ and phase $S(\boldsymbol{\rho}, t)$:

$$\frac{\partial}{\partial a} \int d^2\rho \left[ S(\boldsymbol{\rho}, t) - \boldsymbol{a}\boldsymbol{\rho} \right]^2 W(\boldsymbol{\rho}) = 0 \tag{4.67}$$

and in the case of a symmetrical weighting function

$$\boldsymbol{a} = \frac{\int d^2\rho S(\boldsymbol{\rho}, t)\rho W(\boldsymbol{\rho})}{\pi \int_0^\infty d\rho W(\rho)\rho^3} \tag{4.68}$$

Application of the Huygens–Kirchhoff principle in the phase approximation [35, 44, 75, 76] for the broad beams ($\Omega \gg 1$) yields an expression for the distribution of the average intensity in the plane $x' = x$:

$$\langle I(x, \boldsymbol{\rho}) \rangle = \left( \frac{k}{2\pi x} \right)^2 \int d^2\rho_1 \exp\left( i\frac{k}{x}\boldsymbol{\rho}_1\boldsymbol{\rho} \right) M_T(\boldsymbol{\rho}_1) \tag{4.69}$$

where

$$M_T(\rho_1) = \int d^2 R \, U_0\left(R + \frac{\rho_1}{2}\right) U_0^*\left(R - \frac{\rho_1}{2}\right)$$

$$\times \exp\left(ik\frac{\rho_1 R}{x}\right)\exp\left[-\frac{1}{2}D_S(R,\rho_1)\right] \qquad (4.70)$$

is the transfer function of the atmosphere and transmitter,

$$D_S(R,\rho) = D_S(\rho) + \langle(a\rho)^2\rangle - 2\left\langle a\rho\left[S\left(R+\frac{\rho}{2}\right) - S\left(R-\frac{\rho}{2}\right)\right]\right\rangle$$

$$= D_S(\rho) - D_1(\rho, R) \qquad (4.71)$$

and $D_1(\rho, R)$ is the variation of the phase structure function due to correction for inclinations.

Calculations carried out by means of the foregoing expressions in the case of a Kármán atmospheric turbulence spectrum have shown that for sufficiently small apertures $a \lesssim L_0$ the correction for random tilts significantly improves the structure of the intensity distribution, whereas for large apertures, $a \gtrsim L_0$, the same correction is ineffectual. The quantitative data obtained on the effectiveness of the given correction evinces the fact that axial intensity in the case of strong fluctuations is increased several decibels by correction, while complete phase compensation makes it possible to obtain [165] an intensity peak roughly half the value in vacuum. In the case of weak fluctuations, tilt correction yields system characteristics close to those associated with diffraction effects. Lawrence [163] has analyzed the limitations of using tilt correction of the phase front of a beam, showing, in particular, that this correction is most effective at distances where the laser beam wanders as a whole without breaking up into a set of separate parts.

Reports have been published recently on the feasibility of using nonlinear optics for the correction of laser beam fluctuations in the atmosphere as well as for the correction of random effects associated with thermal warming of the medium during the propagation of high-energy beams in the atmosphere [174].

In addition to the dynamic correction methods discussed above, there are also *a posteriori* methods, where the corresponding distortion effects are eliminated after completion of an experiment. Both classical optical filtering methods and methods for the solution of ill-posed inverse problems [175] are used in this connection.

## 4.11. Conclusion

As a result of intensive theoretical and experimental research carried out in the last few years on the propagation of laser beams in a turbulent atmosphere, it has recently become possible to make quantitative assessments of the various effects associated with amplitude and phase fluctuations of spatially confined waves, provided that a reliable turbulence model is available. These multivarious effects are discussed in detail in the author's earlier work [4], which does not, however, cover the problems of compensating turbulent distortions of laser beams.

In this chapter, we have attempted within certain space limitations, to present a condensed overview of the most important results pertaining to the given problem. Aspects of the solution of inverse problems of turbulence optics have been left outside the scope of the presentation; they will be considered in Chap. 7. We have also touched only briefly on the influence of a turbulent atmosphere on lidar signals when a laser beam traverses one given layer of the atmosphere twice. This brevity is dictated by the fact that theoretical as well as experimental work in this important area is still in the germinal phase. Only very recently has this research attracted major attention, as may be judged, for example, from the general content of papers presented at the Fourth All-Union Conference on the Propagation of Laser Radiation in the Atmosphere, where relevant papers were accorded the space deserved [176-185].

# 5

# Nonlinear Effects Associated with the Propagation of Laser Radiation in the Atmosphere

## 5.0. Introduction

Nonlinear interactions of laser radiation with the atmosphere significantly alter the laws governing its propagation in the atmospheric medium as treated in the preceding chapters. This circumstance accounts for the considerable interest shown in the investigation of nonlinear effects and the definite progress that has been achieved as a result in the last few years. Although nonlinear interactions of laser radiation with the atmosphere also attend the absorption of radiation by atmospheric gases and its scattering by aerosol particles, as well as propagation in a turbulent atmosphere, we have deemed it appropriate to consolidate their specific discussion in a separate chapter, thereby underscoring not only the specifics, but also the special significance of these phenomena in relation to the propagation of laser radiation in the atmosphere as a whole.

In the ensuing text, we endeavor to analyze the most substantive results of theoretical and experimental research on nonlinear effects in recent times, but because of space limitations, a detailed review of individual problems is not possible here.

## 5.1. Optical Breakdown of Gases

By optical breakdown of gases we understand the process of inception and development of vigorous ionization in gases under the action of powerful laser radiation. The process is accompanied by the occurrence of "laser sparks," the propagation of shock waves and ionization fronts, and shuttering of the laser beam due to strong absorption and nonlinear scattering of light in the generated plasma. The latter effect imposes limitations on the peak optical energy flux that can be transported through the atmosphere.

The optical breakdown of gases has been well studied at a theoretical level and on the basis of laboratory experiments. The fundamental results obtained since the present author's earlier book [1] are covered in books by Raizer [2] and Ready [3] and in survey articles [4–7]. However, direct experiments in the real atmosphere are altogether insufficient. No information has been published on the breakdown of gases in the case of large-aperture beams, as applies to the propagation of laser radiation over long paths in the atmosphere.

The dependence of the breakdown threshold intensity $I_b$ on the laser pulse duration $t_p$ is illustrated schematically in Fig. 5.1. The solid curves characterize the action of radiation in the visible and near-infrared wavelength ranges, and the dashed curves correspond to radiation emitted by a $CO_2$ laser with a wavelength of 10.6 $\mu$m. Curves 1 and 2 correspond to the breakdown of technically pure air and curves 1' and 2' to air containing aerosols and easily ionized impurities.

In the short-wave region of the spectrum, bare electrons capable of initiating cascade ionization of technically pure gases appear as a result of multiphoton ionization of the medium with a process firing time $\lesssim 10^{-12}$ sec. In connection with the propagation of short subpicosecond pulses, or at

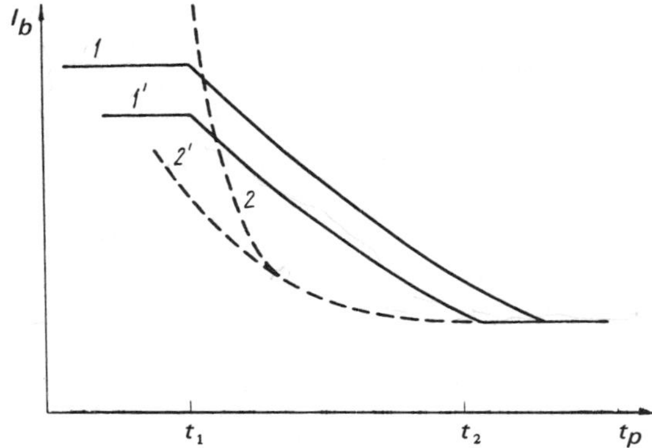

Fig. 5.1. Schematic dependence of optical breakdown threshold intensity on laser pulse duration for visible and near IR wavelengths (solid curves) and for 10.6-$\mu$m radiation (dashed curves). (1, 2) Impurity-free, technically clean air; (1', 2') air containing aerosol and easily ionized impurity particles.

low pressures corresponding to the upper layers of the atmosphere, the bare electrons cannot initiate cascade ionization due to the low probability of collisions with air molecules. The breakdown threshold in this case is determined by photoionization and has a value of $10^{13}$ to $10^{15}$ W/cm$^2$. In Fig. 5.1 this case corresponds to the flat part of the left branch of curve 1.

The following qualitative relation between the breakdown threshold power and the pressure $p$ and pulse duration $t_p$ can be deduced from the condition of complete multiphoton ionization of the medium:

$$P_b \sim \left( p t_p \right)^{-1/n}$$

where $n$ is the multiplicity of multiphoton ionization.

Krasyuk and others [8] have carried out detailed investigations of the optical breakdown of various gases by radiation from a ruby laser with $t_p = 50$ psec over a wide range of pressure variation. Corresponding experiments with a neodymium–glass laser have been conducted by Alcock and Richardson [9]. Breakdown thresholds of the order of $10^{13}$ to $10^{15}$ W/cm$^2$ are obtained for both types of lasers at pressures of the order of $10^2$ Torr in various technically pure gases. At high pressures, the curves corresponding to those shown in Fig. 5.1 acquire a kink, which is attributable to the replacement of multiphoton ionization by a cascade mechanism of laser spark formation.

The presence of traces of easily ionized gas impurities and aerosol particles in the atmosphere acts as a secondary electron source, which promotes a significant reduction in the optical breakdown threshold of air [6, 10, 11]. The breakdown threshold can also be lowered by self-focusing of laser radiation in the atmosphere [12].

Radiation propagating in the atmosphere from a carbon dioxide laser with breakdown of air due to multiphoton ionization is less probable due to the low energy of the quanta. Here an additional possible mechanism for the development of an ion cascade is the photoionization of atoms and molecules previously excited by electron impact.

Cascade ionization of the medium prevails in the air of the atmosphere, where it is sustained by the absorption of laser radiation. The final number density of electrons $N_e$ in cascade ionization breakdown without regard for losses is described by the expression

$$N_e = N_{e0}\exp(\nu_i t) = N_{e0}2^k \tag{5.1}$$

in which $N_{e0}$ is the density of bare electrons, $\nu_i$ is the average frequency of ionizations produced by the entire electron spectrum, and $k$ is the number of electron generations in the cascade. For $N_{e0}=10^6 \mathrm{cm}^{-3}$ and $N_e=10^{19} \mathrm{cm}^{-3}$, we have $k \approx 43$.

The cascade theory of optical breakdown of pure gases is described in Raizer's book [2]. In the rigorous formulation, the problem entails finding a solution of the quantum difference equation for the electron energy spectrum; this equation can be reduced to a differential equation that approximately describes the breakdown of a gas by laser variation in the visible and infrared ranges. When recombination losses, spatial diffusion, and the capture of electrons by heavy molecules are taken into account, this equation has the form

$$dN_e/dt = \phi(t) + (\nu_i - \nu_a)N_e - \nabla^2(DN_e) - \beta N_e^2 \tag{5.2}$$

where $\phi(t)$ is a function characterizing the intensity of the sources of bare-electron generation, $\nu_a$ is the frequency of attachments of electrons to heavy molecules as a result of capture, and $D$ and $\beta$ are the coefficients of spatial diffusion and recombination, respectively. The expression for the average ionization frequency is written in the form

$$\nu_i = \frac{e^2 E_0^2 \nu_m}{2m\left(\nu_m^2 + \omega^2\right)I_i} \tag{5.3}$$

where $e$ and $m$ are the electron charge and mass, $\omega$ and $E_0$ are the frequency and rms strength of the laser electric field:

$$E_0 = \left(\frac{8\pi I}{c\varepsilon_0^{1/2}}\right)^{1/2} \tag{5.4}$$

$\varepsilon_0$ is the permittivity of the medium, $I$ is the radiation intensity, $c$ is the speed of light, $I_i$ is the particle ionization energy, and $\nu_m$ is the frequency of elastic collisions of electrons with neutrals.

From (5.2) and (5.3) we readily obtain an expression for the threshold intensity of radiation $I_b$ in the absence of losses:

$$I_b = \frac{c\varepsilon_0\left(\nu_m^2 + \omega^2\right)mI_i}{4\pi e \nu_m} \frac{\ln\left(N_a/N_{e0}\right)}{t} \tag{5.5}$$

Expression (5.5) corresponds to an intermediate region of the curves shown in Fig. 5.1; $N_a$ is the density of neutral particles, and $N_{e0}$ is the density of bare electrons.

For air at atmospheric pressure, $\nu_m \sim 10^{13}$ sec$^{-1}$, which is much lower than $\omega$ for the visible and near-infrared regions. In this case, we obtain from (5.5) $I_b \sim \omega^2/t\nu_m \sim \omega^2/t_p$; thus, the threshold intensity for a cascade mechanism of breakdown in the steady state is inversely proportional to the air pressure and the wavelength squared of the laser radiation.

For broad laser beams propagating in the atmosphere, the main losses are attributable to the capture of electrons by oxygen molecules and, to a lesser extent, recombination, diffusion, and reradiation processes. It follows from the results of calculations [6] of the breakdown threshold for 10.6-$\mu$m laser radiation in pure air as a function of the pulse duration with losses due to the electron capture by $O_2$ molecules that the threshold intensity in the steady-state development of the cascade process for pulses with durations greater than $10^{-5}$ sec is $4 \times 10^9$ W/cm$^2$. The threshold for shorter pulses increases inversely as the duration.

Experimental studies of the optical breakdown thresholds of molecular gases and air under the action of ruby and neodymium–glass lasers with pulse durations of 40 nsec at various pressures have shown that the values of the thresholds for 0.69-$\mu$m radiation are roughly an order of magnitude higher than for a wavelength of 1.06 $\mu$m for all the gases investigated ($N_2$, $O_2$, $CO_2$, and air). At a pressure of 1000 Torr, the threshold intensities for air are approximately $7 \times 10^{10}$ and $2 \times 10^{11}$ W/cm$^2$ for neodymium–glass and ruby lasers, respectively. Corresponding experiments conducted under the same conditions with atmospheric gases (Xe, Ne, Ar) have disclosed lower breakdown thresholds for those gases [6] because the development of the cascade process in the case of molecular gases is complicated by additional electron energy losses due to the nonionizing excitation of molecular oscillations. Also, this effect is promoted by the presence of low electron-excitation levels in the molecules.

Experiments with a 10.6-$\mu$m laser with a pulse duration of 160 nsec at various air pressures have yielded values for the breakdown threshold at a pressure of 1000 Torr that fall in the interval from $1 \times 10^9$ to $6 \times 10^9$ W/cm$^2$ as the focal length of the lens is varied between 5 and 15 cm. As mentioned earlier, the presence of dust particles in the atmosphere lowers the optical breakdown threshold by 1 or 2 orders of magnitude. This result, for example, has been obtained in [13] for a 10.6-$\mu$m laser with a pulse duration of 35 to 40 nsec. In experiments with a $CO_2$ laser having a pulse duration of 200 nsec [14], the breakdown threshold for purified air is at least $10^{10}$ W$\cdot$cm$^2$, whereas in ordinary air containing microscopic dust particles, breakdown is observed at a radiation intensity of $2 \times 10^9$ W/cm$^2$. Dust particles with a diameter of 20 $\mu$m lower the threshold to $10^8$ W/cm$^2$.

Laser sparking in the atmosphere radically disrupts the usual pattern of propagation of laser radiation insofar as, on the one hand, spark generation consumes a sizable fraction of the radiation energy and, on the other, the medium of the spark itself has low transparency for laser radiation. For this reason, we briefly discuss the problems of laser spark dynamics and the transparency of its plasma.

The breakdown of air by $Q$-switched pulses is accompanied by expansion of the breakdown region in the direction of the focusing lens. The initial rates of expansion in this case are of the order of $10^7$ cm/sec [2]. The initial density of electrons after the formation of breakdown, $N_e \gtrsim 10^{19}$ cm$^{-3}$, corresponds to single ionization of the gas in the focal volume. The absorption coefficient of an optical wave in the breakdown plasma is given by the expression [2]

$$\alpha_\omega [\mathrm{cm}^{-1}] = \frac{4\pi e^2 N_e \nu_m}{mc(\omega^2 + \nu_m^2)} \tag{5.6}$$

and in the case of a singly ionized gas is of the order of 100 km$^{-1}$, corresponding to the value of the volume extinction coefficient in a water cloud with average microphysical parameters and a visibility of 40 m in its interior.

Under the action of hard ultraviolet and soft x-ray radiation emitted by the central part of the spark, partial ionization takes place in the surrounding gas volume with a radius of the order of 10 cm [15–17]. This effect is referred to as the "ionization aureole" [15].

Several mechanisms have been described in the literature for the motion of the plasma front. The optical detonation mechanism is based on the hypothesis of transformation of a detonation wave into a shock front after cessation of the action of the laser pulse, at which time the ionization aureole can play a significant part in the expansion of the plasma. This mechanism can account for the possible formation of a long spark [4]. Raizer and others [18, 19] describe a "breakdown wave" mechanism, whereby weak focusing of a beam in the atmosphere produces visible motion of the spark boundary due to nonsimultaneous attainment of the threshold electron densities along the path. The velocity of the breakdown wave in this case increases with the power of the laser and can exceed the optical detonation threshold. Bunkin and others [20] have discovered a mechanism such that the laser spark discharge front propagates with velocities of several tens of meters per second, i.e., the so-called "slow-burning" mechanism. The laser spark in this case is forcibly "ignited" by the generation of a "primer" plasma from an external source. This state corresponds to the flat portion on the right-hand sides of the curves in Fig. 5.1.

The threshold intensities of laser radiation for the sustainment of "optical burning" are 2 to 3 orders of magnitude lower than for initial spark ignition. Figure 5.2 gives experimental data on the threshold power density radiated by a $CO_2$ laser for plasma maintenance as a function of the beam cross-sectional area [21]. The plasma consisted of a bright core immediately in front of the focal point of the focusing system and a surrounding, somewhat fainter blue sheath with a diameter of a few centimeters. The experimental data indicated in the figure by the various kinds of points refer to cases in which the primer plasma is obtained by electrical discharge. The star-point indicates the result obtained in the irradiation of a steel target.

The processes of plasma formation and propagation by the breakdown of gases near solid targets due to radiation from a $CO_2$ laser with a microsecond pulse duration have been systematically investigated [7, 22–25] with the development of a physical model of the process of initiation of low-threshold breakdown of a gas due to the vaporization of a film adsorbed on a solid target. The analytical and experimental results give values of the breakdown threshold intensity equal to $(5–10) \times 10^6$ W/cm$^2$. The measured thresholds for the maintenance of the breakdown plasma turn out to be roughly equal to the thresholds for maintenance of a plasma on the surface of metals.

The foregoing discussion indicates that the thresholds for optical breakdown of the atmosphere by powerful laser radiation vary between widely separated limits as a function of the wavelength, beam diameter,

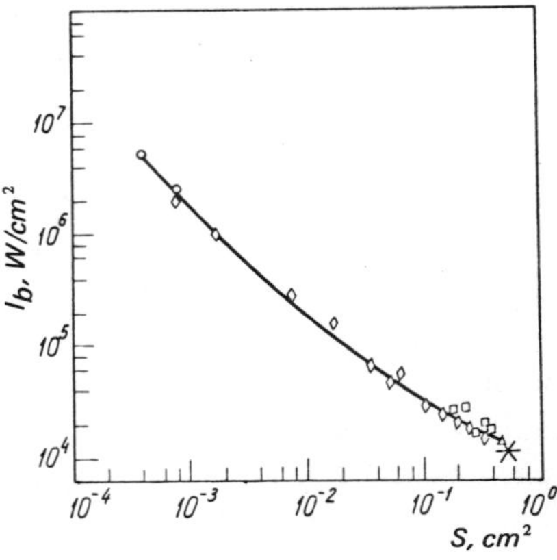


Fig. 5.2. Radiation intensity necessary for plasma maintenance versus beam cross section. Different point symbols correspond to different techniques for recording the optical breakdown event with excitation of the primary plasma by an electrical discharge; the star-point corresponds to plasma initiation with irradiation of a steel target.

lasing regime, and state of the atmosphere. The lowest thresholds should be expected for broad $CO_2$ laser beams in the presence of atmospheric dust particles or near-solid surfaces. The limiting intensities for the stable propagation of radiation from these lasers in the real atmosphere for pulses with durations $t_p \lesssim 10^{-6}$ sec and continuous (quasicontinuous) emission are $\sim 10^7$ to $10^8$ W/cm$^2$ and $10^4$ to $10^5$ W/cm$^2$, respectively.

## 5.2. Nonlinear Spectroscopic Effects in Gas Media

In linear spectroscopy, given a low spectral density of emission sources and a linear dependence of the polarization of the medium on the amplitude of the light field acting on it, the propagation of light beams in the medium is described by means of the spectral optical parameters (absorption coefficient and refractive index), which determine only the structure and state of the medium [26].

If the radiation field interacting with the medium is comparable with the fields governing intra- and intermolecular interactions, i.e., with the fields determining the quantum transition probabilities in the molecules as well as relaxation processes, the methods of linear spectroscopy become inapplicable for description of the processes of interaction of radiation with a molecular medium [27].

The interaction of powerful radiation with a medium is described in its most general form by the self-consistent solution of the Maxwell equations and the equations for the components of the density matrix of the medium. Here the spectral optical parameters are introduced only in certain special cases. The most complex situation arises in connection with the propagation of high-power (in particular, pulsed) radiation in gas media in which the relaxation times of the populations (distribution of molecules among the energy states) and polarization of the states are commensurate, while transitions in the optical region of the spectrum are easily subjected to various electrical perturbations [27].

Powerful laser radiation propagating in a gas medium produces variations of the quantum and statistical properties of the molecules, splitting of the energy levels, mixing of states, and changes of the orientation and time of interaction of the molecules, the trajectories of their motion, and the molecular interaction potential, as well as the stimulation of chemical reactions and, hence, variation of the rates of relaxation processes, transition probabilities, and spectra of the molecular systems [27–29].

As in linear spectroscopy, the greatest information about the processes of interaction of powerful laser radiation with the medium is contained in the contour of the absorption line. Four nonlinear effects are paramount in the problem of the absorption line contour in a strong field: (1) the spectroscopic saturation effect; (2) the dynamic Stark effect; (3) effects of the field on the molecular interaction potential; (4) the stimulation of molecular chemical activity [27–30, 38–42].

## 5.2.1. Spectroscopic Saturation

The spectroscopic saturation effect is related to population equalization of the molecular levels between which resonance transitions take place. Its action has the effect of decreasing the absorption coefficient at the line center and broadening the line due to the greater rate of population equalization under the action of absorption at the center of the line than in the wings. The radiation intensity at which the saturation effect is observed is [30]

$$I_s = \frac{c\hbar^2}{2|\mu|^2 T_1 T_2} \tag{5.7}$$

where $|\mu|^2$ is the square of the matrix element of the dipole moment of transition, $T_1$ is the relaxation time of the level populations, and $T_2$ is the phase relaxation time.

The spectroscopic saturation effect has been studied in detail theoretically [1, 30–33]. Experimental data have been obtained on the saturation of the centers of lines associated with transitions in $CO_2$, $SF_6$, and $BCl_3$ [31–34], exhibiting satisfactory agreement with the theoretical. For example, Ryabov [34] found that the absorption coefficient at the center of the line for $SF_6$ at a partial pressure of 20 Torr in a mixture with argon at a total pressure of $10^3$ Torr is diminished by one-half for a laser output intensity of $1.2 \times 10^6$ W/cm² with a pulse duration of 120 nsec. The theoretical value of the intensity $I_s$ for this case is $10^6$ W/cm².

Detailed experimental investigations of the inception of the spectroscopic effect in the shape of the absorption line for water vapor with center at 694.38 nm ($4_{-3}$–$5_4$ transition of the 000–103 band) in connection with its broadening by air, $N_2$, and $CO_2$ are reported in our work [35–37]. Figures 5.3 and 5.4 give the results of investigations of the line shape obtained for a relative air moisture content of 40% at room temperature and pressures of 730 and 270 Torr ($H_2O$ partial pressures of 7 and 3 Torr, respectively) with

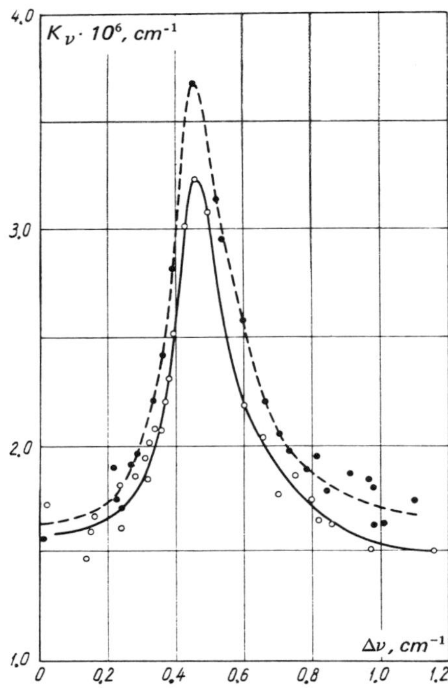

Fig. 5.3. Absorption in air, $p = 730$ mm Hg, $T = 290°$K, $\alpha = 40\%$. (1)●–●, $I_{1\,\mathrm{las}} = 5$ MW/cm$^2$; (2) ○–○, $I_{1\,\mathrm{las}} = 35$ MW/cm$^2$.

a ruby laser emitting at intensities of 5 and 35 MW/cm$^2$. The values of $I_s$ determined from the experimental data for pressures of 730 and 270 Torr are equal to 180 and 43 MW/cm$^2$, which are in good agreement with the values calculated according to expression (5.7): 200 and 55 MW/cm$^2$. We note that $I_s$ is interpreted as the intensity value at which the absorption coefficient decreases by one-half.

The measured values of the absorption line half-width conflicts with the theoretical predictions; according to the theory of the half-width of absorption lines in a strong field, it should vary as $(I + I/I_s)^{1/2}$ and so it should increase with the intensity. In our case, the calculations yield 10 and 12.5% increases in the half-width of the line at pressures of 730 and 270 Torr as the intensity is increased from 5 to 35 MW/cm$^2$. Experimentally, the line narrows by 9.4 and 9.0%, respectively. The indicated fact clearly implies that the behavior of the absorption line shape is determined not only by the saturation effect, but also by the variation of the molecular interaction potential in the field, possibly as a result of a growth in the number of excited molecules during irradiation and of the orientation of dipole molecules in the field.

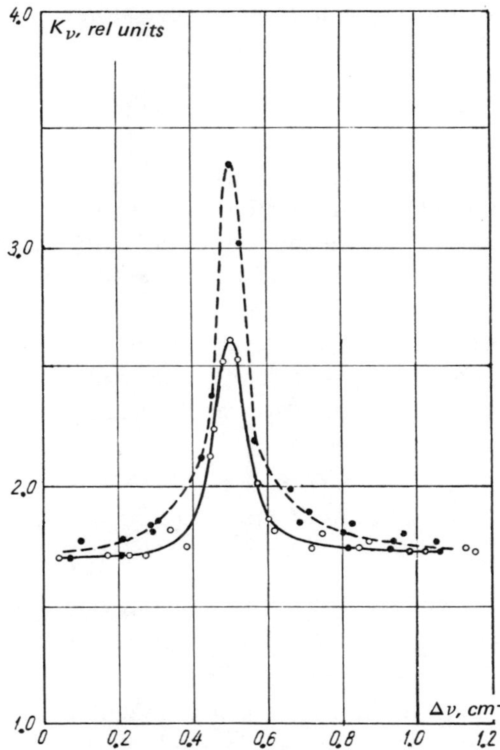


Fig. 5.4. Absorption in air, $p = 270$ mm Hg, $T = 290°K$, $\alpha = 40\%$. (1) -●-, $I_{las} = 5$ MW/cm$^2$; (2) -O-, $I_{las} = 35$ MW/cm$^2$.

Investigations of the behavior of the shape of the $H_2O$ line broadened by $N_2$ and $CO_2$ at radiation intensities of 5 and 35 MW/cm$^2$ yield the following results: In the case where the broadening gas is $N_2$ at a partial pressure of 150 Torr and the partial pressure of the $H_2O$ is 7 Torr, the absorption coefficient at the center of the line is observed to decrease by 0.67, while the absorption in the wings changes only slightly. The pattern changes abruptly in a mixture of $H_2O$ at 6 Torr with $CO_2$ at 290 Torr, namely, the center absorption remains unchanged, while the absorption in the wings changes more with increasing distance from the center of the line.

## 5.2.2. Dynamic Stark Effect

The dynamic Stark effect induces a shift of the transition frequency in a light field, resulting in broadening of the absorption line by an amount comparable with its usual value at intensities [38]

$$I_{St} = \frac{c\hbar^2}{|\mu|^2 T_2^2}$$

(5.8)

The theoretical study of this effect is in the nascent phase. It has been shown [39] that the Stark shift in molecules of the HCl and CO type with a transition dipole moment of order $10^{-19}$ cgs esu, depending on the type of transition, amounts to 1 to 3 $Hz/(W/cm^2)$ and can increase by an order of magnitude or more in the event of an equidistant vibrational structure between resonance levels in the molecules. Theoretical calculations and estimates for more complex molecules are lacking so far. Also unavailable are experimental data for molecular transitions in the optical wavelength range.

### 5.2.3. Effects of the Radiation Field on the Molecular Interaction Potential

The variation of the molecular interaction potential under the action of a strong light field is attributable to the orienting action [28] of the field on molecules possessing a dipole moment.

A strong field not only orients polar molecules, it also inhibits their disorientation in collisions with other molecules. Consequently, the effective cross section for collisions that contribute to line broadening is diminished. Theoretical estimates of the magnitude of the critical field (radiation intensity) show that narrowing of the rotational lines is to be expected when the field-squared addition to the molecular interaction potential $A \sim \alpha E^2$, where $\alpha$ is the polarizability of the molecule, no longer satisfies the condition [28]

$$B_0 \gg A$$

(5.9)

where $B_0$ is the rotational structure constant.

A second cause of variation of the molecular interaction potential is associated with the increase in the number of excited molecules per unit volume due to a strong field and the resulting fact that the broadening of the line is now determined by collisions of molecules of the broadening gas with molecules of the absorbing gas in both the ground and in the excited states.

Finally, one other cause of the influence of a strong light field on the molecular interaction potential is dictated by the influence of the field on the dynamics of the collision process between absorbing and broadening molecules. The critical fields for this effect are given by the expression [40]

$$2V\tau_c = \frac{2|\mu|E}{\hbar}\tau_c \sim 1 \qquad (5.10)$$

where $\tau_c$ is the characteristic collision time of the molecules.

The influence of a strong light field on the molecular interaction potential is such as to decrease the effective collision cross section of the molecules and to narrow the collisional shape of the absorption lines. The resultant absorption line shape is determined by the sum total of the mechanisms indicated above, and the nature of its broadening can be extremely complex.

The given effect has been analyzed theoretically in simple models (two-level system—alkali metals) [28, 30, 38–42]. The existing estimates show that the variation of the molecular interaction potential must be taken into account at optical intensities of $10^7$ W/cm$^2$ or higher. The resultant action of the field is manifested in narrowing of the collisional line shape and in a reduction of the absorption coefficients in the far wings [40, 41, 43]. Kochanov and others [44] have obtained experimental confirmation of this inference in observations of the variation of the width of narrow resonances within the Doppler contour of $CO_2$ due to a corresponding variation of the effective collision cross section.

## 5.2.4. Stimulation of Chemical Activity of Molecules

The stimulation of chemical activity of molecules by a strong light field under definite conditions can induce effects that are impossible to ignore in quantitative estimates of the absorption of laser radiation by atmospheric gases. One reason for the given effect has to do with the capability of a strong field to enhance the content of gas molecules in the excited state, resulting in a substantial increase in the efficiency of chemical reactions. For example, the cross section of the reaction $O_3 + NO \rightarrow NO_2^* + O_2$ is increased twentyfold if vibrations of ozone at the fundamental frequency $\nu_3$ are excited by a $CO_2$ laser [45]. Reactions involving $CO_2$ and $N_2O$ are stimulated analogously.

In the pumping of the fundamental mode $\nu_3$ in pure $CO_2$ and $N_2O$, which have equidistant level spacings, the threshold power of a continuous $CO_2$ laser for the initiation of an appreciable increase in the reaction yield is approximately $3.2 \times 10^{-2}$ W/cm$^{-2}$ Torr, while in the pumping of CO modes it is $2 \times 10^{-4}$ W/cm$^{-2}$Torr$^{-2}$ [29].

Moving into the near-infrared and visible regions of the spectrum, we find that the quantum energy increases, as does the energy imparted to the molecule in excitation, so that the efficiency of stimulation of chemical reactions can increase accordingly.

The theory of the stimulation of chemical reactions in gases in connection with the selective action of laser radiation on the molecular bonds is mainly based on stepwise excitation in an equidistant vibrational spectrum in the emission region of a $CO_2$ laser. The existing experimental work refers to pure gases at low pressures. The processes of laser-stimulated chemical reactions in gases of the real atmosphere have not been studied either theoretically or experimentally.

## 5.2.5. Modification of the Characteristics of Laser Radiation in a Resonance-Absorbing Molecular Medium

The propagation of powerful laser radiation in a molecular-gas medium is accompanied not only by the nonlinear spectroscopic effects discussed above, but also by a variation of the spectral energy characteristics of the radiation itself. The variation of the corresponding parameters of a powerful laser pulse in this case is determined by the relationship between the pulse duration $t_p$ and the relaxation times $T_1$ and $T_2$ [42]. For gases at pressures of 0.1 to 1 atm, i.e., under typical atmospheric conditions, the interaction of radiation emitted by lasers with $t_p \sim 10^{-8}$ sec satisfies the condition $t_p \gg T_2$, i.e., is incoherent. The analysis of the variation of the amplitude and phase characteristics of the radiation pulse in this case entails the solution of a system of equations [42] containing the transition dipole moment matrix element and the relaxation times $T_1$ and $T_2$, which is valid for the two-level approximation. If the indicated characteristics are known, then for any relations between $t_p$ and $T_1$ the given system of equations can be solved analytically or numerically [46].

The corresponding calculations show that propagation in a resonance-absorbing medium with an optical density $\tau_0 \sim 5$ is attended by shortening of the laser pulse, a variation in the shape of its edges, broadening of the spectrum, and a variation of the polarization characteristics [42, 46–50]. The two-level system approximation proves inadequate in the analysis of the interaction of laser pulses with complex molecular systems. The dynamics of the evolution of the pulse characteristics in this case poses an extremely complex problem, which does not yield even to numerical analysis [46].

The majority of the experimental work in which distortion of a pulse and modification of its spectral composition have been observed refers to the interaction of radiation with condensed media. An experimental study of the distortion of a radiation pulse emitted by a $CO_2$ laser and propagating in gaseous $SF_6$ indicates an increase in the slopes of the leading and trailing edges of the pulse as well as a two-thirds decrease in its duration for an optical density $\tau_0 \sim 3\text{--}4$ [51].

Lopasov and others [52, 53] have conducted experimental investigations of the distortion of a ruby laser pulse and the variation of its spectrum during propagation in an atmosphere of molecular iodine vapor. At a radiation intensity of 120 MW/cm$^2$, the pulse spectrum broadens 40%, while the pulse duration is shortened only 12%. An investigation of the propagation of a dye laser pulse with a duration of 20 nsec and intensity of 10 MW/cm$^2$ in a resonance-absorbing potassium vapor indicates an increase in the radiation spreading from $10^{-2}$ to $10^{-1}$ rad due to interaction with the $K$ line, for which the transition dipole moment would be $\sim 10^{-18}$ cgs esu. In the case of the absorption lines of water vapor, a reduction of the indicated effect by 2 orders of magnitude should be expected due to the correspondingly smaller values of the transition dipole moments. However, it can prove substantial over long paths in the atmosphere. Direct investigations of the given effects in the real atmosphere have not been carried out to date.

## 5.3. Thermalization of a Molecular Gas in Resonance Excitation by Laser Radiation

In the sum total of self-induced thermal effects of laser radiation propagating in a gaseous medium (see the preceding section), special status is held by the self-induced thermal effect in resonance-absorbing media. In this case, the formation of nonlinearity of the refractive index of the medium is governed by the thermalization dynamics or the process of evolution of the gas temperature of a resonance-excited molecular gas. Transient cooling of the gas can take place in this situation in connection with intermode absorption of laser radiation, i.e., the kinetic cooling effect [54].

Akhmanov and others [54] have surveyed the current status of the effect and reported their own original results of theoretical and experimental investigations of the cooling kinetics of molecular-gas mixtures $CO_2$–$N_2$–$O_2$ and $N_2O$–$N_2$ during the absorption of radiation emitted by a $CO_2$ laser. The content of the present section rests by and large on the cited survey.

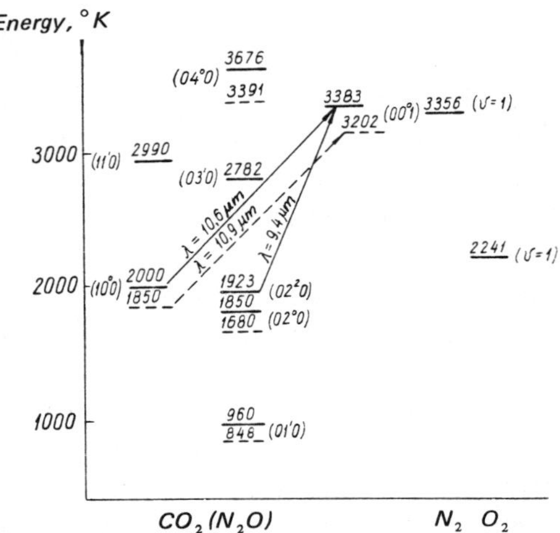


Fig. 5.5. Diagram of lower vibrational levels of $CO_2$, $N_2O$ (dashed line), $N_2$, and $O_2$ molecules.

The kinetic cooling effect may be summarized as follows. The resonance absorption of $CO_2$ laser radiation by a molecular-gas mixture $CO_2$–$N_2$–$O_2$ takes place at the transitions $CO_2(02^00) \rightarrow CO_2(00^01)$ and $CO_2(10^00) \rightarrow CO_2(00^01)$, which correspond to wavelengths $\lambda = 9.4$ and 10.6 $\mu$m (see Fig. 5.5). The radiation from an $N_2O$ laser with a wavelength of 10.9 $\mu$m is resonance absorbed at the transition $N_2O(10^00) \rightarrow N_2O(00^01)$. At the initial instant, the $CO_2$ or $N_2O$ laser radiation, on being absorbed at the indicated intermode vibration–rotation transitions, upsets thermodynamic equilibrium, increasing the population of the $00^01$ level and decreasing the population of the $10^00$ or $02^00$ level. The population of the lowest $CO_2$ (or $N_2O$) level $01^10$ is lowered by vibration–rotation energy–exchange processes associated with molecular collisions.

After disruption by the above-indicated processes, thermodynamic equilibrium is restored by nonresonance vibration–translation (V–T) relaxation and intermode vibration–vibration (V–V) relaxation processes, which induce a redistribution of energy between the vibrational and translational degrees of freedom (DOF) of the gas. Thus, a reduction of the temperature of the gas is possible in a time interval shorter than the characteristic times of vibrational energy dissipation of the $01^10$ and $00^01$ levels. The subcooling $\Delta T$ can be estimated on the basis of the energy conservation principle according to the expression

$$\Delta T = T_\infty - T \approx \frac{1}{5k}(E_{100} - E_{001})\exp\left(-\frac{E_{100}}{kT_0}\right) \tag{5.11}$$

in which $T_\infty$ and $T$ are the temperatures of the gas before and after interaction with the radiation field, $k$ is the Boltzmann constant, and $E_{001}$ and $E_{100}$ are the energies of the upper and lower levels participating in the absorption of laser radiation.

From (5.11) we obtain the subcooling for molecular $CO_2$ at $T = 300°K$ ($E_{100} = 2000°K$, $E_{001} = 3380°K$): $\Delta T \approx 0.4°K$. A similar estimation for molecular $N_2O$ ($E_{100} = 1850°K$, $E_{001} = 3220°K$) yields $\Delta T \approx 0.6°K$. To obtain data on the influence of the parameters of the molecular system (composition of the mixture and various relaxation times) and characteristics of the laser radiation (pulse shape and radiation intensity) on the thermalization of a gas, the authors of [54] have carried out an appropriate detailed theoretical investigation. Analyzing the possible relaxation processes in the investigated molecular-gas mixtures, they formulate the proper kinetic equations for the quantities $E_i$ representing the stored energy of vibrational quanta in the $i$th mode per single molecule. The thermalization equation is then obtained from the kinetic equations and the heat-conduction equation.

The numerical calculations of the kinetic equations and the thermalization equation were carried out varying the peak intensity of the radiation pulse, its shape, and the $CO_2$ partial pressure in the interval from 0.01 to 1 atm at a total pressure of 1 atm; the fundamental results may be summarized as follows.

As the $CO_2$ partial pressure is varied from 0.01 to 1.0 atm, the duration of the kinetic cooling effect decreases roughly from $10^{-3}$ to $10^{-5}$ sec, while the time to attain maximum cooling varies approximately from $2 \times 10^{-5}$ to $5 \times 10^{-6}$ sec. The normalized cooling "depth" has a characteristic maximum, which in the case of a mixture of gases with $CO_2$ is juxtaposed against a value of the partial pressure $\approx 0.3$ atm, and in the case of a mixture with $N_2O$ it occurs at a value of the $N_2O$ partial pressure $\approx 0.5$ atm., i.e., far beyond the limits of concentrations of these gases in the real atmosphere.

Calculations of the dependence of the cooling temperature on the radiation intensity $I$ have shown that for $I < 10^3$ W/cm² the kinetic cooling effect does not occur in a gas mixture $CO_2 + N_2$. In the interval of $I$ from $10^4$ to $10^6$ W/cm², the cooling "depth" $\Delta T$ increases with $I$, reaching saturation at $I = 10^6$ W/cm², a fact that is explained by luminous excitation of the transition $00°1 \rightleftharpoons 10°0$ or $02°0 \rightleftharpoons 00°1$. Appropriate calculations have clarified the role of molecular oxygen in the kinetic cooling effect, namely, that of increasing the cooling time and decreasing its depth as the $O_2$ partial pressure is increased.

A study of the influence of the pulse shape and duration on the kinetic cooling effect has shown that a longer pulse makes the cooling depth $\Delta T$ and cooling time $t_c$ greater, while the variation of the slope of the leading edge of the radiation pulse can be controlled by the parameters of the cooling effect. With a decrease in the slope of the leading edge of the laser pulse, the value of $t_c$ increases while $\Delta T$ decreases.

All other conditions being equal, the cooling depth for a radiation wavelength of 9.4 $\mu$m is approximately one-third the value for 10.6-$\mu$m radiation.

The experimental data obtained to date exhibit satisfactory agreement with the analytical results presented above.

We conclude this section with a brief discussion of acoustical phenomena associated with the absorption of radiation in a molecular-gas medium. It is noted in [54] that the density of a molecular gas subjected to nonequilibrium heating by resonant laser radiation is established by the excitation of acoustic waves, which are a potential source of error in estimating the effects of kinetic cooling of a vibrationally excited gas. Thus, the temperature of a gaseous medium irradiated by a laser source varies with the rate of V–T relaxation processes, while the variation of the density and the associated variation of the refractive index may lag the temperature. This lag is attributable to the pressure buildup process within the limits of the laser beam. Consequently, hydrodynamic processes affect both the amount of variation of the refractive index and the process of its evolution.

Calculations have shown [54] that different situations will occur, depending on the relationship between the gas cooling time $t_c$ and the transit time of sound across the laser beam $\tau_s$. For $t_c > \tau_s$, the transient buildup of the density follows the buildup of the temperature. For $t_c \approx \tau_s$, the rate of change of the density falls substantially behind the rate of change of the temperature, and finally for $t_c \ll \tau_s$, this process is greatly magnified.

As for the time $t_c$ itself, with an increase in the intensity of laser radiation resonance absorbed by a molecular-gas medium, the rate of V–T relaxation in the medium must increase, and so the time $t_c$ decreases. Experimental studies of the interaction of a $CO_2$ with molecular $SF_6$ gas [54] indicate that the V–T relaxation time is shortened by one-half to one-fifth as the laser intensity is increased from $5 \times 10^3$ to $2 \times 10^6$ W/cm$^2$.

The kinetic cooling effect discussed in this section for molecular gases will unquestionably occur in the real atmosphere in connection with the resonance absorption of laser radiation by various molecular-gas components. However, the necessary data have not yet been obtained for appropriate quantitative estimates.

## 5.4. Self-Induced Thermal Effects of Laser Beams

The self-induced thermal effects of laser beams propagating in the atmosphere are caused by the absorption of radiant energy by atmospheric gases and a concomitant variation of the density of the medium in the beam channel. The indicated density variation results in the formation of thermal lenses in the gas. The attendant self-induced effects are of practical significance insofar as they are characterized by rather low thresholds. With this fact in mind, we discuss the effects in more detail.

Several characteristic situations can arise, depending on the relations between the characteristic times of the heat-transfer processes and the optical irradiation time:

$$\frac{R_0}{u_s} \ll t \ll \frac{R_0}{v_\perp}, \frac{R_0^2}{4\chi} \tag{5.12}$$

$$\frac{R_0}{u_s} \ll \frac{R_0}{v_\perp} \lesssim t \tag{5.13}$$

$$t \lesssim \frac{R_0}{u_s} \ll \frac{R_0}{v_\perp}, \frac{R_0^2}{4\chi} \tag{5.14}$$

$$\frac{R_0}{v_\perp} \lesssim t \lesssim \frac{R_0}{u_s}, \frac{R_0^2}{4\chi} \tag{5.15}$$

where $R_0$ is the radius of the laser beam, $u_s$ is the sound velocity in the medium, $v_\perp$ is the lateral component of the relative velocity of the medium and the beam due to the wind, beam slewing, or photoabsorptive convection, and $\chi$ is the thermal diffusivity of air. It is assumed in every case described by relations (5.12)–(5.15) that the irradiation time is much greater than the thermalization time of optical energy in the medium.

Below we consider the laws of nonlinear interaction of laser beams with the atmosphere under various propagation conditions.

### 5.4.1. Transient Thermal Self-Defocusing of a Laser Beam in the Atmosphere

The atmospheric propagation of a cylindrically symmetrical beam with pulse duration satisfying conditions of the type (5.12) and (5.14) is accompanied by the formation in the medium of a transient gas lens, which has axial symmetry and induces nonlinear angular spreading of the beam [55–63].

In the field of a radiation source with complex amplitude $E(x, \mathbf{r}_\perp, t)$, where $x$ is the coordinate along the beam axis and $\mathbf{r}_\perp(y, z)$ is the radius vector in the cross section (transverse), the dynamics of the permittivity is described by the system of thermohydrodynamic equations [64]

$$\rho T \frac{\partial S}{\partial t} = \kappa_T \nabla^2_{\mathbf{r}_\perp} T + q_a \tag{5.16}$$

$$\rho \frac{\partial \mathbf{V}}{\partial t} = -\nabla_{\mathbf{r}_\perp} p + \nabla_{\mathbf{r}_\perp} p_s \tag{5.17}$$

$$\frac{\partial \rho}{\partial t} = \mathrm{div}(\rho \mathbf{V}) \tag{5.18}$$

$$S = C_v \ln T - C_v(\gamma - 1)\ln \rho + \mathrm{const} \tag{5.19}$$

$$p = R_b \rho T, \qquad \varepsilon = \varepsilon_0 + \frac{\partial \varepsilon}{\partial \rho}(\rho - \rho_\infty) \tag{5.20}$$

where $\nabla_{\mathbf{r}_\perp} = \mathbf{y}\,\partial/\partial y + \mathbf{z}\,\partial/\partial z$, $\mathbf{y}$ and $\mathbf{z}$ are orthogonal unit vectors, $S$ is the entropy, $T$ is the temperature, $\kappa_T$ is the molecular thermal conductivity, $C_v$ is the isochoric heat capacity, $\gamma$ is the adiabatic exponent, $\mathbf{V}$ is the hydrodynamic velocity vector of the medium, $p$ is the pressure, $R_b$ is the specific gas constant, $\delta\rho = \rho - \rho_\infty$ is the deviation of the air density $\rho$ from the equilibrium value $\rho_\infty$, $p_s = (1/16\pi)(\rho\,\partial\varepsilon/\partial\rho)|E|^2$ is the pressure due to electrostriction, $q_a = (c\varepsilon_0^{1/2}/8\pi)k_\nu|E|^2$ is the energy flux imparted to the medium by the absorption of laser radiation, $c$ is the velocity of light in vacuum, and $k_\nu$ is the molecular absorption coefficient of air. Expressions (5.16)–(5.20) take account of the nonadiabatic nature of energy transport in the medium due simultaneously to heat conduction and the hydrodynamic mechanism. For small superheats of the medium, such that $(T - T_\infty)/T_\infty \ll 1$, the system (5.16)–(5.20) is linearized and serves as the basis of consolidation of a single equation for the variation of the permittivity of the medium $\delta\varepsilon = \varepsilon - \varepsilon_\infty$:

$$\frac{\partial^2}{\partial t^2}\delta\varepsilon = u_s^2 \nabla^2_{\mathbf{r}_\perp}\delta\varepsilon + \gamma\chi\frac{\partial}{\partial t}\nabla^2_{\mathbf{r}_\perp}\delta\varepsilon - u_s^2\chi\int_0^t dt_1\,\nabla^4_{\mathbf{r}_\perp}\delta\varepsilon$$

$$+ \frac{\partial\varepsilon}{\partial\rho}(\gamma - 1)\int_0^t \nabla^2_{\mathbf{r}_\perp}q_a\,dt' - \frac{\partial\varepsilon}{\partial\rho}\nabla^2_{\mathbf{r}_\perp}p_s + \frac{\partial\varepsilon}{\partial\rho}\gamma\chi\int_0^t \nabla^4_{\mathbf{r}_\perp}p_s\,dt' \tag{5.21}$$

Equation (5.21) satisfies equilibrium initial and boundary conditions. The last two terms on its right-hand side are related to the ponderomotive action of the radiation on the medium. Estimates show [65] that effects elicited by the absorption of light in the atmosphere prevail over the electrostriction mechanism of nonlinearity, beginning with an optical irradiation time

$$t\,[\sec] = \frac{\rho\,\partial\varepsilon/\partial\rho}{c\varepsilon_0^{1/2}k_\nu(\gamma-1)} \approx \frac{0.5\times10^{-14}}{k_\nu\,[\mathrm{cm}^{-1}]}$$

Thus, for radiation from a $CO_2$ laser with $k_\nu = 10^{-6}$ $\mathrm{cm}^{-1}$, the thermal nonlinearity mechanism prevails over the electrostriction mechanism, beginning with $t \gtrsim 5$ nsec.

Equation (5.21) admits simple analytical solutions [66] in the extreme cases of "short" and "long" light pulses satisfying the respective conditions (5.14) and (5.12):

$$\delta\varepsilon = \frac{k_\nu c\varepsilon_0^{1/2}(\gamma-1)}{8\pi u_s^2}\frac{\partial\varepsilon}{\partial\rho}\int_{x/c}^{t}\frac{t_1^2}{2}\nabla_{\mathbf{r}_\perp}^2|E|^2\,dt_1\left[1+O\left(\frac{t^2}{\tau_s^2}\right)\right] \qquad (5.22)$$

$$\delta\varepsilon = -\frac{k_\nu c\varepsilon_0^{1/2}(\gamma-1)}{8\pi u_s^2}\frac{\partial\varepsilon}{\partial\rho}\int_{x/c}^{t}|E|^2\,dt_1\left[1+O\left(\frac{\tau_s^2}{t^2}\right)\right] \qquad (5.23)$$

where $\tau_s = R_0/u_s$ is the characteristic transit time of sound across the beam.

The form of the solution (5.23) implies that the profile of the permittivity in the propagation of a "long" pulse exactly emulates the time variation of the temperature increase of the medium: $\delta\varepsilon = (\partial\varepsilon/\partial\rho)\delta\rho = (\partial\varepsilon/\partial T)\delta T$, i.e., the process is isobaric. The self-induced thermal action of the beam is maximally efficient in the given situation and is determined by the gradient of the integral energy input to the medium in the beam channel:

$$\nabla_{\mathbf{r}_\perp}\left(k_\nu\int_{x/c}^{t}|E|^2\,dt_1\right)$$

The threshold energy required to attain a nonlinear beam spread equal to the diffraction spread in the case of a collimated beam with a Gaussian intensity profile in the cross section is estimated by means of the simple expression

$$Q_t = \frac{4\pi C_p\rho\varepsilon_0^{1/2}}{k_\nu k^2|\partial\varepsilon/\partial T|} \qquad (5.24)$$

Thus, for $\lambda = 10.6$ $\mu$m in air at sea level, we have $Q_t \approx 200$ J. In the event that the pulse energy $Q$ greatly exceeds the threshold value, i.e., for $Q/Q_t \gg 1$, the maximum angular spread of the beam is estimated in order of magnitude as

$$\Theta_{\max} \sim \frac{\lambda}{R_0} \left( \frac{Q}{Q_t} \right)^{1/2} \tag{5.25}$$

The theoretical analysis of the propagation of a strong laser beam in an absorbing gaseous medium with thermal nonlinearity is based on a parabolic-type equation for the slowly varying (in comparison with the field frequency $\omega_0$) field amplitude $E$, which is related to the electric vector $\mathbf{e}$ by the equation

$$\mathbf{e}(\mathbf{r}, t) = \mathbf{j} E(\mathbf{r}, t) \exp(ikx - i\omega_0 t)$$

in which $\mathbf{j}$ is a unit vector characterizing the polarization state, $k = 2\pi/\lambda$, and $x$ is the coordinate measured along the beam axis at the boundary of the medium. The equation mentioned above has the form

$$2ik \frac{\partial E}{\partial x} + \nabla_{\mathbf{r}_\perp}^2 E + k^2 \left( \delta\varepsilon - i \frac{k_\nu}{k} \right) E = 0 \tag{5.26}$$

It is closed by the appropriate system of constitutive equations for the calculation of $\delta\varepsilon$, for example, of the form (5.16)–(5.20). The validity of Eq. (5.26) is limited by the conditions

$$\frac{|\delta\varepsilon|}{E_0}, \frac{k_\nu}{k}, k_\nu R_0, \frac{R_0}{x} \ll 1$$

A great many publications have been devoted to the development of methods for solving the problem of the self-induced thermal action of a beam on the basis of the quasioptical equation (5.26). The simplest expressions are obtained in the nonaberration approximation and correspond to a class of solutions of the form

$$E(x, \mathbf{r}_\perp, t) = \frac{E_0}{f} \exp\left[ - \frac{r_\perp^2}{2R_0^2 f^2} + \frac{ikr_\perp^2}{2F} + i\varphi \right] \tag{5.27}$$

in which $f$, $F$, and $\varphi$ are parameters depending on $x$ and $t$. The distribution of the field at the boundary of the medium corresponds to a single-mode laser beam with a Gaussian intensity profile, an effective radius $R_0$, $f=1$, and a square-law phase distribution with radius of curvature of the phase front $F=F_0$.

The simplified equations for $f$, $F$, and $\varphi$ corresponding to the best approximation of expression (5.27) to the solution of the initial parabolic equation for the case of a weakly absorbing medium have the form [106]

$$F(x,t)=f/f'_x k \tag{5.28}$$

$$\varphi'_x=R_d^{-1}\left[f^{-2}+\tfrac{3}{2}\exp(-\tau_0)\int_0^{D_0}f^{-2}\,dD_0\right] \tag{5.29}$$

$$f''_{xx}=R_d^{-2}\left[f^{-3}+f\exp(-\tau_0)\int_0^{D_0}f^{-4}\,dD_0\right] \tag{5.30}$$

where $R_d=kR_0^2$, $\tau_0=\int_0^x k_\nu\,dx'$ is the optical thickness of the absorbing medium, and

$$D_0=\frac{1}{Q_t}\frac{cR_0^2\varepsilon_0^{1/2}}{8}\int_{x/c}^t dt_1|E_0|^2$$

For $D_0\ll 1$ and $\tau_0\ll 1$, Eq. (5.30) is solved by separation of variables [106]:

$$f(x,t)=f(x,0)\exp(\tfrac{1}{4}D_0)$$

where $f(x,0)$ is the dimensionless width of the beam in a linear medium:

$$f(x,0)=\left(1+\frac{x}{F_0}\right)^2+\left(\frac{x}{R_d}\right)^2$$

For an arbitrary value of $D_0$, the behavior of the dimensionless effective beam width is described by the asymptotic expressions [68]

$$f=\left(1+\frac{x}{F_0}\right)\psi(\xi)$$

$$\psi(\xi)=\begin{cases}(1+\xi)^{1/2}, & \xi\leqslant 1\\[2mm]\dfrac{1}{2^{1/2}}\xi^{3/4}(1+\xi^{-1}), & \xi>1\end{cases} \tag{5.31}$$

$$\xi=D_0^{-1/2}\frac{(x/R_d)^2}{(1+x/F_0)(1+R_d^2/F_0^2)}$$

The corresponding expression for the pulse energy density on the beam axis $q_0 = (c\varepsilon_0^{1/2}/8\pi)\int_{x/c}^{t} dt_1 |E(x,0,t_1)|^2$ has the form

$$q_o = \frac{Q_t}{\pi R_0^2}\left(1 + \frac{R_d^2}{F_0^2}\right)\left(\frac{R_d}{x}\right)^2 \begin{cases} \ln(1+\xi), & \xi < 1 \\ \left(\ln 2 + 1 - \dfrac{2\xi^{1/2}}{1+\xi} + 2\tan^{-1}\xi^{1/2} - \dfrac{\pi}{2}\right), & \xi > 1 \end{cases}$$

$$(5.32)$$

Numerical modeling of the initial equation (5.26) with a Gaussian beam at the boundary of the medium

$$E(0,\mathbf{r}_\perp,t) = E_0\exp\left(-\frac{r_\perp^2}{2R_0^2} + \frac{ikr_\perp^2}{2F_0}\right) \tag{5.33}$$

has been carried out in a number of papers (e.g., [66, 69–73]). The results of calculations of the distortion of the initial beam profile under the conditions of the transient self-induced effect [66] subject to the constraints (5.14) are given in Fig. 5.6.

The curves in Fig. 5.6 correspond to different values of the ratio $t/\tau_s$ in the interval from 0 to 2.3 for $x/R_d = 0.07$ and $k_\nu P_0\tau_s = 7.52$ J/cm, where $P_0$ is the power of the beam.

Calculations [74] of the self-defocusing of a "long" pulse obeying condition (5.12) show that during propagation in a medium with a self-induced thermal lens an initial Gaussian beam is transformed into a beam with a complex aberration structure (see Fig. 5.7). The aberration in this case is most pronounced for a thin gas lens [59] for which the domain of the effective self-induced action of the beam is much shorter than the total propagation path.

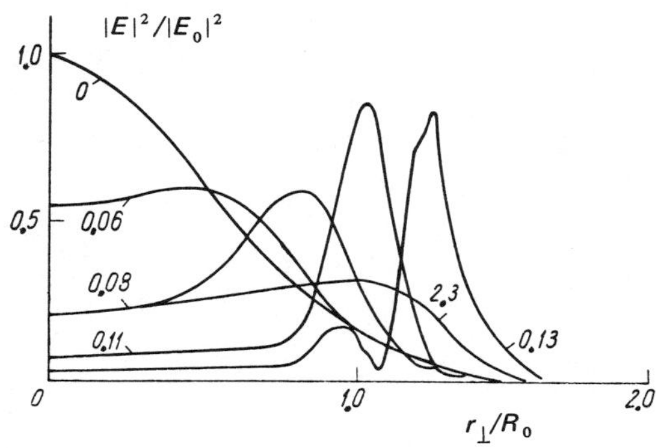


Fig. 5.6. Evolution of intensity profile in cross section of a collimated Gaussian beam in a thermally nonlinear medium. The curves correspond to different values of the parameter $t/\tau_s$ for $x/R_d = 0.07$, $k_\nu P_0\tau_s = 7.52$ J/cm.

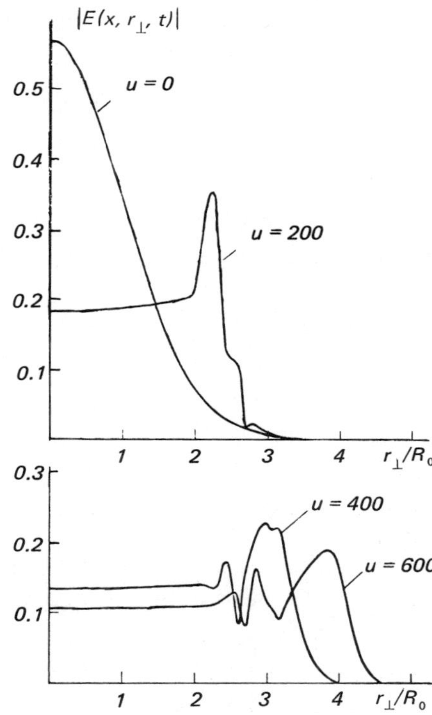



Fig. 5.7. Transverse distribution of field amplitude in a beam in a nonlinear medium for various excesses of the energy above threshold. Analytical parameters: $x/R_d = 0.1$, $t/\tau_s \gg 1$, $u = Q/Q_t$.

## 5.4.2. Bending and Thermal Blooming of Laser Beams in the Atmosphere Due to Crosswind or Beam Slewing

Two special attributes of the self-induced action of a strong laser beam moving relative to an absorbing medium are nonlinear wind deflection of the beam and modification of the beam shape (thermal blooming) [69–72, 75–94]. These effects are caused by disruption of the axial symmetry of the gas lens due to variation of the heat-transfer regime in the medium. The distribution of the permittivity in the beam channel with allowance for wind-induced heat transfer in the domain corresponding to conditions (5.14) is described by the heat-conduction equations [75]:

$$\frac{\partial T}{\partial t} - (\mathbf{V}\nabla_{\mathbf{r}_\perp})T = \chi \nabla^2_{\mathbf{r}_\perp} T + \frac{k_\nu I}{\kappa_T} \tag{5.34}$$

$$\delta\varepsilon = \frac{\partial \varepsilon}{\partial T}(T - T_\infty), \qquad I = \frac{c\varepsilon_0^{1/2}}{8\pi}|E|^2 \tag{5.35}$$

The solution of (5.35) and (5.34) is conveniently written in the form of a series expansion near the beam axis:

$$\delta\varepsilon(\mathbf{r}_\perp, t) = \frac{k_\nu I}{4\kappa_T}\frac{\partial\varepsilon}{\partial T}\left[\frac{2\varepsilon_y y}{R_0} + \frac{\varepsilon_{zz}z^2}{R_0^2} + \frac{\varepsilon_{yy}y^2}{R_0^2} + \cdots\right] \qquad (5.36)$$

where $\varepsilon_{ik}$ denotes the coefficients of the expansion, which have the following form for a Gaussian beam (5.33) [75]:

$$\varepsilon_y = \mathrm{Pe}\,\exp(2\,\mathrm{Pe}^2)\left[K_0(2\,\mathrm{Pe}^2) - K_1(2\,\mathrm{Pe}^2)\right] + \frac{1}{2\,\mathrm{Pe}}$$

$$\varepsilon_{zz} = -\frac{1}{2\,\mathrm{Pe}^2} + K_1(2\,\mathrm{Pe}^2)\exp(2\,\mathrm{Pe}^2) \qquad (5.37)$$

$$\varepsilon_{yy} = -\left[4\,\mathrm{Pe}^2\,K_0(2\,\mathrm{Pe}^2) - (4\,\mathrm{Pe}^2 - 1)K_1(2\,\mathrm{Pe}^2)\right]\exp(2\,\mathrm{Pe}^2) + (2\,\mathrm{Pe}^2)^{-1}$$

where $K_0$ and $K_1$ are Macdonald functions and $\mathrm{Pe} = v_\perp R_0/4\chi$ is the Péclet number. The $y$ axis is aligned with the direction of the lateral component of the wind velocity: $v_\perp = v_y$. The inclusion of only those terms written in the expansion in the solution for $\delta\varepsilon$ corresponds to the nonaberration description of the thermal lens. The term $\varepsilon_y$ in this case determines the upwind inclination of the beam as a whole; $\varepsilon_{zz}$ and $\varepsilon_{yy}$ characterize its defocusing along each axis.

Calculations have shown [75] that beam defocusing effects decrease monotonically with increasing crosswind. The defocusing in the direction of the $y$ axis decreases more rapidly in this case than in the perpendicular direction. As a result of nonuniform defocusing, the beam acquires the shape of an ellipse oriented across the wind. The wind deflection of the beam as a whole attains a maximum at $\mathrm{Pe} \approx 0.3$. For larger values of Pe, $\varepsilon_y \sim \mathrm{Pe}^{-1}$.

In the nonaberration description of the wind distortion of a Gaussian beam, its intensity is written in the form [94]

$$I(x,\mathbf{r}_\perp, t) = \frac{I_0}{f_1(x,t)f_2(x,t)}\exp\left\{-\tau_0 - \frac{z^2}{R_0^2 f_1^2} - \frac{[y - Y(x,t)]^2}{R_0^2 f_2^2}\right\}$$

$$f_1|_{t=0} = f_2|_{t=0} = 1 + \frac{x}{F_0} + \left(\frac{x}{R_d}\right)^2 \qquad (5.38)$$

where $f_1$ and $f_2$ are the dimensionless widths of the beam along each axis in its cross section and $Y$ is the wind displacement of the beam center. In this case, the effective phase front $\varphi = \int_0^x \delta\varepsilon_{\mathrm{ef}}\, dx'$ represents a second-order surface:

$$\varphi = \varphi_0 - \Theta_y(y - Y) + \frac{z^2}{2}\frac{df_1}{dx} + \frac{y^2}{2}\frac{df_2}{dx} \tag{5.39}$$

Making use of the expansion of the permittivity, we have

$$\Theta_y = \frac{dY}{dx} = 4\int_0^x \frac{k_\nu I \varepsilon_y}{\kappa_T}\left|\frac{\partial\varepsilon}{\partial T}\right| \tag{5.40}$$

$$f_{1,2} = 4\int\int_0^x dx'\, dx'' \frac{k_\nu I}{\kappa_T}\varepsilon_{zz,yy}\left|\frac{\partial\varepsilon}{\partial T}\right| \tag{5.41}$$

The parameters entering into the integrands in (5.40) and (5.41) may include a dependence along the path in the event of, say, slant or vertical beam propagation. Also, the quantity $v_\perp$ will be a function of the path in the case of beam slewing. An analytical solution of the system (5.38),(5.40),(5.41) can be obtained by successive iterations with respect to the light field acting on the medium. In particular, for large Péclet numbers, such that heat conduction is insignificant, the solution for the upwind angular displacement of the beam as a whole in the specified-field approximation $I = I|_{t=0} = I_0$ for a homogeneous path has the form

$$\Theta_y(x,t) = -\frac{2R_0 F_0}{L_T^2}\left\{1 - \left(1 + \frac{x}{F_0}\right)^{-1} + \exp(-k_\nu F_0)\right.$$

$$\left.\times\left[Ei(k_\nu(x + F_0)) - Ei(k_\nu F_0)\right]\right\} \tag{5.42}$$

where $Ei$ is the integral exponential function and $L_T$ is a characteristic length of self-induced thermal action of a collimated Gaussian beam in a homogeneous medium:

$$L_T = \left(\frac{2C_p\rho v_\perp R_0}{k_\nu I_0|\partial\varepsilon/\partial T|}\right)^{1/2} \tag{5.43}$$

In the case of a collimated beam,

$$\Theta_y = \frac{2R_0}{k_\nu L_T^2}[1 - \exp(-\tau_0)] \tag{5.44}$$

The slewing of a laser beam in the atmosphere has been investigated by Vorob'ev [93]. Allowance for slewing is equivalent to the consideration of an inhomogeneous medium in which the components of the transverse component of the wind velocity relative to the beam are determined by the relations

$$v_y = v_\perp \cos\psi + \omega x, \qquad v_z = v_\perp \sin\psi \tag{5.45}$$

in which $\psi$ is the angle between the slewing plane and the vector transverse component of the wind velocity and $\omega$ is the angular velocity of slewing. The $y$ axis is situated in the slewing plane. The results of numerical calculations of the angular displacements of a collimated Gaussian beam along the $y$ and $z$ axes in the nonaberration approximation [93] show that the self-induced action of a beam is most efficient for $\psi \to \pi$, in which case there is a "rest zone" $x_r = v_\perp /\omega$, where the beam is motionless relative to the medium. We note that for $\psi = \pi$ downwind heat transfer is absent in the plane $x = x_r$, and for the correct solution of the "self-action" problem it is necessary to consider higher-order heat-transfer mechanisms associated with molecular heat conduction, atmospheric turbulence, or photoabsorptive convection.

In the event of rapid slewing of a strong beam, such that the linear velocity of the beam is commensurate with the velocity of sound, $\omega x \approx u_s$, the formation of the gas lens is controlled by the hydrodynamic processes in the medium, and in the case of a one-dimensional beam [84, 85] with Mach numbers $M = v_\perp /u_s \sim 1.1$ to $1.3$, shock waves can be initiated as a result of absorbed radiant energy. Experimental [85] and theoretical [87–89] studies with two-dimensional beams have shown that anomalies in the transonic range are less evident in comparison with estimates for a one-dimensional beam; the behavior of the medium in the subsonic and supersonic ranges is asymmetrical.

Following Vorob'ev [88] we give the results of calculations of the stationary distribution of permittivity perturbations in a Gaussian beam channel

$$\delta\varepsilon(x, y, z=0) = -a_0 \left\{ \frac{M}{(1-M^2)^{1/2}} b\left(\frac{y}{R_0}\right) + \frac{\sqrt{\pi}}{2M}\left[1 + \phi\left(\frac{y}{R_0}\right)\right] \right\}, \quad M < 1,$$

$$\tag{5.46}$$

$$\delta\varepsilon(x, y, z=0) = a_0 \frac{\sqrt{\pi}}{2} \left\{ \frac{\exp(-y^2 M^2/R_0^2)}{(M^2-1)^{1/2}} \left[1 + \phi\left(\frac{My}{R_0}(M^2-1)^{1/2}\right)\right] \right.$$

$$\left. - M^{-1}\left[1 + \phi\left(\frac{y}{R_0}\right)\right] \right\}, \qquad M > 1 \tag{5.47}$$

where $\phi$ is the probability integral and

$$b(\xi)=\exp\left(-\xi^2\right)\int_0^{\xi}\exp\left(\xi^2\right)d\xi, \qquad a_0=\frac{\partial\varepsilon}{\partial\rho}\cdot\frac{k_\nu I_0 R_0}{C_p T_\infty u_s}$$

The solution has a singular point in the vicinity of $M\approx1$, where it is required to take into account higher-order heat- and mass-transfer mechanisms and to go over to the nonlinear, nonsteady hydrodynamical equations.

The distribution of the refractive index along the axis in the beam channel at transonic slewing velocities is shown in Figs. 5.8(a) and 5.8(b). We see that a deflection of the beam in the slewing direction is expected for $M<1$, whereas for $M>1$ a gas lens focusing in the plane $z=0$ is formed in the medium.

Advances in the development of numerical techniques for the exact solution of the nonlinear parabolic equation (5.26) with the use of high-speed computers have made it possible to calculate the aberration structure of the radiation and to analyze the singular features of the self-induced thermal action of beams having a complex initial profile [73, 90]. Annularly defined beams are of considerable interest from the standpoint of the realization of conditions for the self-focusing of radiation in the atmosphere.

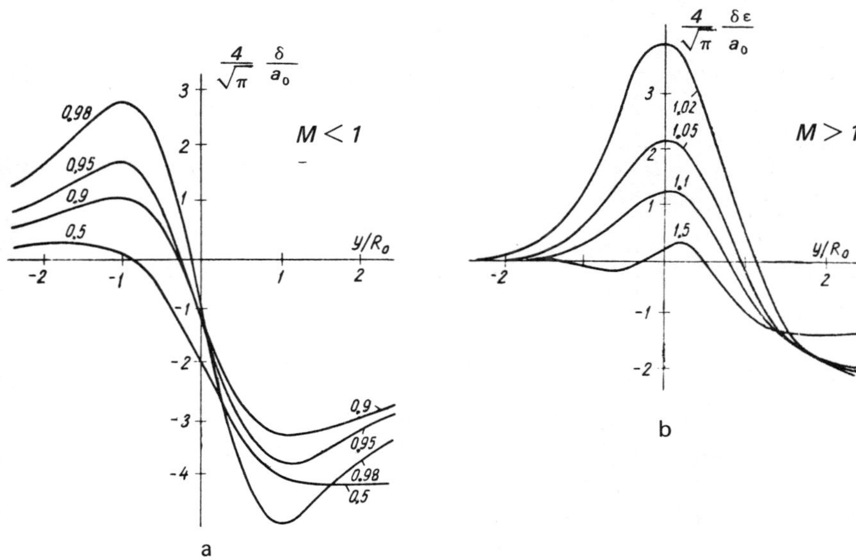

Fig. 5.8. (a, b) Variation of permittivity of the medium in the beam cross section for transonic slewing velocities of the latter. The curves correspond to different values of the Mach number: $M=v_\perp/u_s$.

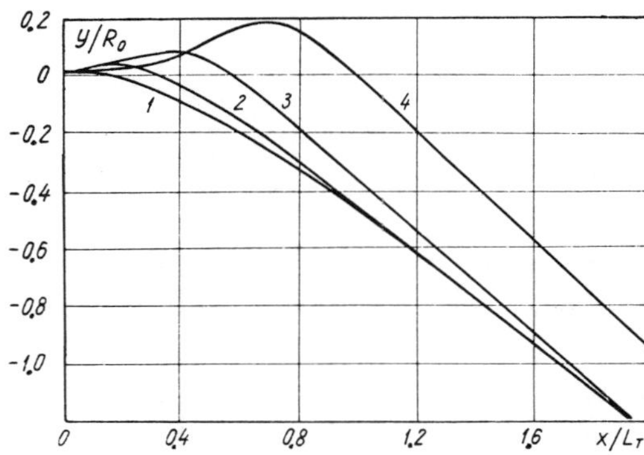

Fig. 5.9. Displacement of energy center of beam in a moving medium. (1) Gaussian beam, $L_T/R_d=0.12$; (2, 3, 4) annular beams, $L_T/R_d=0.12$, $R_{02}/R_{01}=$ 0.125, 0.25, 0.5.

By contrast with a Gaussian beam, a convergent lens is formed in nonsteady heating of a medium by a beam with an intensity trough in its center [73, 76, 77]. We note that an analogous effect is possible for a Gaussian beam subjected to collinear slewing of its axis in a circle with a radius of the order of the initial beam radius $R_0$ [95]. Figure 5.9 gives the results of calculations [73] of the steady wind displacement of the center of a Gaussian beam of the form (5.33) for $F_0=\infty$ and of an annularly defined beam having a boundary with the medium in the form of the difference between two Gaussian beams:

$$E(0,\mathbf{r}_\perp,t)=E_0\left[\exp\left(-\frac{r_\perp^2}{2R_{01}^2}\right)-\exp\left(-\frac{r_\perp^2}{2R_{02}^2}\right)\right] \qquad (5.48)$$

where $R_{01}$ and $R_{02}$ are the inside and outside radii. The displacement of the center of the beam is given by the expression

$$Y=\frac{\displaystyle\int_{-\infty}^{\infty} dy\,y|E|^2}{\left(\displaystyle\int_{-\infty}^{\infty} |E|^2\,dy\right)_{y=0}} \qquad (5.49)$$

Calculations have shown that as a Gaussian beam propagates through a moving medium ($\mathrm{Pe}\gg1$) it acquires a crescent shape and its center is deflected by the wind (curves 1 and 2 in Fig. 5.9). The crescent shape transforms into an almost-elliptical configuration with increasing value of Pe, and then, as $\mathrm{Pe}\to\infty$, it recovers its unperturbed form without the self-induced effect. In an annular beam with $R_{02}/R_{01}=0.5$, only the downwind part of the beam acquires a crescent shape, while the upwind

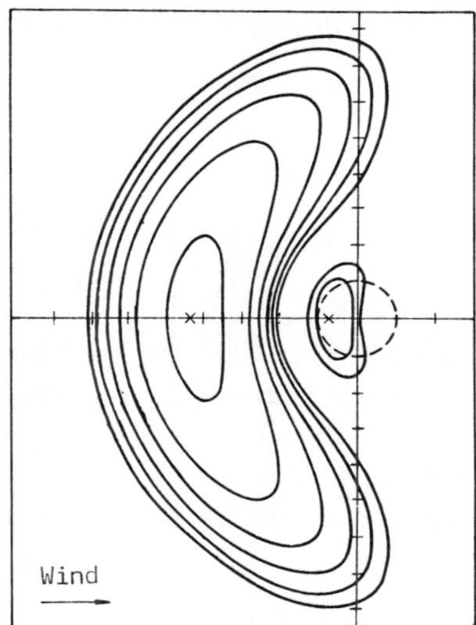


Fig. 5.10. Wind distortion of a strong Gaussian beam in the atmosphere. The curves correspond to lines of equal intensity in the beam cross section at levels of 0.09, 0.14, 0.23, 0.36, 0.57, and 0.9 of the peak intensity, the position of which is indicated by a cross in the large part of the beam. The calculated displacement of the intensity peak is $Y/R_0 = 4.4$. The dashed curve represents the $e^{-1}$ line of the initial beam.

part is elongated in the direction of the wind. With an increase in the path length, for $x \gtrsim L_T$ the beam is separated into two parts: a larger cross section downwind and a smaller one upwind. It is inferred from Fig. 5.9 that the deflection of the centroid of beams with an annular profile is smaller than for Gaussian beams and, unlike the latter, the displacement of annular beams along the initial parts of the path takes place in the opposite direction—downwind. Figure 5.10 illustrates the wind distortion of a collimated Gaussian beam (5.33) [92] in the atmosphere for an absorption coefficient $k_\nu = 0.7 \times 10^{-6}$ cm$^{-1}$, $v_\perp = 200$ cm/sec, $x = 2 \times 10^3$ cm, $\lambda = 10.6$ $\mu$m, $R_0 = 14.15$ cm, and a power $P_0 = 10^5$ W. Pearson and others [90] have also performed a numerical analysis of the wind distortion of multimode beams with an intensity trough at the center. Others [64, 81] have investigated problems in the interaction and "self-action" of a train of power laser pulses.

It is essential to note that self-induced bending of the axis of a laser beam can also take place in a medium initially at rest due to the formation of a deflecting gas lens in connection with nonuniform heating of a nonaxisymmetrical beam as well as due to the inception of convective motion of the medium in the zone of the laser beam. The photoabsorptive convection phenomenon has been investigated in several papers [96–105]. Gerasimov and others [103–104], using dimensional analysis, have obtained simple estimates for the average velocity of photoabsorptive convection in a beam propagating along a horizontal path:

$$v_\phi = \frac{c_1 \beta g R_0^4 k_\nu I_0}{\kappa_T \nu}, \qquad \mathrm{Pe} \leqslant 1 \qquad\qquad (5.50)$$

$$v_\phi = c_2 \left( \frac{\beta g R_0^2 k_\nu I_0}{c_p \rho} \right)^{1/3}, \qquad \mathrm{Pe} \gtrsim 1 \qquad\qquad (5.51)$$

Here $\beta$ and $\nu$ are the coefficients of thermal expansion and kinematic viscosity of air, $g$ is the acceleration of gravity, and $c_1$ and $c_2$ are constants of the order of unity. An analysis of the results indicates that steady-state convective motion evolves in the weak convection regime (5.50) with a rise time $R_0^2/4\chi$ and in the fully developed convection regime (5.51) with a rise time $R_0/v_\phi$.

### 5.4.3. Experimental Investigations of Self-Induced Thermal Effects of Laser Beams

Experimental research on the nonlinear effects associated with absorption of laser radiation in gaseous and liquid media has been carried out in a large number of papers [55–63, 68, 78–81, 83, 86, 92, 96–98, 100, 102, 105–107]. Corresponding measurements have been performed under model laboratory conditions in air contaminated with definite absorbing gases or in cells containing absorbing liquids as well as in air over a relatively long path of length 195 m. Thermal defocusing effects, the influence of wind and beam slewing in the medium, and the photoabsorptive convection effect have been investigated. We now give certain illustrations of the results.

Figure 5.11 [68] gives the dependence of the nonlinear angular spread of a $CO_2$ laser beam on the incident power in steady-state heating of a gaseous medium, subject to constraints of the form $t \geqslant R_0^2/4\chi$. The experimental conditions include an absorption coefficient $k_\nu = 0.03$ cm$^{-1}$, $R_0 = 0.2$

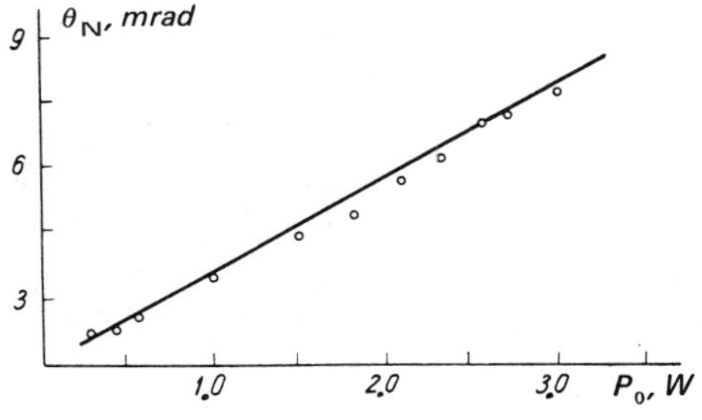


Fig. 5.11. Nonlinear spread of a $CO_2$ laser beam versus incident power.

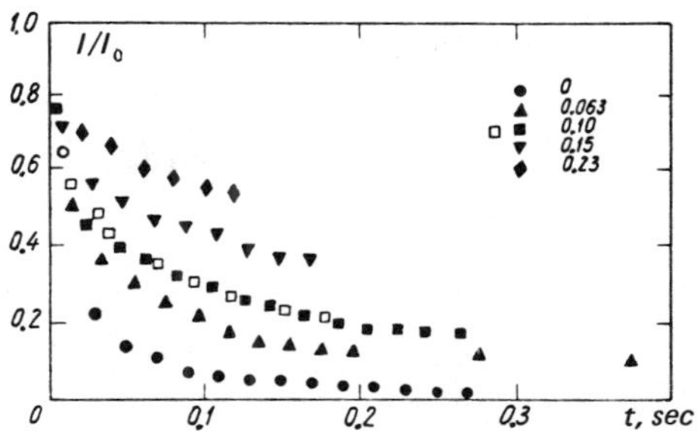


Fig. 5.12. Relative intensity on the axis of a focused $CO_2$ laser beam during slewing of the medium relative to the beam at various angular velocities (values in $\sec^{-1}$ indicated in the figure).

cm, and $x=70$ cm. The absorption in air is increased by small additives of propane ($C_3H_8$). The solid curve represents the results of a theoretical calculation in the nonaberration approximation.

The results of experimental measurements of the relative intensity on the unperturbed axis of a focused $CO_2$ laser beam with rotation of the gas cell with various angular velocities for $x=103$ cm, simulating the process of slewing relative to the medium, are given in Fig. 5.12 [106]. The measurements were performed with a laser power $P_0=10$ W and $R_0=0.32$ cm. The detector was placed in the focal plane of the focused beam. The pressure of the $CO_2$ gas in the cell was 10 atm, which yielded an absorption coefficient $k_\nu=0.42$ m$^{-1}$. It is seen that the "self-action" of the beam is substantially diminished with increasing angular velocity of relative motion of the medium.

Miller and others [86] have conducted an experiment with a $CO_2$-laser over a 195-m path. When measures were taken to shield the beam against crosswind, the experimentally observed radiation intensity in the focal plane of the receiving lens was reduced to one-half the value along a path with steady wind.

On the basis of an analysis of the results of laboratory experiments and numerical calculations of the self-action of laser radiation in a moving gaseous medium, Gebhardt [92] has proposed a simple model relating the steady-state nonlinear variation of the peak intensity $I_m$ in the beam cross section to its value $I_m^{(0)}$ in a linear medium:

$$I_m(x)=I_m^{(0)}(x)f_N \qquad (5.52)$$

where $f_N$ is an empirical function of the parameter $N$: $f_N=(1+0.0625N^2)^{-1}$. The parameter $N$ for a collimated Gaussian beam in a weakly absorbing medium ($\tau_0 \lesssim 1$) has the form $N=2x^2/L_T^2$. The relative variation of the peak intensity in the cross section of a beam propagating in a gaseous medium with crosswind is plotted in Fig. 5.13 on the basis of Gebhardt's data [92].

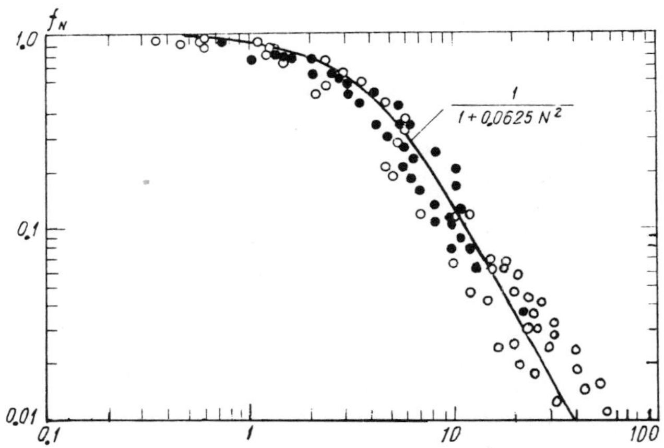



Fig. 5.13. Relative peak intensity in the cross section of a beam propagating in a gaseous medium with crosswind, according to experiment (light circles), numerical solution of the nonlinear parabolic equation (dark circles), and the empirical model $(1+0.0625N^2)^{-1}$.

It is seen that the proposed simple model (5.52) agrees satisfactorily with the results of measurements.

Acceptable consistency between the above-described theory of the self-induced action of a laser beam propagating in an absorbing gaseous medium and the corresponding results of measurements has also been obtained in photoabsorptive convection studies [59, 61, 96–98, 100, 105, 106].

## 5.5. Self-Induced Thermal Effects of Laser Beams in Atmospheric Aerosols

### 5.5.1. General Status of the Problem

The absorption of powerful laser radiation by aerosol particles can produce heating, vaporization, and disintegration of the particles and, as a result, a change in the optical characteristics of both the particles themselves and the surrounding medium. The earliest papers in this area were concerned with the surface evaporation conditions of radiation-heated droplets and solution of the nonlinear transport equation in a cloud with a radiation-distorted droplet-size spectrum [108–112].

The transport of radiation in disperse liquid-droplet media has been studied in several papers [110, 111, 113, 114]. The problem of the surface evaporation of droplets has been solved in approximations consistent with low power densities on the part of the disturbing radiation ($\lesssim 10$ W/cm$^2$) in the presence of diffuse mass and heat transfer from the surface of the evaporating droplet [115].

Experimental studies have shown [116–118] that the quasisteady approximation, which is applicable to the majority of the calculations, yields satisfactory results for an effective radiation power density up to 200 W/cm$^2$ and droplets with radii of $10^{-3}$ to $10^{-2}$ cm.

Investigations of the transient phase of evaporation as well as the influence of kinetic, hydrodynamic, thermal-diffusion, and other effects [109, 117–120] have produced results close to those obtained in the above-cited works.

The investigation of the thermal action of laser radiation on disperse media is progressing toward the study of the explosive vaporization regimes predicted by Kuzikovskii [109]. The first experiments in this direction were performed by Kuzikovskii and others [117, 121], who observed the explosive vaporization of droplets. The threshold bounds of this regime have been determined under the condition that the substance at the center of the droplet attains near-critical and critical states [122, 123]. The first investigations of the motion of droplets under the action of diverse types of forces arising in an optical field have been carried out [124–130]. A number of authors have investigated effects that promote self-induced modifications: recondensation [131, 132], melting of crystalline particles [133, 134], etc.

The interaction of a laser beam with solid aerosol particles produces nonlinear scattering of radiation by thermohydrodynamic perturbations of the density of the medium in the vicinity of absorbing centers. Related studies are reported in several papers [135–147].


## 5.5.2. Classification of Nonlinear Thermal Effects in Aerosols

The simplest classification of nonlinear thermal interactions of strong optical radiation with an aerosol is devised by comparing the characteristic times of the processes of propagation of thermal and acoustic disturbances in the cross section of a beam of radius $R_0$ and in the space between absorbing centers with a number density $N$ (Fig. 5.14). The dashed lines 7 and 5 in Fig. 5.14 correspond to the rise times of quasisteady heat transfer in a medium across the boundary of a radiation-absorbing particle and the heating time of the particle to its maximum temperature. Here $\chi$ is the molecular thermal diffusivity of the medium, $C_p\rho$ and $C_p^a\rho_a$ are the volumetric isobaric heat capacities of the medium and the particle, and $a$ is the

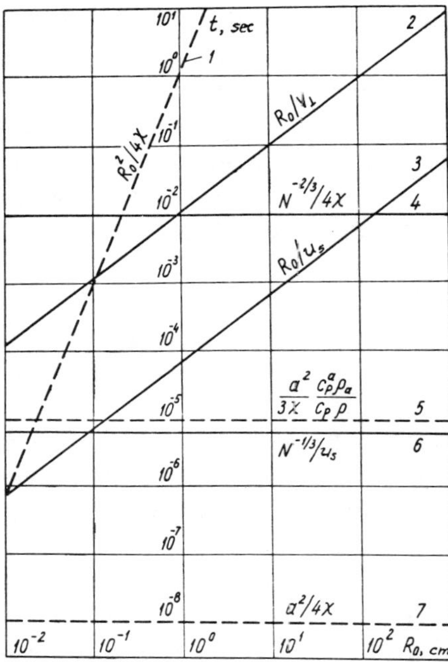

Fig. 5.14. Characteristic times of relaxation processes in a laser beam channel with absorbing aerosol particles.

particle radius. The solid lines 4 and 6 characterize the average overlap time of the thermal and acoustic aureoles from individual absorbing centers. The sloping lines 2 and 3 describe the variations of the transit times of the wind, $R_0/v_\perp$, and sound, $R_0/u_s$, across the beam away from its radius, $v_\perp$ is the lateral component of the wind velocity, and $u_s$ is the velocity of acoustic disturbances in the medium. The dashed line 1 indicates the dependence on $R_0$ of the temperature relaxation time in the space scales of the beam due to molecular heat conduction. The curves are plotted for representative values of the parameters of an atmospheric aerosol: $a=1$ $\mu$m; $C_p^a \rho_a/C_p \rho = 10^3$; $N = 10^3$ cm$^{-3}$; $v_\perp = 10^2$ cm/sec.

The following situations are the most important relation to the propagation of pulsed radiation:

$$t \lesssim \frac{R_0}{u_s}, \quad \begin{cases} t \ll \left(4N^{2/3}\chi\right)^{-1}, \quad \left(u_s N^{1/3}\right)^{-1} & (5.53) \\ \left(u_s N^{1/3}\right)^{-1} \ll t \ll \left(4N^{2/3}\chi\right)^{-1} & (5.54) \end{cases}$$

$$t \gtrsim \frac{R_0}{u_s}, \quad \begin{cases} t \ll \left(4N^{2/3}\chi\right)^{-1} & (5.55) \\ t \gtrsim \left(4N^{2/3}\chi\right)^{-1} & (5.56) \end{cases}$$

For continuous radiation of duration $t_r \gtrsim R_0/v_\perp$, the time $t$ of optical irradiation of the medium in (5.53)–(5.56) must be interpreted as the characteristic time $R_0/v_\perp$ corresponding to displacement of the medium relative to the beam in slewing or crosswind. The characteristic heat-conduction time in the channel $R_0^2/4\chi$ for real atmospheric conditions can almost always be neglected.

Below we describe briefly the most important results of theoretical and experimental work on the self-induced effects of powerful laser radiation in model aerosol media.

### 5.5.3. Optical Effects on Isolated Particles

#### 5.5.3.1. Subexplosive Evaporation of Water Droplets

The evaporation of a water droplet in the field of laser radiation has been thoroughly studied both theoretically [108, 109, 119, 146, 148] and experimentally [116–118, 122].

The rate of evaporation of a droplet in a radiation field is determined [109, 122] on the assumption of homogeneity of the optical field in the droplet. The dissipation time of optical into thermal energy is assumed to be small in comparison with the droplet relaxation time. The external fields of the temperature and partial vapor pressure are determined in the quasi-steady approximation on the basis of the Chapman–Enskog theory of inhomogeneous gases with regard for diffusion, heat conduction, and Stefan heat and mass transfer. The quasisteady approximation is applicable here for practically any evaporation conditions since the stabilization times of the fields in the vapor–gas medium are much smaller than the characteristic evaporation time of the droplet.

In this setting, the following system of equations is applicable to the external temperature and partial vapor pressure fields [122]:

$$\frac{\partial p_v}{\partial t} = \frac{1}{R}\frac{\partial}{\partial R}\left[\frac{D\mu_1}{R_bT^e}R^2\left(1+\frac{\mu_1}{M}\frac{p_v}{P-p_v}\right)\frac{\partial p_v}{\partial R}\right]$$

$$C_p^e\rho_e\frac{\partial T^e}{\partial t} = \frac{1}{R^2}\frac{\partial}{\partial R}\left[\lambda^e R^2\frac{\partial T^e}{\partial R} - R^2 C_p^e T^e m\right]$$

$$m = -\frac{D\mu_1}{R_bT^e}\left(1+\frac{\mu_1}{M}\frac{p_v}{P-p_v}\right)\frac{\partial p_v}{\partial R} \tag{5.57}$$

$$M = \mu_2 - (\mu_2 - \mu_1)p_v/P$$

Here $T^e$ is the temperature of the vapor–gas mixture, $p_v$ and $P$ are the pressures of the vapor and the mixture, $\mu_1$ and $\mu_2$ are the molecular weights of the vapor and atmospheric gases, $D$ is the diffusion coefficient, $\rho_e$ is the density of the vapor–gas mixture, $R_b$ is the gas constant, $\lambda^e$ and $C_p^e$ are the thermal conductivity and specific heat of the mixture, and $R$ is the distance from the center of the drop.

The temperature field in the interior of the droplet is described by the heat-conduction equation

$$\frac{\partial T^a}{\partial t} = \chi_a \frac{1}{R^2} \frac{\partial}{\partial R}\left( R^2 \frac{\partial T^a}{\partial R} \right) + \frac{3IK_a}{4C_p^a \rho_a a} \qquad (5.58)$$

in which $a$ is the radius of the droplet, $I$ is the radiation energy flux density, $t$ is the time, $K_a$ is the absorption efficiency factor, and $C_p^a, \rho_a, \chi_a$ are the specific heat, density, and thermal diffusivity of the liquid, respectively.

The system (5.57), (5.58) is subject to Dirichlet conditions of arbitrary form at the moving boundary of the droplet and standard initial conditions [109], and the system is then solved. A unique solution is found by matching the temperature and pressure fields outside and inside the droplet by the condition of continuity of the heat flux at the droplet surface in conjunction with the gaskinetic relations between the surface temperature of the droplet and the vapor pressure and temperature of the mixture at the bounding surface.

The results obtained by the scheme described above make it possible to classify the evaporization regimes of a spherical particle as shown in Fig. 5.15, in which the product $IK_a$ is plotted along the horizontal and the particle radius on the vertical axis. Regimes 1–3 in the figure describe steady-state particle evaporation processes. Regime 1, investigated in [115], is characterized by relatively large heat losses associated with the thermal conductivity of the medium and by a practically linear dependence of the

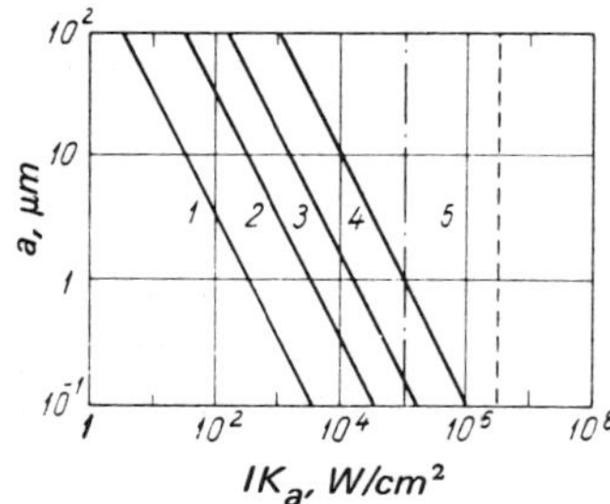


Fig. 5.15. Diagram of the evaporation regimes of a spherical water droplet in an optical field.

diffusion flux of the vapor on the droplet surface temperature. For evaporation in the second steady-state regime, the flux exhibits strong nonlinear growth with the temperature so that the heat losses due to thermal conduction in the gas become comparatively small. The third steady-state evaporation regime is highly favorable in the energy aspect because of the very low heat losses associated with the thermal conductivity of the gas. The hydrodynamic flow of vapor from the surface of the droplet plays an important role in the heat- and mass-transfer processes of evaporation in the third regime.

The evaporation rates in the first three regimes are described by the expressions

$$\frac{da}{dt} = -\frac{IK_a}{4\rho_a\left[Q_1 + \left(\lambda^e R_b^2 T_\infty^3 / D\mu_1^2 p_\infty L\right)\right]}\,; \qquad Q_1 = L + C_p^e T_\infty \qquad (5.59)$$

$$\frac{da}{dt} = -0.496\left(IK_a\right)^{1.102} \qquad (5.60)$$

$$\frac{da}{dt} = -\frac{IK_a}{4Q_2\rho_a}\,; \qquad\qquad Q_2 = L + C_p^e \frac{D}{\left(D/T^e\right)} \qquad (5.61)$$

Here $T_\infty$ is the temperature of the medium in which the droplet is located.

Regime 4 is characterized by the emergence of a nonsteady state on the part of the temperature field inside the droplet and mobility of its boundary. In this regime, the evaporation process is realized predominantly by hydrodynamic mass and heat transfer from the droplet. The evaporation rate in the indicated region is written

$$\frac{da}{dt} = -\frac{3IK_a}{2\pi^2 Q_2\rho_a} \sum_{n=1}^{\infty} \frac{1}{n^2}\left[1 - \exp\left(-\frac{\pi^2 n^2 \chi_a}{a^2}t\right)\right], \qquad t \leqslant \frac{a_0^2}{6\chi_a} \qquad (5.62)$$

$$\frac{da}{dt} = -IK_a \Big/ \left(4Q_2\rho_a - \frac{4}{15}\frac{IK_a a}{\chi_a} - \frac{1}{15}\frac{Ia^2}{\chi_a}\frac{dK_a}{da}\right), \qquad t > \frac{a_0^2}{6\chi_a} \qquad (5.63)$$

where $a_0$ is the initial radius of the droplet.

Regime 5 corresponds to explosion of the droplet, at the center of which almost-critical parameters of the substance are attained in heating.

The dot–dash line in the regime diagram (Fig. 5.15) separates the domain of diffusion and hydrodynamic vapor and heat transfer and the gasdynamic domain. The dashed line represents an estimate of the boundary of the evaporation regime in which the contribution of the vapor kinetic energy to the energy balance at the surface of the droplet is significant [149]. For the droplet sizes realized in clouds, however, this regime cannot be attained, since their explosion sets in even for small values of $IK_a$.

The results of experimental investigations of the evaporation rate of water droplets of various sizes, including those with a radius less than or equal to 20 $\mu$m, indicate satisfactory agreement of the data with the results of a calculation carried out on the assumption of homogeneity of the optical field inside the particle.

Numerical calculations of the evaporation of water droplets with allowance for Stefan flow, based on the complete system of thermohydrodynamical equations [119, 148, 150], yield results that differ only sightly from the results of calculations in the quasisteady approximation for the time dependence of the particle radius. For example, according to either theory, the particle radius varies from 10 to 0.5 $\mu$m over times that disagree at most by 20%.

### 5.5.3.2. Fragmentation and Gasdynamic Explosion of Water Droplets in Strong Optical Fields

When the intensity of laser radiation is increased, the surface regimes of evaporation of aerosol droplets are replaced by violent ejection of part of the mass of the droplet due to the attainment of near-critical parameters of the liquid in isolated zones of the particle volume. The process causes vapor and finely disperse liquid fractions to be present simultaneously in the explosion products. The explosive evaporation regime of droplets irradiated with laser radiation has been observed experimentally [117, 121].

The cause of metastable superheating of local zones is associated with the finite heat-conduction time, which is aggravated by the nonuniform distribution of the optical field in the particle interior. Pertinent calculations based on the formulas of Mie theory have been carried out [151–155].

The distribution of the temperature fields in a droplet has been investigated [156] with regard for the inhomogeneity of internal sources associated with the nonuniformity of the electromagnetic field distribution when a water droplet is acted upon by radiation with $\lambda = 10.6$ $\mu$m and a high radiation power density $\sim 10^4$ W/cm$^2$. This study indicates that a very sharp but spatially confined maximum of the radiation intensity distribution inside the droplet is observed near the shadow surface (away from the radiation source) of the droplet at the initial instant. As time passes, the maximum of the temperature distribution shifts into the zone of the illuminated (toward the source) hemisphere due to the presence of a maximum of the power of the heat sources in this zone, which encompasses a sizable portion of the droplet volume.

Calculations [156] have shown that in droplets with an initial radius $a_0 \lesssim 8$ $\mu$m the temperature maximum is attained near the center, while for larger droplets, $a_0 > 10$ $\mu$m, it occurs near the illuminated surface, and the temperature distribution inside the droplet is strongly nonuniform and depends on the droplet sizes, the power of the disturbing radiation, and its spatial distribution. For high-intensity laser sources, the temperature inhomogeneities induced by heat transfer and particle optics can serve as zones of localization of superheated (metastable) states of the droplet substance.

Experimental investigations of the mechanisms by which water droplets are affected by laser radiation with sharply differentiated spectral and temporal characteristics have shown that they will explode when definite energy thresholds are attained.

Two models of the process can be discerned according to the nature of the absorption of radiant energy incident on the particle and the distribution of the internal optical field in the droplet: (1) heating of the particle volume; (2) heating of the liquid exclusively in local zones of the droplet volume.

Uniform heating with allowance for surface evaporation at the demarcation between evaporation regimes 4 and 5 has been investigated [109, 122]. With this kind of heating, the inhomogeneity of the internal sources is attributable to heat transfer associated with surface evaporation so that almost the entire volume of the particle is in the superheated state and the center is heated to the temperature of the limit of absolute thermodynamic instability. The resulting development of homogeneous nucleation of the boiling process propagates throughout the entire volume of the droplet. The bubbles generated and growing at the center of the droplet are unstable with respect to small oscillations of the surface [123], and the growing (with time) disturbance can lead to rupture of the droplet.

The possibility of the existence of superheated states in droplets is a consequence both of the purity of its substance and of its heating conditions. At normal pressures, the temperature limit of absolute instability for water ($T_t^a$) is approximately equal to 320°C [123, 157]. In order to estimate the threshold intensity for attainment of $T_t$ at the center of the droplet, it is sufficient to set the expression obtained in [109] for the temperature of the center of a particle with heat transfer away from the free surface equal to the value of the indicated threshold temperature $T_t$:

$$2 \sum_{n=1}^{\infty} (-1)^n \int_0^t \left( J_0 - \frac{\partial T^a}{\partial t'} \right) \exp\left[ -\frac{\pi^2 n^2 \chi_a}{a^2}(t-t') \right] dt' - T_0^a = T_t^a$$

$$(5.64)$$

where $T^a$ is the temperature of the droplet surface,

$$J_0 = \frac{3IK_a}{4C_p \rho_a a_0} \tag{5.65}$$

$K_a$ is the efficiency factor for absorption of radiation by a spherical particle and is specified by the expression [158]

$$K_a = \exp\left\{ -0.2\left[ (n_a^2 + \mathrm{K}_a^2)^{1/2} - 1 \right] \right\} \left[ 1 - \exp\left( -\frac{8\pi \mathrm{K}_a a}{\lambda} \right) \right] \tag{5.66}$$

in which $n_a$ and $\mathrm{K}_a$ are the components of the complex refractive index of the particle. The solution (5.64) does not exist for every intensity level. We consider some asymptotic cases deduced from (5.64). They are determined from the relationship between the characteristic stabilization time of the temperature field field $\tau_1$ and the adiabatic heating time $\tau_2$ to the threshold temperature.

In the case of large intensities ($\tau_2 \ll \tau_1$), the consequence of (5.64) will almost always be adiabatic heating of the droplet, and the time at which the threshold temperature is reached is $\tau_2$. In the case $\tau_2 \gg \tau_1$ (for example, due to smallness of $a_0$), the threshold temperature is attained in the stabilization time of the temperature field inside the droplet $\sim a_0^2/\chi$, and the corresponding threshold intensity is

$$I = \frac{b\chi}{a_0^2}(T_t^a - T_\infty) \tag{5.67}$$

This value then determines the droplet explosion threshold in the evaporation regime diagram published in [122].

A numerical analysis of the behavior of the threshold intensities resulting in the explosion of small droplets in the radiation field of a $CO_2$ laser within the framework of the physical model discussed here has been carried out [159], along with estimates of the time to attain the threshold temperature at the center of a droplet.

In connection with the analysis of the mechanisms of explosion of weakly absorbing droplets, it is practical to estimate the quantities characterizing the energy balance of a droplet in the explosion process. These quantities include the energy of formation of the free surface, the kinetic energy of the explosion products, the energy of evaporation, and the energy absorbed up to the initiation of explosion. Estimates have shown that bursting of a droplet can take place with energy inputs several orders of magnitude smaller than the evaporation energy. Optical breakdown of the substance of the droplet emerges as the droplet rupture mechanism in this case.

The results of experimental studies of the conditions of explosion of transparent droplets under the action of radiation from a Q-switched ruby laser [160] indicate the decisive role of the optical breakdown of water at points of maxima of the optical field in the droplet in the explosion mechanism. The rupture of particles with diameters of 50 to 200 $\mu$m takes place at a radiant energy density of 0.1 J/cm$^2$ and a pulse duration of $2 \times 10^7$ sec. Optical breakdown could also account for the earlier experimental results of Barinov and Sorokin [121]. For an average peak intensity of $10^8$ W/cm$^2$ in an individual laser beam, the power density in "hot spots" of the droplet with allowance for diffraction maxima of the optical field is $\sim 2.5 \times 10^{10}$ W/cm$^2$, which exceeds the breakdown threshold for water [161–163].

If the laser radiation intensity is lower than the optical breakdown threshold of the droplet substance, then rupture of the latter is associated with superheating of the droplet, i.e., with thermal effects. The energy required for bursting of the droplet in this case is determined by the evaporation energy.

The inhomogeneities of the intensity distribution of the field in a droplet exert a significant influence on the duration of the rupture process and its dynamics. The presence of intensity maxima in local zones of the droplet turns these zones into centers of local ejections of finely disperse particles, and rupture of the particle takes place as a multistage process.


### 5.5.3.3. Vaporization of Spherical Solid Particles

The vaporization of solid particles has a number of singular aspects stemming from the need to consider the temperature dependence of the thermophysical characteristics of a particle and the medium due to the very large heating effects involved, processes of thermal dissociation of molecular substances, and a number of other phenomena.

The initial system of equations for the quasisteady superheating of a particle by radiation and the diffusion mechanism of heat and mass transfer [147] in the medium can be written in the form

$$-\rho_a \frac{da}{dt} = B\exp\left(-\frac{L\mu_1}{R_b T^a}\right) - \alpha v \rho_v^a \tag{5.68}$$

$$\frac{\partial T^a}{\partial t} = \frac{3}{4}\frac{IK_a}{C_p^a \rho_a a} + \frac{3\lambda^e}{C_p^a \rho_a a}\times\left.\frac{\partial T}{\partial R}\right|_{R=a} + \frac{3L}{aC_p^a}\times\frac{da}{dt} \tag{5.69}$$

$$-\lambda^e \left.\frac{\partial T}{\partial R}\right|_{R=a} = \frac{2}{3}\frac{\lambda_0^e T_\infty}{a}\left[\left(\frac{T^a}{T}\right)^{3/2}-1\right] \tag{5.70}$$

$$(\rho_v^a - \rho_a)\frac{da}{dt} = -D\left.\frac{\partial \rho_v}{\partial R}\right|_{R=a} = -\frac{D_0(T^a/T_\infty)^{3/2}-1}{\ln(T^a/T_\infty)} \tag{5.71}$$

where $\rho_a$ is the material density of the particle, $\rho_v$ is the vapor density, $\rho_v^a$ is the vapor density at the particle boundary, $a$ is the particle radius, $T^a$ is the temperature of the particle, $T$ is the temperature of the medium, $L$ is the heat of vaporization, $\mu_1$ is the molecular weight of the vapor, $\alpha$ is the accommodation coefficient, $V=(R_b T^a/2\pi\mu_1)^{1/2}$ is the effective reflux velocity, $D=D_0(T/T_\infty)^{3/2}$ and $\lambda^e=\lambda_0^e(T^a/T_\infty)^{3/2}$ are the diffusion coefficient and thermal conductivity of air [164], $C_p^a$ is the heat capacity of the particle material, $B$ is the rate coefficient, and $\rho_\infty, T_\infty$ are the values of $\rho_v$ and $T$ in the medium far from the particle.

The system (5.68)–(5.71) takes into account the jump of the vapor density near the interface, providing an additional criterion for delineating the class of small particles with $\alpha\ll1$, and it also takes into account the mobility of the interface during evaporation. From Eqs. (5.68) and (5.71), neglecting $\rho_\infty$ in comparison with $\rho_v$, we obtain an equation for $a(t)$, which in combination with (5.69) forms a closed system:

$$\frac{da}{dt} = \frac{\alpha v}{2} + \frac{\tilde{D}}{2a} - B\exp\left(-\frac{L\mu_1}{R_b T^a}\right)$$

$$-\left[\left(\frac{\alpha v}{2}+\frac{\tilde{D}}{2a}\right)^2 + \frac{B^2}{4\rho_a^2}\exp\left(-\frac{2L\mu_1}{R_b T^a}\right) + \frac{\tilde{D}-\alpha va}{2a\rho_a}B\exp\left(-\frac{L\mu_1}{R_b T^a}\right)\right]^{1/2},$$

$$\tilde{D}=D_0\frac{(T^a/T_\infty)^{3/2}-1}{\ln(T^a/T_\infty)^{3/2}} \tag{5.72}$$

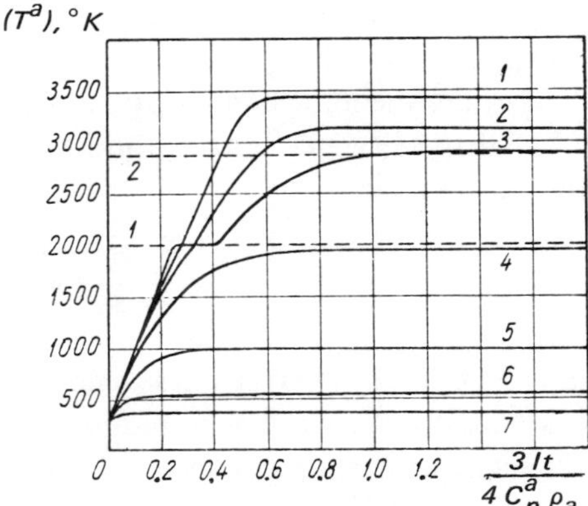

Fig. 5.16. Temperature of particle ($a_0 = 1$ $\mu$m) versus time for various values of the incident radiation power $I_0 K_a$: (1) $3.2 \cdot 10^5$ W/cm$^2$; (2) $10^5$; (3) $6.5 \cdot 10^4$; (4) $3.2 \cdot 10^4$; (5) $10^4$; (6) $3.2 \cdot 10^3$; (7) $10^3$ W/cm$^2$

The given theory is valid for the vaporization of substances that do not undergo thermal decomposition under the action of radiation. The system of equations (5.69), (5.72) has been solved numerically, with the absorption efficiency factor $K_a$ calculated according to the approximation formula (5.66). The variations of the particle temperature, vapor density at its surface, and reduced radius have been calculated for a quartz particle with an initial radius $a_0 = 10^{-4}$ cm under the action of square pulses from a $CO_2$ laser with an emission wavelength $\lambda = 10.6$ $\mu$m and pulse duration of 3 $\mu$sec. Figure 5.16 gives certain results of a calculation of the time dependence of the particle temperature for various incident radiation power values. We note that the effective heat of vaporization is evaluated in these calculations with allowance for dissociation effects.

We note in conclusion that for substances with a small accommodation coefficient ($\alpha = 0.022$ for quartz) the vapor pressure near the particle surface turns out to be less than atmospheric, even with superheating well above the boiling point $T_b$. For example, calculations show that in the case described above the saturated vapor pressure above a particle is attained at a temperature 1.12 times greater than $T_b$.

### 5.5.4. Action of Strong Laser Radiation on a Polydisperse Water Aerosol

The effects of laser radiation on a water aerosol have been the subject of numerous theoretical and experimental studies, a comprehensive bibliography of which may be found in our survey article [165]. We confine the present section to a very brief sketch of the most important results, drawing on the cited survey.

In the theoretical description of the action of strong laser radiation on a polydisperse water aerosol, the size spectrum of the latter can be described by the equation

$$\frac{\partial f}{\partial t} + \frac{\partial}{\partial a}(\dot{a}f) + v_\perp \frac{\partial f}{\partial y} = 0 \tag{5.73}$$

in which $y$ is the transverse coordinate of the beam, $\dot{a}$ is the rate of evaporation of a droplet of radius $a$, and $v_\perp$ is the component of the wind velocity transverse to the beam. Considering $v_\perp$ to be positive, we write the boundary conditions in the form

$$f(a, y, 0) = f\left(a, -(R^2 - z^2)^{1/2}, t\right) = f_0(a) \tag{5.74}$$

where $R(x)$ is the radius of the beam, $x$ is the coordinate measured along the beam axis, and $z$ is the transverse coordinate.

We wish to examine those situations in which the droplet evaporation rate is proportional to the radiation power flux $I$:

$$\dot{a} = -\varphi(a, a_0)I(y, t) \tag{5.75}$$

According to our classification [122], expression (5.75) is strictly satisfied in regimes 1 and 3 and approximately so in regimes 2 and 4, i.e., it satisfactorily describes the rate of evaporation of droplets in the range of cloud sizes for effective radiated power densities up to $10^3$ or $10^4$ W/cm$^2$.

The solution of (5.73) is written in the form

$$f(a, y, t) = f_0\left[a_0(a)\right] da_0/da \tag{5.76}$$

where $a_0(a)$ is the function obtained by inversion of the solution of the Cauchy problem

$$da/d\xi = -\varphi(a, a_0)I(\xi, \eta), \qquad a(\pm\eta) = a_0 \tag{5.77}$$

where $\xi$ and $\eta$ are new variables defined according to the expressions

$$t = \xi + \eta, \qquad y + \frac{(R^2 - z^2)^{1/2}}{v_\perp} = \xi - \eta$$

Integration of (5.77) gives

$$\int_a^{a_0} \frac{da}{\varphi(a, a_0)} = \int_{\pm\eta}^{\xi} I(\xi', \eta)\, d\xi \tag{5.78}$$

where the plus sign is taken at points where $y' = y + (R^2 - z^2)^{1/2}/v_\perp \leqslant t$. The droplet-size spectrum is therefore a function of the integral on the right-hand side of (5.78). This quantity, which is proportional to the energy absorbed by a fixed droplet up to the given time, may be referred to as the energy variable. Also dependent on it is the polydisperse extinction coefficient for an evaporating fog, as implied by the definition

$$a(i) = \pi N_0 \int_0^\infty a^2 f(a, i) K_0(a)\, da \tag{5.79}$$

where $N_0$ is the number density of droplets and $K_0$ is the radiation extinction efficiency factor. If the source is stationary and the power is uniformly distributed over its aperture, then, independently of $x$, the energy variable has the form

$$i = \begin{cases} \int_0^{y'} I(y'')\, dy'', & y' \leqslant t \\[2ex] \int_0^t I(t')\, dt', & y' > t \end{cases} \tag{5.80}$$

Thus, in the region occupied by the radiation we can discern a stationary and a nonstationary part, which are equivalent in terms of their mathematical description.

The propagation of a light beam under conditions such that it is acting on an aerosol can be described by the equation

$$-\operatorname{div} I\mathbf{n} = I\big[\alpha(i) + K_\nu\big] \tag{5.81}$$

in which $\mathbf{n}$ is the unit vector in the direction of propagation of radiation and $K_\nu$ is the volume absorption coefficient of the atmospheric gases.

It can be shown by suitable transformation of (5.81) that an energy variable of the form (5.80) obeys the following equation in the case of plane wave propagation:

$$-\frac{\partial i}{\partial x} = \int_0^i \alpha(i')\, di' \tag{5.82}$$

where $\alpha(i')$ is an integrable function which vanishes at $i = i_c \leqslant \infty$.

Under the condition $i(0)=I_0(t)$, we have

$$\int_{I_0 t}^{i} \frac{di''}{\int_0^{i''} \alpha(i')\,di'} + x = 0 \tag{5.83}$$

This quadrature formula determines the dependence of the energy variable on distance and time. An expression for $I$ can be obtained by differentiating $i$ with respect to the time.

It follows from (5.82) that the velocity of points at which $i$ (and, hence, $\alpha$ and $I$) is constant is given by the expression

$$\frac{dx}{dt} = I_0 \Big/ \int_0^{I_0 t} \alpha(i)\,di \tag{5.84}$$

It is clear, therefore, that in a time equal to $i_c/I_0$ a transition zone is formed, in which the extinction departs from exponential and which then moves into the depth of the layer with a velocity

$$V_3 = I_0 \Big/ \int_0^{\infty} \alpha(i)\,di \tag{5.85}$$

The front of a zone of total illumination exists in the tail of the transition zone.

The spatial intensity distribution in the stationary region is obtained by replacing the time with the coordinate $y'$.

The formation of a transition zone in the illumination channel, its characteristics, and the error of the approximations used to solve Eq. (5.81) have been tested in our experimental work with radiation wavelengths of 1.06 $\mu$m.

The results of the test indicate satisfactory agreement of the various results.

We now consider the propagation of a stationary beam from a $CO_2$ laser with a Gaussian profile in a polydisperse water fog transported with a constant velocity [114].

Equation (5.78) enables us to calculate the limiting value of the energy variable at $x=0$:

$$i(0) = \frac{R_0\sqrt{\pi}}{2v_\perp} I_0 \exp\left(\frac{-z^2}{R_0^2}\right) \left\{ \Phi\left[ \frac{v_\perp}{R_0}(\xi-\eta) - \frac{(R^2-z^2)^{1/2}}{R_0} \right] \right.$$

$$\left. - \left[ -\frac{v_\perp}{R_0}\binom{0,\quad \eta\geqslant 0}{2\xi,\quad \eta<0} - \frac{(R^2-z^2)^{1/2}}{R_0} \right] \right\}, \tag{5.86}$$

where $\Phi$ is the probability integral, $I_0$ and $R_0$ are the radiated energy flux density on the axis and the effective radius of a Gaussian beam with profile

$$I(0)=I_0\exp\left(-\frac{y^2+z^2}{R_0^2}\right) \tag{5.87}$$

at the entrance to the aerosol layer.

The alternative in (5.86) signifies the existence of a stationary and a nonstationary region in the active zone. The corresponding boundary $\eta=0$, as is apparent from (5.77), moves with the wind velocity $v_\perp$.

A numerical calculation of $(i)$ shows that a good approximation for large-droplet fogs is provided by the exponential function

$$\alpha(i)=\alpha_0\exp\left(-\beta k_0 i\right) \tag{5.88}$$

in which $\alpha_0$ is the unperturbed value of $\alpha$, $\beta$ is an approximation parameter, which is determined by means of the least-square deviation criterion, and $k_0$ is a parameter characterizing the droplet evaporation regime [122].

Proceeding from (5.83) and taking (5.88) into account, we can write the distribution of the energy variable in the region occupied by radiation in the form

$$i=\frac{1}{\beta k_0}\ln\left(1+\exp\left(-\tau_0\right)\left\{1-\exp\left[\beta k_0 i(0)\right]\right\}\right) \tag{5.89}$$

where $\tau_0=\alpha_0 x$ is the optical thickness of the path. The distribution of the radiated power flux can be obtained from (5.89) according to either of the expressions

$$I=\frac{\partial i}{\partial \xi}, \qquad I=I(0)\exp\left(-\int_0^x\alpha(i)\,dx'\right) \tag{5.90}$$

The result has the form

$$I=\frac{I(0)\exp\left[\beta k_0 i(0)\right]}{\exp\left[\beta k_0 i(0)\right]+\exp\left(\tau_0\right)-1} \tag{5.91}$$

where $i(0)$ and $I(0)$ are given by expressions (5.86) and (5.87).

The latter relation completely describes the self-induced action of a collimated Gaussian beam in a fog transported with a constant velocity. In the case investigated here, unlike the problem treated in [133], the asymptotic nature of $\alpha(i)$ is such that the active zone is not divided into a

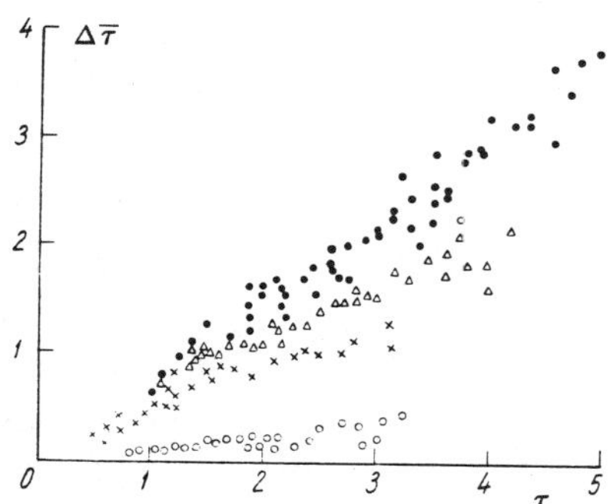

Fig. 5.17. Variation of optical thickness of an artificial fog under the action of continuous $CO_2$ laser radiation versus initial optical thickness. Peak power densities $P_0$ of incident radiation: (1) ●, 485 W/cm², $v=0$; (2) ▽, 211 W/cm², $v=0$; (3) ×, 100 W/cm², $v=0$; (4) ○, 211 W/cm² under the action of crosswind $v=70$ cm/sec.

transition region and a region of total illumination for arbitrary finite time of thermal action.

Experimental studies of the effects of $CO_2$ laser radiation on a polydisperse artificial water fog have been carried out on the basis of measurements of the microstructure and optical thickness of the fog in the active zone. Figure 5.17 shows the variation of the optical thickness $\Delta\tau$ of the investigated fogs as a function of the initial optical thickness for various laser powers. Also shown in the figure is the effect of crosswind with a velocity of 70 cm/sec. A comparison of the experimental data in Fig. 5.17 with the calculated results indicated good agreement between them.

Investigations of the shape of the enhanced-transmittance zone of a fog under the action of a $CO_2$ laser in the horizontal and vertical planes have shown that the shape is symmetrical in the horizontal plane about the center of a powerful beam in the absence of crosswind. In the vertical plane, owing to the settling of fog particles and the resulting warm-up of upward convection flows, the enhanced-transmittance zone has a maximum transmittance at the lower boundary of the zone of action of the powerful beam, indicating the predominant influence of particle settling on the shaping of the zone in comparison with convection flows.

### 5.5.5 Influence of Recondensation Processes on the Evaporation of a Water Aerosol under the Action of Laser Radiation

The results described in the preceding section have been obtained on the assumption that all the evaporation products of particles situated in the channel of the acting laser beam are in the vapor state. In reality, some of those products, depending on the conditions in the beam channel, participate in recondensation processes, which lead to the formation of secondary cloud or fog particles. Recondensation problems have been investigated in several papers [131, 132, 166–168] in which the nucleation and growth of secondary particles near evaporating droplets in various lasing regimes are analyzed in detail, heat- and mass-transfer processes between the primary and secondary condensed aerosol fractions are investigated, and results characterizing the conditions for the initiation of radiation-induced recondensation are obtained. However, in order to describe the clearing process it is necessary to have solutions of the self-consistent problem involving the nonlinear radiation transport equation, which do not exist. The indicated problem can be solved on the basis of the theory set forth below.

We first of all take into consideration the fact that in analyzing the kinetics of evaporation of an isolated droplet it is no longer permitted to assume that the temperature $T_\infty$ and concentration $\rho_v(T_\infty)$ in the region of sinks (formally at an infinite distance from the droplet) are constant. In the given quasisteady-state problem, we start with the energy balance equation

$$IK_a a = 4\lambda^e (T^a - T_\infty) + 4DL\left[\rho_v(T^a) - \rho_v(T_\infty)\right] \tag{5.92}$$

in which $I$ is the radiated power density, $K_a$ is the absorption efficiency factor, $a$ is the particle radius, $\lambda^e$ is the thermal conductivity, $T^a$ is the temperature of the droplet surface, $L$ is the specific heat of vaporization, $D$ is the vapor diffusion coefficient in air, and $\rho_v(T)$ is the saturated vapor concentration corresponding to the temperature $T$.

Linearizing (5.92), we expand the dependence of $\rho_v$ on $T^a$ into a series in the neighborhood of the point $T_e$ representing the initial value of the temperature of the droplet and medium, which in the general case does not coincide with $T_\infty$.

Restricting the expansion to linear terms in $T^a - T_e$ and making use of the relations between the droplet characteristics and the sink characteristics, we can write the evaporation kinetic equation, which can then be integrated for a sufficiently transparent droplet to yield the expression

$$a^2 = \exp\left(-\frac{8}{3}n_a\frac{D}{\gamma_L}\kappa_a\eta\int_0^t Idt'\right)\left\{-\frac{2D}{\gamma_L}\int_0^t dt'\left[\xi T_\infty + (\xi-1)\rho_v(T_\infty)+\theta\right]\right.$$
$$\left. \times\exp\left(\frac{8}{3}n_a\frac{D}{\gamma_L}\kappa_a\eta\int_0^{t'} Idt''\right)+a_0\right\} \tag{5.93}$$

in which $a_0$ and $\kappa_a$ are the initial radius and absorption coefficient of the droplet, $n_a$ is the refractive index of its material,

$$\xi = \rho_v(T_e)E\beta, \qquad \theta = \rho_v(T_e)E\chi - \rho_v(T_e)ET_e + \rho_v(T_e),$$

$$E = \frac{L\mu_1}{R_b T_e^2}, \qquad \alpha = \left[4\lambda^e + 4LD\rho_v(T_e)E\right]^{-1}, \qquad \beta = 4\lambda^e L,$$

$$\gamma_L = 4LD\alpha, \qquad \eta = \rho_v(T_e)E\alpha, \qquad \chi = 4LD(ET_e - 1)\rho_v(T_e)\alpha$$

$R_b$ is the gas constant, and $\mu_1$ is the molecular weight of the vapor.

The time dependence of the temperature and concentration of the vapor at infinity in (5.93) must be determined by solving the evaporation problem for a set of particles. However, it is already implicit in the evaporation kinetic equation that in the presence of supersaturation there is a critical droplet radius such that the smaller droplets will grow in radiant heating, while the more sizeable droplets will evaporate. The critical radius is given by the expression

$$a_c = \left[-\left(\xi T_\infty + (\xi-1)\rho_v(T_\infty) + \theta\right)\left(\tfrac{4}{3}n_a\kappa_a\eta I\right)^{-1}\right]^{1/2} \tag{5.94}$$

The evaporation of a set of droplets is described by the system

$$\frac{\partial f}{\partial t} + \frac{\partial}{\partial a}\left(f\frac{da}{dt}\right) = 0 \tag{5.95}$$

$$\frac{\partial \rho_v(T_\infty)}{\partial t} = 4\pi D\int_0^\infty f(a)a\left[\rho_v(T^a) - \rho_v(T_\infty)\right]da \tag{5.96}$$

$$C_p\rho\frac{\partial T_\infty}{\partial t} = 4\pi\lambda^e\int_0^\infty f(a)a(T^a - T_\infty)\,da \tag{5.97}$$

Here $f(a)$ is the droplet-size spectrum, $C_p$ is the specific heat of vapor–gas mixture at constant pressure, and $\rho$ is its density. To close the given system of equations it is required to augment it with relations between the droplet and sink characteristics as well as the droplet evaporation kinetic equation. Then, once the initial values of $f$, $\rho_v(T_\infty)$, and $T_\infty$ have been specified, the time variations of these quantities can be determined.

Inasmuch as the equation for the evaporation rate $da/dt$ is integrable [expression (5.93)], the integral of Eq. (5.95) can be constructed as follows:

$$f(a,t) = f_0\left[a_0(a)\right]\left|da_0/da\right| \tag{5.98}$$

where $f_0(a_0)$ is the initial probability density function of the droplets with respect to their sizes and $a_0(a)$ is the function obtained by inversion of

(5.93). The integrals with respect to $a$ on the right-hand sides of (5.96) and (5.97) can be convoluted by means of (5.98).

Let us consider the case in which the initial spectrum has the form

$$f_0(a_0) = N\delta(a_0 - a_m) + N_i\delta(a_0 - a_i) \qquad (5.99)$$

where $N$ and $a_m$ are the number density and radius of droplets in the main large-droplet fraction and $N_i$ and $a_i$ are the density and radius of the nuclei. The spectrum of nuclei is introduced to account for recondensation in the case of supersaturation. It may be assumed that $a_i = 0$. Irrespective of this assumption, the last stage of condensation will be correctly described when the droplets grow as a result of diffusion.

As a result of convolution of the right-hand sides of (5.96) and (5.98), we obtain a system of integrodifferential equations for the determination of $\rho_v(T_\infty)$ and $T_\infty$, which describes the variation of the vapor concentration and temperature as a result of both evaporation and condensation. These equations go over to integral equations on the assumption of dynamic equilibrium of the large-droplet fraction with the small-droplet fraction. The solution of these equations [131] by the method of successive approximations makes it possible to obtain data on the evaporation kinetics of water droplets with recondensation.

Pertinent calculations have shown that, as a result of recondensation, the secondary particles grow to sizes adequate for optical activity from the point of view of the values of the volume extinction coefficients.

Thus, under the action of a powerful laser beam directed into a polydisperse water aerosol, two competing processes take place in the zone of the beam: (1) evaporation of large droplets; (2) nucleation of secondary small particles. After attaining the maximum sizes for the given lasing conditions, the condensed water particles are subjected anew to radiation. The role of recondensation is therefore tantamount to a corresponding slowing down of the clearing process in the channel occupied by the laser beam. This conclusion is also valid when the assumption of dynamic equilibrium between the fractions of water aerosol particles is lifted.


### 5.5.6 Nonlinear Scattering of Laser Radiation by Thermal and Acoustic Aureoles in the Vicinity of Absorbing Particles

The absorption of laser energy by solid aerosol particles with large values of the imaginary part of the complex refractive index results in the formation of acoustic and thermal aureoles and perturbations of the density of the medium in the vicinity of the particles.

The principal mechanism of the self-induced action of the laser beam in this case must be attributed to nonlinear scattering of light at hydrodynamic density perturbations of the medium in the vicinity of the absorption centers [143, 146, 169–172].

The system of thermohydrodynamical equations describing the spatial distribution of the pressure $p$, density $\rho$, hydrodynamic velocity $\mathbf{v}$, and temperature $T$ in the medium in the approximation of uniform heating of a spherical particle of radius $a$ has the form

$$C_p\rho\frac{\partial T}{\partial t} = \nabla(\lambda^e\nabla T) + \frac{\partial p}{\partial t}, \qquad |\mathbf{r}-\mathbf{r}_n| > a \tag{5.100}$$

$$\frac{\partial T^a}{\partial t} = \frac{3}{4aC_p^a\rho_a}\left[\left|\frac{cK_n}{8\pi}|\mathbf{E}|^2 + 4\lambda^e\nabla T\right|_{|\mathbf{r}-\mathbf{r}_n|=a} - 16\sigma b_\lambda(T^a)^3(T^a-T_\infty)\right]$$

$$\tag{5.101}$$

$$\partial\mathbf{v}/\partial t + (\mathbf{v}\nabla)\mathbf{v} = -\rho^{-1}\nabla\rho \tag{5.102}$$

$$\partial\rho/\partial t + \mathrm{div}(\rho\mathbf{v}) = 0; \qquad p = R_b\rho T \tag{5.103}$$

The boundary conditions are as follows:

$$T|_{|\mathbf{r}-\mathbf{r}_n|=a} = T^a; \qquad T|_{t=0} = T^a|_{t=0} = T_\infty$$

$$\rho|_{t=0} = \rho_\infty; \qquad p|_{t=0} = p_\infty; \qquad \mathbf{v}|_{t=0} = \mathbf{v}|_{\mathbf{r}-\mathbf{r}_n=a} = 0 \tag{5.104}$$

All the functions satisfy the unperturbed boundary conditions at infinity. In the system (5.100)–(5.104), $T^a$ is the warm-up temperature of the particle, $t$ is the time, $T_\infty, p_\infty, \rho_\infty$ are the unperturbed values of the temperature, pressure, and density of the medium, $\lambda^e$ is the molecular thermal conductivity of air, $C_p$ and $R_A$ are its isobaric specific heat and specific gas constant, $c$ is the speed of light in air, $C_p^a\rho_a$ is the volume specific heat, $\sigma$ is the Stefan–Boltzmann constant, $b_\lambda$ is the grayness index, $K_a$ is the efficiency factor for absorption of light by the particle at wavelength $\lambda$, $\mathbf{E}$ is the electric field in the light wave, and $\mathbf{r}_n$ and $\mathbf{r}$ are the radius vectors of the center of the $n$th particle and the observation point. The nonlinear variation $\delta\varepsilon_N$ of the permittivity of the medium is related to its thermodynamic characteristics by the Lorentz–Lorenz relation.

In the simplest case, the propagation of thermal and acoustic disturbances in the medium can be taken into account within the framework of linear acoustics and the quasisteady-state heat transfer in the medium across the particle of the boundary; this state is realized for an optical irradiation time $t \gg a^2/\chi$, $a^2/\chi_a$, where $\chi = \lambda^e/C_p\rho$ and $\chi_a$ are the thermal diffusivities of the medium and the particle, respectively.

In this case, the real source can be replaced by a point source [146] and the system (5.100)–(5.103) consolidated into a single linearized equation for the total density perturbation in the medium $\delta\rho = \rho - \rho_\infty$:

$$\left( \frac{\partial^3}{\partial t^3} - \gamma\chi \nabla^2 \frac{\partial^2}{\partial t^2} - u_s^2 \nabla^2 \frac{\partial}{\partial t} + \chi u_s^2 \nabla^4 \right) \delta\rho = (\gamma-1)\pi a^2 K_a I \nabla^2 \delta(\mathbf{r}-\mathbf{r}_n)$$

$$(5.105)$$

subject to the boundary conditions

$$\delta\rho\Big|_{t=0} = \frac{\partial\delta\rho}{\partial t}\Big|_{t=0} = \delta\rho\big|_{|\mathbf{r}-\mathbf{r}|\to\infty} = 0$$

Here $\gamma$ is the adiabatic exponent, $I$ is the radiation flux density, $u_s$ is the speed of sound in air, and $\delta(\mathbf{r})$ is the delta function. A solution of Eq. (5.105) is found by the method of integral transforms. It is inferred from an analysis of the solution that the total density perturbation of the medium in the linear acoustics setting comprises the additive contribution of isobaric thermal expansion of the air and the acoustic disturbance.

For $t \gg \chi/u_s^2$, the temperature distribution near the particle with radiant heat losses has the form

$$T(\mathbf{r}, t) = T_\infty + \frac{a^2 c K_a}{8\pi^{1/2}\chi^{1/2}\left(\lambda^e + 4\sigma b_\lambda a T_\infty^3\right)} \int_0^t (t-t_1)^{-3/2}$$

$$\times \exp\left[-\frac{|\mathbf{r}-\mathbf{r}_n|}{4\chi(t-t_1)}\right] I(t_1)\, dt_1 \left[1 + O\left(\frac{a^2}{3\chi t}\frac{C_p^a\rho_a}{C_p\rho}\right)\right]$$

$$(5.106)$$

The characteristics of light scattering by an optical inhomogeneity with a given permittivity distribution $\varepsilon(\mathbf{r}, t)$ for an absorbing particle of arbitrary radius are subsequently investigated in the "soft-particle" approximation: $|\varepsilon - 1| \ll 1$. In this case, the smoothly varying complex amplitude $\mathbf{E}$, which is related to the electric field $\mathbf{e}$ by the expression $\mathbf{e} = \mathbf{E}\exp(i\omega_0 t)$ ($\omega_0$ is the emission frequency) is given by the following expression in the wave zone

$|\mathbf{r}-\mathbf{r}_n|\gg 4k\chi t, ku_s^2 t^2$ [173]:

$$\mathbf{E}(\mathbf{r},t)=\mathbf{E}_0\exp(-i\mathbf{k}\mathbf{R})+\frac{\exp(-ikR)}{R}\big[\mathbf{n},[\mathbf{E}_0,\mathbf{n}]\big]S(\omega,t) \quad (5.107)$$

where $\mathbf{k}$ is the wave vector, $k=|\mathbf{k}|=2\pi/\lambda$, $\mathbf{R}=\mathbf{r}-\mathbf{r}_n$, $\mathbf{n}=\mathbf{R}/R$, $\mathbf{E}_0$ is the amplitude of the incident field, $S(\omega,t)$ is the amplitude of the scattering function for light scattered by the inhomogeneity:

$$S(\omega,t)=-\frac{ik}{2\pi}\iint_{-\infty}^{\infty}dR_1'dR_2'\exp(-ik\mathbf{R}_\perp\omega_\perp)$$

$$\times\left\{1-\exp\left[-\frac{ik}{2}\iint_{-\infty}^{\infty}dR_3'(\varepsilon(\mathbf{R}',t)-1)\right]\right\} \quad (5.108)$$

$\omega=\mathbf{k}/k-\mathbf{R}/R$, and $\omega_\perp$, $\mathbf{R}_\perp(R_1,R_2)$ are the components of the corresponding vectors in the plane normal to $\mathbf{k}$. We note that it is unnecessary for the "softness" condition to be satisfied in the limiting cases $ka\varepsilon_a''\gg 1$ and $ka\ll 1$ ($\varepsilon_a=\varepsilon_a'-i\varepsilon_a''$ is the complex-valued permittivity of the particle).

Simple analytical expressions can be obtained in the scalar approximation for the efficiency factor for light scattering by the inhomogeneity

$$K_s=2a^{-2}\int_0^\pi d\theta\sin\theta\big|s[2\sin(\theta/2)]\big|^2$$

and the angular scattering function $B(\omega,t)=4(a^2K_s)^{-1}|s(\omega,t)|^2$, where $2\sin(\theta/2)=|\omega|$, if the second term in the exponent inside the braces, which describes the phase lead of a plane wave within the limits of the induced density perturbation, has a small absolute value in comparison with unity and the absolute value of the first term. In particular, the expression for $K_s$ in the case of a step pulse acting on an absorbing particle ($ka\varepsilon_a''\gg 1$) has the form

$$K_s=K_s^{(0)}+\frac{\ln 2}{2\chi}t\left(\frac{aK_akI_0(\gamma-1)}{2u_s^2}\frac{\partial\varepsilon}{\partial\rho}\right)\left[1-{}_1F_1\left(1,\frac{3}{2};-\frac{u_s^2 t}{2\chi\gamma}\right)\right]$$

$$(5.109)$$

where ${}_1F_1$ is the confluent hypergeometric function and $K_s^{(0)}$ is the efficiency factor for light scattering by the undisturbed particle.

The expression for $K_s$ is the case of an arbitrary function $I(t)$ and $t\gg\chi/u_s^2$, such that only nonlinear scattering by the thermal aureole (region of isobaric thermal variation of the density near the heated particle) is significant, has the form

$$K_s = K_s^{(0)} + \frac{1}{\chi} \left( \frac{\pi a K_a k}{4 C_p \rho} \frac{\partial \varepsilon}{\partial T} \right)^2 \iint_{a^2/4\chi}^{t} \frac{dt_1 \, dt_2 \, I(t_1) I(t_2)}{2t - t_1 - t_2} \tag{5.110}$$

An analysis of relations (5.108), (5.109), and (5.110) shows that in the event of radiation acting on a particle with large absorption ($ka\varepsilon_a'' \gg 1$) and low superheats of the medium, the processes of scattering by the particle and hydrodynamic perturbation of the density are independent; acoustic density perturbations yield an appreciable contribution to the variation of the scattering cross section of the inhomogeneity in comparison with the thermal aureole for optical irradiation times $t \lesssim 10^{-6}$ to $10^{-7}$ sec.

In the case of optical radiation acting on Rayleigh ($ka \ll 1$) and weakly absorbing ($ka\varepsilon_a'' \lesssim 1$) aerosol particles, the additivity condition fails. Then, because of the opposite signs of the phase variation of the wave within the limits of the particle and the thermal aureole ($\partial \varepsilon / \partial T < 0$ for air), partial mutual compensation of the linear and nonlinear terms is possible in the expression for the amplitude scattering function, thereby serving as the cause of a new "aureole" mechanism of self-clearing of a turbid medium. The effect is most pronounced in the case

$$\overline{\delta T} (\chi t)^{1/2} \left| \frac{\partial \varepsilon}{\partial T} \right| \approx (\varepsilon_a - 1) a \tag{5.111}$$

or

$$\beta \, \overline{\delta T} (\chi t)^{1/2} |\mathrm{Im} \, \varepsilon_0| \approx a |\mathrm{Im} \, \varepsilon_a| \tag{5.112}$$

where $\beta$ and $\varepsilon_0$ are the coefficient of thermal expansion of the heated air and the complex permittivity of air and $\overline{\delta T}$ is a characteristic variation of the temperature in the thermal disturbance region.

Experimental studies of the self-induced action of millisecond pulses from ($\lambda = 0.69$ $\mu$m) and neodymium–glass ($\lambda = 1.06$ $\mu$m) lasers have been carried out [138, 144]. The scattering media were cement dust, talc, nickelous oxide, and wood smoke. The particles had a spherical shape, or nearly so, in every case. Figure 5.18 gives some of the results of measurements of the time dependence of the nonlinear variation of the weighted-mean angular spread during the action of the radiation pulse in various scattering media. It is evident from the figure that the nonlinear angular

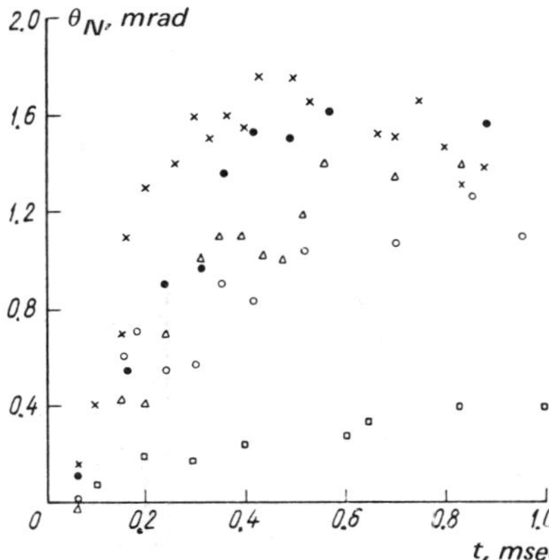

Fig. 5.18. Results of measurements of the non-linear weighted-mean angular spread of a probe beam during the action of a millisecond pulse on various polydisperse media. ($\times$, $\bullet$) Cement suspension, laser wavelength $\lambda = 0.69$ $\mu$m, pulse energy $Q = 40$ J; ($\bigcirc$) suspension of talc particles, $\lambda = 0.69$ $\mu$m, $Q = 40$ J; ($\square$) wood smoke, $\lambda = 1.06$ $\mu$m, $Q = 150$ J.

spread observed in the measurements attains several milliradians and so the given effect can induce significant changes in the law of propagation of laser beams in an atmosphere filled with the corresponding solid particles.

An analysis of the radiant power profiles in the focal plane of the objective in the investigation of nonlinear light scattering by localized thermal inhomogeneities indicates the following:

a. Stratification of the beam into an undisturbed part, an amplitude-attenuated part, and a part scattered by optical density perturbations with a characteristic scattering angle $\theta \sim [2k(\chi t)^{1/2}]^{-1}$, where $k$ is the wave number, takes place in the initial stage of interaction of the light pulse with the aerosol. After a time $t \approx 0.6$ msec, the amplitudes of the scattered and transmitted radiation becomes practically commensurate.

b. The radiant power profile is randomized, acquiring a small-scale statistical structure.

c. After transmission of a strong pulse, the relaxation of the optical properties of the medium in the beam channel discloses two characteristic time scales $T_1$ and $T_2$. The time $T_1$ is of the same order of magnitude as the characteristic averaging time $(4\chi N^{2/3})^{-1}$ of thermal inhomogeneities in the space between particles; the second time scale is of the order $T_2 \approx 10^2$ msec and is governed by heat-conduction processes in the beam space scales and by turbulent blurring of the optical channel.

A quantitative comparison of the experimental results with a theoretical calculation of the self-broadening effect of optical pulses on the basis of a solution of the nonlinear radiation transport equation in the small-angle approximation has been carried out for a medium consisting of a suspension of nickelous oxide particles [144]. The results of the comparison indicate satisfactory agreement between the data for a pulse energy not exceeding the critical value of 30 J corresponding to a change of the state of aggregation of the radiation-heated aerosol particles.

### 5.5.7. Nonsteady Acoustic Self-Focusing of Laser Radiation in a Gaseous Medium Containing Absorption Centers

We now examine the propagation of short laser pulses of duration $t \lesssim R_0/u_s$, where $R_0$ is the beam radius and $u_s$ is the sound velocity in a gaseous medium containing center of hydrodynamic density perturbations. It is readily perceived that corresponding conditions are realizable in the real atmosphere. The most important situation in this case [50] arises when the acoustic density perturbations intersect in the space between particles and regions of isobaric expansion of the medium (thermal aureoles) exist as localized inhomogeneities occupying a small volume of the medium, i.e.,

$$\left(u_s N^{1/3}\right)^{-1} \ll t \ll \left(4\chi N^{2/3}\right)^{-1}$$

Taking into account the additivity of the contributions to the density variation of the medium around a particle from the thermal perturbation $\delta\rho_T$ and acoustic perturbation $\delta\rho_s$ in the linear acoustics setting, we can write the density variation in a discretely absorbing medium in the form

$$\delta\rho(\mathbf{r}, t) = \sum_n \delta\rho'_T(\mathbf{r}-\mathbf{r}_n, t) + \left\langle \sum_n \delta\rho_s(\mathbf{r}-\mathbf{r}_n, t) \right\rangle + \sum_n{}' \delta\rho_s(\mathbf{r}-\mathbf{r}_n, t)$$

$$(5.113)$$

The second term in (5.113) describes the statistical-mean profile of the acoustic perturbation in the medium, and the third term characterizes the random deviations from the statistical mean at a fixed point of the medium; $\mathbf{r}_n$ is the radius vector of the center of the $n$th particle.

It follows from (5.113) that the dynamics of the optical beam due to nonlinear variation of the permittivity $\delta\varepsilon = (\partial\varepsilon/\partial\rho)\delta\rho$ is determined by two competing processes: self-broadening due to nonlinear scattering by localized thermal aureoles and acoustic density fluctuations, and self-focusing on the statistical-mean acoustic profile of the density perturbation in the medium, as described by the second term in (5.113). We discuss the analysis of this term in closer detail. It can be shown that when the centers of the particles are statistically independent the spatial acoustic density fluctuations form a generalized Poisson process. The averaging in (5.113) is then easily performed by means of the expression for the characteristic functional of a generalized Poisson process. In the interval $t \ll R_0/u_s$ we obtain

$$\left\langle \sum_n \delta\rho_s \right\rangle = \delta\tilde{\rho}_s = -\frac{\beta\alpha_a}{C_p} I_0 t \tag{5.114}$$

where $C_p$ and $\beta$ are the specific heat and coefficient of thermal expansion of air, $\alpha_a$ is the volume absorption coefficient of the aerosol, $T$ is the temperature of the medium, and $I_0$ is the radiation intensity. For an arbitrary relation between the times $t$ and $\tau_s = R_0/u_s$, where $u_s$ is the sound velocity, the dynamics of the function $\delta\tilde{\rho}_s$ can be analyzed on the basis of the linearized acoustical equations. In particular, for a beam with a Gaussian distribution in the cross section and a time-constant intensity on its axis, the solution for $\delta\tilde{\rho}_s$ has the form

$$\delta\tilde{\rho}_s = -\frac{\beta\alpha_a I_0}{C_p} t \exp\left(-\frac{t^2}{\tau_s^2}\right)$$

$$\times \left[ {}_1F_1\left(\frac{1}{2}, \frac{3}{2}; \frac{t^2}{\tau_s^2}\right) - \frac{r_\perp^2}{R_0^2} {}_1F_1\left(-\frac{1}{2}, \frac{3}{2}; \frac{t^2}{\tau_s^2}\right) + \cdots \right] \tag{5.115}$$

where $r_\perp(y, z)$ is the cylindrical coordinate and $R_0$ is the beam radius. For a pulse with a smooth leading edge, the acoustic density profile is proportional to $(\partial T/\partial t)\tau_s$. For a negative intensity gradient, the perturbation $\delta\tilde{\rho}_s$ acquires the opposite sign.

Next we consider the analysis of the optical beam dynamics. We note first of all that in the case $x \gg u_s t$, which usually occurs, the fluctuations of the phase lead along the ray path $\int_0^x d\xi \Sigma'_n \delta\rho_s(\xi - \xi_n, \mathbf{r} - \mathbf{r}_n, t)$ can be close to Gaussian by the integral limit theorem. The beam broadening due to scattering by acoustic density fluctuations is then readily estimated on the basis of the parabolic equation for the field in the approximation of inhomogeneities delta correlated along the path [174]. The estimates indicate a negligible role of scattering by acoustic density fluctuations associated with the third term in (5.113) in comparison with broadening of the beam in connection with scattering by thermal aureoles for $t \gg \chi/u_s^2 \approx 10^{-9}$ sec. The influence of the other two terms in (5.113) is taken into account on the basis of the small-angle transport equation for a medium with regular refraction. In particular, the expression for the effective beam cross section in the approximation of a weakly nonlinear medium for a Gaussian beam in the interval $\tau_0 \ll 1$ is obtained in the form

$$\Omega = \Omega_0 + \Omega_s\left[1 - \tfrac{1}{5}(\eta x)^2\right] - \pi(\eta x)^2\left[R_0^2 + \left(\frac{1}{k^2 R_0^2} + \frac{R_0^2}{F_0^2}\right)\frac{x^2}{3} + \frac{2}{3}\frac{x R_0^2}{F_0}\right]$$

where $\eta^2$ is the coefficient of the squared term in the expansion of $\tfrac{1}{2}(\partial\varepsilon/\partial\rho)\delta\tilde{\rho}_s$ into a series with respect to $r_\perp$ for the axial zone of the beam and characterizes the degree of focusing of the radiation, $\Omega_s$ is the broadening of the beam at the thermal aureoles, $F_0$ is the initial radius of curvature of the phase front of the Gaussian beam, $\tau_0$ is the initial optical thickness of the aerosol, and $\Omega_0$ is the broadening of the beam in the nonlinear medium.

An assessment of the acoustic self-focusing effect according to the theory described here indicates the possibility of its occurrence in connection with atmospheric propagation. For example, in the interval of values of the parameters $t/\tau_s < 1$ self-focusing predominates over beam broadening due to aureole scattering at distances

$$x \gtrsim (ak)^2 P_0 K_a \frac{\ln 2}{8\pi\chi}\frac{1}{C_p\rho}\left|\frac{\partial\varepsilon}{\partial T}\right|$$

where $P_0$ is the radiant power in the beam.

Bukatyi and others [175] have observed the acoustic self-focusing effect in experimental studies of the action of the leading edge of a millisecond laser pulse of wavelength $\lambda = 0.69$ $\mu$m and energy $Q = 5$ J with $R_0 = 0.7$ cm on cement dust particles. The results of these measurements exhibit satisfactory agreement with the given theory. This effect can play a significant role in the real atmosphere because the laser beams used there have large cross sections ($R_0 \sim 10^1$ to $10^2$ cm), such that the transit time of sound across the beam $\tau_s = R_0/u_s = 0.3$ to 3 msec and large pressure differences can be formed between the medium in the beam channel and in the free atmosphere.

## 5.6. Propagation of Laser Radiation in Nonlinear Randomly Inhomogeneous Media

To treat the combined influence of atmospheric turbulence and the nonlinear action of light with the atmosphere is of immense importance in connection with the propagation of powerful laser beams over long paths.

Turbulent broadening of a beam in the atmosphere can attenuate the self-induced effects of radiation, and, in turn, the presence of nonlinearity in the medium can alter the nature of the interaction between the beam and turbulent inhomogeneities, both as a result of the formation of a regular guided-wave channel in the medium and due to the randomization of the medium in the field of a strong randomly modulated wave.

A great many theoretical studies have already been devoted to the self-induced processes of strong radiation in a turbulent atmosphere [93, 140, 142, 176–188]; we discuss the main results below.


### 5.6.1. Self-Induced Effects of Laser Beams in a Randomly Inhomogeneous Medium with a Fast Nonlinearity Mechanism

The permittivity in the investigated situation is described by the expression [176]

$$\varepsilon = \varepsilon_0 + \varepsilon_1(\mathbf{r}) + \varepsilon_2 |E|^2 + \cdots \qquad (5.116)$$

in which $\varepsilon_0$ is the regular part and $\varepsilon_1$ the fluctuating part of the permittivity of the undisturbed air, $\varepsilon_0 \approx 1$, $\langle \varepsilon_1 \rangle = 0$, and $\varepsilon_2 |E|^2$ is the field-squared increment to the permittivity of air.

The starting expression for this problem is the parabolic equation for a medium with large-scale inhomogeneities:

$$2ik(\partial E/\partial x) + \Delta_{\mathbf{r}_\perp} E + k^2 \varepsilon_1 E + k^2 \varepsilon_2 |E|^2 E = 0 \qquad (5.117)$$

in which $x$ is the axial coordinate and $\mathbf{r}_\perp(y, z)$ is the two-dimensional radius vector in the cross section of the beam.

Bespalov and others [176] have obtained a solution of Eq. (5.117) for the case of a plane wave in the approximation of weak nonlinearity of the medium. This equation has been used as the basis for an investigation [178–180] of the broadening of a laser beam with neglect of fluctuations of the nonlinear part of the permittivity. For the model of inhomogeneities delta correlated along the path, closed equations for the various moments of the field have been obtained from (5.117) in this case [174]. An approximate solution of the equation for the second-order coherence function for a Gaussian beam has led to the conclusion that self-focusing and broadening due to scattering by turbulent inhomogeneites contribute additively to the variation of the beam cross section in the case of weak nonlinearity.

Vlasov and others [179, 180] have also analyzed the effect of turbulence on the collapse of a beam in the atmosphere due to self-focusing ($\varepsilon_2 > 0$) on the basis of an analysis of the weighted-mean beam cross section calculated in a moving coordinate system fixed at the beam centroid. For a Kolmogorov spectrum of atmospheric turbulence, $\Phi_\varepsilon(\kappa) = 0.033 C_\varepsilon^2 \kappa^{-11/3} \exp(-\kappa^2/\kappa_m^2)$, the collapse condition is specified by the relation

$$\beta_c = \frac{P_c}{P_{\text{sf}}} = 1 + \tfrac{3}{4} k^2 R_0^{8/3} (4.38)^{2/3} l_0^{-2/3} c_\varepsilon^{4/3} \left\{ 1 - \left[ 1 + 17.5 \left( \frac{R_0}{l_0} \right)^2 \right]^{-1/3} \right\}^{2/3}$$

(5.118)

where $P_c$ and $P_{\text{sf}}$ are the power values for collapse and self-focusing, $k$ is the wave number, $R_0$ is the beam radius, $l_0 = 5.9/\kappa_m$ is the inner turbulence scale, and $C_\varepsilon^2$ is the structure constant for the permittivity fluctuations.

It follows from (5.118) that for $R_0 = 1$ cm, $C_\varepsilon^2 = 10^{-15}$ cm$^{-2/3}$, and $l_0 = 0.1$ cm, the collapse condition for a beam in a turbulent atmosphere corresponds to a twelvefold excess of its power over the critical self-focusing power in a homogeneous medium, i.e., $\beta_c \geqslant 12$.

Vorob'ev [181] has developed two approximate methods for treating fluctuations of the nonlinear part of the permittivity of the medium: (1) a perturbation method with respect to the nonlinear term; (2) a variational energy method. In the first method, the problem can be handled analytically on the basis of an approximation of the fluctuation part of the permittivity by the model of random wedges, which rotate the beam as a whole. In the indicated approximation, which is valid for narrow beams such that their radius is smaller than or of the same order as $l_0$, an expression is derived for the average intensity on the axis of an initially Gaussian collimated beam.

The variational energy method [181] makes it possible to deal with a fairly strong nonlinearity of the medium when the beam power is of the order of the self-focusing threshold. For a Gaussian beam, at the boundary of the medium, a solution is sought in this case in the form (5.27), where $f$, $F$, and $\varphi$ are the effective beam parameters, representing random functionals of $\varepsilon_1$. The fluctuating part of the permittivity is described by the model of random lenses. An analysis of the expression derived for the mathematical expectation of the dimensionless beamwidth squared leads to the conclusion that random broadening in the focusing medium decreases as the beam power is increased.

Armand [182] has analyzed the propagation of a laser beam with regard for the height dependence of the permittivity (5.116). The model problem of scattering by random permittivity inhomogeneities during beam propagation in a guided-wave channel has been investigated in several papers [178, 181, 184].

### 5.6.2 Thermal Interaction of Powerful Laser Radiation with an Absorbing Turbulent Medium

In the case of thermal nonlinearity of the medium, the field dependence of the permittivity is given by the functional

$$\varepsilon = \varepsilon_0 + i\varepsilon_0' + \varepsilon_1(\mathbf{r}) + \varepsilon_2(t, |E|) \tag{5.119}$$

where $i\varepsilon_0'$ and $\varepsilon_1$ are the imaginary and fluctuating parts of the complex permittivity of air.

The nonlinear increment $\varepsilon_2 = (d\varepsilon/dT)\delta T$ for the propagation of continuous radiation is determined by solving the heat-conduction equation for the temperature deviation:

$$\frac{\partial}{\partial t}\delta T + \mathbf{v}_\perp \nabla_{\mathbf{r}_\perp}\delta T - \chi\nabla_{\mathbf{r}_\perp}^2\delta T = \frac{k_\nu}{C_p\rho}\frac{c\varepsilon_0^{1/2}}{8\pi}|E|^2 \tag{5.120}$$

where $\mathbf{v}_\perp$ is the wind velocity vector in the plane of the beam cross section, $\chi$ is the molecular thermal diffusivity of air, $C_p\rho$ is its volume specific heat, and

$$k_\nu = \frac{k}{\varepsilon_0}\left[\varepsilon_0' + \mathrm{Im}\,\varepsilon_1(\mathbf{r})\right]$$

Resolving the solution (5.120) into the sum of a regular and a fluctuation part, $\delta T = T_0 + T'$, and assuming corresponding deviations from the mean $\mathbf{v}_\perp'$, $k_\nu'$, $E'$ of the random variables $\mathbf{v}_\perp$, $k_\nu$, $E$, we arrive at the array of equations for the small perturbation method.

Vorob'ev [187] has investigated the elementary case of a regular guided-wave channel in the absence of wind ($v_\perp = 0$) in the nonaberration approximation on the basis of the parabolic equation for $E$, approximating $\varepsilon_1$ by the random-wedge model.

An analysis of the results indicates that the nonlinear increment to the variation of the scattering increases with focusing of the beam, and the presence of a defocusing guided-wave channel produces additional beam broadening due to scattering by turbulent inhomogeneities.

Vorob'ev [183] and Alferness [186] have investigated the mechanism of initiation of thermal fluctuations in connection with the loss of regularity of the temperature profile in the beam as a result of wind-velocity fluctuations. A simple expression is obtained [183] for the variance of the temperature fluctuations on the beam axis:

$$\langle T'^2 \rangle = \left( \frac{\langle k_\nu \rangle R_0 I_0}{C_p \rho} \right)^2 \frac{\langle v_\perp^2 \rangle}{\langle v_\perp \rangle^4} \tag{5.121}$$

where $k_\nu$ is the absorption coefficient and $I_0$ is the beam power density.

Calculations according to expression (5.121) for various values of the parameters in it have shown that the variation of the temperature fluctuations associated with turbulent motion can be significant in the case of beam propagation along the average wind or in the "rest zone" when the beam slewing rate is equal to the average crosswind velocity.

Vorob'ev [93] has developed an approach based on application of the heat-transfer equation in a medium characterized by an effective turbulent thermal conductivity, arriving at a similar conclusion that the influence of turbulence on the average temperature profile can be significant as $\langle v_\perp \rangle \to 0$.

In [183], the smooth perturbation method is used to analyze the influence of heating of the atmosphere on the intensity fluctuations induced by its turbulence. The results of this analysis indicate that the fluctuations in a thermally nonlinear medium are lower in comparison with the conditions in a linear medium.

Theoretical studies of the fluctuations of the log-amplitude in a discretely absorbing medium with strong thermal nonlinearity have been carried out [188] on the basis of a self-consistent numerical solution of the given problem. A numerical analysis of the correlation function is carried out in the first smooth-perturbation approximation with the use of the linear terms of the expansion of the solution for the induced refractive-index variation of air into a functional series near its regular values.

The effect of randomization of the medium in radiant heating as a result of the abrupt transition of laminar to turbulent-induced convection has been investigated in experimental work [177, 185, 189, 190].

The experimentally measured critical Reynolds numbers for randomization of the convection flow in the vertical propagation of a laser beam in an absorbing gas fall in the interval [190]

$$3 < \mathrm{Re}_c < 180$$

$\mathrm{Re} = 2\rho R_0 V_\Phi / \eta$, where $\eta$ is the dynamic viscosity of air and $V_\Phi$ is the average photoabsorptive convection rate. We note that the indicated values of $\mathrm{Re}_c$ are 2 or 3 orders of magnitude lower than the corresponding values at which "demarcation" of the airflow into tubes takes place.

Summarizing the foregoing, we note that if we exclude the case in which the laser beam propagates along the average wind velocity or its slewing rate is equal to the average crosswind velocity, then the qualitative pattern of the combined action of thermal nonlinear effects and turbulence exhibits a mutually compensating influence. Thus, the heating of a turbulent atmosphere by a laser beam occurs nonuniformly. Accordingly, in regions where light-wave antinodes occur, there is additional heating and defocusing gas lenses are formed; conversely, wherever the intensity is minimal, thermal nonlinearity incurs focusing. Consequently, turbulent mixing in the atmosphere tends to smear the temperature profile associated with laser heating and therefore abates the influence of thermal nonlinear effects [93, 191, 192].

It is important to note, on the other hand, that a number of aspects of the problem in question have yet to be solved. For example, the interaction of short laser pulses with atmospheric turbulence under the conditions of hydrodynamic motion of the radiation-heated atmosphere has not been investigated to date. Fluctuation effects associated with resonance cooling of the atmosphere have not been studied. Nor are there any experimental data on the variation of the statistics of strong laser radiation propagating in the real atmosphere. Finally, we are compelled to mention the conspicuous lack of data from experimental work on all the known nonlinear thermal effects under natural field conditions.

## 5.7. Self-Focusing of Laser Radiation Due to the Kerr and Electrostriction Effects

The nonlinear permittivity of air in the case of fast Kerr and electrostriction effects is written as a power series in the electric field $\mathbf{E}$ [193]:

$$\varepsilon = \varepsilon_0 + \tfrac{1}{2}\varepsilon_2 |E|^2 + \frac{3}{8}\varepsilon_4 |E|^4 + \frac{15}{16}\varepsilon_6 |E|^6 + \cdots \tag{5.122}$$

where $\varepsilon_2, \varepsilon_4, \varepsilon_6,\ldots$ are nonlinear coefficients, and the fractions in front of them account for averaging of the response of a medium with a finite relaxation time, which is usually much greater than the period of the intruding optical wave.

Exclusive of the vicinity of caustics, in self-focusing Eq. (5.122) can be restricted to the squared term. In the case of a cylindrically symmetrical beam with maximum field on the axis and a field-negative nonlinearity of the medium ($\varepsilon_2 < 0$), rays are refracted toward the periphery of the beam. For $\varepsilon_2 > 0$, clearly, the reverse self-focusing effect takes place. A suitable candidate for the parameter characterizing the efficiency of nonlinear refraction is the self-focusing threshold power $P_{sf}$, which is determined from the condition of cancellation of the diffraction spreading of a collimated beam in a nonlinear medium and has the form

$$P_{sf} = \frac{c\varepsilon_0^{1/2}}{k^2|\varepsilon_2|^2} \tag{5.123}$$

In this instance, beam collapse in a medium with $\varepsilon_2 > 0$ will be observed at a distance

$$x_c \approx \frac{kR_0^2}{[(P/P_{sf})-1]^{1/2}} \tag{5.124}$$

where $R_0$ is the initial beam radius and $P$ is its power.

The temporal transience of the power of a laser pulse can have the singular effect of moving the foci along the beam axis. In the case of Q-switched laser pulses, the foci can move at velocities attaining $\approx 10^9$ cm/sec. If the beam power is much greater than the self-focusing threshold, the beam cross section can become stratified into separate waveguides.

A systematic theory of the propagation of strong optical radiation in a medium with a nonlinear permittivity of the form $\frac{1}{2}\varepsilon_2|E|^2$ is set forth in two survey papers [194, 195]. Its discussion is beyond the scope of our problem. In this connection, we proceed with a brief description of the Kerr and electrostriction effects.

It is generally known that the Kerr effect is associated with orientation of the dipole moments of molecules in the direction of a strong electric field, essentially due to the almost-instantaneous inception of anisotropy in the properties of a refractive medium. The electrostriction effect is typified by the incursion of an additional pressure in a strongly irradiated region.

The value of the permittivity $\varepsilon_2$ in air in the case of Kerr nonlinearity is equal to $8 \times 10^{-16}$ cgs esu for oxygen and $2.8 \times 10^{-16}$ cgs esu for nitrogen; in the electrostriction case, it is equal to $10^{-14}$ cgs esu. The rise times to a steady-state value of the nonlinearity differ more substantially, amounting to $3 \times 10^{-14}$ sec for the Kerr effect and $R_0/u_s \sim 10^{-3}$ to $10^{-5}$ sec for electrostriction, where $u_s$ is the sound velocity in the medium.

The self-focusing threshold power $P_{sf}$ is roughly proportional to the nonlinear permittivity $\varepsilon_2$, the value of which is small in the case of the investigated Kerr and electrostriction effects, and so the values of $P_{sf}$ are large. The generation of refractive-index nonlinearities by these effects in the real atmosphere is masked in the majority of circumstances by the self-induced nonlinear thermal effects discussed in the preceding sections of this chapter.

## 5.8. Effects of Stimulated Scattering of Strong Radiation in the Atmosphere

During the propagation of high-intensity laser radiation in the atmosphere, stimulated scattering effects can occur in connection with the driving up of small spontaneous thermal oscillations as a result of incident and scattered waves acting on them. The stimulated scattering process can be regarded as the power amplification of incipient noise $p = p_N \exp(M)$ with a gain (growth rate) $M$, which depends on the initial beam power $P$ according to the equation

$$M = \frac{P}{\pi R_0^2} \int_0^x g(x') \, dx' \tag{5.125}$$

in which $R_0$ is the beam radius, $x$ is the path length, and $g$ is a proportionality factor (incremental gain).

The threshold value of the total gain $M_t$ is determined by the spontaneous (incipient) noise level, and for the atmospheric ground layer it is assumed to be $M_t \approx 30$. The corresponding threshold radiation intensity is calculated in terms of the incremental gain $g$ and $M_t$ according to the equation

$$I_t = \frac{M_t}{\displaystyle\int_0^x g(x') \, dx'} \tag{5.126}$$

In stimulated scattering, not only the spectral composition, but also the energy diagram of the radiation in the beam varies, causing the energy state and propagation conditions of strong radiation to vary as well.

Several types of stimulated scattering are discerned, depending on the type of nonlinearity of the medium [196]:

1. stimulated Raman scattering of light (SRS) with the excitation of vibration–rotation transitions of the molecules;
2. stimulated Brillouin (Mandel'shtam–Brillouin) scattering (SMBS) by acoustic waves;

3. stimulated temperature scattering (STS) by isobaric temperature disturbances;
4. stimulated Rayleigh-wing scattering (SRWS) due to interaction of the field with anisotropically polarizable molecules or electron-shell deformation effects;
5. stimulated concentration scattering of light (SCS) by fluctuations of the molecular concentration.

Several other hybrid types of stimulated scattering with higher thresholds are also possible.

For the separate treatment of all the stimulated scattering effects, the equations for the scattered field in the quasioptical approximation may be written in the form [197–198]

$$\left( \frac{1}{c}\frac{\partial}{\partial t} \pm \frac{\partial}{\partial x} \pm \frac{i}{2k}\nabla^2_{\mathbf{r}_\perp} + \frac{k_\nu}{2} \right) E_s = \frac{ikb}{4\varepsilon_0} E_0 l \tag{5.127}$$

where $t$ is the time, $x$ is the axial coordinate, $\varepsilon_0$ is the unperturbed permittivity, $\mathbf{r}_\perp(y, z)$ is the radius vector in the beam cross section, and $k_\nu$ is the absorption coefficient. The parameter $b$, depending on the type of stimulated scattering, is equal to $\partial\varepsilon/\partial Q$ for SRS, $\partial\varepsilon/\partial N_a$ for SMBS, $\partial\varepsilon/\partial T$ at constant pressure for STS, $\partial\varepsilon/\partial N_a$ for SCS, or $b=1$ for SRWS. The plus sign refers to forward stimulated scattering, i.e., in the direction of the disturbing radiation, and the minus sign refers to back stimulated scattering. The quantities $\rho$, $T$, $N_a$, and $Q$, depending on the type of stimulated scattering, are interpreted as, respectively, the density, temperature, molecular concentration, and optical phonon coordinate (for SCS) in the medium. The complex amplitudes $E_0$, $E_s$, and $l$ correspond to the representation of the electric fields $\mathbf{e}_0$ and $\mathbf{e}_s$ of the incident and scattered waves and the perturbations of the medium $l$ in the form

$$\mathbf{e}_0 = \mathbf{j}_0 E_0 \exp(i\mathbf{k}_0\cdot\mathbf{r} - i\omega_0 t) \tag{5.128}$$

$$\mathbf{e}_s = \mathbf{j}_s E_s \exp(i\mathbf{k}\cdot\mathbf{r} - i\omega t) \tag{5.129}$$

$$l = l\exp\left[ i\Omega t - i(\mathbf{k} - \mathbf{k}_0)\cdot\mathbf{r} \right] \tag{5.130}$$

where $\omega_0$ is the pump frequency, $k_0 = \omega_0/c$, $c$ is the speed of light, $\omega$ is the frequency of the scattered field, $k = \omega/c$, and $\mathbf{j}_{0,s}$ denotes unit vectors.

The value of $\omega$ is chosen equal to $\omega = \omega_0 - \Omega$, where $\Omega$ is the frequency of variations of the perturbations in the medium and depends on the particular type of stimulated scattering. For SCS, irrespective of the scattering direction, $\Omega = \Omega_0$, where $\Omega_0$ is the optical phonon frequency. In back

SMBS, $\Omega=2ku_s$, where $u_s$ is the speed of sound in the medium. In back SRS, SRWS, and SCS, it is convenient to let $\Omega=0$ (the slight shift of the maximum of the scattered-field spectrum can be taken into account by appropriate frequency modulation in the complex amplitude $E_s$ of the scattered wave).

The solution of Eq. (5.129) in conjunction with suitable constitutive equations for the medium [197–204] makes it possible to determine the scattered radiation field as a function of the characteristics of the medium and the driving field.

The lowest-threshold stimulated-scattering effects capable of significantly affecting the propagation of laser beams in the atmosphere are [196]: SMBR; SCS with excitation of vibrational levels of nitrogen molecules (VSCS); SCS with excitation of rotational levels of nitrogen and oxygen molecules (RSCS). Vibrational SCS is strongest at transitions of the Q branch of nitrogen molecules (2330 cm$^{-1}$). Vibration–rotation interaction of molecules greatly complicates the structure of the Q branch and the dependence of that structure on the partial pressures of the gas. An analysis of SMBS in a gas has been carried out in several studies [196, 201, 204, 205] over a wide range of pressures, making it possible to deduce theoretical relations for the gain and relaxation time as a function of the pressure. Figure 5.19 gives curves, plotted according to the theory, for the threshold power $P_t$ of steady-state VSCS and SMBS effects in the case of focused single-mode monochromatic beams ($\lambda=0.53$ $\mu$m) as a function of the pressure in nitrogen. The abscissa parameter $\rho$ represents the ratio of the product $N_a\mu_a$ (where $N_a$ is the number density of nitrogen molecules and $\mu_a$

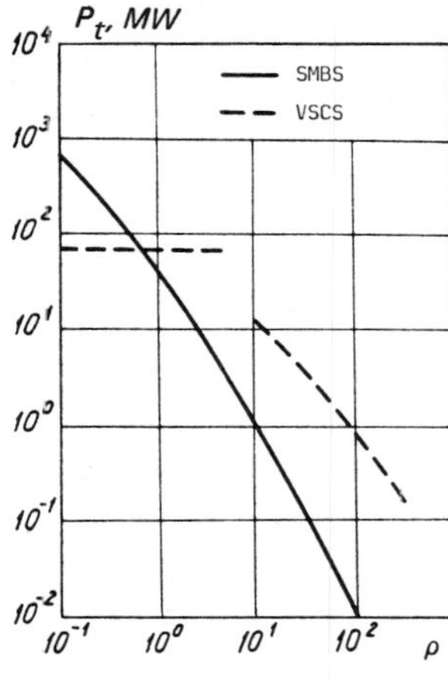


Fig. 5.19. Threshold powers of steady-state SMBS (—) and VSCS (- -) effects in nitrogen for a coherent focused laser beam.

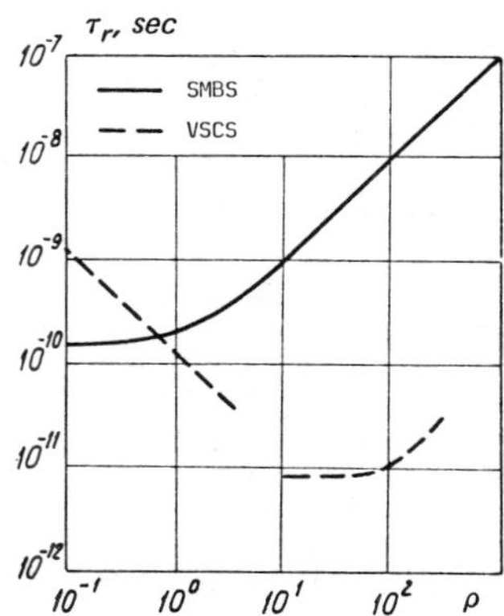



Fig. 5.20. SMBS (—) and VSCS (- -) relaxation times in nitrogen versus relative pressure.

is the molecular weight) to the same product for a standard atmosphere. Figure 5.20 gives the corresponding relaxation times $\tau_r$ for the same effects.

In the case of short pulses with $t \lesssim \tau_r$, the stimulated scattering is of a nonsteady nature and for SCS is predominantly in the forward direction (forward SCS).

Exceeding the thresholds of steady-state SMBS and SCS in the first case causes transfer of a sizable fraction of the incident radiation power in the direction opposite to propagation of the pump wave; and in the second case energy is transferred into the scattered wave in both the forward and backward directions.

The incremental gain for the above-noted low-threshold RSCS and VSCS effects in air, according to theoretical estimates [196], is $g = 0.5 \times 10^{-5}$ cm/MW, and for all other types of stimulated scattering we have $g \leqslant 10^{-8}$ cm/MW.

The scattering spectrum for RSCS in nitrogen contains two relatively strong lines of roughly equal intensity, shifted into the Stokes region by 76 and 90 cm$^{-1}$, and in oxygen it contains a single line with a 70-cm$^{-1}$ Stokes shift. The VSCS spectrum for nitrogen without RSCS contains only one line, shifted 2330 cm$^{-1}$ relative to the pump.

Stimulated scattering processes depend strongly on the pump statistics. Thus, for the excitation of stimulated scattering by incoherent beams, in which case the width of the temporal spectrum of the incident field exceeds the spontaneous-scattering linewidth, the stimulated-scattering threshold can prove to be very much higher than that under the action of coherent radiation.

Bearing in mind that the SCS and SMBS threshold power values in air are considerably higher than for thermal nonlinear effects, it is readily understood that the occurrence of stimulated-scattering effects in connection with the propagation of strong laser radiation in the real atmosphere will be masked by self-induced thermal effects.

## 5.9. Conclusion

It is clearly revealed by the content of the present chapter that enormous strides have been made in recent years in the study of nonlinear effects accompanying the propagation of power laser radiation in the atmosphere. This progress is particularly noticeable in the related theoretical work, which has made it possible at the present time to estimate in approximate quantitative terms the state of all known effects for a given model of the atmosphere. At the same time, however, it is necessary to underscore the conspicuous deficit of experimental data, especially under the conditions of the real atmosphere.

In light of the foregoing, the prime task of the next phase of research on nonlinear interactions of laser radiation with the atmosphere must be viewed as the implementation of systematic experimental investigations under natural conditions, along with the necessary battery of measurements of the physical parameters of the atmosphere in the channel of a laser beam and in the nearby surroundings during the course of its action.

The multivariety of effects of nonlinear interaction of laser beams with the atmospheric medium enormously complicates the already complex problem of propagation of laser radiation in the atmosphere. On the other hand, that same multivariety will doubtless open up impressive new possibilities for the practical utilization of these effects for, as a concrete example, the investigation of atmospheric phenomena and processes with the application of techniques for the long-range laser monitoring of the profiles of atmospheric parameters.

# 6

# Optical Background Noise in the Atmosphere

## 6.0. Introduction

The propagation of optical waves and, in particular, laser radiation in the atmosphere under any conditions is accompanied by an enormous set of complex phenomena involving interaction of the radiation with the atmospheric medium. The understanding of these phenomena, which we have discussed in the first five chapters of the present book, is of decisive significance in the design of various effective laser systems for operation in the atmosphere. However, this entire fund of knowledge is insufficient for any quantitative assessment of the efficiency of operation of a particular system in the atmosphere without access to data on optical atmospheric interference effects, which impart a noise component to the useful information-carrying signal of any laser system. In the final analysis, the efficiency, reliability, and life of the system are determined by the signal-to-noise ratio.

The sum total of all atmospheric optical noise effects can be divided into two groups: (1) noise generated by the propagation of an optical wave in the atmosphere; (2) noise from sources that exist independently of the presence of a propagating wave in the atmosphere. The first group includes noise associated with aerosol (particulate), molecular, and Raman scattering and with other processes of interaction between optical waves and the atmosphere. The second noise category is a result of radiation from the sun, planets, stars, and a variety of artificial sources interacting with the atmosphere. Also included in this group are the self-radiations of the atmosphere and the underlying surface, as well as radiation emitted by primary sources and reflected from the latter surface.

315

We have discussed the noise accompanying the propagation of laser radiation in the atmosphere in the preceding chapters. In this chapter, therefore, we summarize the fundamental results of theoretical and experimental research on atmospheric optical noise of phonon origin, adhering by and large to the book [1].

## 6.1. General Description of Optical Background Noise in the Atmosphere

Table 6.1 lists quantitative data on the power of various sources whose emitted radiation is responsible for optical background noise in the atmosphere along with the ratios of that power to the power of solar radiation. The data given in the table characterize the indicated sources from the standpoint of total radiated energy. On the other hand, to determine the main quantity of interest, namely the signal-to-noise ratio, in application to laser sources, it is required to know the noise levels in a narrow spectral interval centered at the emission wavelength of a particular laser. Consequently, the most important objective is to know the spectral power distribution of the sources covered in the table or, more precisely, the spectral distribution of the noise created by these and other sources in the atmosphere.

We first consider the purely qualitative picture of the spectral behavior of daytime background noise. The main sources of background noise in this case are atmospheric scattering of solar radiation and thermal radiation by the earth's surface and the atmosphere. The role of each of these sources depends strongly on the state of the atmosphere, the observation conditions, the position of the sun, etc. It may be approximately assumed, however, that in the visible and near-infrared regions of the spectrum, roughly up to wavelength $\lambda = 3$ $\mu$m, solar radiation scattering, with a maximum in the vicinity of wavelength 0.55 $\mu$m, is dominant. For wavelengths $\lambda > 4$ $\mu$m, on the other hand, the intrinsic self-radiation of the atmosphere and earth's surface, with a maximum around 10 $\mu$m, prevails. The minimum noise level is observed in the vicinity of 3 or 4 $\mu$m.

Under nighttime conditions, along with the self-emitted radiation of the atmosphere and ground and radiation from other nonselective sources (see Table 6.1), another important potential noise source is the airglow, particularly in isolated narrow parts of the spectrum including the emission lines of atmospheric gases.

**Table 6.1.** Power of Various Radiation Sources Producing
Atmospheric Optical Noise

| Radiation source | Power | |
|---|---|---|
| | in watts | relative to sun |
| Sun | $1.76 \times 10^{17}$ | 1 |
| Moon | $3.09 \times 10^{12}$ | $1.76 \times 10^{-5}$ |
| Clouds | $1.60 \times 10^{12}$ | $9.09 \times 10^{-6}$ |
| Starlight | $2.61 \times 10^{10}$ | $1.48 \times 10^{-7}$ |
| Bright auroras | $2.53 \times 10^{10}$ | $1.44 \times 10^{-7}$ |
| Cosmic rays | $1.63 \times 10^{10}$ | $9.26 \times 10^{-8}$ |
| Meteors | $1.44 \times 10^{10}$ | $8.18 \times 10^{-8}$ |
| Night airglow | $1.12 \times 10^{10}$ | $6.37 \times 10^{-8}$ |

A rough idea of the magnitudes of maximum luminance of the background near 1 and 10 $\mu$m from various sources may be gained from Table 6.2.

Together with the spectral and angular distributions of various background noise levels in the atmosphere and their polarization properties, it is often important in practice to know their fluctuation characteristics, which also vary between wide limits, depending on the nature of the noise. Thus, solar radiation in the spectral interval $\lambda \leqslant 2$ $\mu$m reflected by a water surface is the main type of daytime noise, which has a considerable variance of luminance fluctuations. Luminance irregularities of a cloudy sky present a significant interference for scanning receiving systems.

The nature of atmospheric background noise in the optical wavelength range is extremely complex because in the majority of cases this noise owes its formation to the simultaneous occurrence of a great many processes of interaction between radiation from a noise source and the atmosphere. The description of each of these processes requires the appropriation of complex

**Table 6.2**

| Nature of background noise | Maximum background luminance $W/cm^2 \ sr \cdot \mu m$ | |
|---|---|---|
| | $\lambda = 1 \ \mu m$ | $\lambda = 10 \ \mu m$ |
| Reflection of solar radiation by water surface | $10^{-1}$ | $10^{-5}$ |
| Scattering of solar radiation by atmosphere (luminance of clear sky) | $10^{-2}$ | $10^{-7}$ |
| Scattering of solar radiation by clouds (luminance of cloudy sky) | $10^{-3}$ | $10^{-7}$ |
| Thermal radiation of atmosphere | $10^{-7}$ | $10^{-3}$ |
| Airglow | $10^{-10}$ | $10^{-6}$ |

theories and relevant experiments. We need merely recall the enormous set of intra- and intermolecular interaction processes as well as the effects of macrophysical parameters (pressure, composition of the gaseous mixture, temperature), that must be considered in analyzing the fine structure of the absorption spectra of atmospheric gases. The correct treatment of aerosol scattering effects must take into account the particle-size spectra, concentration, geometry, and components of the complex refractive index of the particles. Accordingly, exact calculations of the characteristics of background noise in the atmosphere are generally impossible. That is why the bulk of the present chapter comprises related experimental data.

## 6.2. Background of Scattered Solar Radiation

### 6.2.1. Spectral Composition of Scattered Radiation

The intensity of scattered solar radiation in the atmosphere depends strongly on the wavelength. In the case of a Rayleigh atmosphere, this dependence is uniquely described by the $\sim\lambda^{-4}$ law. A unique relationship does not exist for particulate scattering because the scattering coefficients are determined by the microphysical parameters of the particles, and these vary extensively in the atmosphere. It is a reasonable assertion, however, that the intensity of aerosol scattering exhibits a wavelength dependence weaker than $\sim\lambda^{-4}$. Moreover, the spectrum of direct solar radiation exerts a significant influence on the spectral behavior of the intensity of radiation scattered by both Rayleigh and aerosol mechanisms.

Figure 6.1 gives the spectral composition of scattered solar radiation in the case of a cloudless sky for comparatively strong turbidity of the

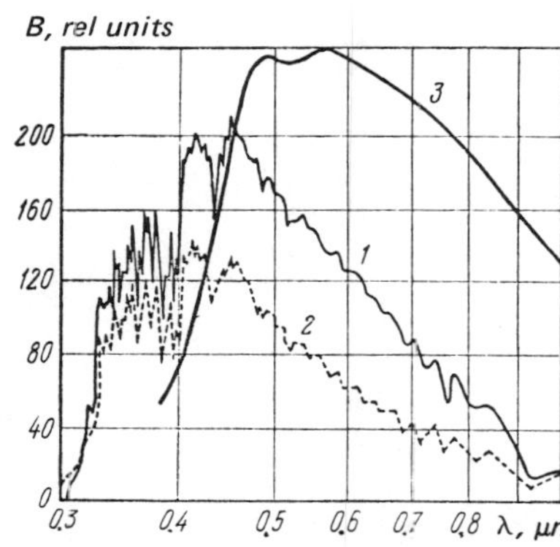


Fig. 6.1. Spectral intensity of scattered solar radiation for a clear sky at the zenith (curve 1) and at the minimum-luminance point of the sky (curve 2).

atmosphere [2]. Also shown in this figure for comparison is the envelope of the direct solar radiation spectrum measured from the ground (curve 3). The principal features of the variation of the scattering spectrum are visible in the figure: a shift of its maximum toward shorter wavelengths in comparison with the direct solar spectrum and an appreciable relative increase in the intensity of short-wave radiation.

The spectral composition of the scattered radiation varies considerably according to the position of the sun and the viewing angle relative to the sun [3]. The spectral behavior of scattered solar radiation for various angular distances $\varphi$ from the sun and the same atmospheric conditions as in Fig. 6.1 is shown in Fig. 6.2, borrowed from Kondrat'ev [2].

Figures 6.1 and 6.2 disclose a sharp drop in the intensity of scattered solar radiation with increasing wavelength, beginning approximately at 0.5 $\mu$m. This result is attributable to the fact that both the Rayleigh scattering coefficient and the volume scattering coefficient of hazes as well as the emission spectrum of the sun decay with increasing wavelength in the indicated interval. The same behavior persists in the near-IR region, as we see in Fig. 6.3, which gives the spectral luminances of the sky in the wavelength interval from 0.55 to 1.8 $\mu$m at various heights above sea level under cloudless-sky conditions for a high meteorological visibility range [4]. The flat segments of the curves correspond to the transmission band half-widths of the light filters used in the measurements. The height of the measuring instrument (photometer) $H$ in km is given in the caption. The photometric measurement point in the sky has the following coordinates relative to the ground: angle above the horizon $\xi = 30°$; azimuth relative to solar vertical 165°. With increasing height of the photometer, the height of the sun above the horizon changes, corresponding to 13, 14.5, 17.5, and 19° for the curves indicated in the figure. The data of Fig. 6.3 were obtained for

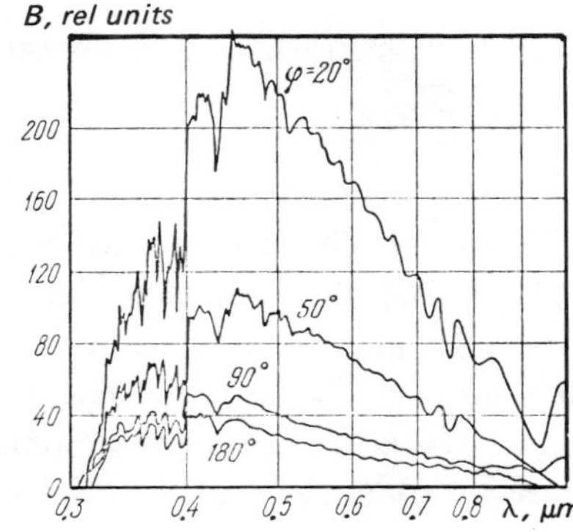


Fig. 6.2. Spectral intensity of scattered solar radiation at various points of the almucantar (angular distances from the sun are indicated in the figure).

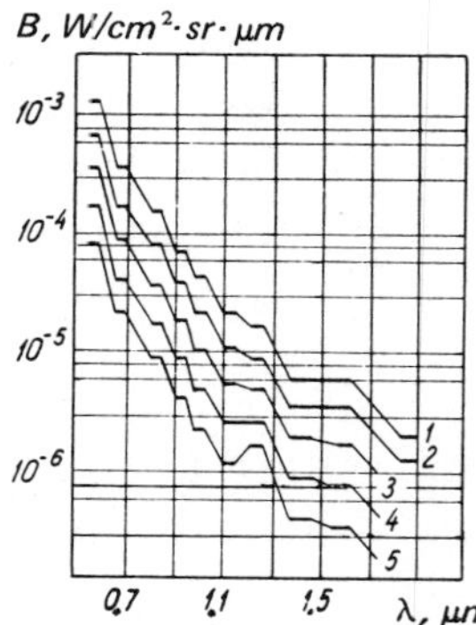



Fig. 6.3. Spectral luminance of clear sky (W/cm² sr·μm) for various heights and viewing angles above the horizon. (1) $H=4$ km, $\eta_\odot=13°$; (2) $H=8$ km, $\eta_\odot=14.5°$; (3) $H=12$ km, $\eta_\odot=16°$; (4) $H=16$ km, $\eta_\odot=17.5°$; (5) $H=20$ km, $\eta_\odot=19°$.

the maximum luminance in the part of the spectrum around 0.58 $\mu$m, i.e., $9.7\times10^{-2}$ W/cm²sr·$\mu$m.

It is evident from Fig. 6.3 that the luminance of scattered solar radiation in the cloudless atmosphere decreases almost by 3 orders of magnitude as the wavelength is varied from 0.55 to 1.8 $\mu$m. With a further increase in the wavelength, such an abrupt decrease in the luminance of the cloudless sky is not observed because Rayleigh scattering is no longer significant here, and the scattering in hazes has a very different spectral behavior from that in the visible region (see Chap. 3). For example, if the haze particles are assumed to be water, scattering maxima are observed in the vicinity of the absorption bands of liquid water with centers at 2.9 and 6.0 $\mu$m. However, in the interval $\lambda>2$ $\mu$m, the determinant role in the spectral behavior of scattered solar radiation in the atmosphere must be ascribed to the solar emission spectrum, implying a long-wave limit of the scattered solar radiation background in the vicinity of 3 or 4 $\mu$m; beyond this limit, the thermal radiation of the atmosphere and ground begin to play the dominant part.

## 6.2.2. Luminance and Polarization of the Daytime Cloudless Sky

The luminance and polarization of the daytime cloudless sky is amenable to usefully precise calculation only in the case of a Rayleigh atmosphere. The most complete data of calculations of the Stokes parameters with allowance for polarization and multiple-scattering effects are found in the tables of Coulson and others [5]. The calculations rest on the following assumptions: The atmosphere represents plane-parallel layers totally in the gaseous state; the scattering is isotropic; fluorescence and absorption are absent; the underlying surface diffusely reflects radiation according to the Lambert law with an albedo equal to 0.00, 0.25, and 0.80.

A comparison of the calculated data for a Rayleigh atmosphere with the experimental results for the real atmosphere shows [6] that only sometimes in the ultraviolet region is good agreement observed between the data (with the exception of small scattering angles). In the visible and more so in the IR regions of the spectrum, where aerosol scattering plays a strong or governing role, the observed luminances of the daytime sky differ appreciably from the calculated values for a Rayleigh atmosphere.

We now describe some of the most representative results of quantitative experimental studies of the luminance of the daytime cloudless sky. Figures 6.4 and 6.5 give isophots obtained at wavelengths of 0.7 and 2.42 from the data of Glushko and others [7]. The isophots represented in the figure were obtained under conditions corresponding to the observation of maximum luminance values at 0.7 $\mu$m and minimum values at 2.42 $\mu$m. It is evident from the figures that the actual luminance values measured for the points of minimum luminance at the two wavelengths can differ by a factor of more than 2000. The ratio between the luminances at these two wavelengths is not as great in other situations and depends on the angular distance from the sun, diminishing as the latter is approached. The clear-sky distribution of the luminance in the atmospheric window from 1.8 to 2.5 $\mu$m has been investigated [8]. Figure 6.6 gives measurement data borrowed from that work for two typical days with high and low brightness. Also reported in the cited study are measurements of the luminance of the sky with clouds present, which significantly distort the spatial structure of the clear-sky background. These distortions occur even in the presence of tenuous cirrus clouds.

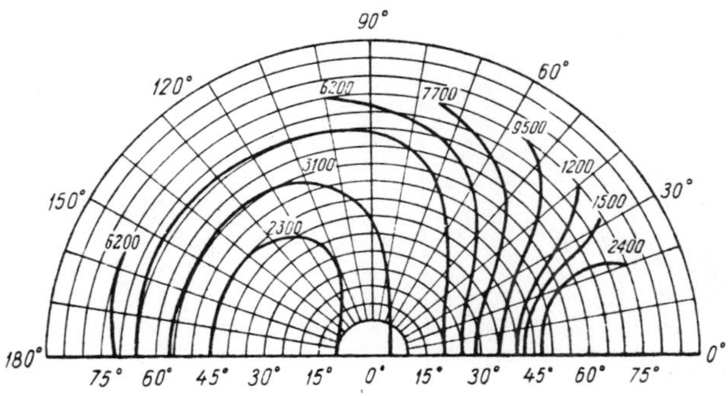


Fig. 6.4. Sky luminance distribution (W/cm$^2$ sr·$\mu$m) at a wavelength of 0.7 $\mu$m (zenith angle of sun: 60°).

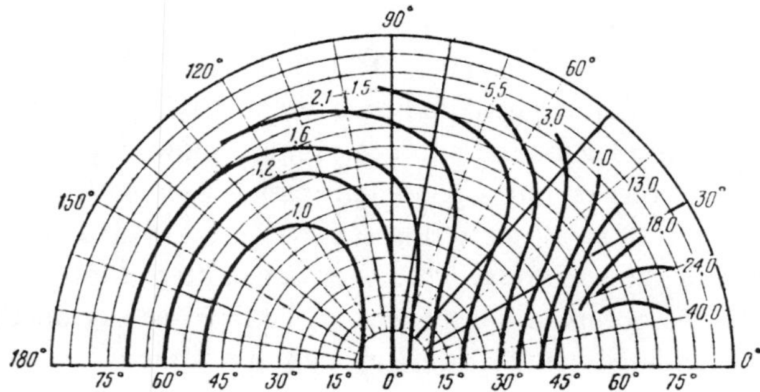

Fig. 6.5. Sky luminance distribution (W/cm² sr·µm) at a wavelength of 2.42 µm (zenith angle of sun: 60°).

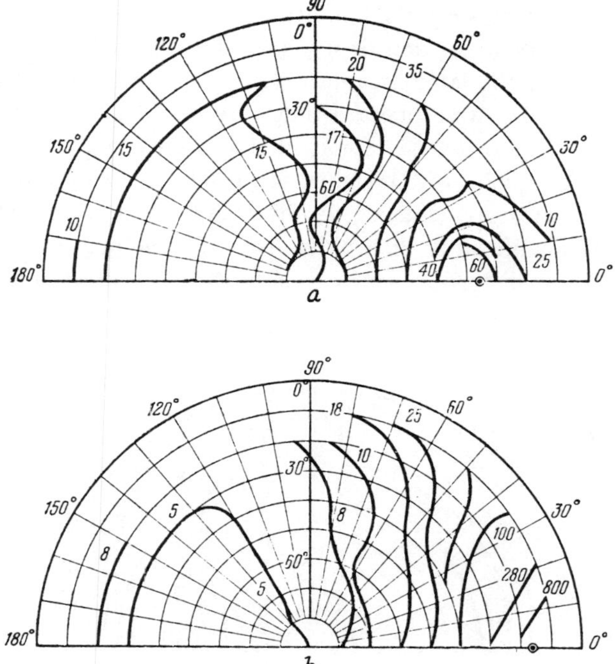

Fig. 6.6. Clear-sky luminance distribution (µW/cm² sr) in wavelength interval 1.8–2.5 µm for two typical days.

The variation and distribution of the luminance are also affected by the underlying surface. Measurements conducted at a fixed optical thickness and a wavelength of 1.01 $\mu$m, but with different albedos (0.67 and 0.36) [7] show that the ratio of the observed luminances, depending on the angular distance and azimuth relative to the sun, can vary from 0.92 to 1.28, i.e., by more than 30%.

On moving into the longer-wavelength part of the spectrum, we find that the role of the background created by scattered solar radiation diminishes, while the role of atmospheric thermal radiation increases. The result is that the spatial luminance distribution of the sky acquires concentric isophots. Only close to the sun is the luminance of the sky enhanced appreciably by scattered radiation. In all other directions, the luminance displays a regular increase from the zenith to the horizon. Figure 6.7 gives experimental data for the distribution of the luminance for the clear sky in the interval from 3.9 to 4.2 $\mu$m during the morning and dusk hours of one

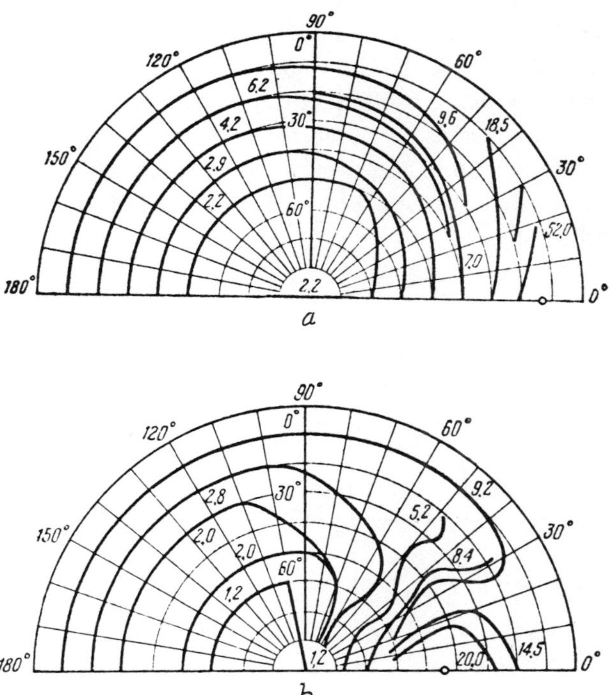

Fig. 6.7. Clear-sky luminance distribution ($\mu$W/cm$^2$ sr) in wavelength interval 3.9–4.2 $\mu$m in morning and dusk hours of one day.

day [9]. An important attribute of the indicated spectral interval, as well as the longer-wave part (4.5 to 5.2 $\mu$m), is the fact that the angular dependence of the luminance at angles of elevation above 70° (near the zenith) and at large azimuths relative to the sun can be completely neglected [9].

In many practical situations, the scattered solar radiation background level can be diminished by the use of polarizing devices in the receiving system. We now describe certain data of interest from this point of view on the polarization characteristic of scattered radiation in the daytime sky. Figure 6.8 illustrates typical points in the solar vertical [6, 10]. The maximum degree of polarization is observed near minimum-luminance points at an angular distance from the sun $\varphi \simeq 90°$. The position of this maximum varies between 3 and 5°, and its value does not exceed 0.88, falling usually between 0.5 and 0.7, depending on the optical properties of the atmosphere and the underlying surface. Other characteristic points with variable positions between 12 and 30° are the Babinet, Brewster, and Arago neutral points and a "topside-observed point," all with zero degree of polarization. For viewing directions between the neutral points and the sun, as well as between Arago's point and the antisolar point, negative polarization is observed (the plane of oscillation of the electric vector is situated in the plane of the solar vertical). In the visible and IR regions of the spectrum, a common power-law increase is observed in the degree of polarization with distance from the sun, up to angles of order 90°, after which it decreases [7]. The foregoing portrays in rough terms the spatial polarization pattern of the daytime cloudless sky.

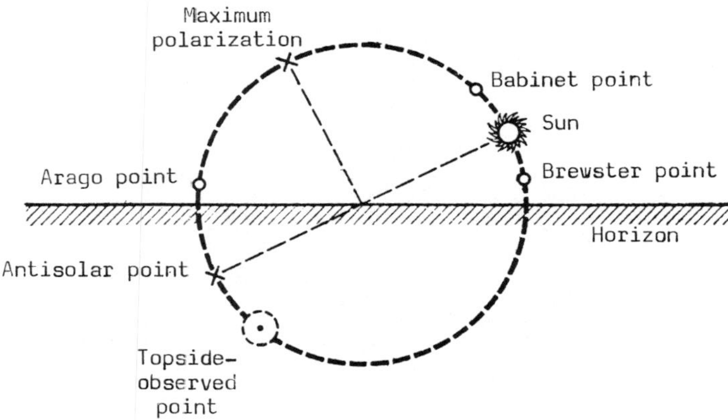


Fig. 6.8. Positions of polarization maximum and neutral points on the solar vertical.

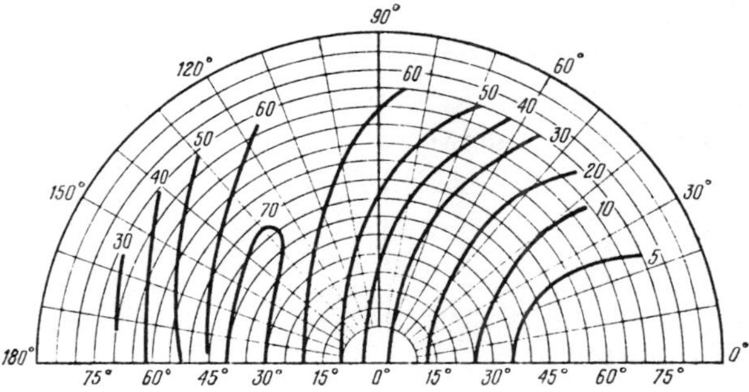

Fig. 6.9. Distribution of the degree of polarization in the sky (%) at a wavelength of 0.70 $\mu$m (zenith angle of sun: 60°).

Horizontal inhomogeneities of the atmosphere and underlying surface, which play the major role in the formation of the scattered background, effect significant variations in both the polarization pattern of the sky and the plane of polarization. For a very turbid atmosphere, elliptical polarization with semiaxis ratios to 0.1 can be observed [6]. Specific examples of the distribution of the degree of polarization in the sky at wavelengths of 0.7 and 2.16 $\mu$m are given in Figs. 6.9 and 6.10 [7]. These examples correspond to the observed maximum degrees of polarization at 0.7 $\mu$m and minimum values at 2.16 $\mu$m. It is seen in the figures that the maximum degree of polarization varies from 70 to 18%. On the whole, the degree of polarization is characterized by a decrease with increasing wavelength. This behavior can be attributed to the diminishing influence of Rayleigh scattering.

Molecular absorption, which tends to diminish multiple scattering and radiation reflected by the underlying surface, exerts a strong influence on

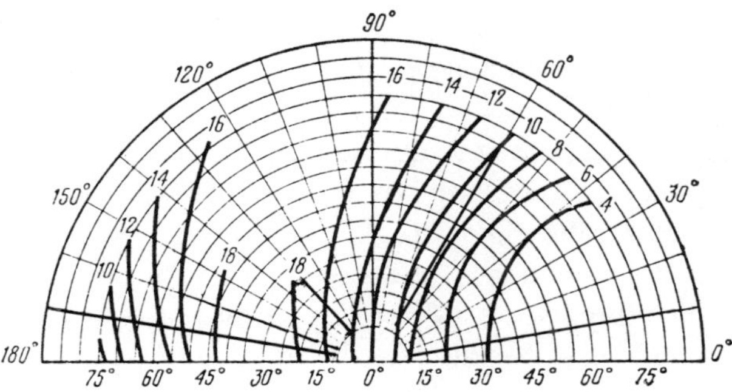

Fig. 6.10. Distribution of the degree of polarization in the sky (%) at a wavelength of 2.16 $\mu$m (zenith angle of sun: 60°).

the distribution and value of the degree of polarization. Observations indicate [7] a systematically higher degree of polarization in the absorption band in comparison with adjacent parts of the spectrum. For example, absorption in the 0.94-$\mu$m water-vapor band produces a 10 to 15% increase in the degree of polarization at isolated points in comparison with the 1.01-$\mu$m region.

### 6.2.3. Statistical Structure of the Luminance of the Cloudy and Cloudless Skies

The presence of both temporal and spatial variations of the luminance of the sky necessitates the use of statistical methods for their description. In the majority of cases, the appropriate characteristics are chosen on the basis of the hypothesis of isotropicity and homogeneity of the radiation fields and a normal distribution of the luminance values. For the quantitative description of the luminance variations of the sky, therefore, it is customary to use only functions of the first and second moments.

Current experimental studies [11] indicate, however, that the distribution functions of the luminance variations of cloud formations can deviate appreciably from normal, changing their character according to the form and congestion of the clouds and, in the case of fractocumulus cloudiness, acquiring a bimodal form. The limits of variation of the standard deviations range from 0.15 for a continuous high- and medium-level cloud cover to 0.48 for a congested cumulus formation.

Aircraft measurement data [12] indicate that the upper limit of the luminance frequency spectrum (with scanning of the cloud surface at a rate of 50 m/sec) falls in the region of 10 Hz, while the lower limit is determined by the largest dimensions of the cloud formations and is situated at hundredths of a hertz. The form of the spatial (or temporal in the case of scanning) spectra of the luminance fields of cumulus, altocumulus, and cirrus clouds depends significantly on the viewing direction. The values of the low-frequency spectra in the direction of the horizon are higher than near the zenith in this case [13] due to the shadowing effect in viewing toward the horizon. We note that the statistical description of cloud formations and the gradation of the cloudy sky with respect to the characteristic statistical properties [14] are of interest not only for the description of background noise, but also for the solution of problems concerning the radiation regime associated with variable cloudiness.

Here we give quantitative data for the spatial luminance spectra of the cloudless and cloudy skies.

In the spectral intervals from 1.8 to 2.5 $\mu$m and from 4.5 to 5.2 $\mu$m, these spectra have been obtained by Kuznechik and Afanas'ev [15] with the use of a radiometer for linear azimuthal scanning between 120 and 360° for an angle of 80° above the horizon and angles of elevation of the sun less than 20°. Figure 6.11 gives the energy spectra of spatial frequencies obtained in [15] with a receiving system having at worst an angular resolution of 0.8° in the interval from 1.8 to 2.5 $\mu$m and of 0.3° from 4.5 to 5.2 $\mu$m. It is evident from the figure that the measured spectrum of spatial luminance inhomogeneities of the clear sky is concentrated in the region up to 1 deg$^{-1}$, i.e., the spatial inhomogeneities have predominantly angular dimensions of 1° or higher. Given the angular resolution and sensitivity of the apparatus used in [15], the spectrum of luminance fluctuations at higher frequencies was not recorded. It follows from a comparison of the spatial luminance spectra for different wavelength intervals that the strengths of the high-frequency harmonic components for the short-wave range are lower than for the long-wave range.

One important statistical characteristic of the cloudy sky is the probability of observing a cloud in the line of sight (at any angle of observation). In meteorology, the cloudiness is described quantitatively relative to the cloudiness characterizing the fraction of obscuration by clouds of an imaginary hemisphere with center at the observation site. The following empirical relation has been derived [16] between the relative cloudiness $n$ and the obscuration at the zenith $n(0)$:

$$n=n(0)+0.5\left[1-n(0)\right]n(0) \tag{6.1}$$

The dependence of the obscuration of the line of sight by clouds on the zenith angle of observation $\Theta$ is described by the expression [17]

$$n(\Theta)=1-\kappa\int_0^\infty P(h)\,dh\int_{h\tan\Theta}^\infty (S-h\tan\Theta)P(S)\,dS \tag{6.2}$$

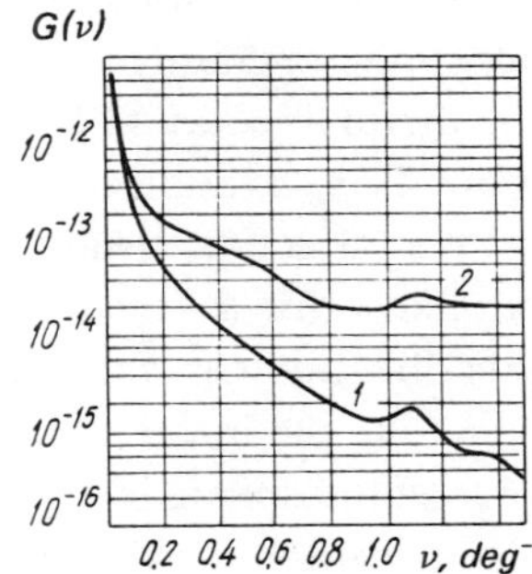


Fig. 6.11. Spatial-frequency spectra $G(\nu)$ [($\mu$W/cm$^2$sr)$^2\cdot$ deg] of the clear sky. (1) Wavelength interval 1.8–2.5 $\mu$m; (2) 4.5–5.2 $\mu$m.

in which $\kappa$ is the cloud frequency (average number of clouds or clearings per unit length), $P(S)$ is the probability density function of clearings between clouds, and $P(h)$ is the probability density of the vertical congestion of individual clouds. The quantities $\kappa$, $P(S)$, and $P(h)$ are determined experimentally from ground-based and airborne measurements.

Calculations performed [16, 17] according to expressions (6.1) and (6.2) yield satisfactory qualitative consistency with the experimental work of the same authors.

## 6.3. Self-Radiation Background of the Atmosphere

Problems of the self-radiation of the earth's atmosphere constitute an extensive and important branch of physics of the atmosphere. Computational methods, quantitative data, and detailed analyses of the physical foundations of thermal radiation of the atmosphere and earth's surface are presented in a series of fundamental monographs by Kondrat'ev [3, 18, 19]. The most comprehensive description of the physics of processes responsible for the airglow is found in books [20–22] and a survey paper [23]. The intention of this section is to describe the principal quantitative data in a condensed form and to discuss briefly the main laws governing the variation of the brightness characteristics as a function of the optical properties of the atmosphere and the conditions of observation.

### 6.3.1. Thermal Radiation Background of the Atmosphere

Depending on the placement of the receiving–recording system, the thermal radiation background of the atmosphere and the earth's surface gives rise to fluxes in different directions. We note that, according to the established terminology of actinometry [2], thermal radiation of the atmosphere in the direction of the ground is conventionally designated as atmospheric counterradiation (back, descending, incoming radiation). It is the thermal radiation fluxes in this direction that create background noise in ground observations. The thermal radiation of the atmosphere and ground in the direction away from the earth's surface is called ascending or outgoing (for a space observer) radiation. The thermal radiation fluxes in this direction generate background noise in topside viewing.

Like the infrared absorption spectrum, the thermal radiation spectrum of the atmosphere is determined by the optical properties of the gases water vapor, carbon dioxide, ozone, and certain others. The spatial and temporal variability of the content of these gases in the atmosphere is responsible for the variability of the radiation spectra as a function of the meteorological conditions and viewing angles, season, and geographic locale.

The measured energy distributions in the thermal radiation spectrum of the clear-sky atmosphere [2] are given in Fig. 6.12 for the zenith (curve 1) and an angular height of 8° above the horizon (curve 1a). Also shown in this figure for comparison are the ideal blackbody radiation (curve 3) and the calculated distributions for the atmosphere (curves 2 and 2a) at a ground-layer air temperature of 15°C. The spectral resolutions for curves 1 and 2 are indicated in the top part of the figure. We see in Fig. 6.12 that the radiation of the atmosphere is close to the radiation of an ideal blackbody in the spectral intervals from 5.5 to 7.5 $\mu$m and near 15 $\mu$m. The former, of course, contains the water-vapor absorption band with center at 6.3 $\mu$m, while the second includes the absorption band of carbon dioxide. The largest maximum in the radiation spectrum, in the interval of 9 to 10 $\mu$m, is associated with ozone radiation (absorption band with center at 9.6 $\mu$m).

A quantitative analysis of many experimental data shows [3, 18, 24] that the atmosphere radiates as an ideal blackbody throughout the entire spectral range near the horizon for a clear sky and in any direction for a low continuous cloud cover. The influence of continuous cloud cover at various levels on the radiation spectrum of the atmosphere has been calculated by Philipps [25]. The results of these calculations show that the lower the cloud cover, the smaller will be the deviation of atmospheric self-radiation from

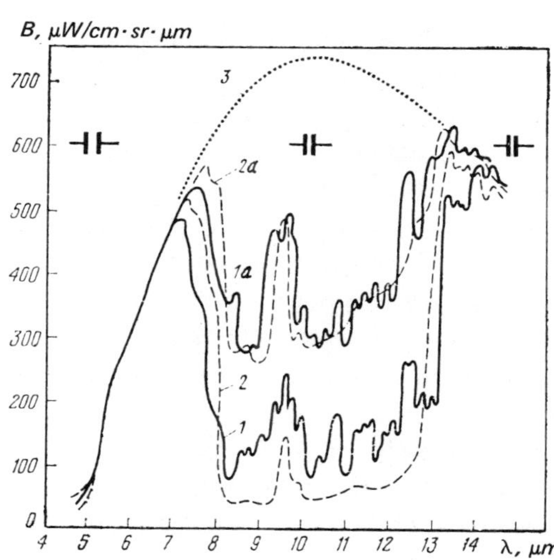


Fig. 6.12. Spectral distribution of thermal radiation intensity of the atmosphere from the zenith and at an angular height of 8° above the horizon. (1, 1a) Results of measurements; (2, 2a) results of calculations; (3) intensity distribution for ideal blackbody radiation.

blackbody radiation in the vicinity of the long-wave atmospheric window from 8.5 to 10.5 $\mu$m.

The changeable stratification of the radiating gases in the atmosphere dictates the transformation of the thermal radiation spectrum with height. A general trend in this case for the interval of 5 to 7 $\mu$m is that the radiation spectrum comes closer to the blackbody spectrum at a temperature equal to the temperature at the corresponding level in the atmosphere as the moisture content is increased. In the atmospheric "window," the thermal radiation flux rapidly decreases with the height. Only the ozone counterradiation depends slightly on the height up to the heights of maximum ozone concentration.

The angular distribution of the thermal radiation of the atmosphere in the vicinity of strong absorption bands for the clear sky and completely overcast sky is characterized by slight dependences on the azimuth and zenith angles. In the daytime, only in parts of the sky close to the sun is any appreciable angular anisotropy observed due to strong forward scattering.

The angular distribution for the clear and overcast skies in atmospheric windows does not depend on the azimuth angle. The variation of the optical thickness of the atmosphere with the zenith angle causes the thermal radiation flux to depend on that angle. The dependence of the thermal radiation intensity of the atmosphere on the zenith angle differs in different spectral intervals. This fact greatly confounds any possibility of simple calculations. Only for the angular distribution of the total fluxes do we find fairly simple approximate expressions that are consistent with experiment [18].

Partial cloudiness exerts the greatest influence on the angular distribution of atmospheric thermal radiation insofar as it imparts a statistical structure to the sky luminance. In the vicinity of absorption bands, the angular variations of the luminance cannot be large because the thermal radiation flux evolves from the warmer thinner strata of the atmosphere near the ground and the luminance of the sky is practically independent of the state of the higher atmospheric layers. In the windows, on the other hand, sizable angular variations of the sky luminance are to be expected. The possible luminance differences of the cloudy sky at various zenith and azimuth angles, according to the experimental data [16], can attain factors of 3 or 4.

Quantitative data on the spectra of spatial (temporal in the case of angular scanning) frequencies of the cloudy-sky luminance (daytime and nighttime) in the wavelength interval from 8.4 to 12.5 $\mu$m have been obtained [26, 27] by means of a high-speed radiometer with high angular resolution ($4 \times 4$ ft) with circular scanning of the sky. Approximation expressions have been found for the spatial spectra:

$$G(\nu) = \frac{G(\nu_1)}{\nu^{S_0 + S_1 \log \nu}} \tag{6.3}$$

where $G(\nu_1)$ is the power of the first harmonic, $S_0$ and $S_1$ are empirical constants for the given type of cloud cover, and $\nu_1 = 1.8$ periods/rad. Table 6.3 gives the values of the constants for the average spectra and various cloudinesses.

It follows from the table that the difference between the average luminance spectra for various types of cloud cover is quite appreciable, a result that is of practical significance from the standpoint of objective identification of the cloud cover at various times of the 24-h cycle.

Along with the relatively slow space–time variations, the sky luminance associated with thermal radiation of the atmosphere also experiences rapid fluctuations. A suitable analysis [28, 29] shows that the statistical characteristics of these fluctuations are highly consistent with the characteristics of the temperature field of the atmosphere up to time intervals of 1 sec.

## 6.3.2. Airglow Background of the Atmosphere

In view of the fact that the excitation mechanisms of many emissions have not been thoroughly investigated to date, all we have is a kind of nominal delimitation of the phenomena responsible for the selective airglow. It is customary to distinguish [21] the polar auroras, night airglow, twilight, and day airglow. The polar auroras are usually interpreted as sporadic electromagnetic radiation emitted by the upper layers of the atmosphere, where it is stimulated by solar corpuscular fluxes. The temporal variability of the polar aurora is one of its distinctive features in contrast with the relatively constant airglow. For the latter, the principal mechanisms responsible for the high selectivity of atmospheric radiation are luminescence

Table 6.3

| Cloud cover | Average luminance, $10^{-3}$ W·cm$^{-2}$ sr$^{-1}$ (at local angles) | $\log G$ | $S_0$ | $S_1$ |
|---|---|---|---|---|
| Cu | 0.8–1.6 ($\geqslant 15°$) | $-7.35$ | 2.27 | $+0.16$ |
| Ac | 0.6–1.3 ($\geqslant 20°$) | $-7.97$ | 2.09 | $+0.10$ |
| Ci, Cc | 0.15–0.7 ($\geqslant 30°$) | $-8.9$ | 2.24 | $-0.096$ |
| Instrument noise | $(1–5)\cdot 10^{-3}$ | $-11.7$ | 1.73 | $-0.28$ |

Table 6.4

| Emission | $(W/cm^2)\cdot10^{-8}$ | Wavelengths of strongest lines, $\mu m$ |
|---|---|---|
| $N_2^+$ | 0.85 | 0.3582; 0.3884; 0.3914; 0.4278; 0.4237; and others |
| $N_2$ | 1.8 | 0.3371; 0.3577; 0.3755; and others |
| $O^+$ | 0.36 | 0.5577 |
| $O^+$ | 0.16 | 0.630–0.636 |
| $H\alpha$ | 1.65 | 0.656 |
| $O_2$ | 1.0 | 0.860; 0.845; 0.768; and others |
| $N_2$ | 4.0 | 1.051; 0.891; 0.872; 0.854; and others |
| $N_2^+$ | 5.0 | 1.614; 1.511; 1.452; 1.104; 0.915; and others |
| $O_2$ | 1.3 | 1.466 |

and resonant scattering. The zodiacal light created by scattering beyond the limits of the geocorona, where the nature of the scatterers is still a matter of debate, as well as the direct and scattered radiation from cosmic bodies and stars altogether account for as much as one-fourth of the total illumination of the moonless sky. However, the smearing of the emission spectrum of these sources renders their contribution inconsequential in any spectral interval.

The spectral composition of the nonthermal radiation of the atmosphere is characterized by a set of emission lines. Table 6.4 lists the strongest lines and bands in the polar aurora spectrum [30]. Analogous lines are also observed in the nightglow and dayglow spectra.

The nightglow spectra in the intervals of 6200–6420, 6760–7000, and 9610–10,000 Å are given in Fig. 6.13 according to data of Nefed'eva [31]. The radiation intensity is plotted on the vertical axis in $mR/\mu m$, where the Rayleigh $(R)$ is a unit such that $1\ R/\text{Å} = 10^3 h\nu\ W/cm^2\ \mu m$, $h$ being the

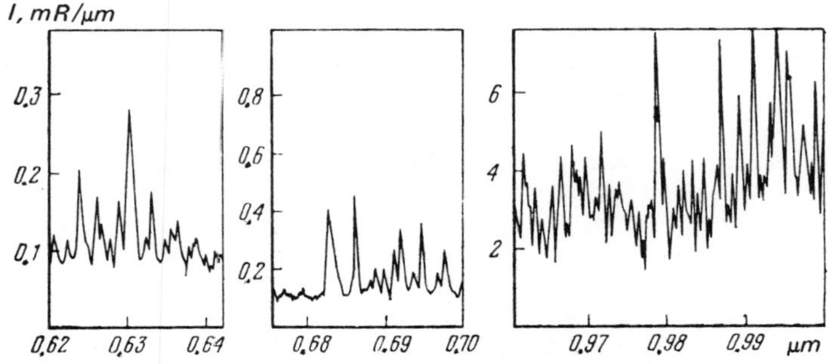

Fig. 6.13. Selected intervals of the nightglow spectrum.

Planck constant and $\nu$ the emission frequency. The airglow luminance increases in transition from the ultraviolet to the infrared region.


## 6.4. Characteristics of the Outgoing Radiation of the Earth–Atmosphere System

In viewing from negative angular positions (topside viewing), background noise is generated by thermal radiation from the earth's surface, atmospheric radiation, and the reflection of radiation by the atmosphere and ground. These background noise sources then determine the characteristics of the ascending (outgoing) radiation in both the long-wave ($\lambda > 4\ \mu$m) and the short-wave ($\lambda < 4\ \mu$m) regions of the spectrum.

In this section we give a brief portrayal of the main characteristics of ascending radiation from the earth. A comprehensive bibliography and detailed analysis of the results of theoretical and experimental research in this area may be found in several books [3, 18, 19, 24, 32].


### 6.4.1. Spectral Composition

The basic laws governing the spectral distribution in the long-wave ascending radiation flux are illustrated by analytical data taken from Niilisk and Noorma [33] and presented in Fig. 6.14. The calculations were carried out for summer conditions at middle latitudes with a high relative humidity and at various heights in nadir viewing. The influence of the atmosphere is absent at the ground level, and the ascending radiation spectrum represents the smooth radiation spectrum of the underlying surface. The influence of the atmosphere increases with ascent. In the vicinity of the strong absorption band of water vapor at 6.3 $\mu$m and of ozone at 9.6 $\mu$m, distinct radiation minima are formed at great heights. The positions of the minima and maxima in the ascending radiation spectrum are interchanged in comparison with the counterradiation spectrum.

The main features of the spectral composition of the long-wave ascending radiation persist at great heights [34].

Intensive satellite investigations of the outgoing radiation spectra in recent years have made it possible to perform a statistical analysis of the results [32]. Figure 6.15, borrowed from Andrianov and others [32], gives the results of statistical processing of data obtained by means of scanning diffraction spectrometers on board the Kosmos 45 and Kosmos 65 satellites,

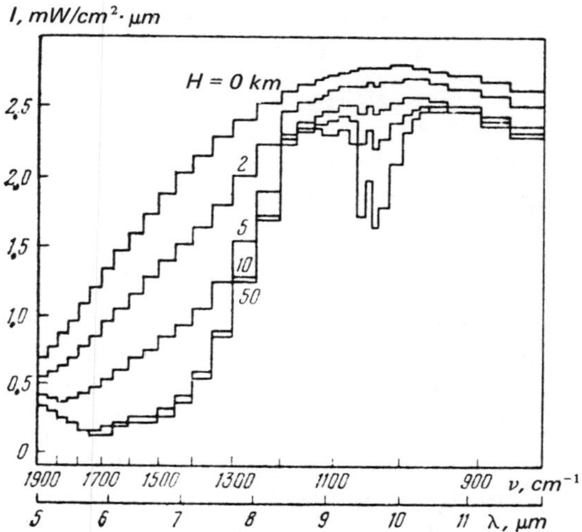


Fig. 6.14. Spectral intensity of summer ascending radiation at middle latitudes and various heights (indicated in the figure).

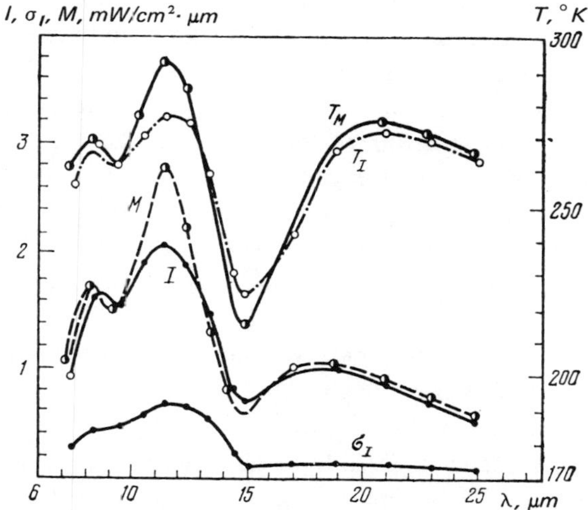


Fig. 6.15. Generalized statistical characteristics of the spectral intensity of earth radiation versus wavelength.

with 1200 measurements at latitudes from 65°N to 65°S. The spectral resolution of the instruments and the angle of the instantaneous field of view were 1.1 to 1.4 $\mu$m and $1°46' \times 2°20'$. The average altitude of the satellites in flight was 250 km. Figure 6.15 gives the spectral distributions of the average radiation intensity $I$, the standard deviations of the intensity $\sigma_I$, the modes of the random intensity $M$, and the values of the radiation temperatures $T_{\bar{I}}$ (right scale), as well as the temperature $T_M$ calculated from the modal value. The statistical characteristics in the figure are global, without differentiation into the ensembles of radiation on the shaded or illuminated sides, the cloudy or clear sky, dry land or marine, etc.

The short-wave ascending radiation flux is determined by radiation from the underlying surface and scattering of solar radiation in the atmosphere. Consequently, the spectral composition and its variability, as in the case of descending radiation, depend in a complex way on the optical properties of the atmosphere and the underlying surface, on the height and position of the sun, on the presence and nature of clouds, etc. The fundamental laws for these dependences are similar to those given for the descending radiation spectrum. A new aspect of the short-wave ascending radiation spectrum is the stronger influence of the ground albedo, which asserts itself in the magnitude of the flux to a greater degree than in the spectral composition.

Calculations have shown [19] that, as in the case of the descending radiation, the spectral intensity of the ascending radiation diminishes rapidly with increasing wavelength; at $\lambda = 2.75$ $\mu$m, the outgoing radiation intensity is lower by 3 orders of magnitude than at $\lambda = 0.7$ $\mu$m. The rather sparse experimental data on the spectral dependence of the short-wave ascending radiation support the main results of the calculations [19].

## 6.4.2. Spatial and Angular Distributions

The spatial and angular distributions of long-wave ascending radiation is characterized by seasonal and latitude dependences. Cloudiness tends to diminish the ascending radiation flux, which in this case is determined by the temperature of the upper cloud layers. Table 6.5 gives calculated data on the average outgoing thermal radiation fluxes from the earth's surface, the troposphere, and the stratosphere [32] in different seasons under average cloudiness conditions.

It is seen in the table that the main contributor to the outgoing thermal radiation in all seasons is the troposphere. In regard to the seasonal

Table 6.5

| Radiating medium | Average thermal radiation flux, $10^{-3}$ W/cm$^2$ | | | | |
| --- | --- | --- | --- | --- | --- |
| | Winter | Spring | Summer | Autumn | Annual average |
| Earth's surface (in atmospheric "windows") | 2.0 | 2.0 | 1.8 | 1.8 | 1.9 |
| Troposphere | 19.3 | 19.2 | 20.5 | 19.7 | 19.7 |
| Stratosphere | 0.8 | 1.1 | 1.3 | 0.7 | 1.0 |
| Total outgoing radiation | 22.1 | 2.3 | 23.6 | 22.2 | 22.6 |

dependence of the ascending radiation fluxes, it is insignificant. Similar calculations indicate quite a different pattern in the case of the latitude dependence of the ascending radiation fluxes. For example, the flux in polar regions under average conditions has a typical value of $13.9 \times 10^{-3}$ W/cm$^2$, whereas in the subtropics it is typically $25.4 \times 10^{-3}$ W/cm$^2$.

A characteristic pattern of the angular distribution of the long-wave ascending radiation is a slow decline of the intensity with variation of the viewing angle from the nadir to the limb of the earth. Near the latter, the intensity decays rapidly (infrared darkening toward the horizon). The nature of the underlying surface injects certain corrections into the indicated pattern.

The laws occurring in the angular distribution of the long-wave outgoing radiation are similar to those noted above for the ascending radiation. Figure 6.16 gives the results of measurements of the angular distribution of the outgoing radiation in absolute units from on board the Kosmos 65 satellite [32] with the use of a diffraction spectrometer, the main characteristics of which are described above. The measurement program was geared primarily for horizon observations at wavelengths of 9.6, 11, 12, 15, 18, and 20 $\mu$m. Simultaneous monitoring of the cloudiness at an undersatellite point (at the nadir) indicated the presence of clouds over all parts of the satellite trajectory used in processing of the data. A quantitative analysis of the data in Fig. 6.16 indicates that the effective limb of the earth at a wavelength of 15 $\mu$m is approximately 27 km higher than at other wavelengths, in correspondence with theoretical notions. Also consistent with present-day theoretical notions are other laws in the angular distribution of the long-wave earth-to-space radiation, but quantitative comparison of the experimental and calculated data requires an exceedingly difficult—and so far impractical for calculations—consideration of the specific meteorological conditions, above all the total cloud condition.

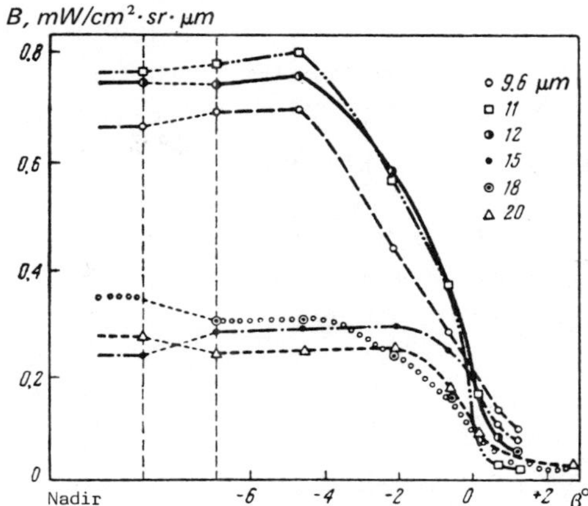



Fig. 6.16. Intensity of outgoing radiation versus viewing angle for certain spectral intervals (indicated in the figure).

The short-wave outgoing radiation field is determined by the scattering of direct solar radiation in the atmosphere, the reflection of direct and scattered radiation by the underlying surface, and the scattering of reflected solar radiation. Such a complex assortment of processes necessitates incorporation of the angular scattering functions, the scattering and absorption coefficients, the vertical distributions of these optical characteristics in the atmosphere, the reflecting properties of the underlying surface, the curvature of the atmosphere, and the polarization and refraction of radiation into the calculations. Naturally, the inclusion of all these factors in the calculations by various methods can be implemented only under certain simplifying assumptions.

## 6.5. Characteristics of the Reflection of Optical Radiation by the Underlying Surface

The reflective properties of the underlying surface are characterized by such energy variables as the albedo and luminance factor. We recall that the albedo is defined as the ratio of the radiant flux reflected by a given surface in all directions of the contiguous hemisphere to the incident flux on that surface. We are primarily concerned with the spectral albedo $A$, i.e., the albedo in a narrow wavelength interval. The angular distribution of the intensity of reflected radiation (unnormalized angular reflection function) is characterized by the concept of the luminance factor of reflected radiation. For the purpose of this discussion, we are mainly interested in the quantitative measure of this factor in a definite spectral interval, i.e., the spectral luminance factors $R_\lambda$. For the rigorous treatment of polarization effects in connection with reflection, it is necessary to determine the above-indicated quantities in terms of the Stokes parameters [35, 36], but the discussion of these problems can usually be confined to just the degree of polarization.

The reflective properties of the underlying surface have been most thoroughly investigated for the visible region of the spectrum. For example, Krinov's book [37] gives pertinent data for 370 objects. The reflective properties of mainly geological formations are given in [38]. The characteristics of the reflection of optical radiation by the underlying surface in the infrared part of the spectrum have received less attention [3, 9, 39].

### 6.5.1. Spectral Albedo

The most detailed measurements of the spectral albedo for soils, road pavements, vegetation covers, and snow, in the spectral range from 0.4 to 1 $\mu$m are reported in [3]. Figure 6.17, which is taken from [3], shows the spectral dependence of the albedo for certain types of underlying surface. It is evident from the figure that the albedo for soil and vegetation increases in the near-IR region of the spectrum in comparison with the visible region. On the other hand, a reduction of the albedo in the IR region is observed for snow covers and water surfaces. This tendency toward reduction for the indicated surfaces, as will be evident from the results of measurements for the luminance factor, continues into the longer-wave part of the spectrum.

The experimental data show that diffuse reflection by real surfaces is largely nonorthotropic and differs from reflection by surfaces for which the

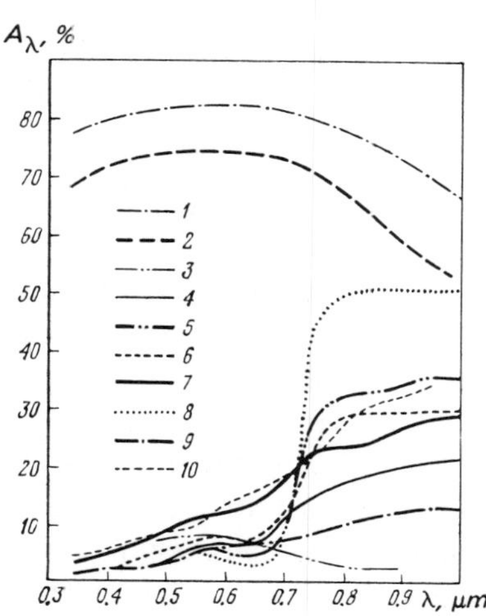


Fig. 6.17. Spectral albedo of various natural underlying surfaces. (1) Ice-crusted snow (zenith angle of sun during measurements: (38°); (2) wet coarse-grain snow (37°); (3) water surface of lake; (4) soil after snow thaw (24°); (5) silage corn (54°); (6) high green corn (56°); (7) yellow corn (46°); (8) Sudan grass (52°); (9) black earth (chernozem) (50°); (10) grain stubble (35°).

angular distribution is described by Lambert's law. As a result, the albedo of the underlying surface depends both on the illumination conditions (position of the sun) and on the viewing direction. In particular, it is a well-known fact [3] that the minimum albedo occurs during midday (with the sun at high points). According to the results of soil and vegetation measurements [40], the spectral albedo can vary by as much as 50% from its maximum value, depending on the position of the sun.

The albedo of thick clouds is completely determined by their optical properties and the properties of the overlying layers of the atmosphere. The albedo of clouds has been successfully calculated by approximate methods of radiation transport theory [41] as well as by more accurate numerical methods [42]. The numerical data indicate that the albedo in the visible spectrum has a value of 60 to 90%, depending on the form and height of the clouds. The IR albedo, as in the case of outgoing radiation, is characterized by a selective wavelength dependence [41] with a general tendency to decrease toward longer wavelengths. Indirect estimates for the interval of 8 to 12 $\mu$m [3] show that the average albedo for water clouds is 3–4% and for mixed clouds (containing ice crystals) it is 8–9%. The sparse available experimental data are qualitatively consistent with calculations [3].

The results of calculations of the spectral albedo of water surfaces [36] exhibit an appreciable windspeed dependence of the albedo values for all wavelengths, including the visible and IR ($\lambda \lesssim 17$ $\mu$m) regions of the spectrum; this dependence becomes stronger for zenith distances of the sun greater than 70°. On the other hand, the wind velocity has scarcely any effect on the spectral behavior of the albedo.

## 6.5.2. Spectral Luminance Factors

Other imported quantities from the standpoint of estimating background noise are the angular distribution (angular reflection function) and spectral behavior of the luminance factor. The angular distribution of the luminance factors of the majority of natural formations is characterized by symmetry about the plane of the solar vertical. The angular distributions in the plane of the solar vertical for various types of underlying surfaces tend to be elongated both in the direction of incidence of the solar rays and in the direction of specular reflection angles. An analysis of the wavelength-integrated angular reflection functions given in [3] indicates that the coefficient of the angular dependence in the range of viewing angles from 0 to 85° for various azimuths relative to the sun does not exceed a value of 3 for road pavements and vegetation covers. For water and snow surfaces and mixed forestation, the indicated coefficient can attain a value of 10 or more. Measurements of the spectral angular reflection functions at wavelengths of 2.2, 2.4, and 3.7 $\mu$m in the range of angles from 0 to 50° for certain types of underlying surface [43] have shown that the coefficient of the angular dependence does not exceed 1.8. This limit of variation of the angular dependence may be regarded as small since the variations of other conditions (such as the humidity) account for at least comparable variations of the spectral luminance factor.

The pronounced elongation of the angular reflection function for water and snow surfaces is explained by the major role of the specular component. For a snow cover, this component depends strongly on the state of the cover, and for water it depends on the surface wave state. In the latter case, as calculations indicate [36], for a low position of the sun the spectral luminance factor can be close to unity in the direction of specular reflection angles, creating a zone of enhanced luminance known as the light trail.

The temporal variability of water surface waves imparts a statistical character to the luminance of the reflected radiation. Considering the importance of the statistical properties of water-reflected radiation and the high luminance level in the region of the light trail, we consider the characteristics of this kind of background noise in more detail below.

Direct solar radiation reflected from water and snow surfaces is completely or partially polarized, the degree of polarization depending on the zenith distance of the sun and the viewing angles. According to calculated data [36], the degree of polarization for a water surface does not depend on the wind velocity. It attains its maximum value of 100% at reflection angles (angle between the direction to the sun and the viewing angle) of about 106° and decreases to 0% with a decrease or increase in the reflection angle from that value.

The spectral variation of the luminance factor for various natural formations is currently investigated for the most part in the spectral range up to 2.5 $\mu$m. The results of measurements of the spectral luminance factors for various types of underlying surface are compiled in Fig. 6.18, taken from [36]. The decrease of the luminance factor along the given curves for certain surfaces in the vicinity of 1.5 and 2.0 $\mu$m is attributable to the influence of the absorption bands of water; this influence lessens as the surface becomes drier. Certain data for the luminance factors in the indicated spectral range may also be found in [44]. Data on the spectral variation of the reflection coefficients over a wide range of wavelengths (up to 100 $\mu$m) are given in [45]. Some of these data are presented in Fig. 6.19.

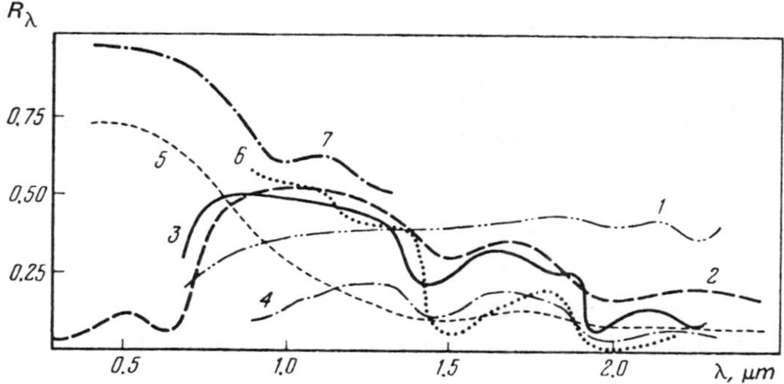

Fig. 6.18. Spectral reflection coefficients of various surfaces in the interval up to 2.5 $\mu$m. (1) Fine sand; (2) plant foliage; (3) tree leaves (newly fallen); (4) black peat (wet); (5) snow (old); (6) snow (fresh); (7) analytical curve for snow.

Borisov [43] has conducted measurements of the luminance factors at wavelengths of 2.2, 2.4, and 3.7 $\mu$m for 14 types of surfaces. These measurements indicate a strong dependence of the spectral luminance factors on the moisture content of the surface. The luminance factors of dry and wet sand, for example, differ roughly by a factor of 4, and the same is true for the luminance factors of dry and green grasses. A wet surface has smaller values of the reflection coefficients. Laboratory measurements of the reflection coefficients of pure water and sea water in the wavelength intervals of 2 to 22 $\mu$m and 1.1 to 2.1 $\mu$m are reported in [46]. It turns out that the reflection spectra of sea water scarcely differ from those of pure water.

The spectral behavior of the luminance factor for cloud formations have essentially already been discussed in the preceding section. Here it suffices to note that appreciable variations in the spectral behavior of the luminance factor are observed for different types of cloud formations, where the clearcut emergence of absorption bands is typical for the liquid–droplet phase (in cumulus clouds) and for the solid phase (in cirrus clouds). This feature, which is largely typical of the infrared region of the spectrum, is used extensively at the present time in aircraft and rocket soundings. If

Fig. 6.19. Spectral reflection coefficients of various specimens in the interval 0.7–100 $\mu$m. (1) Sand; (2) soil; (3) asphalt.

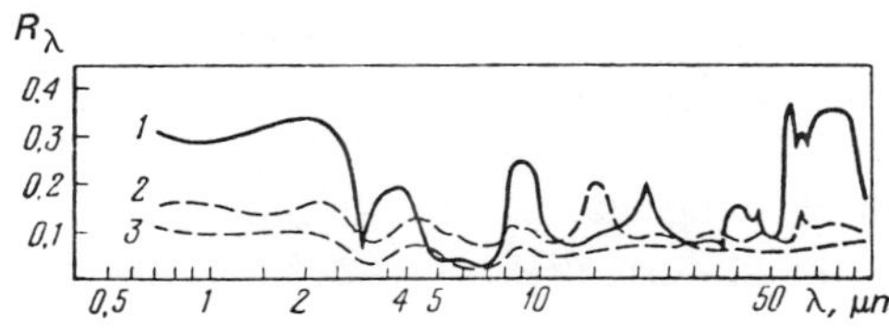

wavelength-tunable lasers are used, the indicated feature can also be utilized to advantage for the laser probing of cloud formations both from the ground and from airborne equipment.

### 6.5.3. Fluctuation Characteristics of the Luminance of a Rough Water Surface

For a complete description of the background noise induced by the reflection of solar radiation from water surfaces and for the development of techniques for the long-range probing of marine layers of the atmosphere and water surfaces, it is necessary, in addition to the time-average values, to know the statistical characteristics of the reflected radiation. Here we describe certain results of measurements [47] of the averages, variances, distribution functions, and correlation functions, as well as the spike characteristics of the fluctuating luminance of water surfaces.

Measurements in the region of the light trail, which is distinguished by the maximum average luminance, have been carried out on Lake Baikal, which has a considerable depth and, hence, a characteristic sea-wave state. The statistical characteristics of the luminances of the water surface were investigated by means of a photometer with a 3-ft angular field of view for the spectral interval around 1.06 $\mu$m and in the interval of frequencies up to 20 Hz. The measurements were performed at various zenith angles of the sun in the interval from 40 to 88°, wind azimuths from 60 to 120°, and an approximately uniform sea height of 2 points. Altogether 120 samples of the luminance of the water surface in the azimuth plane and 50 samples in the plane of the angle of elevation were recorded. For the majority of the samples, the univariate probability distribution functions were obtained, and the conformity of the calculated distribution with a log–normal function was tested. In the event of a sizable deviation from that function, the distribution was further tested for conformity with a normal, Rayleigh, or exponential distribution function. An analysis of the resulting distribution functions in the azimuth plane shows that they obey a log–normal law for azimuths of observation up to $+12°$, zenith angles of the sun $\Theta = 50$ to $60°$, and wind azimuths $\alpha_V = 60$ to $120°$. For a value of $\alpha_V$ from 18 to 30° and for $\Theta = 80$ to $88°$, significant deviations from all the tested distributions occur for all values of $\alpha$.

Following are the main results of the measurements of the statistical characteristics in the azimuth plane. The maximum values of the luminance and the unnormalized variance are observed at angles of about 6°, i.e., are shifted in the direction of the wind. Another luminance maximum, about

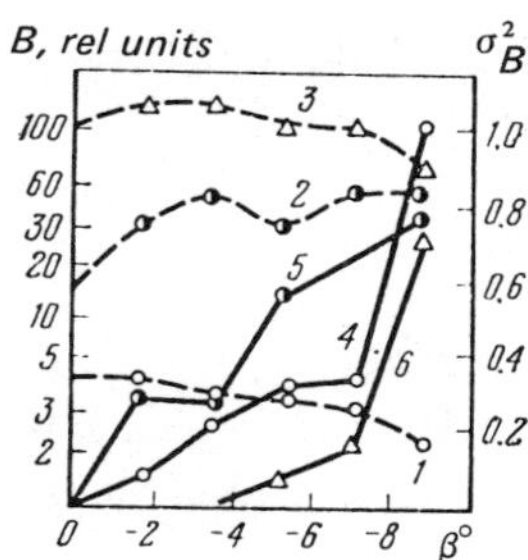

Fig. 6.20. Average luminance of a water surface (a, - - -) and normalized variance of fluctuations (b, —) versus angles of elevation at the center of the light trail for various solar zenith angles: (1,4) 5°; (2,5) 68°; (3,6) 84°.

half the strength of the main one, appears at the center of the light trail. With increasing zenith angles of the sun, the maximum variance shifts to the center of the light trail and diminishes in value. Figure 6.20 gives the dependence of the average luminance in relative units and the normalized variance on the angles of elevation (relative to the center of the light trail) for various solar zenith angles, without regard for the different averagings of the receiving system for different angles of elevation $\beta$.

The autocorrelation functions of the luminance fluctuations in the azimuth plane exhibits an oscillatory behavior at the observable center of the light trail (near 6°) and a decaying trend in the peripheral regions. In the plane of angles of elevation, unlike the azimuth plane, periodic oscillations (with the period of the surface waves) of the autocorrelation functions are observed only in the central zone (close to the specular reflection angle).

Some of the recorded samples distinguished by the greatest degree of variation of the luminance were further processed by the methods of outlier theory. Figure 6.21 gives data pertaining to the mean intervals $\overline{\Theta}$ between

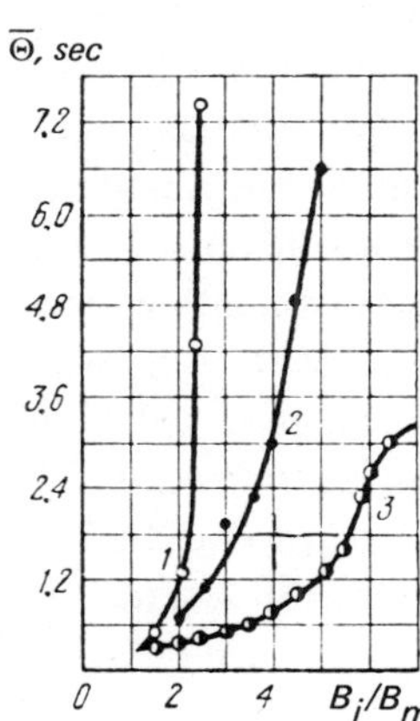

Fig. 6.21. Mean intervals between outliers. (1) Azimuth angle $\alpha = 0°$, angle of elevation $\beta = 3.6°$; (2) $\alpha = 18°$, $\beta = -7.2°$; (3) $\alpha = 0°$, $\beta = -7.2°$.

outliers (spikes), determined according to the expression

$$\overline{\Theta} = \frac{T_{av} - T_{tot}}{N}$$

in which $T_{av}$ is the averaging time (50 sec), $T_{tot}$ is the total time in which the luminance $B_i$ exceeds a fixed level, and $N$ is the number of spikes of $B_i$ above the median level $B_m$. The median signal level was adopted as the normalization level. The data given in Fig. 6.21 indicate a complex distribution of the statistical characteristics of the luminance in the light trail itself and close to it. This result is a consequence of the complex statistical structure of the rough water surface, whose reflected radiation contains both specular and diffuse components.

## 6.6. Conclusion

The quantitative material presented in this chapter in regard to various background-noise effects provides a tool in many instances for determining the noise component of an optical signal carrying a particular parcel of useful information and, hence, to estimate the operational effectiveness of a particular laser system in the atmosphere. It must be recalled in this connection, however, that the actual pattern of the background-noise field will undoubtedly deviate from those obtained experimentally with corresponding spectral, temporal, and spatial averaging.

In application to laser systems, this disparity may prove most significant in relation to the corresponding spectral averaging because the width of the laser emission line differs by several orders of magnitude from the spectral resolution of the instruments used to measure various background noise processes. On the other hand, this disparity will prevail most of all in situations where the laser-emitted radiation falls in the vicinity of the central part of the absorption line of a particular atmospheric gas. If, however, the laser radiation falls in an atmospheric window and does not coincide with the central part of any of the faint absorption lines that are generally present in all windows, then the spectral resolution of the instruments measuring background noise will not play a major role if the mildly selective aerosol and molecular scattering processes are responsible for the main contribution to the noise level.

A similar situation arises in the nighttime operation of laser systems, where the selective nightglow can exert a significant influence on the formation of the noise component of a useful optical signal.

Continued research on the spatial, temporal, and spectral distributions of various background-noise effects in the optical wavelength range unquestionably remains a timely objective, the auspicious solution of which will eventually yield more accurate and more reliable data, which are needed for many scientific and practical problems, including the problem of determining the operational effectiveness of various laser systems in the real atmosphere.

# 7

# *Laser Applications in Atmospheric Research*

## *7.0. Introduction*

Close in the wake of the first lasers were the first studies aimed at the practical utilization of these remarkable light sources for investigations of the atmosphere. This activity was largely motivated by two paramount considerations: (1) the practical need for the development of devices for the long-range sensing and monitoring of atmospheric parameters; (2) the awesome capabilities of laser methods in regard to atmospheric research.

The practical need for the development of devices for long-range monitoring of the parameters of the atmosphere was dictated by the fact that existing standard methods for the measurement of these parameters, although still used extensively even today throughout the worldwide network of hydrometeorological stations, cannot produce the vast space–time data arrays essential to the solution of important problems such as the long-term weather-prediction problem. The following are among the primary shortcomings of standard methods: (1) the necessity of obtaining data from direct measurements, making it technically infeasible to acquire such data with the required spatial and temporal resolution on a planetary scale; (2) the restricted set of measurable parameters (measurables: pressure, temperature, humidity, wind; immeasurables: aerosols, concentrations of gases that absorb solar radiation, other than water vapor); (3) the limited ceiling and nonreal-time character of monitoring based on the most accessible and widely used radiosonde method. These difficulties are surmountable through the development of methods and means for long-distance monitoring of those atmospheric parameters that are significant in the evolution of weather-formation processes.

*347*

The laser approach holds a special rank among all presently known methods for long-range monitoring of the atmosphere, particularly insofar as we have been first-hand witnesses to its swift progress practically from the genesis of the first lasers and the first laser–radar, or lidar (light detection and ranging), systems. The first published report, in 1963, of the use of a ruby laser to probe aerosol stratification is well known [1].

The advantages of the laser method for investigations of the atmosphere are related to the existence of a sizable body of phenomena involving the interaction of optical waves with the atmosphere and exhibiting large cross sections. Typical are the effects of molecular, resonance, and aerosol (particulate) scattering, spontaneous and stimulated Raman and resonant Raman scattering, fluorescence and resonant fluorescence, molecular absorption, Doppler and collision broadening of the absorption lines of atmospheric gases, Doppler frequency shift, amplitude and phase fluctuations induced by atmospheric turbulence, and an entire series of nonlinear effects accompanying the propagation of laser radiation for definite values of the power and pulse duration.

These methods also possess very important assets in the high performance indices attainable by their means: real-time acquisition of data; high temporal and spatial resolution of data; very large probing distances with respect to many important parameters of the atmosphere; high sensitivity in the detection of minute impurities. Laser methods, in principle, afford the possibility of investigating atmospheric processes on a real-time scale. The measurement information obtained by these methods in "encoded" form reaches the receiving equipment with the speed of light, and once "decoding" methods are known, i.e., once the corresponding inverse problems have been solved, the final result will be obtained in a time interval directly related to the capabilities of the processing electronic computer hardware.

Every laser pulse, generally speaking, carries information about the profiles of physical parameters of the atmosphere. The spatial resolution of the results is determined by the duration of the probe pulse. Thus, the usual durations of tens of nanoseconds automatically ensure a spatial resolution of a few meters, provided, of course, that the receiving and processing equipment has compatible speed.

Lasers now exist, with pulse durations of the order of $10^{-8}$ sec, which are capable of generating $10^3$ to $10^4$ pulses per second. The application of such lasers opens the way to the acquisition of monitoring data with spatial resolutions of the order of 1 and with temporal resolutions up to $10^4$ profiles per sec.

Laser methods are enjoying enormously broad applications in studies of atmospheric pollution by aerosols and gases of industrial origin. Their ability to compete with other known methods in this area is unquestionable, most particularly in regard to the investigation of the dynamics of atmospheric contaminations.

While quite a large array of equipment and apparatus has emerged since the very first publication of the results of laser probing of the atmosphere and although a great many monitoring results have been obtained and several books and survey papers have been published [2–14] on the use of lasers for the investigation of atmospheric parameters, the fact remains that this problem is still in the stage of vigorous development, which is scarcely expected to slow down in the immediate future. Accordingly, the systematization and generalization of the vast material accumulated to date pose a timely problem. In the present chapter, which is devoted to such a generalization, we focus particular attention on the results of investigations carried out in the most recent times and on problems for which solutions are still pending. A special place is reserved in the chapter for methods of long-range laser monitoring of the parameters of the atmosphere. Definite attention is also given to the applications of frequency-tunable lasers for determining the concentrations of atmospheric gases by laser-spectroscopic methods.

## 7.1. Fundamentals of Methods for Laser Probing of the Atmosphere; the Lidar Equation

The basic idea of laser probing of the atmosphere may be summarized as follows. If a laser pulse of duration $\tau$ and beam spread $\varphi_0$ is sent into the atmosphere, at every instant $t$ it will occupy an essentially cylindrical volume in space. The generatrices and cross section of the cylinder are uniquely determined by the specification of $\tau$, $\varphi_0$, and $t$. The pulse interacts with the atmosphere over its entire path of propagation and, hence, at every instant $t$. The nature of the interaction depends on the properties of the probed volume of the atmosphere and the properties of the pulse. Depending on the composition of the atmosphere, as characterized by the appropriate physical parameters (pressure, temperature, gas constituency, aerosol characteristics, etc.), different processes of interaction of light with the atmospheric medium (molecular and aerosol scattering, molecular absorption, etc.) will be manifested in varying degrees. These interactions show up in the form of photons that have the same frequency as the probe pulse and are scattered or absorbed by the probed volume, or in the form of frequency-shifted photons, etc.

At every instant $t$, the corresponding volume of probed atmosphere responds in all directions to its interaction with the laser pulse. This response or, better, the laser signal echo pulse carries information about the physical parameters of the atmosphere, and it can be recorded by a suitable receiving device. If the latter is conjoined with the transmitting device or is situated next to it, the laser probing or monitoring configuration is said to be monostatic. If the transmitter and receiver are separated by an appreciable distance (large baseline), we have a bistatic probing configuration.

In the ensuing discussion, without detracting from its generality, we consider monostatic configurations. In this case, considering only single pulse–atmosphere interaction events, we obtain the basic equation for laser probing of the atmosphere, customarily known as the atmospheric lidar equation:

$$P_r(r) = \eta P_0 A r^{-2} \left( \frac{c\tau}{2} \right) \beta_\pi(r) \exp\left[ -2 \int_0^r \alpha(r')\, dr' \right] \qquad (7.1)$$

in which $P_r(r)$ is the power of the echo signal arriving at the receiver, $P_0$ is the power of the probe pulse, $A$ is the area of the receiving antenna, $r$ is the distance from the lidar apparatus to the probed volume, $c$ is the speed of light, $\tau$ is the pulse duration, $\beta_\pi(r)$ is the cross section of interaction in the backward direction, the factor $\exp[-2 \int_0^r \alpha(r')\, dr']$ characterizes the total attenuation (extinction) of radiation in the atmosphere over the path from transmitter to probed volume to receiver, $\alpha(r')$ is the volume extinction coefficient, which accounts for the attenuation due to all possible causes and mainly due to aerosol and molecular scattering and molecular absorption by atmospheric gases, and $\eta$ is a calibration constant.

In the most common situation, where only three interaction processes are taken into account, namely, molecular scattering, aerosol attenuation, and molecular absorption, we can write the expressions

$$\beta_\pi(r) = \beta_\pi^R(r) + \beta_\pi^M(r) \qquad (7.2)$$

$$\alpha(r) = \alpha_R(r) + \alpha_M(r) + \alpha_a(r) \qquad (7.3)$$

in which $\beta_\pi^R$ and $\beta_\pi^M$ are the volume coefficients of Rayleigh and aerosol backscattering, $\alpha_R(r)$ and $\alpha_M(r)$ are the volume coefficients of Rayleigh and aerosol scattering, $\alpha_a$ is the volume coefficient of absorption by atmospheric gases, which in general is represented by the sum

$$\alpha_a(r) = \sum_i \alpha_a^i(r) \qquad (7.4)$$

and $\alpha_a^i(r)$ is the absorption coefficient of the $i$th line contributing to the absorption at a given frequency (wavelength). We note that all quantities in expressions (7.1)–(7.4) except $A$ and $r$ depend on the wavelength of the probing radiation.

## 7.2. Quantitative Interpretation of the Lidar Equation

Expressions (7.1)–(7.4) apply to the case of one-frequency laser probing, with which we begin our discussion of the problem, bearing in mind that the quantities $P_r$, $P_0$, $\beta_\pi$, $\eta$, $\beta_\pi^R$, $\beta_\pi^M$, $\alpha_R$, $\alpha_M$, and $\alpha_a$ depend on the wavelength. In the case of multifrequency probing, expressions (7.1)–(7.4) are written out as many times as there are frequencies used. We shall discuss this case later.

It is evident from (7.1)–(7.4) that for single-frequency laser probing, in which case it is required to take into account molecular scattering, aerosol attenuation, and molecular absorption, we cannot obtain information about any of the unknowns in these expressions without recourse to *a priori* information about them or to suitable supporting assumptions. The usual procedure is as follows. The vertical profile of the volume Rayleigh scattering coefficient $\alpha_R(r)$ and, hence, the profile of the volume Rayleigh backscattering coefficient $\beta_\pi^R(r)$ are considered to be known since a one-to-one relationship exists between $\alpha_R(r)$ and $\beta_\pi^R(r)$. (Rayleigh scattering has a unique normalized angular scattering function.) Data on the $\alpha_R(r)$ profile are taken from the standard model of a Rayleigh atmosphere. It is also assumed that the transmittance of the atmospheric layer between the transmitting–receiving system and the probed volume is known or can be regarded as close to unity and ignored. This quantity can also be determined in the course of atmospheric probing, as we shall discuss later.

Under the given assumptions, we use the results of single-frequency probing to arrive directly at the profile of the volume aerosol extinction coefficient in the backward direction $\beta_\pi^M(r)$ at the probing frequency (wavelength) since all quantities entering into (7.1) are now known (the calibration constant $\eta$, which accounts for light-reflection losses in the optical sections of the receiving and transmitting systems and the quantum efficiency of the receiver are presumed to be known beforehand). The $\beta_\pi^M(r)$ profile provides a concept of the stratification of aerosol layers in the atmosphere and a qualitative picture of the corresponding distribution of the aerosol mass.

The most interesting data pertain to the profiles of the volume aerosol extinction coefficient $\alpha_M(r)$ and the microphysical parameters of aerosols (concentration, size spectrum, shape, and refractive index of the particles). All of these data are contained in the quantity $\beta_\pi^M(r)$, and their extraction requires the adoption of additional assumptions or suitable independent measurements.

The values of $\alpha_M(r)$ can be obtained from the values of $\beta_\pi^M(r)$ if the ratio between these quantities, called the lidar ratio, is known:

$$b(r) = \frac{\beta_\pi^M(r)}{\alpha_M(r)} \tag{7.5}$$

It is understood that every aerosol angular scattering function (see Chap. 3) is matched by a particular value of the ratio $b$, so that the problem of obtaining the $\alpha_M(r)$ profiles from data on the $\beta_\pi^M(r)$ profiles with single-frequency probing turns out to be far from unambiguous, and it becomes important to know the values of the lidar ratios. We shall discuss this problem separately below. At this point, we merely note that it is customary to assume for the acquisition of data on the $\alpha_M(r)$ profiles from the $\beta_\pi^M(r)$ profiles that the ratio $b$ does not vary along the probing path and that its numerical value can be determined from appropriate measurements in the ground layer of the atmosphere.

In order to obtain data on the profiles of the number of aerosol particles per unit volume or the mass concentration of particles from the results of single-frequency laser probing, it is necessary to invoke an additional assumption about the size distribution, complex refractive index, and shape of the particles. The particles in this case are assumed to be spherical so that the results of Mie theory can be used in solving the stated problem.

Despite the many assumptions used, the data obtained in single-frequency laser probing on the profiles of the volume aerosol extinction coefficient, number of particles per unit volume, and mass concentration of particles yield a qualitatively correct picture of the processes. Not much can be said, of course, about the quantitative consistency of the results with reality. It is important, therefore, not only to analyze the foregoing assumptions, but also to develop methods for laser probing of the atmosphere whereby the use of *a priori* information can be eliminated altogether or at least restricted in volume. The ensuing sections of the chapter are concerned specifically with these problems.

## 7.3. Separation of the Aerosol and Molecular Components of Echo Signals

The reasonably accurate separation of a laser echo signal ("lidar return") into the components associated with aerosol attenuation and Rayleigh scattering is of fundamental importance, first, insofar as it obviates the need for any hypothesis about the known Rayleigh component and, second, because knowledge of the latter automatically solves the problem of acquiring data on the atmospheric density profiles since $\alpha_R$ and $\beta_\pi^R$ are related one-to-one with the number of molecules per unit volume. Knowledge of the density, in turn, provides us with information on the pressure and temperature because these three quantities are interrelated by two well-known equations: the equation of state and the hydrostatic equation.

The problem of separating the components of an echo signal can be solved on the basis of laser probing methods equipped for the reception of several echo signals. The latter can be, for example, signals obtained at the probing frequency and at the Raman scattering frequency of one of the gaseous components of the atmosphere with an already known scattering cross section and profile, say $N_2$. Aspects of the theory of separation of an echo signal for this case are discussed in detail in our paper [15]. However, the indicated systems have an essential shortcoming in that the small value of the Raman scattering cross section imposes a low monitoring ceiling. Multifrequency laser monitoring systems, for which we have developed a corresponding theory [16], appear more promising. Following is a brief outline of that theory.

Let us consider the case of probing of the atmosphere by pulses with two different wavelengths $\lambda_1$ and $\lambda_2$, for which the lidar equations are written in the form

$$P_r(r,\lambda_1)=\eta(\lambda_1)P_0(\lambda_1)Ar^{-2}\left(\frac{c\tau}{2}\right)$$

$$\times\left[\beta_\pi^R(r,\lambda_1)+\beta_\pi^M(r,\lambda_1)\right]T_R(r,\lambda_1)T_M(r,\lambda_1) \qquad (7.6)$$

$$P_r(r,\lambda_2)=\eta(\lambda_2)P_0(\lambda_2)Ar^{-2}\left(\frac{c\tau}{2}\right)$$

$$\times\left[\beta_\pi^R(r,\lambda_2)+\beta_\pi^M(r,\lambda_2)\right]T_R(r,\lambda_2)T_M(r,\lambda_2) \qquad (7.7)$$

where

$$T(r,\lambda)=\exp\left[-2\int_{r_1}^{r_2}\alpha(r,\lambda)\,dr\right] \tag{7.8}$$

and the rest of the notation is the same as in (7.1)

For the system (7.6)–(7.7) to be determinate for a pair of characteristics $\beta_\pi^R$ and $\beta_\pi^M$, we introduce additional coupling relations of the form

$$\beta_\pi^R(\lambda_1)=k_1\beta_\pi^R(\lambda_2);\qquad \beta_\pi^R(\lambda_1)=k_2\alpha_R(\lambda_1);\qquad \alpha_R(\lambda_1)=k_3\alpha_R(\lambda_2) \tag{7.9}$$

$$\beta_\pi^M(\lambda_1)=b_1\beta_\pi^M(\lambda_2);\qquad \beta_\pi^M(\lambda_1)=b_2\alpha_M(\lambda_1);\qquad \alpha_M(\lambda_1)=b_3\alpha_M(\lambda_2) \tag{7.10}$$

In the latter relations, the coefficients $k_1, k_2$, and $k_3$ are uniquely determined by the theory of Rayleigh scattering, while $b_1$, $b_2$, and $b_3$ are similarly determined by the theory of light scattering by polydisperse aerosols (Mie theory for spherical particles). For known wavelengths $\lambda_1$ and $\lambda_2$, the coefficients $k_1$, $k_2$, and $k_3$ have unique values and are determined from the well-known Rayleigh equation, whereas the coefficients $b_1$, $b_2$, and $b_3$ can assume different values, depending on the microphysical parameters of the aerosol. These coefficients can be selected on the basis of statistically supported data from appropriate experimental studies, to be discussed in the next section.

For the solution of the system (7.6)–(7.7), an iterative algorithm has been developed, similar to the one described in our earlier work [15].

The condition for convergence of this algorithm is the relation

$$\frac{\beta_\pi^R(\lambda_1)}{\beta_\pi^R(\lambda_2)}\neq\frac{\beta_\pi^M(\lambda_1)}{\beta_\pi^M(\lambda_2)} \tag{7.11}$$

which is practically always fulfilled. Accordingly, the proposed method is aptly called the method of functional separation of the components of an echo signal by atmospheric constituents since it is based on the diverse spectral behavior of the optical characteristics of the gaseous and aerosol constituents. The effectiveness of the method improves as the number of wavelengths is increased. If the number of wavelengths is greater than two, the corresponding system of equations can be solved by the method of least squares.

Laser systems used for probing of the upper atmosphere operate by storing the number of received photons from specific layers of the atmosphere. In this case, the system of equations (7.6)–(7.7) is conveniently written in discrete form with the following as measurable quantities:

$$I_i = \int_{r_1}^{r_{i+1}} \frac{P_r(r)r^2}{P_0\eta}\,dr \tag{7.12}$$

where $i$ is the index enumerating the probed layer. In the case of two-wavelength probing, the system (7.6)–(7.7) takes the following form for the $i$th layer:

$$\frac{I_{i,1}}{T_{i-1,i}h_i} = \left[\beta_\pi^R(r_i,\lambda_1) + \beta_\pi^M(r_i,\lambda_1)\right]Q(\tau_{i,1}) \tag{7.13}$$

$$\frac{I_{i,2}}{T_{i-1,2}h_i} = \left[\beta_\pi^R(r_i,\lambda_2) + \beta_\pi^M(r_i,\lambda_2)\right]Q(\tau_{i,2}) \tag{7.14}$$

where

$$h_i = r_{i+1} - r_i, \qquad T_{i-1,j} = \exp\left[-2\sum_{n=1}^{i-1}\tau_{n,j}\right],$$

$$Q(\tau) = 1 - \frac{e^{-2\tau}}{2\tau}, \qquad \tau_{i,j} = h_i\alpha_i(\lambda_j), \qquad j=1,2$$

An illustration of the influence of the measurement errors and errors of specification of $b_1$, $b_2$, and $b_3$ on the accuracy of determination of the components $\beta_\pi^R$ and $\beta_\pi^M$ is given in [16] for two- and three-frequency probing of the atmospheric layer up to a height of 10 km and for two-frequency probing of the atmospheric layer from 10 to 50 km. The same paper indicates a number of inaccuracies in [17–19], which discuss the method of two-frequency probing for separation of the echo-signal components into aerosol and gaseous constituents.

The use of two-frequency laser probing of the atmosphere for separation of the echo signal into atmospheric constituents is also proposed in [20–22].

## 7.4. Investigations of the Lidar Ratio

The ratio of the volume aerosol backscattering coefficient to the volume aerosol scattering coefficient is uniquely determined by the polydisperse angular scattering function, which varies between very wide limits as a function of the nature of the aerosols, their past history, the stage of development of atmospheric moisture, and other characteristics. To the complete determination of the lidar ratio, of course, it suffices to know the polydisperse angular scattering functions. Consequently, all existing data on the latter can be recruited for the determination of the quantity $b$, and new measurements can similarly be based on the use of investigations of the angular scattering function. This procedure, however, is too complex and is unwarranted solely for the purpose of obtaining information about the lidar ratio.

The lidar ratio can be determined with the simultaneous application of lidar and a transmittance meter in the ground layer of the atmosphere or on board an aircraft in a cloudy medium, or even by means of two lidar systems. It is extremely important in this case, in conjuction with the determination of this ratio, to also measure such atmospheric parameters as the humidity, temperature, and wind, which data make it possible to interpret correctly the results of investigations. Requirements of this type are met in recent studies [23–33].

Balin and others [23–24] have investigated the relationship of the lidar ratio to the relative humidity in the ground layer. The measurements were performed at the field base station of the Main Geophysical Observatory at Voeikovo, below Leningrad. The volume aerosol scattering coefficient $\alpha$ and average value of the volume aerosol backscattering coefficient $\beta_\pi^M$ were measured simultaneously along a 940-m baseline. The coefficient $\alpha_M$ was determined by the basic method, and $\beta_\pi^M$ was determined by means of lidar with the use of a ruby laser ($\lambda = 0.6943$ $\mu$m). The results of a correlation analysis of 53 samples are given in Table 7.1, where the majority of the measurement samples (70%) were obtained for a meteorological visibility range $V_M = 15$ km. In Table 7.1, $f$ is the relative humidity.

It is evident from the table that an increase in the relative humidity is accompanied by an increase in the volume aerosol extinction coefficient, whereas the lidar ratio varies appreciably only in the interval of relative humidities $f < 70\%$. The cross-correlation coefficient $R_{b/f}$ is equal to 0.96 in the humidity interval from 35 to 70% and to 0.06 in the interval from 70 to 95%. For the high humidities characteristic of the presence of strong haze

Table 7.1.

| $f,\%$ | 35–39 | 40–49 | 50–59 | 60–69 | 70–79 | 80–89 | 90–95 |
|---|---|---|---|---|---|---|---|
| $\bar{\alpha},\mathrm{km}^{-1}$ | 0.09 | 0.12 | 0.21 | 0.28 | 0.42 | 0.59 | 0.75 |
| $\bar{b}$ | 0.052 | 0.042 | 0.036 | 0.029 | 0.025 | 0.024 | 0.026 |

and light fog (4 km$\leqslant V_M \leqslant 10$ km), the average value of the lidar ratio is in good agreement with the calculated results of Gol'dberg [34]. On the whole, the behavior of the function $b=b(f)$ is qualitatively consistent with the values calculated on the basis of Mie theory [35]. The average value $\bar{b}$ for the humidity interval from 35 to 70% agrees with the value proposed by Hamilton [36] for all hazes.

Least-squares processing of the experimental data yields the approximate expression

$$b(f)=0.0039+1.6f^{-1}+4f^{-2} \tag{7.15}$$

We note that relation (7.15) has been obtained for an air mass with a stable prevailing northerly wind from inland. This relation no longer holds with the appearance of a new air mass blowing from the sea.

Toropova and Ten [25] have analyzed data obtained on the influence of the relative humidity on the value of the lidar ratio from corresponding measurements in various geographical regions and at different times. The analysis shows that a reduction of the lidar ratio with increasing relative humidity is observed in every case. The reduction is more pronounced, the shorter the meteorological range. In the case of high transmittance, situations occurred in which the value of the lidar ratio did not change with variation of the relative humidity from 34 to 87%.

Summarizing the problem of the influence of relative humidity on the lidar ratio in the ground layer of the atmosphere, we note that the data obtained by different authors, while supporting the general trend of a reduction in the lidar ratio with increasing relative humidity, still evince a considerable scatter of the points in this relation. This fact is illustrated by Fig. 7.1, which is taken from the cited paper [25]. In future studies of this problem, it would be very desirable to perform complex experiments with simultaneous measurements of the lidar ratio, relative humidity, wind, and microphysical parameters of the aerosols. By carrying out such measurements with certain representative aerosol ensembles (for example, at least with separation of the aerosols into overland and overwater types), it should be possible to obtain appropriate correlation relations with maximum values of the cross-correlation coefficients $R_{b/f}$. High values of the coefficients $R_{b/f}$ are to be expected, for example, in the atmospheres over large open-pit operations, where the aerosol is generated by a source that varies little with time.

Several studies [26–33] have been devoted to the vertical profile of the lidar ratio, for which it is important to have data in connection with the

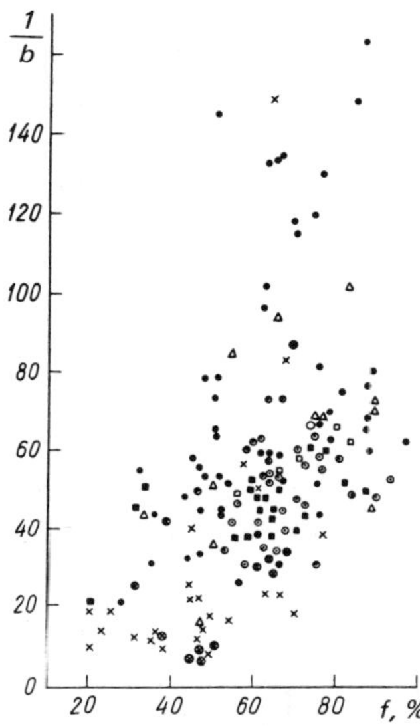

Fig. 7.1. Experimental data on the quantity $1/b$ for various values of the relative humidity.

interpretation of the results of laser probing of aerosols with the use of single-frequency lidar. The vertical profiles of the lidar ratio were obtained by the simultaneous application of two lidars using ruby lasers ($\lambda = 6943$ Å), one situated on the ground for sensing of the atmosphere in the vertical direction and the other on board an aircraft flying through the sensing zone of the first lidar at various heights. The airborne lidar was used to determine the volume aerosol backscattering coefficient $\beta_\pi^M$ at the corresponding heights. The values obtained for $\beta_\pi^M$ were substituted into the lidar equation, from which the volume aerosol scattering coefficient was then determined. The measurements of $\beta_\pi^M$ were carried out from atmospheric volumes roughly 100 m from the aircraft, permitting the attenuation of the atmospheric layer from the lidar to the probed volume to be neglected.

Simultaneously with the determination of $\beta_\pi^M$, measurements were performed on the standard meteorological parameters by means of radiosondes as well as from an aircraft. Figure 7.2 gives one illustration of the results obtained, clearly exhibiting the height dependence of the lidar ratio and its correlation with the relative humidity at heights from 200 to 1500 m. An analysis of the results of investigations of $b(r)$ and $\alpha_M(r)$ with the simultaneous application of ground-based and airborne lidars during the spring of 1975 near the city of Tomsk indicates the presence of a frequently encountered layered structure in the vertical distribution of atmospheric aerosols, the greatest temporal and spatial variations of this structure taking

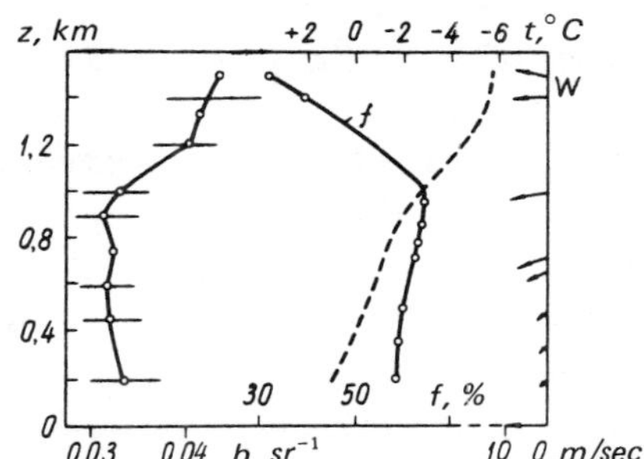

Fig. 7.2. Height variations of the lidar ratio (left curve), relative humidity $f$, temperature (dashed curve), and wind velocity vector **W**.

place in the bottom 1-km layer. However, despite the structural inhomogeneity of the atmosphere when it is in a relatively stable state, the lidar ratio does not experience large variations with height. An exception is found in height intervals characterized by temperature inversion, which is clearly manifested in the vertical variation of $b(r)$.

To obtain data on the vertical profile of the lidar ratio in the boundary layer of the atmosphere, Balin and others [28, 33] have proposed the application of two ground-based lidars operating simultaneously in reception and transmission and located in such a way that their optical axes intersect at a 135° angle. Each lidar in this case records echo signals from the total scattering volume at angles of 45 and 180°, and so it is possible to write a system of four lidar equations, the solution of which yields the following expression for the lidar ratio:

$$b = \frac{K}{4\pi}\left[\frac{P_1(h)P_2(h)}{P_1'(h)P_2'(h)}\right]^{1/2} \tag{7.16}$$

where $K$ is evaluated by the nephelometric method of determining the volume aerosol extinction coefficient

$$\sigma = 4\pi K^{-1}\sigma(45°) \tag{7.17}$$

$P_1(h)$, $P_2(h)$, $P_1'(h)$, and $P_2'(h)$ are the echo signals from the scattering volume at height $h$ at angles 180 and 45°. For the majority of situations encountered in the atmosphere, the quantity $K$ is equal to 1.45 within 10% error limits [37, 38].

By successively varying the angular positions and azimuths of both lidars in such a way as to keep the angle between their optical axes constant, it is possible to investigate the height variation of the lidar ratio. The height interval in this case depends both on the potentials of the lidars and on their separation. The higher the frequencies at which it is required to obtain the values of $b(h)$, the greater must be the lidar potentials and the baseline between them.

The method described above has been used to determine the profiles of the lidar ratio at two wavelengths, 0.69 and 0.53 $\mu$m (ruby laser and the second harmonic of a neodymium–glass laser) in the boundary layer of the atmosphere (height to 260 m, lidar baseline equal to 1300 m). The spatial resolution in the measurements was not worse than 4 m. An analysis of the results of the investigations leads to the following conclusions: The most marked variations of $b(r)$ and $\alpha_M(r)$ with height are observed in the bottom 100-m layer of the atmosphere. The growth of the lidar ratio indicates a corresponding rearrangement of the aerosol particle-size spectrum. At heights above 100 m, in the absence of temperature inversions, a further decrease takes place in the volume aerosol extinction coefficient, whereas the lidar ratio essentially remains constant, evincing the fact that the microphysical composition of the aerosols is essentially invariant, only the particle concentration changing. This result is consistent with the theoretical prediction of the height variation of the parameters of finely disperse aerosols [39].

When temperature inversion layers are present in the atmosphere, they are clearly evinced in the height profiles of $b(r)$ and $\alpha(r)$, where either profile exhibits extrema in the inversion zone; the maxima of $\alpha_M(r)$ are juxtaposed with the minima of the height variation of the lidar ratio. The method makes it possible to determine the linear dimensions of the inversion layers, which turn out to be of the order of 50 m. The particle-size distribution in these layers differs from the distribution in the upper and lower contiguous layers. The indicated laws are observed for both wavelengths of the probe pulses.

We conclude this section with an illustration of the correlation between the volume backscattering coefficient and the volume extinction coefficient in a fog at various stages of its development, during which the particle-size spectrum undergoes substantial variations. Figure 7.3 gives the results of corresponding measurements carried out by Alan and Bateman [40] and reported at the Seventh International Laser Radar Conference in November 1975 at the Stanford Research Institute. The quantity $n$ in this figure represents the constant in the empirical formula

$$\beta_\pi^M = \mathcal{Q}[\alpha(r)]^n \tag{7.18}$$

in which $\mathcal{Q}$ is an empirical constant.

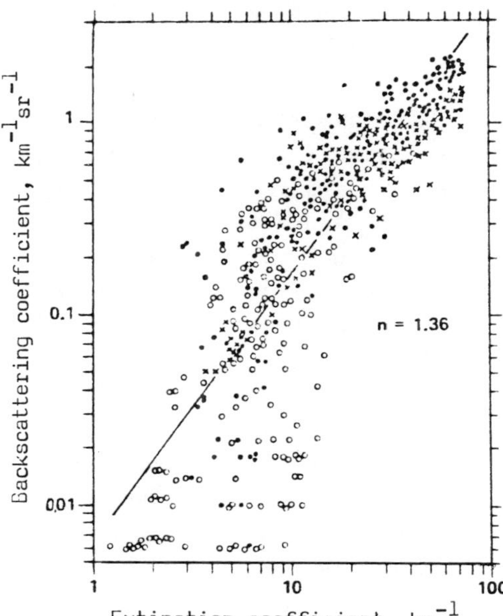



Fig. 7.3. Correlation between the backscattering and extinction coefficients in fog during a 2 h 30 min period on Feb. 24, 1975. (○) First 50 min; (·) second 50 min; (×) third 50 min.

The curve in Fig. 7.3, as noted in [40], is not typical. In the majority of cases, the authors observed a much stronger correlation between $\beta_\pi^M$ and $\alpha(r)$ than is represented in this figure. The quantity $n$ in (7.18) in this case varies from 1.1 to 1.5 (the most typical value is 1.4), and for an arbitrary standard value $\alpha(r)=20$ $km^{-1}$ the coefficient $\beta_\pi^M$ varies from 0.1 to 0.8 $km^{-1}$ (the most typical value is 0.3).

Thus, many interesting data have been obtained in recent years on the behavior of the lidar ratio under various atmospheric conditions. However, the final resolution of this problem requires still greater diligence on the part of researchers, which will doubtless promote the new research techniques developed in recent years and described in this section. As already emphasized above, it is extremely important to accompany these investigations with a determination of the microphysical parameters of the atmospheric aerosol and to carry them out for definite types of aerosol ensembles. Serious attention must be given to studies of the height variation of the lidar ratio in various characteristic zones, particularly insofar as this variation is a conclusive indication of the transformation of the particle-size spectra with height in the atmosphere.

## 7.5. Influence of Multiple-Scattering Effects on Probing Results

The atmospheric lidar equation (7.1) has been derived with only the consideration of single events of interaction between the probe pulse and the atmospheric layers. However, in optically dense media (such as clouds) or in connection with the transmission of a pulse through larger optical thicknesses, multiple-scattering effects can yield a significant contribution to the amplitude of the echo signal and thus influence the probing results obtained on the basis of expression (7.1).

The multiple-scattering contribution depends on the optical thickness of the medium traversed by the probe pulse, the geometrical parameters of the lidar transmitting and receiving systems, the scattering coefficient and angular function, and the distance to the probed volume. In this connection, the multiple-scattering contribution depends most strongly on the distance $r$ to the probed volume, the angular aperture of the receiver $\varphi$, and the volume aerosol extinction coefficient $\alpha_M$. For the sake of generality, it is convenient to consolidate the three indicated factors into a single dimensionless parameter $\tilde{\eta}$:

$$\tilde{\eta} = r\alpha_M \tan\varphi \qquad (7.18a)$$

Detailed studies of the indicated relations have been carried out [41–45]. The most effective method of investigation in this case is found to be the Monte Carlo approach, which makes it possible to obtain data concerning the influence of any scattering multiples on the echo signals for any set of parameters affecting the echo signal. Table 7.2 gives the results of a calculation of the role of multiple-scattering effects according to the Monte Carlo method.

The first column of the table lists the optical thicknesses of the probed layer. The other columns give the values of $(I_{ms}/I_{ss})\times 100\%$, which characterizes the ratio between the signal levels generated solely as a result of the multiple-scattering background $I_{ms}$ and due to single scattering $I_{ss}$ as a function of the parameter $\tilde{\eta}$ characterizing the geometry of the experiment.

It is sufficient in many practical situations to limit the consideration to double-scattering effects [45]. Accordingly, a number of authors have obtained appropriate expressions [46–55] and have estimated the roles of double scattering in the formation of laser echo signals under various probing conditions. We now summarize some of those results.

The most general expression for the results of lidar studies in the atmosphere in the double-scattering approximation with allowance for

**Table 7.2.** Role of Multiple-Scattering Effects in the Formation of Laser-Pulse Echo Signals: The Quantity $(I_{\mathrm{ms}}/I_{\mathrm{ss}}) \times 100\%$ as a Function of $\tau$ and $\tilde{\eta}$.

| | $\tilde{\eta}$ | | | | | | |
|---|---|---|---|---|---|---|---|
| $\tau$ | 0.0029 | 0.00582 | 0.00873 | 0.0174 | 0.0262 | 0.0436 | 0.0654 |
| 0.3 | 1.1 | 2.1 | 7.2 | 15.0 | 33.8 | 44.3 | 70.8 |
| 0.6 | 1.5 | 3.2 | 10.0 | 20.3 | 36.6 | 53.7 | 78.1 |
| 0.9 | 1.9 | 4.8 | 12.9 | 24.1 | 41.3 | 62.2 | 86.3 |
| 1.2 | 2.2 | 5.3 | 15.1 | 26.4 | 43.0 | 66.3 | 89.8 |
| 1.5 | 2.8 | 6.9 | 16.7 | 28.5 | 45.3 | 69.1 | 95.0 |
| 1.8 | 3.0 | 8.1 | 18.5 | 30.7 | 47.4 | 72.8 | 102.0 |
| 2.1 | 3.2 | 9.8 | 20.0 | 32.1 | 50.5 | 76.1 | 106.2 |
| 2.4 | 3.4 | 11.0 | 21.2 | 34.8 | 54.3 | 80.5 | 110.3 |
| 2.7 | 3.6 | 11.5 | 22.1 | 35.7 | 56.7 | 85.6 | 115.1 |
| 3.0 | 3.8 | 12.2 | 23.0 | 39.0 | 59.1 | 88.3 | 119.8 |
| 3.3 | 4.0 | 13.0 | 24.1 | 41.9 | 61.6 | 92.7 | 125.3 |
| 3.6 | 4.2 | 13.3 | 24.9 | 44.5 | 64.8 | 96.4 | 131.1 |
| 3.9 | 4.4 | 13.9 | 25.5 | 46.6 | 67.8 | 100.0 | 135.6 |
| 4.2 | 4.6 | 14.4 | 26.1 | 48.2 | 70.3 | 104.2 | 140.8 |
| 4.5 | 4.8 | 15.0 | 27.3 | 51.3 | 72.9 | 107.3 | 145.2 |
| 5.0 | 6.2 | 17.8 | 30.1 | 58.2 | 83.2 | 117.4 | 160.7 |

polarization effects has been derived in [51, 55]. In the case of a combined receiving and transmitting lidar device, small spread angles, and short probe pulses, the radiant flux reflected by the scattering medium is written as the sum of the singly and doubly scattered fluxes. Double scattering is represented by the sum of two fluxes, one of which is generated by primary forward-scattered photons, while the second contains photons for which both scattering events are directed into the back hemisphere.

The lidar equation is written in the summation form

$$\mathbf{I} = \mathbf{I}^{(1)} + \mathbf{I}^{(2)} \tag{7.19}$$

where $\mathbf{I}^{(1)}$ is the Stokes vector determined by the lidar equation in the single-scattering approximation, $\mathbf{I}^{(2)}$ is the Stokes vector in the double-scattering approximation, for which the following expression has been obtained for an arbitrary type of scattering matrix:

$$\mathbf{I}^{(2)}(r) = 2P_0 \Delta r \alpha_M(r) \exp\left[-2\int_0^r \alpha_M(r')\,dr'\right] \int_0^{2\pi} d\psi \int_0^{\pi/2} d\theta$$

$$\times \int_{x(\theta)}^r \sin\theta\,\hat{K}(\psi)\hat{f}(\theta')\hat{f}(\theta)K(\psi)\mathbf{S}^0\alpha_M(x)\,dx \tag{7.20}$$

$\theta$ is the scattering angle, $\theta' = \pi - \theta + \dfrac{1}{2}\Phi$

$$x(\theta) = r(1 - \tan\theta_0 \cot\theta)$$

$P_0$ is the power of the probe pulse, $2\Delta r = c\tau$ is the geometrical pulse length, $c$ is the speed of light, $\tau$ is the pulse duration, $\alpha_M(r)$ is the volume scattering coefficient, $\psi$ is the angle of rotation about the reference plane representing the origin, $\Phi$ is the angular aperture of the receiver, $K(\psi)$ is the matrix operator of rotation of the reference plane, $\hat{f}(\theta)$ is the scattering matrix, and $\mathbf{S}^0$ is the dimensionless Stokes vector.

Equation (7.20) is next written for the Mie scattering matrix, i.e., for an ensemble of spherical particles. The initial scattering matrix in this case is taken to be

$$\hat{f}(\theta) = \begin{bmatrix} f_1(\theta) & f_2(\theta) & 0 & 0 \\ f_2(\theta) & f_1(\theta) & 0 & 0 \\ 0 & 0 & f_3(\theta) & f_4(\theta) \\ 0 & 0 & -f_4(\theta) & f_3(\theta) \end{bmatrix} \qquad (7.21)$$

The scattering matrix is diagonalized to simplify the ensuing transformations:

$$\hat{\lambda}(\theta) = \begin{bmatrix} f_1(\theta) + f_2(\theta) & 0 & 0 & 0 \\ 0 & f_1(\theta) - f_2(\theta) & 0 & 0 \\ 0 & 0 & f_3(\theta) - if_4(\theta) & 0 \\ 0 & 0 & 0 & f_3(\theta) + if_4(\theta) \end{bmatrix}$$

$$(7.22)$$

The elements of this matrix are the eigenvalues of the scattering matrix.

Equation (7.20) is now rewritten for each component $I_i^{(2)}$ corresponding to the vector $I^{(2)}$ in (7.20):

$$I_i^{(2)} = 2P_0 \Delta r \alpha_M(r) \exp\left[-2\int_0^r \alpha_M(r')\,dr'\right] \int_0^{\pi/2} d\theta \int_{x(\theta)}^r dx$$

$$\times \int_0^{2\pi} \alpha_M(x) \sin\theta K'_{ij}(\psi)\lambda_j(\theta')\lambda_j(\theta)K'_{jk}(\psi)R_k^0\,d\psi \qquad (7.23)$$

where $K'_{jk}$ denotes the elements of the operator of rotation of the reference plane, $\lambda_j(\theta')$ and $\lambda_j(\theta)$ are the elements of the scattering matrix, the index $j$ refers to the row and column number since the matrix is diagonal, and $R_k^0$ is the component of the dimensionless Stokes vector in the new basis.

Making use of relation (7.23), we obtain an expression for the degree of polarization of doubly scattered radiation when the medium is irradiated by, for example, linearly polarized light. For two mutually perpendicular components, we obtain from (7.23)

$$I_1^{(2)} = \tfrac{1}{2}\pi P_0 \Delta r \alpha_M(r)\exp\left[-2\int_0^r \alpha_M(r')\,dr'\right]\int_0^{\pi/2}d\theta\int_{x(\theta)}^r \alpha_M(x)\sin\theta$$

$$\times\left\{3\left[\lambda_1(\theta')\lambda_1(\theta)+\lambda_2(\theta')\lambda_2(\theta)\right]-\left[\lambda_3(\theta')\lambda_3(\theta)+\lambda_4(\theta')\lambda_4(\theta)\right]\right\}dx$$

$$(7.24)$$

$$I_2^{(2)} = \tfrac{1}{2}\pi P_0 \Delta r \alpha_M(r)\exp\left[-2\int_0^r \alpha_M(r')\,dr'\right]\int_0^{\pi/2}d\theta\int_{x(\theta)}^r \alpha_M(x)\sin\theta$$

$$\times\left[\lambda_1(\theta')\lambda_1(\theta)+\lambda_2(\theta')\lambda_2(\theta)+\lambda_3(\theta')\lambda_3(\theta)+\lambda_4(\theta')\lambda_4(\theta)\right]dx \quad (7.25)$$

In the case of a homogeneous path, $\alpha(r)=\text{const}$, and expressions (7.24)–(7.25) are simplified. Without writing out these simplified expressions for $I_1^{(2)}$ and $I_2^{(2)}$, we give the final equation for the degree of polarization of doubly scattered radiation, defined in the usual way, for this case:

$$p=\frac{I_1^{(2)}-I_2^{(2)}}{I_1^{(2)}+I_2^{(2)}}=\frac{1}{2}\frac{1-\int_0^{\pi/2}\left[\lambda_3(\theta')\lambda_3(\theta)+\lambda_4(\theta')\lambda_4(\theta)\right]\cos\theta\,d\theta}{\int_0^{\pi/2}\left[\lambda_1(\theta')\lambda_1(\theta)+\lambda_2(\theta')\lambda_2(\theta)\right]\cos\theta\,d\theta}$$

$$(7.26)$$

Estimates by Kaul' and others [45] have shown that the total contribution of higher-order scattering is not more than 10% for an optical thickness $\tau=3$ if the parameter $\tilde{\eta}$ (7.18a) is not greater than 0.01, corresponding, for example, to the case of probing of a cloud from a distance of 1 km with $\alpha_M=20$ km$^{-1}$ (most probable value) and a receiving system with a field of view (f.o.v.) equal to $1'$.

In the probing of hazes, multiple-scattering effects can be taken into account with sufficient practical accuracy in the double-scattering approximation [45].

## 7.6. Inverse Problems of Laser Probing of Atmospheric Aerosols

In the preceding sections, we have discussed problems relating to the extraction of information about the profiles of the volume aerosol extinction coefficients and estimation of the particle concentration from the results of single-frequency laser probing. However, it is most important from the scientific and practical standpoint to obtain data on the microphysical parameters of aerosols: the concentration, size distribution, complex refractive index, and shape of the particles. Unambiguous data on these parameters cannot be obtained from the results of single-frequency probing in a monostatic configuration due to the restricted volume of measurement information. It is quite clear that the greater the amount of data available on the microphysical parameters of aerosols to be obtained, the greater must be the volume of information afforded by the corresponding measurements. It is possible to realize this kind of probing in a monostatic configuration by using several probe frequencies. The use of a bistatic configuration makes it possible to increase the quantity of measurement information as a result of measurement of the echo signals at different scattering angles. Finally, the measurement information can be increased by utilizing the effect of polarization of scattered radiation and other effects.

The solution of inverse problems associated with laser probing of the atmosphere in its present stage of development is particularly important in connection with the fact that only the unambiguous extraction of information on specific monitored parameters will ensure progress in the extensive scientific and practical application of laser methods. We therefore give special attention to this section. The content of the material is mainly based on work carried out under the direction of the author in recent years [56–73]. Reference to individual works will be made as necessary.

### 7.6.1. Methods for Determining the Microstructure of an Aerosol in Multifrequency Laser Probing

Information on the microphysical parameters of an aerosol and, in particular, on the particle-size distribution, extracted from corresponding spectral measurements, is contained in an integral of the form

$$\beta(\lambda) = \int_{a_1}^{a_2} Q(\lambda, a) f(a)\, da \qquad (7.27)$$

in which $f(a)$ is the particle-size distribution function and $Q(\lambda, a)$ is the efficiency factor corresponding to a given experiment; the particles are assumed to be spherical. In laser probing of the atmosphere, $\beta(\lambda)$ can be interpreted as the volume aerosol extinction coefficient in the backward direction $\beta_\pi^M(\lambda, a)$.

It is obvious that the choice of method for solving the inverse problem depends on the "goodness" of the measurement information and the reliability of the initial assumptions. It has been shown in this connection [70] that if the number of probing wavelengths is not greater than four, the optical measurement error falls within the limits of 10–15%, the errors of specification of the real and imaginary parts of the complex refractive index of the aerosol particles do not exceed $\pm 0.05$ and $\pm 0.005$, respectively, and better results are provided by the optimal parametrization method, which has absolute stability in the solution of ill-posed inverse problems, one of which is the problem of inversion of the integral equation (7.27). Given the indicated "goodness" of the initial information, the use of more rigorous and complex methods is not justified.

If the lidar measurement error does not exceed 5% limits and the number of wavelengths used for probing is greater than 6 to 8, the inverse problem can be solved more rigorously, namely, by the use of regularization methods.

### 7.6.1.1. Optimal Parametrization Method

The optimal parametrization method is based on the use of definite *a priori* information about the investigated effect. In particular, for the determination of the particle-size spectrum in the inversion of the integral (7.27), it is assumed, for example, that the analytical form of the distribution $n(a)$ is known. According to this method, the optical characteristic $\beta(\lambda_i)$, measured for several wavelengths, is approximated by a certain model function $\beta_M(\lambda)$ determined by the form of the distribution $n(\alpha_i a)\,da$ and the value of its parameter $\alpha_i$. An algorithm of the optimal selection of the distribution parameters is synthesized on the basis of minimization of functions of several variables in a certain domain of parameter space. We discuss the characteristics of this algorithm in the example of a modified gamma distribution of the number of particles by size, for which we have an analytical expression of the form

$$f(a)\,da = \kappa a^\alpha \exp(-\mu a^\gamma)\,da \tag{7.28}$$

in which $\alpha$, $\mu$, $\gamma$, and $\kappa$ are the distribution parameters, which are related to such characteristics of the distribution as the modal radius $a_s$, the mean radius $a_n$, the number of particles per unit volume $N$, and the particle volume per unit volume of the medium $V$ ($V$ determines the cloud water content $Q_W$) by the expressions [74]

$$\mu = \alpha/\gamma a_n^\gamma \tag{7.29}$$

$$N = \kappa \int_0^\infty a^\alpha \exp(-\mu a^\gamma)\, da = \kappa \gamma^{-1} \mu^{-(\alpha+1)/\gamma} \Gamma\left(\frac{\alpha+1}{\gamma}\right) \tag{7.30}$$

$$V = \tfrac{4}{3}\pi\kappa \int_0^\infty a^{\alpha+3} \exp(-\mu a^\gamma)\, da = \tfrac{4}{3}\kappa\pi\gamma^{-1} \mu^{-(\alpha+4)/\gamma} \Gamma\left(\frac{\alpha+4}{\gamma}\right) \tag{7.31}$$

The optical properties of a polydisperse scattering medium are determined both by the concentration and the sizes of the particles, so that, instead of the distribution $f(a)$, it is useful to work with the distribution of the particles per unit volume by their geometrical cross section $G_p(a)$ with the modal radius $a_s$. In light of the foregoing, in place of the parameter $N = \int_0^\infty f(a)\, da$, we introduce into the optimal parametrization algorithm the parameter $S = \int_0^\infty G_p(a)\, da$, which characterizes the total geometrical cross section of the particles per unit volume. The distribution functions $G_p(a)$ and $f(a)$ are related by the simple equation

$$G_p(a)\, da = \pi a^2 f(a)\, da \tag{7.32}$$

We thus arrive at the new system of parameters $S$, $a_s$, $\alpha$, and $\gamma$, for which

$$S = N\pi a_s^2 \left[\Gamma\left(\frac{\alpha+3}{\gamma}\right) \middle/ \Gamma\left(\frac{\alpha+1}{\gamma}\right)\right]\left(\frac{\gamma}{\alpha+2}\right)^{2/\gamma}; \qquad a_s = a_n\left(\frac{\alpha+2}{\alpha}\right)^{1/\gamma};$$

$$V = \tfrac{4}{3}Sa_s\left(\frac{\gamma}{\alpha+2}\right)^{1/\gamma}\left[\Gamma\left(\frac{\alpha+4}{\gamma}\right) \middle/ \Gamma\left(\frac{\alpha+3}{\gamma}\right)\right] \tag{7.33}$$

We now write the expression for $\beta(\lambda)$ in terms of $S$ and the polydisperse extinction efficiency factor $\overline{Q}(a,\lambda)$ in the new variables:

$$\beta(\lambda) = S\overline{Q}(\lambda) = S\int_0^\infty Q(a,\lambda)\varphi(a)\, da \tag{7.34}$$

where

$$\varphi(a) = \left[\gamma\left(\frac{\alpha+2}{\gamma}\right)^{(\alpha+3)/\gamma}\left(\frac{a}{a_s}\right)^{\alpha+2} \middle/ a_s\Gamma\left(\frac{\alpha+3}{\gamma}\right)\right]\exp\left[-\frac{\alpha+2}{\gamma}\left(\frac{a}{a_s}\right)^\gamma\right]$$

$$\tag{7.35}$$

We represent the minimization function, which determines the degree of proximity between the measured values $\beta(\lambda_i)$ and the model values $\beta_M(\lambda_i)$ ($i=1,2,3,\ldots$) in the form

$$F(S, a_s, \alpha, \gamma) = \sum_{i=1}^{n} \left[ \beta(\lambda_i) - \beta_M(\lambda_i) \right]^2 \qquad (7.36)$$

which is a parabola with respect to the parameter $S$, and so for any fixed values of the parameters $a_s^*, \alpha^*, \gamma^*$ the value of $S$ corresponding to the minimum $F(S, a_s^*, \alpha^*, \gamma^*)$ is given by the expressions

$$S^* = \sum_{i=1}^{n} \beta(\lambda_i) \overline{Q}(\lambda_i, a_s^*, \lambda^*, \gamma^*) \bigg/ \sum_{i=1}^{n} \overline{Q}^2(\lambda_i, a_s^*, \alpha^*, \gamma^*) \qquad (7.37)$$

Accordingly, the minimization of the discrepancy (7.36) in the given case can be carried out separately for the parameter $S$ and for the variables $a_s$, $\alpha$, and $\gamma$. To do so, we go over to the relative values $\beta(\lambda_i)/\beta(\lambda_m)$, where $\lambda_m$ corresponds to the largest measured value of $\beta$. As the minimization function we consider the expression

$$F_1(a_s, \alpha, \gamma) = \sum_{i=1}^{n} \left[ \frac{\beta(\lambda_i)}{\beta(\lambda_m)} - \frac{\beta_M(\lambda_i)}{\beta_M(\lambda_m)} \right]^2 \qquad (7.37a)$$

which does not depend on $S$ and can be rewritten in the form

$$F_1(a_s, \alpha, \gamma) = \sum_{i=1 \, (i \neq m)}^{n} \left[ \frac{\beta(\lambda_i)}{\beta(\lambda_m)} - \frac{\overline{Q}(\lambda_i, a_s, \alpha, \gamma)}{\overline{Q}(\lambda_m, a_s, \alpha, \gamma)} \right]^2 \qquad (7.38)$$

An algorithm for the computation of the optimal distribution parameters is now synthesized as follows.

The method of steepest coordinate descent is used to minimize $F_1(a_s, \alpha, \gamma)$ and to determine $a_s^*$, $\alpha^*$, and $\gamma^*$ and then from the values to calculate $S^*$ by means of (7.37). The function $f(a)$ is calculated from the values obtained for the parameters, and then all the characteristics of the distribution are determined.

The choice of the method of steepest coordinate descent as the minimizing procedure for the function $F_1(a_s, \alpha, \gamma)$ is dictated by the behavior of this function in the neighborhood of the minimum point. The details of the computational procedure are described in [57,60]. Examples of the use of the optimal parametrization method in the laser probing of atmospheric aerosols will be discussed in the description of the probing results.

### 7.6.1.2. Regularization Methods

As in the optimal parametrization method, rather than the size distribution of the number of particles $n(a)\,da$, we consider the distribution of the particles by their geometrical cross section $G_p(a)$. In multifrequency laser probing of an aerosol, the characteristics of the measured quantity $\beta(\lambda)$ are determined in the form of a discrete series of points $\beta_i = \beta(\lambda_i)$ $(i = 1, 2, \ldots, n)$, where $\lambda_i$ belongs to a certain probing interval. The set of values $\{\beta(\lambda_i)\}$ can be treated as a vector $\boldsymbol{\beta}$ in space $R_n$. Then the solution of Eq. (7.27) can also be treated as a certain vector $\mathbf{S}$ in $R_m$. The choice of the number of dimensions of the solution vector $\mathbf{S}$ in the inversion of (7.27) is a crucial consideration and must be made with regard for the information content of the optical measurements [74a]. For example, in the case $m > n$ the solution is indeterminate and requires certain additions, which can be made by one of the regularization methods. In the presence of dependent measurement data, the solution must be regularized even for $m = n$.

The kernel of Eq. (7.27) has a complex analytical form. It is therefore necessary to develop algorithms for obtaining approximate estimates for the distribution function $G_p(a)$, which have practical significance for a vector $\mathbf{S}$ of few dimensions. Below we discuss one variant of the solution of this problem [58].

In place of the distribution $G_p(a)$ we seek a certain step function, or histogram $\overline{G}_p(a)$, the number of dimensions $m$ of which is determined by the values of $\Delta_l^{-1} S_l$, where $S_l = \int_{a'_l}^{a''_l} G_p(a)\,da$ and $\Delta_l = a''_l - a'_l$ is a certain partition of the interval $R(l = 1, 2, \ldots, m)$. Then (7.27) can be written in the form

$$\beta(\lambda) = \sum_l^m Q(\xi_l, \lambda) S_l \tag{7.39}$$

where $\xi_l$ is a certain point of the interval $\Delta_l$, determined by the behavior of both $Q(a, \lambda)$ and $G_p(a)$ in the given interval. The quantities $Q(\xi_l, \lambda_j)$ $(j = 1, 2, \ldots, n;\ l = 1, 2, \ldots, m)$ can be determined once $G_p(a)$ is known. We seek the coefficients $q_{jl}$ in the expression $\sum_l^m q_{jl} S_l$ so that this sum will be close to $\beta(\lambda_j)$ for any $m$. The corresponding quadrature formulas for determination of the coefficients $q_{jl}$ have been formulated by Kostin and others [58]. A numerical check of the quadrature formula

$$\beta(\lambda_i) = \sum_l^m q_{jl} S_l \tag{7.40}$$

indicates good results for integrals with Mie kernels.

For synthesis of the regularizing algorithm, we use the regularization principle of Tikhonov [75]. For the representation of (7.40), we write the regularizing functional in the form

$$F=\left[\sum_{j}^{n}\left(\sum_{l}^{m}q_{jl}S_{l}-\beta_{j}\right)^{2}\right]+\alpha\left[P_{0}\sum_{l}^{m}S_{l}^{2}+P_{1}\sum_{l}^{m-1}(\Delta S_{l,l-1})^{2}\right] \quad (7.41)$$

where $P_0$ and $P_1$ are scale factors.

To determine the effectiveness of the proposed algorithm, we have performed appropriate numerical experiments. Figure 7.4 gives an example of a distribution function of complex form. The corresponding spectral behavior of the coefficient $\beta(\lambda)$ is given in Fig. 7.5. The histogram corresponding to the distribution $G_p(a)$ in Fig. 7.4 for $m=10$ and the reconstructed histogram for $m=10$ and $n=10$ are plotted in Fig. 7.6 on the assumption that the error of determination of $\beta(\lambda)$ falls within $\pm5\%$ limits. It is evident from the figures that 10 probe wavelengths are fully adequate for sufficiently accurate reconstruction of a distribution histogram comprising 10 elements and representing a distinct double-humped distribution. The reconstruction of a simple distribution, for example, of the single-humped type, can be limited to a smaller number of wavelengths, in which case the accuracy requirements of the corresponding measurements are also relaxed.

Practical experience in the application of the proposed regularization algorithm indicates that it is simple to implement on a computer and, in comparison with conventional matrix inversion methods, has a greater stability with respect to oscillating perturbations in the initial data. The

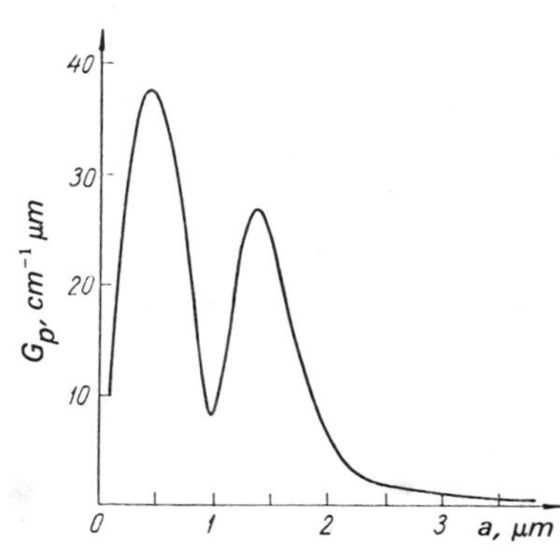


Fig. 7.4. Typical distribution function $G_p(a)$ of complex form.

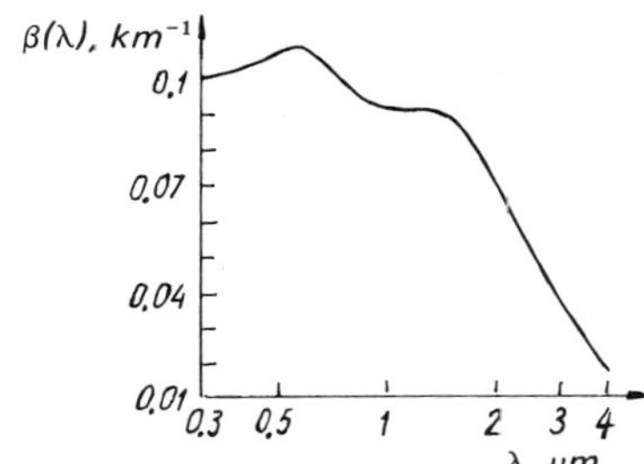

Fig. 7.5. Spectral behavior of the aerosol extinction coefficient $\beta(\lambda)$ for the distribution $G_p(a)$ in Fig. 7.4.

latter result is attributable to the fact that in actual computations this algorithm does not require construction of the inverse operator $Q^{-1}$ for the primary equation $QS=\beta$ or subsequent operations with it. It is similar in structure to the optimal parametrization algorithm, so that the concurrent application of both methods is practical in a number of instances. An example of this approach may be found in [63].

Aspects of the regularization of the solutions of Eq. (7.40) for inversion of the spectral variation of the aerosol scattering coefficient on the basis of the results of prior investigations [65] are discussed in [68].

Kostin and Naats [72] have obtained two other regularization algorithms and have carried out numerical experiments on the basis of them. We now present the fundamental results of this work.

The solution Eq. (7.27) by Tikhonov's method [75,76] is based on minimization of the functional

$$\frac{1}{(\lambda_2-\lambda_1)(R_2-R_1)^3}\int_{\lambda_1}^{\lambda_2}\left[\int_{R_1}^{R_2}Q(\lambda,a)G_p(a)\,da-\beta(\lambda)\right]^2 d\lambda$$

$$+\alpha\left\{\frac{1}{(R_2-R_1)^2}\int_{R_1}^{R_2}G_p^2(a)\,da+\int_{R_1}^{R_2}\left[\frac{dG_p(a)}{da}\right]^2 da\right\}=\min$$

$$(7.42a)$$

where $\lambda_1$ and $\lambda_2$ delimit the range of wavelengths in which the optical characteristics are measured and $\alpha$ is a regularization parameter. The functional (7.42a) is minimized by a function representing the solution of

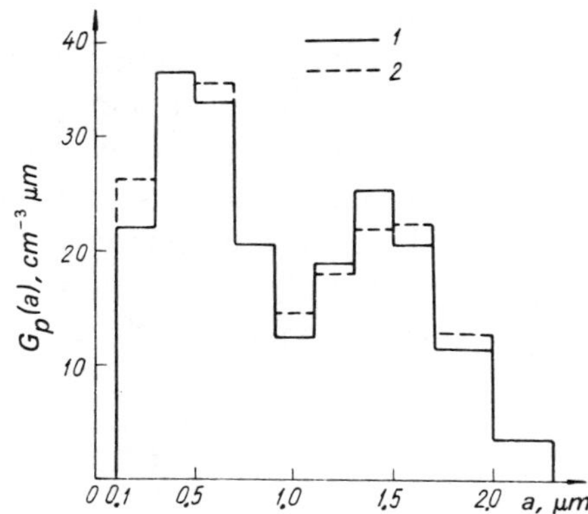



Fig. 7.6. (1) histogram $\overline{G}_p(a)$ corresponding to the distribution $G_p(a)$ in Fig. 7.4 for $m = 10$ and (2), reconstructed histogram for $m = 10$, $n = 10$.

the boundary-value problem for the Euler equation

$$\frac{1}{(\lambda_2 - \lambda_1)(R_2 - R_1)^3} \int_{R_1}^{R_2} \int_{\lambda_1}^{\lambda_2} Q(\lambda, a) Q(\lambda, \xi) G_p(\xi)\, d\lambda\, d\xi$$

$$+ \alpha \left[ \frac{1}{(R_2 - R_1)^2} G_p(a) - \frac{d^2 G_p(a)}{da^2} \right]$$

$$= \frac{1}{(\lambda_2 - \lambda_1)(R_2 - R_1)^3} \int_{\lambda_1}^{\lambda_2} Q(\lambda, a) \beta(\lambda)\, d\lambda$$

$$(7.42b)$$

The numerical solution of Eq. (7.27) by the regularization method is therefore equivalent to solution of the Euler equation corresponding to an algebraic system, which is written in the matrix notation

$$(Q + \alpha \mathcal{D}) S = k\beta \qquad (7.43)$$

The choice of the optimum value of $\alpha$ by the method proposed in [77] provides a stable solution of the system (7.43).

Ordinarily in the construction of the algebraic system the integrals in the Euler equation (7.42b) are replaced by sums on the basis of Simpson's quadrature formula [78]. To ensure the necessary accuracy of solution, it is required to increase the number of dimensions $n$ of the solution vector. The number of usable wavelengths is limited in laser probing of aerosols. Consequently, if we make $m < n$ in compliance with the requirement of keeping the quadrature error small, the matrix $Q$ in (7.43) becomes degenerate, and the solution so obtained is grossly smoothed. In such situations, it is practical to use the quadrature formula (7.40), by means of which the distribution function $G_p(a)$ is calculated at certain stations $a_j$ ($j=1,2,\ldots,n$) consistent with the particular measurements, and then the intermediate values are determined by interpolation. The use of (7.40) to compute the integral on the left-hand side of the Euler equation (7.42b) yields a matrix whose elements are given by the expression

$$Q_{ij} = \frac{1}{(\lambda_2 - \lambda_1)(R_2 - R_1)^3}\left[C_{i,j-1} + B_{ij} + A_{i,j+1}\right] \qquad (7.44)$$

in which

$$C_{i,j-1} = \frac{1}{\Delta_{j-1}} \int_{a'_{j-1}}^{a''_{j-1}} \overline{Q}(a_i, a)\left[a_{j-1}a_{j-2} - (a_{j-1}+a_{j-2})a + a^2\right] da \qquad (7.45)$$

$$C_{i0} = 0$$

$$B_{ij} = \frac{1}{\Delta_j} \int_{a'_j}^{a''_j} \overline{Q}(a_j, a)\left[-a_{j-1}a_{j+1} + (a_{j+1}+a_{j-1})a - a^2\right] da \qquad (7.46)$$

$$A_{i,j+1} = \frac{1}{\Delta_{j+1}} \int_{a'_{j+1}}^{a''_{j+1}} \overline{Q}(a_j, a)\left[a_{j+1}a_{j+2} - (a_{j+2}+a_{j+1})a - a^2\right] da \qquad (7.47)$$

$$A_{i,n+1} = 0$$

$$\overline{Q}(a_j, a) = \int_{\lambda_1}^{\lambda_2} Q(a_j, \lambda) Q(a, \lambda) d\lambda \qquad (7.48)$$

$$\Delta_j = a_j a_{j+1}(a_{j+1} - a_j) - a_{j-1}a_{j+1}(a_{j+1} - a_{j-1}) + a_j a_{j-1}(a_j - a_{j-1}) \qquad (7.49)$$

$$a'_j = \frac{a_j + a_{j-1}}{2}; \qquad a''_j = \frac{a_{j+1} + a_j}{2} \qquad (7.50)$$

The integrals in expressions (7.45)–(7.48) can be computed with a high degree of accuracy. Analogous expressions are readily deduced for the right-hand side of the Euler equation (7.42b).

A second regularizing algorithm can be obtained by transforming the Euler equation as follows:

$$\frac{d^2G}{da^2} - \frac{1}{(R_2-R_1)^2}G_p(a)=f(a) \tag{7.51}$$

where

$$f(a)= \frac{1}{(\lambda_2-\lambda_1)(R_2-R_1)^3\alpha}$$

$$\times\left[\int_{R_1}^{R_2}\int_{\lambda_1}^{\lambda_2}Q(\lambda,a)Q(\lambda,\xi)G_p(\xi)\,d\lambda\,d\xi-\int_{\lambda_1}^{\lambda_2}Q(\lambda,a)\beta(\lambda)\,d\lambda\right]$$

$$\tag{7.52}$$

The boundary-value problem for Eq. (7.51) is solved by the method of Green functions. For the boundary conditions

$$G_p(a)=b_1 \quad \text{at} \quad a=R_1, \qquad G_p(a)=b_2 \quad \text{at} \quad a=R_2 \tag{7.53}$$

the Green function is given by the expression

$$G(\eta,a)= G\left[2\exp\left(-\frac{2R_1}{R_2-R_1}\right)-\exp\left(-\frac{2R_2}{R_2-R_1}\right)\right]^{-1} \tag{7.54}$$

where

$$G=\begin{cases}\left[\exp\left(-\dfrac{\eta}{R_2-R_1}\right)-\exp\left(-\dfrac{2R_2}{R_2-R_1}\right)\exp\left(-\dfrac{\xi}{R_2-R_1}\right)\right] \\ \left[\exp\left(-\dfrac{a}{R_2-R_1}\right)-\exp\left(-\dfrac{2R_1}{R_2-R_1}\right)\exp\left(\dfrac{a}{R_2-R_1}\right)\right], & a\leqslant\eta \\[2em] \left[\exp\left(-\dfrac{\eta}{R_2-R_1}\right)-\exp\left(-\dfrac{2R_1}{R_2-R_1}\right)\exp\left(-\dfrac{\eta}{R_2-R_1}\right)\right] \\ \left[\exp\left(-\dfrac{a}{R_2-R_1}\right)-\exp\left(-\dfrac{2R_2}{R_2-R_1}\right)\exp\left(\dfrac{a}{R_2-R_1}\right)\right], & a\geqslant\eta \end{cases}$$

and the solution of the Euler equation can be written in the form

$$G_p(\eta) + \int_{R_1}^{R_2} G(\eta, a) f(a)\, da = b_1 \frac{dG(\eta, a)}{da}\bigg|_{a=R_1} - b_2 \frac{dG(\eta, a)}{da}\bigg|_{a=R_2}$$

$$(7.55)$$

To estimate the effectiveness of the two given algorithms, corresponding numerical experiments have been carried out, the results of which are given in Fig. 7.7. Curve 1 in the figure corresponds to a certain exact model particle-size spectrum, curve 2 to the solution of the Euler equation, and curve 3 to the solution of Eq. (7.55). A 5% random error was superimposed on the extinction coefficient in the calculations, and the number of wavelengths was chosen equal to 7. It is apparent from the figure that both algorithms yield satisfactory results.

In concluding this section, we note that the particular choice of regularizing algorithm for the inversion of Eq. (7.27) is based on the specifics of the problem, the "goodness" of the measurement information, and the quantity of *a priori* information about the particle-size spectrum. Thus, if a sufficient volume of information about the function $G_p(n)$ is available, the statistical regularization method [79] can be used; but then, on the other hand, the optimal parametrization method affords satisfactory results in this case. A similar analysis of the effectiveness of using various algorithms for the solution of inverse problems associated with multifrequency probing of the atmosphere may also be found in [62–66, 68–70].

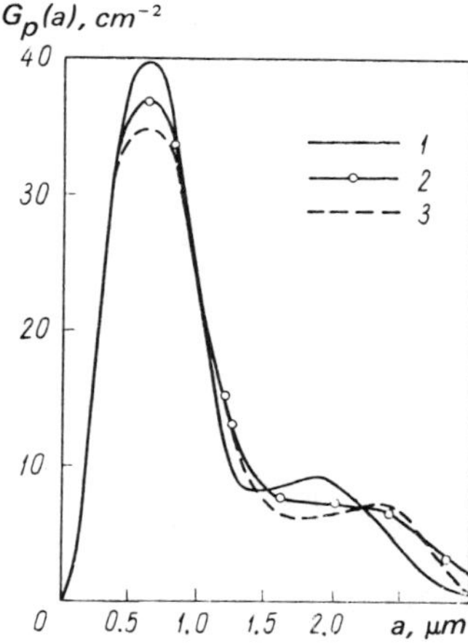


Fig. 7.7. Example of reconstruction of the spectrum of particle sizes with respect to the extinction coefficient.

## 7.6.2. Determination of the Microstructure of Aerosols from the Angular Distribution of Scattered Radiation

Information about the particle-size spectrum of aerosols is contained in the polydisperse angular scattering function. Accordingly, by measuring the intensity of radiation scattered by the aerosol at various angles, it is possible to solve the inverse problem with the data so obtained.

The initial equation in this case takes the form

$$f(\theta_i) = \int_{a_1}^{a_2} Q(\theta_i, a) G_p(a)\, da \tag{7.56}$$

which is analogous to Eq. (7.27). In expression (7.56), $f(\theta_i)$ is the angular scattering function for the angle $\theta_i$ ($i=1,2,\ldots,m$), $Q(\theta_i, a)$ is the scattering efficiency factor determined for spherical particles in the Mie theory, $a_1$ and $a_2$ are the limiting particle radii, and $G_p(a)=\pi a^2 n(a)$ is the distribution of the particles by geometrical cross sections. As in the case of (7.27), the determination of $G_p(a)$ from Eq. (7.56) represents an ill-posed problem of atmospheric optics. It can be solved by one of the methods described above. However, preference should be given to regularization methods because it is far simpler to measure the angular scattering function for many angles than to obtain multifrequency laser probing data. For example, the use of a bistatic laser probing configuration ensures the acquisition of appropriate data on the functions $f(\theta_i)$ with the use of any suitable instrumentation. In what follows, therefore, we shall make use of regularization methods, following Veretennikov and Naats [80]. In the example of solving the problem in question, in particular, we demonstrate the significance of the proper choice of regularization parameter $\alpha$.

In accordance with the general procedure of regularization methods, the solution of the equivalent algebraic system for (7.56), $AS=f$, is given by the expression

$$S_\alpha = (A^T A + \alpha P)^{-1} A^T f \tag{7.57}$$

in which $S_\alpha$ is the solution vector with components $S_i$ ($i=1,2,\ldots,n$), $P$ is a smoothing matrix, the form of which is determined by the constraints on the norm of the solution vector and the solution derivative vector [81], $A$ is the matrix of the algebraic system, $f$ is the vector of measurements, and $\alpha$ is the regularization parameter, the value of which depends on the measurement error; the vector $S$ characterizes the unknown distribution function (DF).

In the foregoing results, the required accuracy of algebraization of Eq. (7.56) for a vector $S$ of not too many dimensions is attained by application of the quadrature formulas in [67]. To estimate the effectiveness of inversion, appropriate numerical experiments have been carried out in which the role of the model distributions is taken by the DF's for hazes $H$ and $M$ [74], for which particle-size intervals of 0.005 to 0.6 $\mu$m and 0.005 to 3 $\mu$m were assumed. The number of angle measurements $m$ was varied from 6 to 18. The wavelength was assumed equal to 0.55 $\mu$m in every case, and the refractive index was $n = 1.56$. Particular attention was devoted to the selection of the regularization parameter $\alpha$ and the search for its optimum value.

The optimization of $\alpha$ is understood to be such that the norm of the deviation $\rho(S_\alpha, S_0)$ of the solution vector $S_\alpha$ from the exact value $S_0$ is a minimum. Figure 7.8 gives the dependence of the quantity $\rho(S_\alpha, S_0)/\|S_0\|$ on $\alpha$, where $\|S_0\|$ is the norm of the exact solution for the case of reconstruction of the haze $H$ particle-size spectrum from the scattering function $f(\theta)$ as the angle $\theta$ runs through values from 90 to 180° with $n = 10$ and $m = 9$, where $n$ is the number of dimensions of the solution vector $S_\alpha$ and $m$ is the number of scattering angles; various values are assigned to the measurement error $\delta$. The figure clearly exhibits the role of the measurement errors in the choice of optimum values of the regularization parameter. In the given case, the optimum value of $\alpha$ varies by more than an order of magnitude for an interval of measurement errors $\delta$ ranging from 1 to 20%. It is also essential to note that the larger the value of $\delta$, the narrower the interval of near-optimum values of $\alpha$. Veretennikov and Naats [80] describe various methods for estimating the optimum values of $\alpha$, which we shall not discuss at length, but merely note that the correct choice of the regularization parameters is extremely important insofar as it significantly affects the accuracy of solution of the corresponding inverse problem.

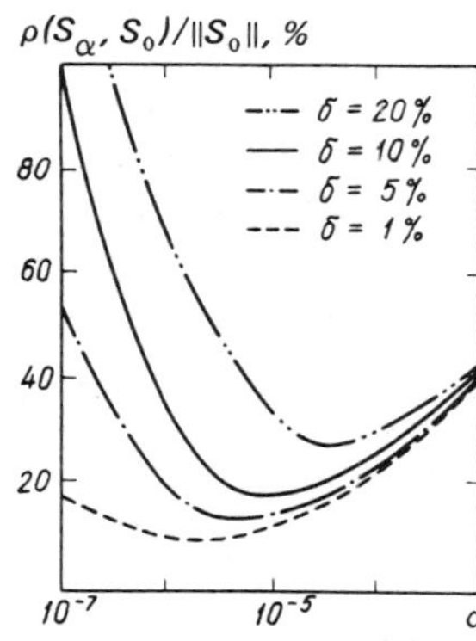


Fig. 7.8.

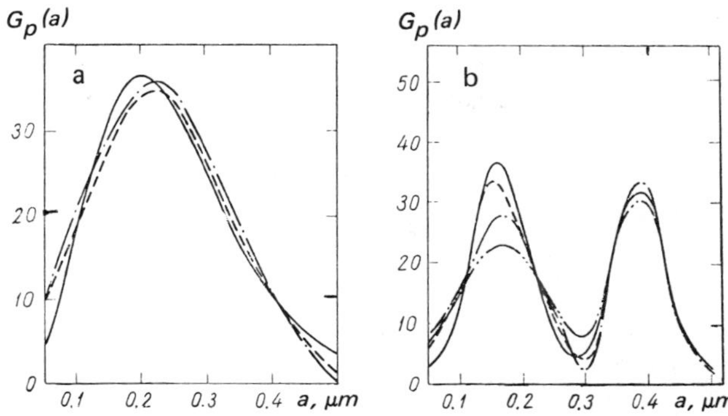

Fig. 7.9. (a) —, Exact; ————, $\delta=5\%$, $\alpha=10^{-2}$; —·—, $\delta=10\%$, $\alpha=5.10^{-2}$. (b) —, Exact; ————, 1%; —·—, 5%; —··—, 10%.

Examples of the reconstruction of the distribution functions $G_p(a)$ from measured values of the scattering intensity at various angles are given in Figs. 7.9(a) and 7.9(b). Figure 7.9(a) gives the results of reconstruction of $G_p(a)$ for haze $H$ according to measurements in the interval of angles from 90 to 180° ($m=9$, $n=10$) as a function of the measurement error and value of the regularization parameters with a constraint on the norm of the derivative. The second figure gives an example of the reconstruction of a double-humped distribution obtained from measurements in the same interval of angles from 90 to 180°, but with a finer partition ($m=18$, $n=10$). A characteristic attribute of this example is the fact that the second maximum of the DF is better reproduced. This result is attributable to the fact that the angular scattering function carries more information about large particles in the interval of angles from 90 to 180°.

In conclusion, we consider the problems of the conditioning of Eq. (7.56) and the errors of reconstruction of $G_p(a)$, which are crucial to the solution of ill-posed inverse problems.

The degree of conditioning of Eq. (7.56) can be characterized by the condition numbers [82], which are related to the "coefficient of initial-data error magnification." The condition number is specified by the quantity $h=(\mu_{max}/\mu_{min})^{1/2}$, where $\mu$ denotes the eigenvalues of the matrix $A^T A$. In

Table 7.3. Condition Numbers for Various Combinations of $a_1, a_2, m, n$, and $\theta$

| $a_1(\mu)$ | $a_2(\mu)$ | $m$ | $n$ | $\theta_{0-90°}$ | $\theta_{90-180°}$ |
|---|---|---|---|---|---|
| 0.005 | 0.6 | 18 | 5 | $1.9 \cdot 10^2$ | $1.1 \times 10^2$ |
| 0.005 | 0.6 | 18 | 10 | $10^7$ | $1.1 \times 10^6$ |
| 0.005 | 3.0 | 18 | 5 | $6.3 \cdot 10^2$ | $1.3 \times 10^1$ |

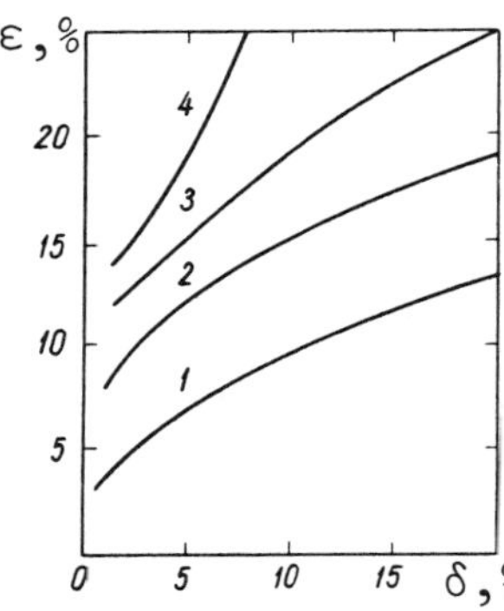

Fig. 7.10. 1. $m=18, n=5$;   2. $m=18$, $n=10$;   3. $m=9$, $n=10$; 4. $m=6$, $n=10$.

other words, this quantity may be interpreted as the ratio of the semimajor to the semiminor axis of the scatter ellipsoid corresponding to the vector whose components are the errors of the unknowns. Table 7.3 gives the condition numbers for various numbers of dimensions of the measured and unknown vectors ($m$ and $n$) as well as various values of $a_1$ and $a_2$ in the intervals of scattering angles from 0 to 90° and from 90 to 180°.

Figure 7.10 gives the results of calculations of the error of reconstruction of the distribution $G_p(a)$ for the haze $H$ model on the basis of scattering intensity data for the interval of angles from 90 to 180° as a function of the optical measurement errors for various values of $m$ and $n$, clearly illustrating the influence of the numbers of dimensions of the measured and unknown vectors as well as the measurement errors on the accuracy of reconstruction of the function $G_p(a)$.

### 7.6.3. Inversion of Polarization Measurements into the Characteristics of an Aerosol

The polarization characteristics of the laser probe echo signal (lidar return) contain a wealth of information about the microphysical parameters of the aerosol, so that the solution of inverse problems on the basis of measurements of the polarization of scattered radiation is of paramount importance in regard to the progress of laser atmospheric-probing methods. We must especially underscore the high sensitivity of this method to the reconstruction of the parameters of the finely disperse aerosol fraction. The polarization characteristics of echo signals can be measured, in general, with the use of monostatic as well as bistatic probing configurations. However, preference must be given to the bistatic configuration here because measurements of the polarization characteristics at different scattering angles unquestionably carry a greater quantity of information.

In the bistatic probing configuration, the principal mathematical relation describing polarization effects is the equation

$$S_i^{(1)}(\theta) = r^{-2} \sum_{j=1}^{4} f_{ij}(\theta) S_j^{(0)} \, dV, \qquad i = 1,2,3,4 \tag{7.58}$$

where $S^{(0)}$ and $S^{(1)}$ are the Stokes parameters of the incident and scattered radiation, respectively, $\theta$ is the scattering angle, $r$ is the distance from the point of observation to the scattering volume $dV$, and $f_{ij}(\theta)$ is an element of the unit-volume scattering matrix, characterizing the scattering properties of the volume $dV$.

The elements $f_{ij}(\theta)$ of the scattering matrix can be represented in the form

$$f_{ij}(\theta) = f_{ij}^R(\theta) + f_{ij}^M(\theta) \tag{7.59}$$

where $f_{ij}^R$ and $f_{ij}^M$ are the Rayleigh and aerosol (particulate) components of element $ij$ of the scattering matrix. The component $f_{ij}^R$ can be estimated on the basis of the standard model of a Rayleigh atmosphere if the separation of $f_{ij}$ into $f_{ij}^R$ and $f_{ij}^M$ does not enter into the probing problem. The component $f_{ij}^M$ depends strongly on the shape, sizes, and complex refractive index of the particles. In the case of spherical particles, the aerosol component can be expressed in terms of the particle-size distribution:

$$f_{ij}^M(\theta) = \int_{a_1}^{a_2} R_{ij}(\theta, \lambda, a) n(a) \, da, \qquad i, j = 1,2,3,4 \tag{7.60}$$

where $a_1$ and $a_2$ are the extreme values of the particle radii and $R_{ij}(\theta, \lambda, a)$ is an element of the Mie scattering matrix for a particle of radius at a probe wavelength $\lambda$ and corresponding refractive index $m$.

Knowing the elements of the matrix $f_{ij}^M(\theta)$, we can solve the inverse problems of aerosol optics. Information about these elements can be obtained from the corresponding lidar equation written for a bistatic probing configuration. Neglecting multiple-scattering effects, we write this equation for the case in which the probe pulse is situated entirely within the field of view of the receiver:

$$S_i^{(1)}(\theta, h) = B(h) T_1 T_2 r_2^{-2} \sin^2\left(\frac{\theta}{2}\right) \sum_{j=1}^{4} f_{ij}(\theta) S_j^{(0)}, \qquad i = 1,2,3,4$$

$$\tag{7.61}$$

where $B$ is a constant of the bistatic system for a given height $h$ and $T_1, T_2$ are the transmittances of the atmospheric layers from lidar transmitter to probed volume and from probed volume to receiver, respectively.

We assume that $T_1$ and $T_2$ are not known. The methods for their determination for laser probing will be discussed later in a separate section. Assuming that the atmosphere is homogeneous in horizontal directions, we can write

$$T_1 T_2 = \exp\left[-\tau(h)\left(\sin^{-1}\gamma_1 + \sin^{-1}\gamma_2\right)\right] \tag{7.62}$$

where $\tau(h)$ is the optical thickness of a vertical column of the atmosphere to height $h$ and $\gamma_1$, $\gamma_2$ are the angles between the horizontal and the optical axes of the transmitter and receiver, respectively.

For known values of the Stokes parameters of the probe pulse $S^{(0)}$ and the received signal $S^{(1)}$, Eq. (7.61) can be rewritten

$$\int_{a_1}^{a_2} Q_i(\theta, a) n(a)\, da = g_i(\theta), \qquad i = 1, 2, 3, 4 \tag{7.63}$$

where

$$g_i(\theta) = S_i^{(1)}(\theta) r_2^2 \sin^{-2}\left(\frac{\theta}{2}\right)(B T_1 T_2)^{-1} - \sum_{j=1}^{4} f_{ij}^R(\theta) S_j^{(0)} \tag{7.64}$$

$$Q_i(\theta, a) = \sum_{j=1}^{4} R_{ij}(\theta, \lambda, a) S_j^{(0)} \tag{7.65}$$

In the case where the incident radiation is linearly polarized at a 45° angle relative to the scattering plane (the vector $S^{(0)}$ has components 1.0, 1.0), the foregoing expressions are simplified, and the elements $Q_i(\theta, a)$ coincide with the elements of the Mie scattering matrix $R_{ij}(\theta, \lambda, a)$, Thus, the determination of the particle-size spectrum in the case of bistatic probing is reducible to the solution of the system of equations (7.63)–(7.65). It is noted at once that this system is an example of an ill-posed inverse problem, the solution of which is stable under initial-data errors, and so it is required to introduce additional information about the unknown solution. Thus, the imposition of a constraint on the norm of the solution or the norm of the derivative of the solution yields an approximate solution of the form [81]

$$n_\alpha = (A^T A + \alpha P)^{-1} A^T g \tag{7.66}$$

where $A$ is the $4m \times l$ matrix of the equivalent algebraic system $An=g$ for Eq. (7.63), $n_\alpha$ is a vector characterizing the unknown distribution at points $[r_1, r_2, \ldots, r_l]$, $g$ is the measurement vector with components $[g_1(\theta_1), \ldots, g_1(\theta_m), g_2(\theta_1), \ldots, g_4(\theta_m)]$, $P$ is a smoothing matrix, and $\alpha$ is the regularization parameters.

By the method proposed in [64] the regularized solution $n_\alpha$ can be sought in the form

$$n_\alpha = (A^T A + \alpha I)^{-1}(A^T g + \alpha \bar{n}) \qquad (7.67)$$

where $I$ is the unit matrix and $\bar{n}$ is a certain known vector belonging to the possible ensemble of solutions.

We note that for $a > \lambda$ the functions $R_{ij}(\theta, \lambda, a)$ oscillate strongly, so that the satisfactory algebraization of Eq. (7.63) with vectors of relatively few dimensions poses a complex computational problem for which specific methods of solution have been proposed [64, 83]. Westwater and Cohen [84] have developed a method for determining the particle-size spectra of aerosols without requiring conversion of the integrals in (7.63) into discrete form but with some sacrifice in accuracy in comparison with the methods described above.

In conclusion, we examine some results of numerical experiments to determine the particle-size spectra from polarization measurements. Figure 7.11 gives the particle-size distribution functions obtained by inversion according to the scheme (7.66) of the results of model bistatic measurements of four elements of the scattering matrix at five scattering angles, from the data of Herman and others [83]. The calculations were carried out for the wavelength of a ruby laser ($\lambda = 0.6943$ $\mu$m), a particle refractive index

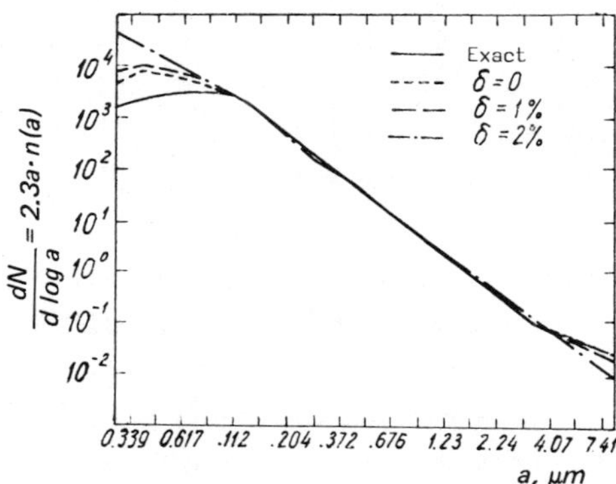


Fig. 7.11.

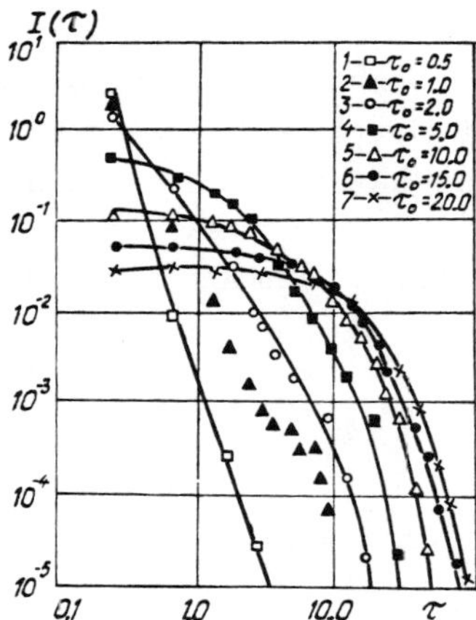



Fig. 7.12.

$n=1.54$, and measurement errors $\delta=0$ to 2%. A modified Young distribution was used as the exact model distribution.

It is evident from Fig. 7.11 that for particle radii $a>0.2$ μm fully satisfactory results are obtained for the solution of the inverse problem. The discrepancies in the interval of small radii $a<0.2$ μm are caused by the fact that the optical contribution of the indicated particles to the total scattering at a wavelength of 0.69 μm is commensurate with the "measurement errors."

Figure 7.12 gives an example of reconstruction of the particle-size spectrum in haze $H$ from six angular measurements of $f_{11}(\theta)$ at wavelength $\lambda=0.6943$ μm for a refractive index $n=1.56$ by the method described in [80]. As in the preceding case, the error of reconstruction of $n(a)$ increases with decreasing particle radius. It is shown in [80] that the error of reconstruction of $n(a)$ depends both on the volume of measurement information and complexity of the shape of the spectrum as well as on the error in the *a priori* selection of the refractive index. It is essential, therefore, to be guided by the objective of solving the problem of simultaneously determining both $n(a)$ and the particle refractive index. The hypothetical feasibility of solving problems of this nature is demonstrated in [71].

## 7.7. Laser Probing of Clouds

The probing of clouds holds a special place in the multivariety of problems in laser monitoring of the parameters of the atmosphere. Its singular status is attributable primarily to the fact that the cloud medium generates strong echo signals (returns), providing a tool for precise investigations of the stratification of cloud layers, in particular for determining the bottom level and water content of clouds in signal-accessible thicknesses. The enormous potential of lidar renders it extremely well suited to such explorations. The solution of the inverse problem for liquid-droplet clouds is greatly simplified in light of the fact that the complex refractive index of the particles is known beforehand for any probe-pulse wavelength, and because the particles are homogeneous and have a spherical geometry. Consequently, the laws of scattering by them are described by Mie theory, and there are only two unknown microphysical parameters: the particle-size distribution and the particle concentration.

For the inversion of optical measurement data in the laser probing of clouds, any of the methods described in the preceding section of the chapter for the solution of inverse problems can be used, including the optimal parametrization method, because the particle-size spectra of clouds in the greater majority of cases are described by skewed single-peak curves of the gamma distribution type, which can be used as *a priori* information.

The strong lidar return pulses from clouds, combined with the high directivity and high repetition rates of the probe pulses, make it possible to investigate the dynamics of rapidly evolving processes in a cloud and to use volumes of the latter as tracers for the assessment of wind and convection movements in the atmosphere.

Quite a number of investigations have been carried out to date on the laser probing of clouds; they have not, however, been generalized to any extent, apart from our previous survey paper [85], in which certain theoretical aspects of the problem are analyzed. Accordingly, the objective of the present section is to try and bridge this gap. We discuss the current status of both theoretical and experimental research.


## 7.7.1. Theoretical Aspects of the Laser Probing of Clouds

The material accumulated thus far on the laser probing, or sounding, of clouds indicates not only the possibility of qualitative-subjective identification of cloud structures [86,87], but also the possibility of quantitative estimation of the volume scattering coefficients, particle concentration, and water content, at least of the bottom of clouds [88,89]. However, the reliability of the results falls off abruptly, often in the processing of the related experimental data, either due to an unsound choice of processing technique or due to some imperfection of that method. The basic difficulties here are associated with the need for correctly assessing the influence of multiple-scattering effects and the small amplitudes of the echo signals returned from great depths in the scattering medium.

Below we discuss various procedures for the laser probing of clouds and present a comparative analysis of the effectiveness and stability of those procedures, as well as modifications of certain ones. We devote special attention to the problems of reconstructing the profile of the volume extinction coefficient. In this endeavor we are guided primarily by [85].

Bearing in mind that in the laser probing of clouds it is permissible, without appreciable error, to neglect all processes of interaction of the probe pulse with the cloud medium, other than aerosol scattering, we write the lidar equation in the form

$$P_r(r) = AP_0 r^{-2}\beta_\pi(r)\exp\left[-2\int_0^r \alpha(r')\,dr'\right] \tag{7.68}$$

where $A$ incorporates all the lidar parameters and, for our convenience, the symbol $M$ is dropped from the volume aerosol backscattering coefficient $\beta_\pi$ and from the volume aerosol total scattering coefficient $\alpha$. The wavelength $\lambda$ is omitted everywhere on the basis of the same considerations. We now turn to specific methods for the solution of Eq. (7.68).

### 7.7.1.1. Log-Derivative Method

The log-derivative method of solution of Eq. (7.68), which has been used in early papers on searchlight probing of the atmosphere [90, 91] and later in a number of laser probing studies [92–96], is based on the following assumptions: (1) The volume aerosol extinction coefficient is equal to the volume aerosol scattering coefficient; (2) the lidar ratio is known and remains invariant within the boundaries of the probed cloud volume.

Under the stated assumptions, the following expression is obtained for the volume extinction (scattering) coefficient:

$$\alpha(r) = \frac{\ln\left[S(r_1)/S(r_2)\right]}{2(r_1 - r_2)} \tag{7.69}$$

where

$$S(r) = P_0 A\beta_\pi(r)\exp\left[-2\alpha(r)r\right] \tag{7.70}$$

and $r_1$ and $r_2$ are points at which discrete readings of the functional $S(r)$ are taken.

Estimates based on the Monte Carlo method have shown that expression (7.69) can be used up to optical thicknesses $\tau \leqslant 3$ for standard lidar apertures. However, the given assumptions greatly restrict the practical utility of this method.

### 7.7.1.2. Slant-Path Method

The slant-path method was proposed by Kano [97] to cope with the difficulties of interpreting the results of laser probing, as noted in [98,99]. The basic idea of this method has been used in [22]. Unfortunately, several errors occur in [97]. The discussion that follows is devoid of those errors.

We formulate the problem of determining $\alpha(z)$ within the limits of an elementary scattering layer $\Delta r$ situated at height $z$. For a signal arriving from $\Delta r$ along two slant paths at angles $\theta_1$ and $\theta_2$ with respect to the vertical, we can write the system of equations

$$S(r_1) = P_0 A \beta_\pi(r_1) \exp\left[-2\int_0^{r_1} \alpha(r)\,dr\right]$$

$$S(r_2) = P_0 A \beta_\pi(r_2) \exp\left[-2\int_0^{r_2} \alpha(r)\,dr\right] \tag{7.71}$$

Assuming that the optical properties of the medium are constant in horizontal directions, i.e., regarding $\beta_\pi$ and $\alpha$ as functions only of the height and $\beta_\pi(r_1) = \beta_\pi(r_2)$, and then transforming to the variable $z = r/\sec\theta$, we obtain from (7.71)

$$\frac{S(z\sec\theta_1)}{S(z\sec\theta_2)} = \exp\left[2(\sec\theta_2 - \sec\theta_1)\int_0^z \alpha(z')\,dz'\right] \tag{7.72}$$

whereupon

$$\alpha(z) = \frac{(d/dz)\ln\left[S(z\sec\theta_1)/S(z\sec\theta_2)\right]}{2(\sec\theta_2 - \sec\theta_1)} \tag{7.73}$$

In the simplest case $\theta_1 = 0°$, $\theta_2 = 60°$, we have

$$\alpha(z) = \frac{1}{2}\frac{d}{dz}\ln\left[\frac{S(z)}{S(2z)}\right] \tag{7.74}$$

$$T(z) = \exp\left[-2\int_0^z \alpha(z')\,dz'\right] = \left[\frac{S(2z)}{S(z)}\right]^{1/2} \tag{7.75}$$

Expressions (7.74) and (7.75) are the working equations of this method. The stability of the latter under the influence of multiple-scattering effects has also been tested by the Monte Carlo method. Despite its stability under these effects, the method has greatly limited applications due to its underlying assumptions.

### 7.7.1.3. Method of Successive Layers

The method of successive layers has been developed in [7, 100] and has been used for analysis of the optical characteristics of the bottoms of clouds. According to this method, the probing path is partitioned into a sequence of layers $\Delta r_i$, in each of which the scattering coefficient and function are considered to be constant. It is also assumed that the extinction coefficient is equal to the scattering coefficient. Then for signals returned from each $i$ th layer, according to (7.68), we write

$$P_r(r_i) = AP_0 r_i^{-2} \alpha(r_i) b(r_i) \exp\left[-2 \sum_{j=1}^{i-1} \alpha(r_j) \Delta r_j\right] \tag{7.76}$$

To solve (7.76) for $\alpha(r_i)$, it is necessary to have *a priori* knowledge of $\alpha(r_1)$ and the sequence $b(r_i)$, where $b$ is the normalized angular scattering function for a 180° angle. The formal solution is written

$$\alpha(r_i) = \frac{P_r(r_i) r_i^2 \exp\left[2 \sum_{j=1}^{i-1} \alpha(r_j) \Delta r_j\right]}{P_0 A b(r_i)} \tag{7.77}$$

For the initial value of $\alpha(r_i)$ it is recommended to use the average value obtained for this coefficient in the undercloud layer from other parallel measurements. Expression (7.77) has been used to process the results of probing of a low stratus raincloud [101]. It was found that the algorithm (7.77) already diverges for $\tau \geqslant 0.5$, clearly as a result of imprecise selection of the initial data on $\alpha$ and $b$ and due to the influence of multiple-scattering effects. In view of this consideration, a numerical experiment was carried out by the Monte Carlo approach. The computational procedure for this method and its capabilities are discussed in detail in our earlier work [102–104]. The purpose of this experiment was to analyze the comparative stability of different methods for the laser probing of clouds under multiple-scattering effects. The calculations were carried out for a ruby-laser wavelength of 0.6943 $\mu$m on the basis of a model of the medium in the form of a plane homogeneous layer with initial characteristics $\alpha^0 = 2$ km$^{-1}$, $b = 0.0355$.

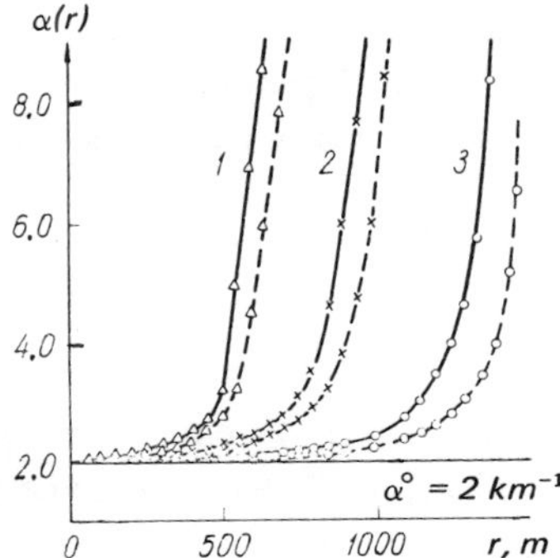



Fig. 7.13. Distorting influence of multiple-scattering background on the accuracy of determination of $\alpha(r)$ by the original (solid curves) and modified (dashed curves) method of successive layers in different receiver apertures: (1) $\phi_d = 1°$; (2) 20′; (3) 3′.

The results of the calculations of the distorting influence of multiple-scattering background on the accuracy of solution of (7.77) under the condition that the apparatus constant $A$ and initial optical parameters are known with perfect precision are given in Fig. 7.13 for three receiver apertures: 1°, 20′, and 3′ (solid curves 1, 2, and 3, respectively). It is evident from the figure that even for a receiver with an angular aperture of 3′ multiple-scattering effects can be neglected in the given method roughly up to an optical thickness $\tau = 1.5$. For larger values of the viewing angle of the lidar receiving system, the values of $\tau$ for which multiple scattering can be disregarded are proportionately lower.

### 7.7.1.4. Modified Successive-Layer Method

We have previously [104, 105] elaborated the method of successive layers in a somewhat modified form that does not require knowledge of any reference value of the scattering coefficient at the beginning of the path. The susceptibility of this modification to multiple-scattering effects is illustrated by the corresponding dashed curves in Fig. 7.13, from which it is inferred that it does not differ very much from the previous case. Accordingly, we now describe still another algorithm, which is considerably more stable under multiple-scattering effects.

If we allow for the fact that the multiple-scattering increment to the signal $P(\Delta r_i)$ is roughly identical in adjacent gating intervals, then, given the same assumptions of invariance of the optical properties of the cloud along the path element $\Delta r_i$, the system of lidar equations can be formulated for the functionals

$$S(\Delta r_i) = \frac{P_r(\Delta r_i)r_i^2}{P_0 A} = b(\Delta r_i)\alpha(\Delta r_i)\exp\left[-2\sum_{j=1}^{i-1}\alpha(\Delta r_j)\Delta r_j\right] \quad (7.78)$$

where $\Delta r_i = r_{i+1} - r_i$, $i = 1, 2, \ldots$, and $S(\Delta r_i) = b(\Delta r_{i+1})\alpha(\Delta r_i)$. We also assume that $b$ changes very little from one layer to the next: $b(\Delta r_i) \cong b(\Delta r_{i+1})$, so that for any two adjacent layer the following relation holds:

$$\frac{S(\Delta r_{i+1})}{S(\Delta r_i)} = \frac{\alpha(\Delta r_{i+1})}{\alpha(\Delta r_i)} T^2(\Delta r_i) \tag{7.79}$$

where $T^2(\Delta r_i) = \exp[-2\alpha(\Delta r_i)\Delta r_i]$.

From (7.79) we deduce the following invertible scheme for processing of the signal $S(r)$ without the requirement of absolute calibration of the signal:

$$\alpha(\Delta r_{i+1}) = \alpha(\Delta r_i) T^{-2}(\Delta r_i) \frac{S(\Delta r_{i+1})}{S(\Delta r_i)}$$

$$\alpha(\Delta r_i) = \alpha(\Delta r_{i+1}) T^{-2}(\Delta r_{i+1}) \frac{S(\Delta r_i)}{S(\Delta r_{i+1})} \tag{7.80}$$

The invertibility of (7.80) means that the reference value of $\alpha^0$ can be its value at any point along the probing path where it is known or has been determined by another means. In particular, the backscattering signal always contains a log–linear part $\Delta r$, where the log-derivative method discussed above is applicable and the value obtained for $\alpha^0$ can be used as the reference value for the iterative scheme (7.80).

The results of a numerical experiment indicate high stability of this method under multiple-scattering noise up to a maximum optical thickness $\tau = 3.8$, including large receiver viewing angles.

### 7.7.1.5. Continuous-Update Method

The continuous-update method is described in [106], but the basic postulates of a similar approach may be found in papers on searchlight probing of the atmosphere [90, 91, 107]. The method is formally constructed on the direct analytical solution of expression (7.68) under the assumptions that the dependence of the lidar ratio on the coordinate $r$ is known and the extinction coefficient is equal to the scattering coefficient. Fernald and others [106] proceed from the stricter requirement of a constant lidar ratio, known *a priori*. In this case

$$T^2(r) = \exp\left[-2\int_0^r \alpha(r')\,dr'\right] = \exp\left[-\frac{2}{b}\int_0^r \beta_\pi(r')\,dr'\right] \tag{7.81}$$

whence

$$\beta_\pi(r) = -\frac{b[d/dr\ T^2(r)]}{2T^2(r)} \tag{7.82}$$

and the lidar equation assumes the form

$$P_r(r) = -\frac{AP_0 b}{2r^2}\frac{d}{dr}T^2(r) \tag{7.83}$$

Separating variables and integrating from 0 to $r$, we obtain the fundamental relation

$$T^2(r) = 1 - \frac{2}{Ab}\int_0^r \frac{P_r(r')r'^2}{P_0}\,dr' \tag{7.84}$$

from which is directly inferred an expression for

$$\alpha(r) = \frac{1}{2}\frac{d}{dr}\ln T^2(r) \tag{7.85}$$

and from the latter we deduce an algorithm for the discrete processing of echo signals:

$$\alpha(\Delta r_i) = \frac{1}{\Delta r_i}\frac{T^2(r_i) - T^2(r_{i+1})}{T^2(r_i) + T^2(r_{i+1})} \tag{7.86}$$

We note that analogous relations have also been obtained in other papers [3, 7, 93, 108].

A numerical experiment carried out for this method has shown that its stability under the influence of multiple-scattering effects is approximately the same as the other methods considered above that are based on utilization of the absolute values of the measured signals. In every case, after the probe signal attains a definite optical thickness, with a further increase in the latter the multiple-scattering contribution increases by a nonlinear law. This fact has also been noted in connection with the processing of experimental probing data [109].

### 7.7.1.6. Parametric Modification of the Continuous-Update Method

To expand the limits of applicability of the continuous-update method, Krekov and others [110] have proposed a modification based on the non-linear relation

$$\beta_\pi(r) = b(r)\alpha(r)\exp[-2\xi\tau(r)] \tag{7.87}$$

in which $\xi$ is a coefficient determined by the conditions of the optical experiment and, in particular, its geometry.

Substituting (7.87) into Eq. (7.68), we obtain

$$P(r)r^2/AP_0 = S(r) = \alpha(r)b(r)T^{(2-\xi)}(r) \tag{7.88}$$

Next, making use of relation (7.82), we obtain a differential equation for the unknown integral characteristic (continuous-update function):

$$\frac{dT^2(r)}{dr} = \frac{2S(r)}{b(r)}T^{2\xi}(r) \tag{7.89}$$

the solution of which has the form

$$T^2(r) = \left\{(1-\xi)\left[C - 2\int_{r_0}^{r}\frac{S(r')}{b(r')}dr'\right]\right\}^{1/(1-\xi)} \tag{7.90}$$

where $C$ is a constant of integration and $r_0$ is the starting point of the probing path. Applying the boundary condition $T^2(r=r_0) = T_0^2$, we evaluate the constant $C$:

$$C = \frac{1}{1-\xi}T_0^{1/(1-\xi)} \tag{7.91}$$

For $T_0^2 = 1$ (zero attenuation of the transmitted laser pulse before the point $r_0$), expression (7.90) can be rewritten in the form

$$T^2(r) = \left[1 - 2(1-\xi)\int_{r_0}^{r}\frac{S(r')}{b(r')}dr'\right]^{1/(1-\xi)} \tag{7.92}$$

It is easily shown that in the integration of the signal $S(r) = S_0(r) + \Delta S_m(r)$, where $\Delta S_m$ is a monotonically increasing function of the multiple-scattering signal, the stability of the solution (7.92) improves with increasing value of the regularization parameter $\xi$. For too large values of $\xi$, however, the solution will deviate from the true value in the other direction. This fact is illustrated by Fig. 7.14, in which the curves are plotted on the basis of results of an appropriate numerical experiment for values of the parameters $\lambda = 0.6943$ $\mu$m, $\beta_t^0 = 2$ km$^{-1}$, $r_0 = 200$ m, and a 1° lidar receiver f.o.v. It is evident from the figure that even with the use of a wide-view receiver the influence of multiple-scattering effects can be eliminated by the proper choice of $\xi$ in the probing of clouds up to large optical depths. Accordingly,

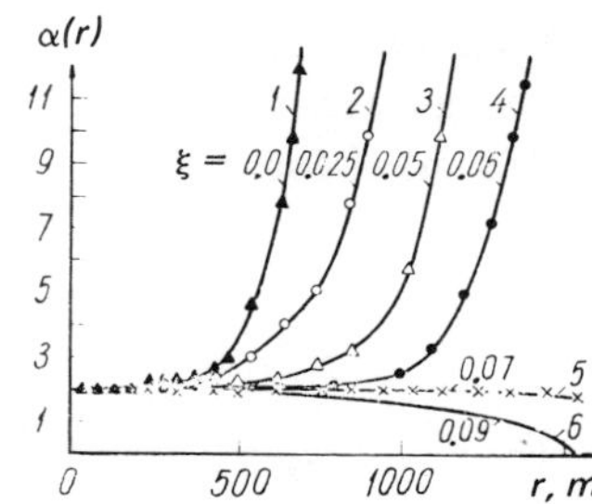


Fig. 7.14. parametric modification of the cumulative integral method, $\lambda = 0.6943$ $\mu$m, $\phi_d = 1°$, $r_0 = 200$ m, $\beta_t^0 = 2$ km$^{-1}$.

the correct choice of regularization parameter poses a particularly vital problem.

Knowing that the contribution of multiple scattering to a lidar echo signal depends not only on the angular aperture of the lidar receiving system, but also on the distance $r_0$ to the cloud, this fact must be taken into account in determining the parameter $\xi$. Appropriate calculations indicate that the parameter governing the multiple-scattering contribution to the echo signal in cloud probing at heights $r_0 \geqslant 200$ m is the dimensionless quantity

$$\eta = r_0 \varphi \alpha (r_0)$$
(7.93)

in which $\varphi$ is the f.o.v. of the lidar receiving system.

According to the same calculations, the quantities $\xi$ and $\eta$ are linearly related, the value $\eta = 0.004$ corresponds to $\xi = 0.08$. This fact enormously facilitates implementation of the proposed parametric modification of the continuous-update method.

### 7.7.1.7. Method of S Functions

The method of $S$ functions is based on application of the following empirical relation between $\beta_\pi$ and $\alpha$:

$$\beta_\pi (r) = k_1 [\alpha (r)]^{k_2}$$
(7.94)

Collis and others [111–114] have made use of the indicated relation, introducing the lidar $S$ function (which we denote by $S_c$ to avoid confusion with the function introduced earlier):

$$S_c(r) = 10 \log \left[ \frac{P_r(r) r^2}{P_r(r_0) r_0^2} \right] = 10 \log \left[ \frac{\beta_\pi(r) T^2(r)}{\beta_\pi(r_0) T^2(r_0)} \right]$$
(7.95)

Differentiating (7.95) with regard for (7.94) and the expression for the one-way transmittance $T(r)$ (7.81), we obtain the nonlinear first-order differential equation

$$\frac{d}{dr}\alpha(r) - C_1 \frac{dS_c(r)}{dr}\alpha(r) - C_2\alpha^2(r) = 0 \tag{7.96}$$

where $C_1 = 1/4.34k_2$ and $C_2 = 2/k_2$. The latter equation is linearized by the substitution $\eta = 1/\alpha$, and the final solution is written in the form

$$\alpha(r) = \frac{\alpha(r_0)\exp[C_1 S_c(r)]}{1 - C_2\alpha(r_0)\int_{r_0}^{r}\exp[C_1 S_c(r)]\,dr} \tag{7.97}$$

We note that the concept of the dimensionless lidar $S_c$ functions with the assumption of a linear relationship between $\beta_\pi$ and $\alpha$ has been used in other studies [115, 116].

We have carried out a numerical experiment on the use of the given method; the results indicate high stability under multiple-scattering effects in comparison with other methods based on absolute echo-signal measurements. However, the multiple-scattering problem still persists here. We have, therefore, undertaken an attempt to modify this method in such a way as to compensate the multiple-scattering contribution to the echo signal, namely, in a relation of the form (7.95) itself. This can be done by adopting as the lidar $S_c$ function, rather than the ratios of the measured signals to the initial reference value $P_r(r_0)$, the ratios of those signals to a sequence of reference values for discrete subintervals, i.e.,

$$S_c(\Delta r_i) = 10\log\left[\frac{P_r(r_i)r_i^2}{P_r(r_{i-1})r_{i-1}^2}\right], \qquad i = 0, 1, 2 \tag{7.98}$$

Now the processing scheme is invertible, and the reference value of $\alpha^0$ can be its value at any point of the path. Also, we have disposed of the troublesome problem of evaluating the integral in (7.97). It can be shown by means of straightforward transformations that the solution of Eq. (7.96) in the iterative scheme so constructed is given as

$$\alpha(\Delta r_i) = \alpha(\Delta r_{i-1})f(\Delta r_i)\left\{1 - \frac{\alpha(\Delta r_{i-1})\Delta r_i}{k_2[1 + f(\Delta r_i)]}\right\} \tag{7.99}$$

where

$$f(\Delta r_i) = \left[ \frac{P_r(\Delta r_i)r_i^2}{P_r(\Delta r_{i-1})r_{i-1}^2} \right]^{1/k_2} \tag{7.100}$$

Inasmuch as the multiple-scattering increment to the echo signal is practically identical on adjacent path elements, a solution in the form (7.99) retains its stability in deep layers of the target cloud.

### 7.7.1.8. Asymptotic-Signal Method

The basic postulates of the asymptotic-signal method are set forth in papers by Kovalev [117–120]. The method provides a rather simple means for eliminating the influence of instrument errors, does not require any assumptions as to the structure or nature of the scattering particles, and makes it possible in large measure to diminish the influence of variations of the angular scattering vector at 180° and to minimize the role of multiple-scattering noise.

The method is based on measurement of a ratio of functionals of the form

$$I(\Delta r_i) = \tfrac{1}{2}Ab_i T_{i-1}^2 \left[ 1 - \exp(-2\alpha_i \Delta r_i) \right] \tag{7.101}$$

for a gating element $\Delta r_i$, $i = 1, 2, 3, \ldots$, and a semiinfinite path segment, i.e.,

$$I_m(\Delta r_i) = \frac{A\bar{b}_m}{2} T_{i-1}^2 \left\{ 1 - \exp\left[ -2\int_{r_i}^{r_m} \alpha(r)\,dr \right] \right\} \tag{7.102}$$

where $\bar{b}_m$ is the mean value of the scattering function on the segment $[r_i, r_m]$. For sufficiently large values of $\alpha(r)$ and $r_m - r_i$, we have $I_m = A\bar{b}_m T_{i-1}^2/2$, and the signal ratio $I(\Delta r_i)/I_m(r_i)$ reduces to the dimensionless function

$$U(\Delta r_i) = \frac{I(\Delta r_i)}{I_m(r_i)} = \left[ 1 - \exp(-2\alpha_i \Delta r_i) \right] \frac{b_i}{\bar{b}_m} \tag{7.103}$$

which is very well suited to practical applications. It can be approximately assumed in a cloud medium that $b_i \cong \bar{b}_m$ and so

$$U(\Delta r_i) = \frac{I(\Delta r_i)}{I_m(r_i)} = 1 - \exp(-2\alpha_i \Delta r_i) \tag{7.104}$$

We note that in the derivation of (7.104), as in the preceding cases, it has been assumed that the aerosol extinction and scattering coefficients are the same. Numerical experiments on multifrequency laser probing of clouds have shown that this assumption is not important and so the asymptotic-signal method with the algorithm (7.104) can also be used in the infrared region of the spectrum [121].

### 7.7.1.9. Influence of Errors of a priori Specification of Aerosol Characteristics on the Accuracy of Interpretation of Lidar Measurements

The preceding sections have been concerned primarily with the stability of various solutions of the lidar equation in the presence of multiple-scattering background. We now turn our attention to the influence of errors in the *a priori* selection of the optical model of the medium on the accuracy of interpretation of lidar echo signals. For this purpose, we isolate a certain interval along the probing path $[r, r+l]$ and assume for simplicity that $b(r)=$ const in this interval, consistent with the assumption that the composition of the aerosol and the parameters of its microstructure remain invariant within the limits of this interval. Under this condition, the lidar equation admits an explicit solution for the profiles of the optical character-istics in the given interval. Thus, we have the following relations for this case:

$$T(r)=1-2I(r)b \tag{7.105}$$

$$\beta_\pi(r)=S(r)/T(r) \tag{7.106}$$

$$\alpha(r)=\beta_\pi(r)b \tag{7.107}$$

where

$$T(r)=\exp\left[-2\int_{r_1}^{r}\alpha(r')\,dr'\right]; \qquad S(r)=\frac{P_r(r)r^2}{AP_0}; \qquad I(r)=\int_{r_1}^{r}S(r')\,dr'$$

We assume that the role of $b$ is taken by a certain $b_0$ in the solution of (7.105)–(7.107). We characterize the error of *a priori* selection by the variance of the possible deviations of $b$ from the true value $b^*$; denoting the variance by $\overline{\Delta^2 b}$, we arrive at the following relation between $b^*$ and $b$:

$$b_0-\theta(\Delta^2 b)^{1/2}<b^*<b_0+\theta(\Delta^2 b)^{1/2} \tag{7.108}$$

where $\theta$ is a certain confidence coefficient [122]. An error in the specified parameter $b$ induces errors in the optical characteristics to be determined, and the formula for finite increments can be used to estimate those errors. In particular, applying this formula to the characteristic $P_r(r)$, we find

$$\frac{\Delta P_r}{P_r} = \frac{1-T}{2T}\frac{\Delta b}{b} \tag{7.109}$$

for all $r$ in the given interval. Applying a suitable averaging technique, we obtain a relation for the rms error:

$$\varepsilon_p = \frac{(1-T)\varepsilon_b}{2T} \tag{7.110}$$

where $\varepsilon_p = (\overline{\Delta^2 P_r})^{1/2}/P_r$ and $\varepsilon_b = (\overline{\Delta^2 b})^{1/2}/b$. Expression (7.110) characterizes the relative error in the determination of $P_r(r)$ from the lidar equation when the constant $b$ is known with error $\varepsilon_b$. Expressions for $\varepsilon_{\beta_\pi}$ and $\varepsilon_\alpha$ are derived analogously:

$$\varepsilon_{\beta_\pi} = \frac{(1-T)\varepsilon_b}{T} \tag{7.111}$$

$$\varepsilon_\alpha = \varepsilon_b/T \tag{7.112}$$

The quantities in front of $\varepsilon_b$ on the right-hand sides of expressions (7.110)–(7.112) may be regarded in a certain sense as the coefficient of "magnification" of the initial error $\varepsilon_b$ due to indeterminacy in the *a priori* information. The smaller the value of this coefficient (which we now denote by $k$), the less the error of *a priori* specification will affect the accuracy of determination of the corresponding optical characteristic. These factors are conveniently treated as functions of the optical thickness $\tau$ of the probed layer. Here, inasmuch as all the factors differ for a given value of $\tau$, it is clear that the lidar equation will carry differing quantities of information about the characteristics $P_r$, $\beta_\pi$ and $\alpha$. Typically, $k_{\beta_\pi}$ is very small for small values of $\tau$. This means that the errors of *a priori* selection of $b$ will scarcely affect the accuracy of determination of $\beta_\pi$. This statement is also true of $P_r(r)$. The following approximate relations hold in the interval of small $\tau$:

$$k_{P_r} \cong \tau; \qquad k_{\beta_\pi} \cong 2\tau; \qquad k_\alpha \cong 1+2\tau \tag{7.113}$$

As the optical thickness is increased, we find that $k_{\beta_\pi} \to k_\alpha$, and all the factors increase abruptly due to the low information yield of laser probing of the scattering medium for large values of $\tau$. As a consequence, the solutions of the lidar equation are highly sensitive to measurement errors and the multiple-scattering background. A reduction of the aperture of the receiving system for large $\tau$ requires a considerable increase in the sensitivity of echo-signal reception, namely, in proportion to the values of $k$. These considerations define the limits of applicability of single-scattering theory in problems of laser probing of the atmosphere.

We now consider the problem of estimating the admissible values of $\varepsilon_b$ for the interpretation of probing results. It can be shown that the error in the determination of $T$ from the lidar equation with allowance for $\varepsilon_b$ and the measurement error $\varepsilon=(\overline{\Delta^2 I})^{1/2}/I$ is given by the expression

$$\varepsilon_T = \frac{(1-T)\left(\varepsilon^2+\varepsilon_b^2\right)^{1/2}}{T} \tag{7.114}$$

With regard for $k_T$, the quantities $\varepsilon$ and $\varepsilon_b$ may be treated as components of the total error $\varepsilon_T$. Accordingly, the error of *a priori* specification of the parameter $b$ can be deemed satisfactory if $\varepsilon_b$ is at least not greater than $\varepsilon$. Otherwise the error in the determination of $T$ is mainly determined by $\varepsilon_b$, rather than by $\varepsilon$, implying ineffective utilization of the measurement information.

We now examine in closer detail the estimation of $\varepsilon_b$ and $b$. The value of $b_0$ can be determined either on the basis of direct experimental measurements or on the basis of the adoption of an appropriate model of the microstructural parameters. In the latter case, in light of the foregoing discussion, the admissible error in the determination of $b$ must satisfy the inequality

$$\left(\overline{\Delta^2 b}\right)^{1/2}\leqslant\varepsilon b_0 \tag{7.115}$$

Bearing in mind that $b_0$ is determined by the microstructural parameters of the probed aerosol, we consider the maximum admissible confidence limits for such parameters as the average radius and $\mu$ in the size distribution $n(r)=\alpha a_n^\mu \exp(-\mu a/a_n)$ of the cloud particles. Curves of $b$ as a

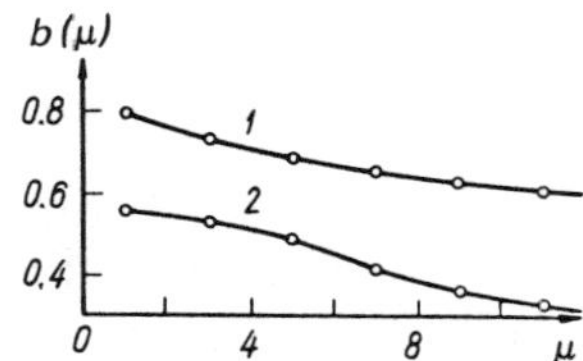

Fig. 7.15. Quantity $b(\mu)$ versus microstructural parameter $\mu$ at two wavelengths: (1) $\lambda=0.6943$ $\mu$m; (2) $\lambda=2.36$ $\mu$m.

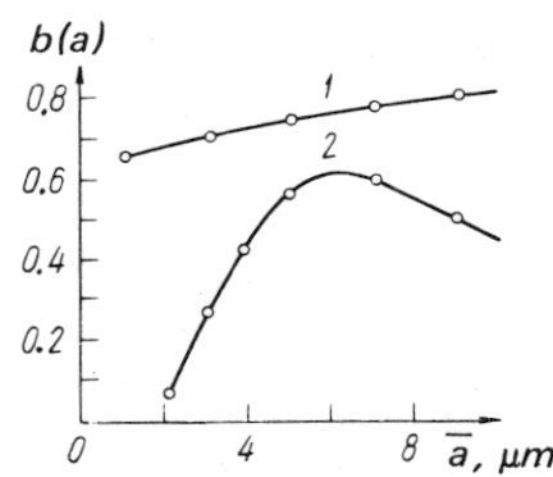


Fig. 7.16. Quantity $b(a)$ versus average radius $\bar{a}$ of cloud particles.

function of the parameters $\mu$ and $a_n$ are given in Figs. 7.15 and 7.16 for wavelengths of 0.6943 $\mu$m (ruby laser) and 2.36 $\mu$m (fluorite–dysprosium laser). The curves in Fig. 7.15 are plotted for $a_n = 4$ $\mu$m, and the curves in Fig. 7.16 for $\mu = b$. Figures 7.15 and 7.16 provide a graphic picture of the admissible variations of the parameters of the particle-size spectrum due to corresponding error in the *a priori* specification of $b$ in the initial lidar equation.

To improve the measurement accuracy automatically imposes requirements on the reduction of error of *a priori* specification of the parameter $b$. In particular, it is virtually meaningless to select $b$ on the basis of model calculations for 2–3% measurement errors because major losses of measurement information are incurred in its interpretation. Consequently, an increase in the accuracy of optical measurements must be accompanied by a concomitant increase in the volume of measurement information to ensure a corresponding reduction in the *a priori* information required.

### 7.7.1.10. Numerical Experiments on Multifrequency Laser Probing of Clouds

Our previously reported [121, 123] numerical experiments on the multifrequency laser probing of clouds are based on the application of the algorithms described in Sections 7.6.1.1 and 7.6.1.2 for the solution of inverse problems. To avoid repetition, we now give an illustration of the results obtained. Figure 7.17 presents cloud $C_1$ particle-size spectra [74] reconstructed by the optimal parametrization method for probing at four wavelengths: 2.36, 3.51, 5.3, and 10.6 $\mu$m. Curve 1 corresponds to the exact solution, and curves 2–5 are plotted for oscillatory ($\varepsilon = 0.1$) and systematic ($\varepsilon = 0.1$) perturbations of the lidar echo pulses.

Table 7.4 give digital results of the reconstruction of the microstructural parameters of a cloud $C_1$ with parameters $\gamma = 1$ and $\alpha = 6$ for the same four-wave probing and application of the optimal parametrization method.

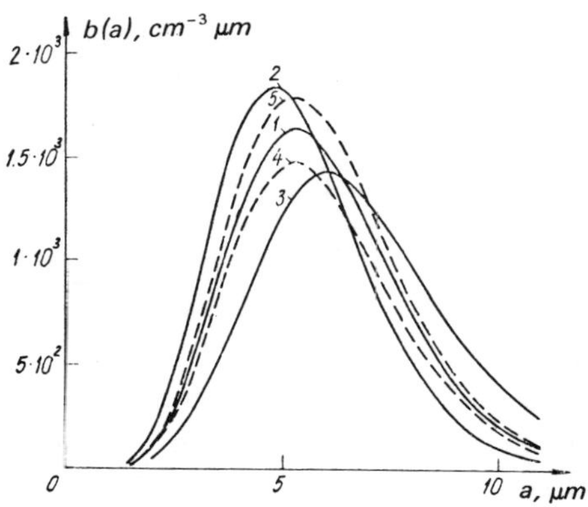


Fig. 7.17. Reconstruction of distribution function $b(a)$ from the optical characteristic $\beta(\lambda)$ (cloud $C_1$ [74]) at wavelengths of 2.36, 3.51, 5.3, and 10.6 $\mu$m with respect to parameters $S$ and $a$, $\gamma=1$, $\alpha=6$. (1) Exact solution; (2,3) solution for oscillatory perturbation, $\varepsilon=0.1$; (4,5) for systematic perturbation, $\varepsilon=0.1$.

In the table, $a_s$ is the particle radius determined by expression (7.32), $G_p$ is the geometrical cross section of the particles per unit volume, $N$ is the number density of particles, $Q_W$ is the water content of the cloud, and $(F_1/n)^{1/2}$ is the discrepancy at the minimum point of the functional (7.38).

It is evident from the figure and the table that if the particle-size spectrum of clouds is described by a gamma distribution function, then the use of four wavelengths for its reconstruction yields fully satisfactory results. The same is true of the other microstructural parameters of clouds. With regard to the validity of the gamma distribution to describe the particle-size distribution in clouds, an analysis of numerous experimental data, discussed in Chap. 3, indicates that this assumption is correct in the majority of situations.

In the general case of multifrequency lidar probing of clouds, where no *a priori* information on the microphysical parameters is used, regularization methods must be used for inversion of the experimental data. Relevant illustrations of their application have been given in Section 7.6.1.2.

Table 7.4. Results of Reconstruction of Microstructural Parameters of Cloud $C_1$ ($\gamma=1, \alpha=6$)

| Microstructural parameters | Systematic perturbation | | | | Oscillating perturbation | | |
|---|---|---|---|---|---|---|---|
| | $\varepsilon=0.01$ | $\varepsilon=-0.1$ | $\varepsilon=0.1$ | $\varepsilon=0.05$ | $\varepsilon=0.1$ | $\varepsilon=0.05$ | $\varepsilon=0.1$ |
| $a_s, \mu$m | 5.3 | 5.3 | 5.3 | 5.7 | 6.1 | 5.1 | 4.9 |
| $G_p,$km$^{-1}$ | 7.82 | 7.04 | 8.61 | 7.76 | 7.69 | 7.92 | 7.99 |
| $N,$cm$^{-3}$ | 100 | 90 | 110 | 88 | 76 | 112 | 123 |
| $Q_W,$g/cm$^3$ | $6.26\times10^{-2}$ | $5.6\times10^{-2}$ | $6.6\times10^{-2}$ | $7.1\times10^{-2}$ | $6\times10^{-2}$ | $6\times10^{-2}$ | $5.8\times10^{-2}$ |
| $(F_1/n)^{1/2}$ | 0.001 | 0.003 | 0.001 | 0.0057 | 0.12 | 0.052 | 0.1 |

### 7.7.1.11. *Polarization Characteristics of Echo Signals in the Laser Probing of Clouds*

Detailed theoretical investigations of the polarization characteristics of backscattering signals in the laser probing of clouds have been carried out in our previous work [89, 124]. The corresponding algorithms have been discussed in Section 7.6.3. We began with a calculation of the characteristics governing the optical model of radiative transfer: the volume scattering and extinction coefficients as well as the components of the scattering matrix for an extensive set of laser wavelengths and types of liquid-droplet clouds obeying a generalized gamma function for the particle-size distribution with various values of the parameters. We then determined the Stokes parameters and degree of polarization of the backscattering signals.

We now present some illustrations of the results of numerical experiments. Figure 7.18 gives echo-signal components, in one of which the polarization coincides with the polarization of the transmitted lidar pulse $I_l(L)$. The second component $I_r(L)$ is cross polarized. The dashed curves in the figure correspond to the results of calculations, and the solid curves to the experimental results for conditions similar to the analytical case. It is evident from the figure that the analytical results agree satisfactorily with the experimental, most particularly at the relative maximum levels $I_l^{\max}(L)$ and $I_r^{\max}(L)$.

Figure 7.19 gives the dependence of the depolarization coefficient $d$ of a backscattering signal on the penetration depth $L$ in the cloud and the angular aperture $\varphi_0$ of the receiving system. For the experimentally realized angle $2\varphi_0$, a quantitative comparison was made between the calculated and

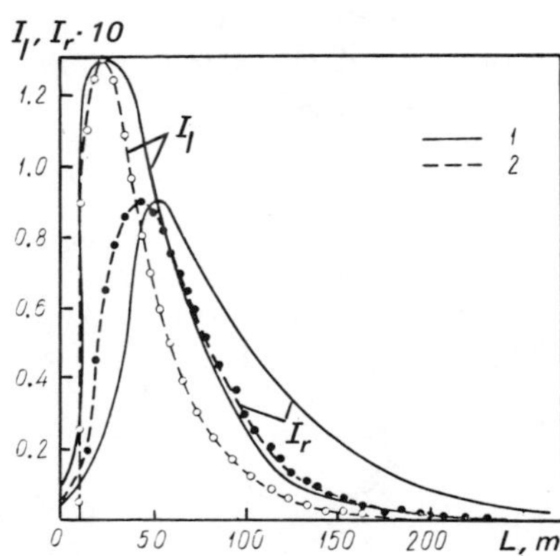


Fig. 7.18. Qualitative comparison of pulse shapes of linearly ($I_l$) and cross-polarized backscattering signals ($I_r$). (1) Experimental, Apr. 25, 1973, $\alpha = 12$ km$^{-1}$; (2) calculated, $\alpha = 16.6$ km$^{-1}$.

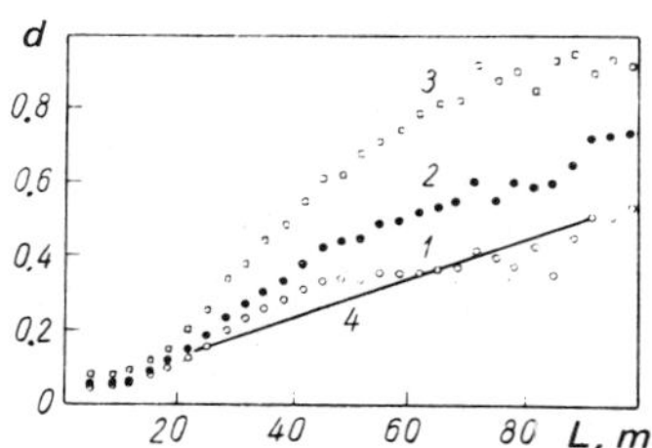

Fig. 7.19. Depolarization coefficient $d$ of backscattering signal versus penetration depth $L$ in the cloud and angular aperture $\theta_d$ of receiver for analytical model of cloud $C_3$ ($\alpha=0.04$ m$^{-1}$) and experiment ($\alpha=0.035$ m$^{-1}$). (1–3) Calculated for apertures $2\theta_d=13'$, $26'$, $180°$; (4) experimental, $2\theta_d=13'$.

experimental data. Their mutual agreement justifies both the experimental procedure and the computational algorithm.

Figure 7.20 gives the dependence of the time lag of $I_r^{\max}(L)$ relative to $I_l^{\max}(L)$ on the volume extinction coefficient, plotted on the basis of calculations and a corresponding experiment. In this case we again observe good agreement between the experimental and analytical data. The fact that the time lag of the cross-polarized component of the echo signal relative to the linearly copolarized component depends on the attenuation is attributable to multiple-scattering effects because the polarization state remains invariant in single backscattering by spherical particles. This effect can be utilized for a direct determination of the volume extinction coefficient in the polarization-lidar sounding of clouds.

Thus, measurement of the polarization characteristics of a lidar return pulse affords considerable information in the probing of clouds. The algorithms described above for the solution of inverse problems in connection with the application of scattering polarization effects yield acceptable results. A similar inference is drawn by analyzing the results of related studies by other authors [125–132].

A number of authors have made repeated use of polarization effects in experimental cloud investigations, the corresponding results of which are discussed below.

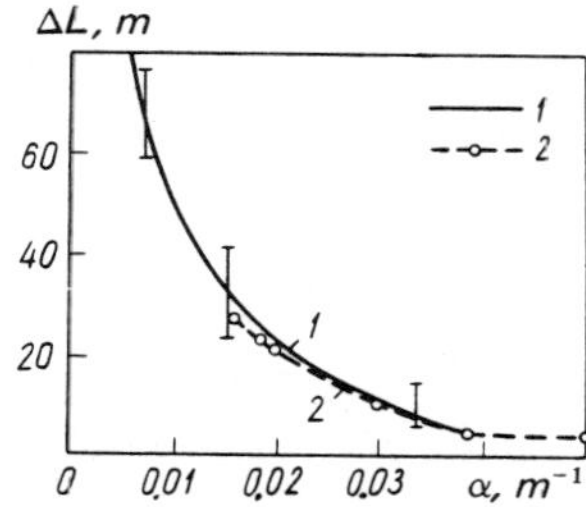

Fig. 7.20. Time lag $\Delta L$ of cross-polarized signal component versus optical density of medium, $\lambda=0.6943$ $\mu$m. (1) Experimental; (2) calculated.

## 7.7.2. Experiments in the Laser Probing of Clouds

Experiments in the laser probing of clouds mainly involve measurements of the polarization characteristics of echo, or return, signals. This situation is explained, on the one hand, by the large information content of those characteristics and, on the other, by the relative simplicity of the corresponding experimental work. Of no small significance, in particular, is the possibility of uniquely determining the phase state of a cloud, namely, by direct measurement of the linearly polarized and cross-polarized components of the echo signal. The same procedure makes it possible to implement the categorical identification of distinct meteorological formations.

Skimming over the details of the experimental procedures, we discuss the most interesting results obtained by different authors in related investigations.

In our own work [133, 134], we have explored the possibility of determining the phase composition of a cloud on the basis of an analysis of the echo-signal polarization characteristics. The experimental lidar was capable of measuring the profiles of the Stokes parameters $\mathcal{F}_l$ and $\mathcal{F}_r$, which were then used to determine the values of the degree of depolarization according to the expression

$$\mathcal{D} = \mathcal{F}r / \mathcal{F}_l \tag{7.116}$$

The high spatial resolution of the lidar enabled us to investigate the behavior of $\mathcal{F}_r$ and $\mathcal{F}_l$ as a function of the depth of the cloud layer. The measurements were performed in relatively homogeneous clouds. Figure 7.21 gives some typical profiles obtained for the degree of depolarization as a function of the depth of penetration of the lidar pulse into the cloud for various values of the volume extinction coefficient. We also investigated the spatial shift $\Delta L$ between maxima of the main and cross-polarized components of the echo signals and the degree of depolarization corresponding to

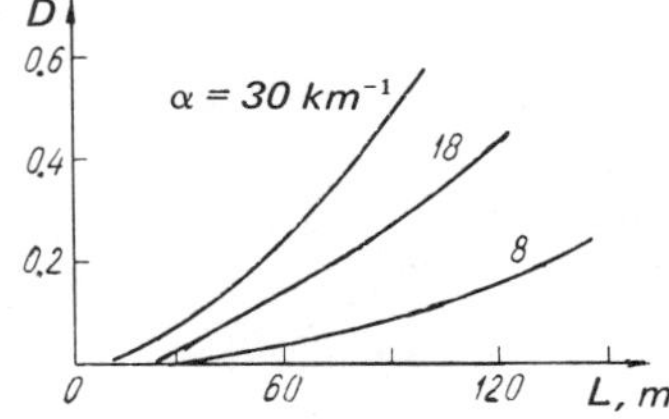


Fig. 7.21. Profiles of degree of polarization with respect to cloud penetration depth.

the extrema:

$$\mathcal{D}_{\mathrm{max}} = \mathcal{F}_r^{\,\mathrm{max}} / \mathcal{F}_l^{\,\mathrm{max}} \tag{7.117}$$

It turned out that a relationship of the parameter $\Delta L$ to the volume extinction coefficient is observed for clouds with a well-delineated bottom (see Fig. 7.20). The parameter $\Delta L$ is related to the depth at which depolarization begins or to the depth at which multiple-scattering effects set in. For less dense clouds, of course, depolarization begins at proportionately greater depths, as is also clearly evident in Fig. 7.21.

The relationship of $\Delta L$ to the volume extinction coefficient $\alpha$ can be approximately written $\Delta L\alpha \cong 0.5$ to $0.35$. The presence of correlation between $\Delta L$ and $\alpha$ suggested a method for determining the volume extinction coefficient of liquid-droplet clouds [135].

The values of $\mathcal{D}_{\mathrm{max}}$ for a given cloud type turned out to depend only slightly on the volume extinction coefficient as the latter varied from 4 to 40 $\mathrm{km}^{-1}$, whereas for other types of cloud structures the value of $\mathcal{D}_{\mathrm{max}}$ varied between the limits 0.05 and 0.35.

In the case of clouds having an indistinctly defined bottom, the above-described laws governing the behavior of the degree of depolarization are distorted by irregularities of the particle concentration, which redistribute the multiple-scattering field in a random fashion, but the shift between maxima of the copolarized and cross-polarized components of the echo signal is preserved.

In the probing of crystal clouds, the cross-polarized component of the echo signal is present in single scattering, the value of $\mathcal{D}$, as a rule, is greater than 0.4, the behavior of the $\mathcal{F}_r$ and $\mathcal{F}_l$ signals is identical, and no appreciable shift between them is observed. In mixed clouds, the degree of depolarization varies between wide limits and, as shown in [136], mirrors the relative concentration of cloud crystals relative to droplets. Appreciable shifts between $\mathcal{F}_r$ and $\mathcal{F}_l$ are not observed in the probing of mixed clouds.

A vast program of aircraft experimental studies on the laser probing of various types of clouds has been carried out by a working group at the Central Aerological Observatory [7, 88, 100, 137–143]. The main object of attention in this work comprised the polarization characteristics of echo signals with a view toward acquiring information about the profiles of the scattering coefficients, the phase state, the particle concentration, and the water content of clouds, as well as performing cloud identification against the background of the underlying ground surface. We now give some of the results of this work.

Shvidkovskii and others [88, 100] have proposed a method for reconstructing the profile of the volume scattering coefficient in such a way as to obtain reliable data from the results of laser probing of clouds up to optical thicknesses $\tau \leqslant 1$. Given definite assumptions concerning the microphysical parameters of a cloud, it is possible to extract information about the cloud particle concentration and water content from the indicated profile. Tyabotov and others [141] have conducted detailed studies of the distortion of lidar echo signals as a function of the volume scattering coefficient. The depolarization and angle of rotation of the polarization plane of lidar echo pulses from various types of clouds and the ground have also been investigated [142].

An analysis of the results of measurements based on the usage of theoretical algorithms which take double-scattering effects into consideration [144] has made it possible to obtain profiles of the particle concentration, water content, degree of depolarization, and volume scattering coefficient in single-frequency laser probing of the bottom of thick clouds. It was found that all of these parameters of the lowest level of a cloud increase very sharply, and then, at depths of 50 to 100 m, their variation becomes smoother. For example, at a depth of 50 to 60 m and at the bottom of a cloud, the volume scattering coefficient has respective values of 50 and 0.8 km$^{-1}$, the particle concentrations at the same points are $4 \times 10^8$ and $1.2 \times 10^7$ m$^{-3}$, and the water contents are 0.3 and $0.8 \times 10^{-3}$ g·m$^{-3}$.

In a series of cloud lidar studies performed by Collis's group at the Stanford Research Institute [86, 87, 145–150], considerable attention was devoted to the characteristics of cirrus clouds, whose comparatively low density makes it possible to determine the bottom and top of a cloud simultaneously with a single laser pulse transmission. Using these clouds as tracers, Collis and his co-workers observed large-scale transport waves in the upper troposphere. A determination of the volume extinction coefficients in cirrus clouds showed that their values are 10 to $10^3$ times the volume Rayleigh scattering coefficients.

Carswell and others [128, 151–153] have obtained a huge quantity of experimental data on the laser probing of clouds, mainly on the basis of echo-signal polarization characteristics. Different types of cloud formations were investigated. A three-channel echo-signal receiving system was used to measure the linearly copolarized, cross-polarized, and 45°-polarized (between the first two) components. Sizable fluctuations were noted both in the degree of depolarization $\mathscr{D}$ as a function of the cloud type and in the variation of $\mathscr{D}$ with penetration of the transmitted pulse into the cloud interior. In the evaluation of the results, optimistic statements were made regarding the feasibility and practicability of using polarization lidars for cloud-diagnostic applications. The authors of the previously cited work [129] arrived at the same conclusion.

A persuasive illustration of the use of lidar to monitor the precipitation of ice crystals in the South Pole region is given in [154]. The application of laser probing for the precise determination of the bottom of clouds is discussed in [155]. We have previously [156] published the results of a successful application of laser probing for the investigation of artificially illuminated clouds by the seeding of condensation nuclei in them. Zhukov and others [157] report the successful outcome of a trial application of two-wave lidar ($\lambda_1 = 0.6943$ and $\lambda_2 = 0.3472$ $\mu$m) in conjunction with short-baseline photometers to determine the microstructural parameters of oil mists in the atmosphere.

Thus, the methods of laser probing of clouds have come to enjoy wide-spread applications in related field studies. They provide a means of ready solution of the problem of identifying the phase composition of clouds without recourse to any *a priori* information; under certain reasonable assumptions regarding the particle-size spectrum, data are obtained on the particle concentration and water content of clouds. In the case of low-density clouds, both the top and bottom boundaries of a cloud can be determined with a high degree of accuracy. As for high-density clouds, the corresponding parameters are reliably determined in the lower part of the cloud without regard for the influence of multiple-scattering effects. Allowance for the latter in accordance with the algorithms described in Section 7.7.1 unleashes possibilities for penetrating into the deeper cloud layers.

In concluding this section, we stress the fact that despite the very marked advances in experimental cloud studies using the laser probing method, many interesting and important problems have yet to be even touched upon, although theoreticians have very recently been able to lay a reasonably good foundation for their solution (see Section 7.7.1). Foremost among these problems are multifrequency laser probing of the bottom of clouds to extract information about their microphysical parameters and, in turn, about their particle-size spectra; laser probing of clouds with measurements of echo-signals at different scattering angles and of the polarization characteristics for the same objective of acquiring data on the microphysical parameters of clouds without the influence of *a priori* information; solution of the above-stated problems for deeper interior layers of clouds with correct adjustment for multiple-scattering effects. It is also essential to underscore the even more complex problem of laser probing of clouds in connection with the extraction of information about the complex refractive index as well as the geometry and orientation of particles in crystal clouds.

## 7.8. Laser Monitoring of Industrial Aerosols

Generally speaking, aerosols of industrial origin coexist with natural aerosols, and the problems related to the determination of either by laser-probe methods scarcely differ from one another. We have nonetheless decided to treat industrial aerosols separately, not only because the problem is of such extreme practical significance, but also in view of the fact that, as a rule, the mass concentration of atmosphere-polluting industrial aerosols are many times, if not orders of magnitude, greater than for natural aerosols.

Systematic studies of aerosols of industrial origin have been in progress during the last five years under the author's direction at the Institute of Optics of the Atmosphere (IOA) of the Siberian Branch of the Academy of Sciences of the USSR (SO AN SSSR) [158–163]. The objective of these studies, on the one hand, is to develop algorithms for the unambiguous extractions of particular aerosol characteristics from probing results and, on the other, to design equipment that can be used to implement the indicated algorithms for relevant experimental research. We have already discussed algorithms for the solution of inverse problems associated with the laser monitoring of aerosols in Section 7.6. In this section, therefore, we turn our attention mainly to describing the main results of experimental work.

The most important characteristic of an industrial aerosol from the standpoint of practical applications is its mass concentration, or the quantity of aerosol matter by weight per unit volume of the medium. The rigorous solution of the problem of determining this characteristic in connection with laser probing poses an extremely complex task requiring the application of whichever of the methods discussed in Section 7.6 will provide the size spectrum and concentration of particles for the ultimate determination of the mass concentration of aerosol matter once the complex refractive index is known. In this connection, it is important to devise a reasonably simple method that will make it possible, on the one hand, to circumvent the stated difficulties and, on the other, to comply with the appropriate accuracy requirements for determination of the given characteristic. One such approach that can be recommended is the direct extraction of information on the mass concentration of aerosols from data on the volume backscattering coefficient.

Our experimental investigations have shown that, with a certain error, these quantities can be assumed to be linearly related. Figure 7.22 gives an example of the correlation between the volume backscattering coefficient $\beta_\pi$ and the mass concentration $M$ of aerosols. The coefficient $\beta_\pi$ was measured by means of a lidar, and $M$ was calculated from direct measurements with the scooping of aerosol samples.

It is quite clear that the correlation coefficient in the dependence of $M$ on $\beta_\pi$ is higher for more homogeneous aerosols in terms of the size spectrum and chemical composition of the particles. Thus, if the aerosol source is the same (such as an industrial carrier in the atmosphere), the indicated method will yield fairly accurate values of $M$ from measurement of $\beta_\pi$. The method is not unconditionally universal. Moreover, for each type of aerosol it is necessary to have a predetermined relation between $M$ and $\beta_\pi$, and in cases where the aerosol mass consists of different aerosol types in proportions that vary in unmonitorable fashion this method can only give crude estimates of the values of $M$. In many practical situations, however, its application is fully justified.

We now show that a linear relationship can be derived between the mass concentration of an aerosol and the volume extinction coefficient in the backward direction under definite assumptions. We assume that the aerosol has a single common origin and is characterized by a definite particle-size spectrum and, hence, a definite polydisperse angular scattering function. We choose the wavelength of the laser probe pulse in such a way

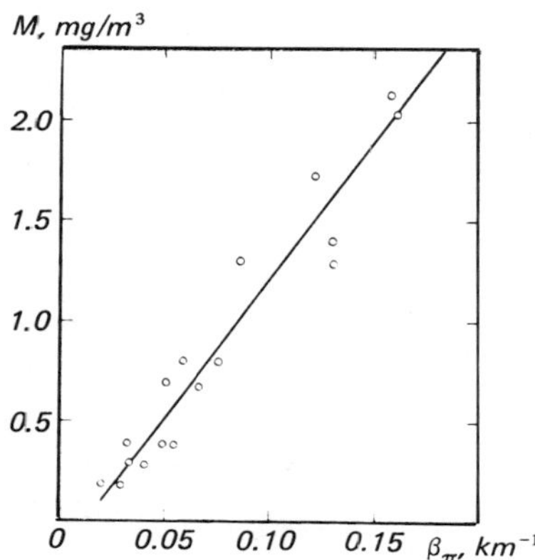

Fig. 7.22. Mass concentration of aerosol versus backscattering coefficient of radiation from lidar observations with simultaneous scooping of aerosol samples.

as to be many times the modal radius of the aerosol particle-size distribution. Then the following relation holds:

$$\frac{\int_0^{a_1} a^3 n(a)\,da}{\int_0^{\infty} a^3 n(a)\,da} \cong 1 \tag{7.118}$$

where $a$ is the particle radius, $n(a)$ is the particle-size distribution function, and $a_1$ is the limiting value of the particle radius.

In the case of a homogeneous monodisperse aerosol, the mass concentration $M$ is related to the volume extinction coefficient by the expression

$$M = \tfrac{4}{3} C \frac{a\alpha(\lambda, a)}{Q(\chi, m)} \tag{7.119}$$

in which $C$ is a constant of the particle material, $\alpha$ is the volume extinction coefficient, $Q$ is the extinction efficiency factor, and $\chi$ is the Mie parameter.

For a polydisperse aerosol, we can write

$$M = \tfrac{4}{3} C \sum_{i=1}^{n} \frac{a_i \alpha_i}{Q(\chi_i)} \tag{7.120}$$

In the interval of small values of $\chi$ in the interval $0 \leqslant \chi \leqslant \chi_1$, where $\chi_1 = 2\pi a_1/\lambda$, $Q(\chi)$ can be approximated by the linear function

$$Q(\chi) = ka \tag{7.121}$$

where $k$ is a coefficient depending on the type of aerosol. Substituting (7.121) into (7.120), we obtain

$$M = \frac{4}{3} \frac{C\alpha}{k} \tag{7.122}$$

In the given case, therefore, the quantity $M$ turns out to depend linearly on $\alpha$ and, hence, on the volume backscattering coefficient $\beta_\pi$ since the lidar ratio has a fully defined value according to the assumptions stated above.

In the general case of industrial aerosol monitoring, information on the mass concentration of particles and certainly on the microphysical parameters of aerosols can be obtained on the basis of a solution of the inverse problems by the algorithms discussed in detail in Section 7.6.

We now present some illustrations of our results of laser monitoring of industrial aerosols. Figure 7.23 gives an example of the use of lidar to obtain a horizontal section of the values of the volume extinction coefficient under the conditions of an urban atmosphere heavily contaminated with aerosols over a $3\times3$ km area with horizontal slewing of the optical axis. The isolines representing equal values of $\ln\alpha$ bound domains with corresponding values of the mass concentration of aerosols. The symbol $S$ marks the lidar site.

Figure 7.24 gives the variation of the vertical aerosol distribution in the period from 2124, August 24, 1972, to 0525, August 25, 1972, in the same urban atmosphere. As a visual aid, each successive curve is shifted one unit along the horizontal axis. It is distinctly clear from the figure how the layer of increased turbidity existing at the beginning of the measurement period at a height of about 2 km, its formation being possibly influenced by light overhead cloudiness (see the upper part of the figure), subsequently decays concurrently with disappearance of the cloudiness. The top of the monitored layer is clearly registered in the $\beta_\pi$ profile and decreases continuously during the measurement period, while at the same time the mass aerosol concentration in the boundary layer of the atmosphere increases accordingly.

Figure 7.25 illustrates two typical vertical profiles of the volume extinction coefficient, obtained in an atmosphere of a coarse polymetallic carrier to a depth of about 100 m. Curve 1 refers to the case of an unstable state of the atmosphere, with good aeration of the carrier, resulting essentially in an exponential decay of the mass concentration with height. Curve 2 illustrates the presence of a heavy aerosol layer, the maximum of which roughly corresponds to the surface of the carrier. Measurements of the temperature profile indicated that a pronounced temperature inversion took

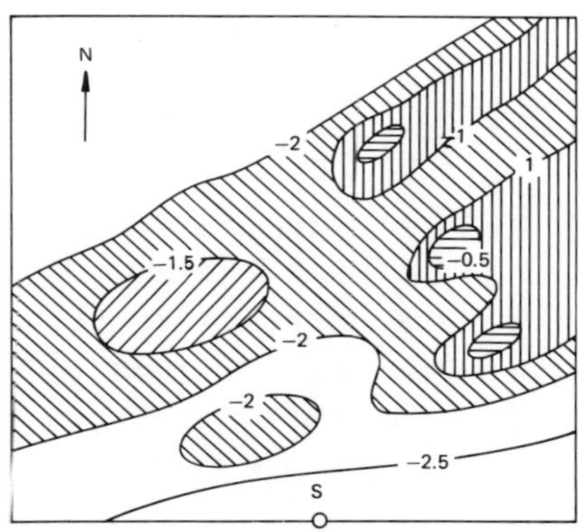


Fig. 7.23. Example of aerosol environment determined by scanning in a horizontal plane. The solid curves represent isolines of the quantity $\ln\alpha$. Frame dimensions: $3\times3$ km; point $S$ denotes the site of the lidar.

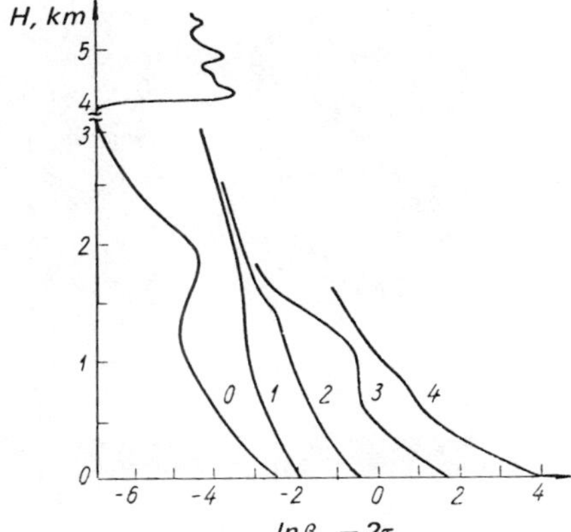

Fig. 7.24. Variation of vertical aerosol distribution from 2124, Aug. 24, 1972, to 0525, Aug. 25, 1972 (each successive curve is shifted one unit along the horizontal axis; the true abscissa value is obtained by subtracting the curve number).

place in the vicinity of the maximum of the aerosol layer, inhibiting aeration of the carrier space. These illustrations unequivocally evince the considerable promise of laser monitoring techniques in application to industrial aerosols.

A similar conclusion stems from the results of other investigations, of which the most important is the work of Collis's group, a major contribution to the investigated problem [164–170]. The originality of this series of investigations lies primarily in the design of a unique automated measurement technique, which ensures the acquisition of monitoring data with high temporal and spatial resolution. Figure 7.26 illustrates the capabilities of this apparatus. The measurement time is plotted along the horizontal axis and the height on the vertical axis. Each of the vertical lines corresponds to

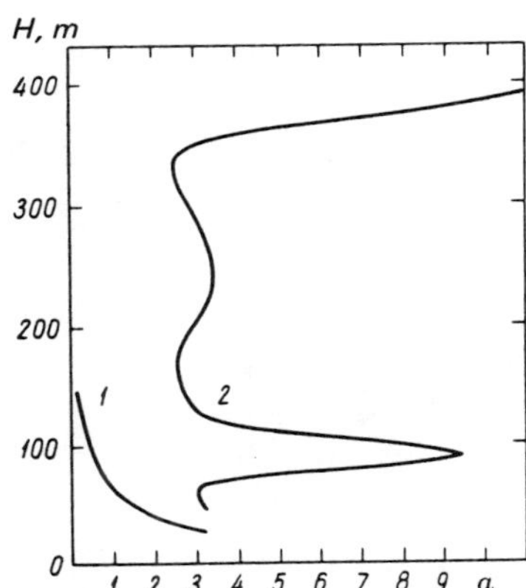

Fig. 7.25. Height dependence of scattering coefficient above carrier in different meteorological situations. (1) Unstable atmosphere (good aeration of carrier); (2) aeration impeded by the presence of inversion. The scattering coefficient is given in relative units.

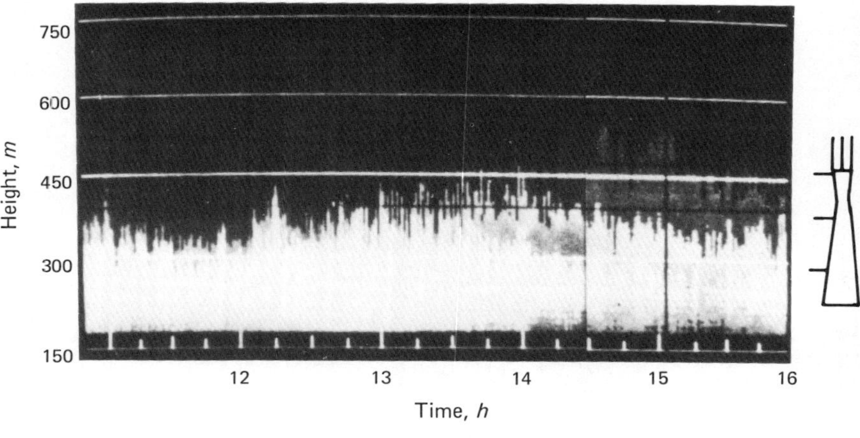

Fig. 7.26.

the results of a single monitor-pulse transmission, the profiles of whose echo signals are processed and plotted with the aid of a computer. The same apparatus makes it possible to obtain vertical and horizontal sections of the volume backscattering coefficients, which can be inverted to obtain the values of the volume scattering coefficients and mass concentrations of an aerosol. Figure 7.27 gives a vertical section of the mass aerosol concentration obtained by means of the automated lidar in stack effluents. The numbers alongside the isolines correspond to the value of $10 \log(M/M_0)$, where $M$ is the concentration in the stack effluent and $M_0 = 100$ mg/m$^3$ is the reference mass concentration far from the effluent.

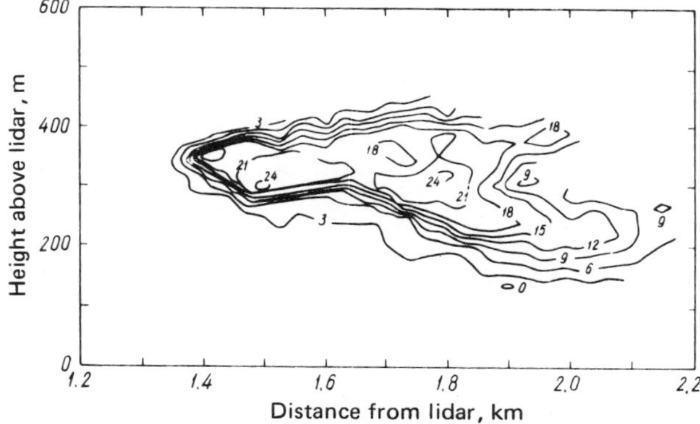

Fig. 7.27.

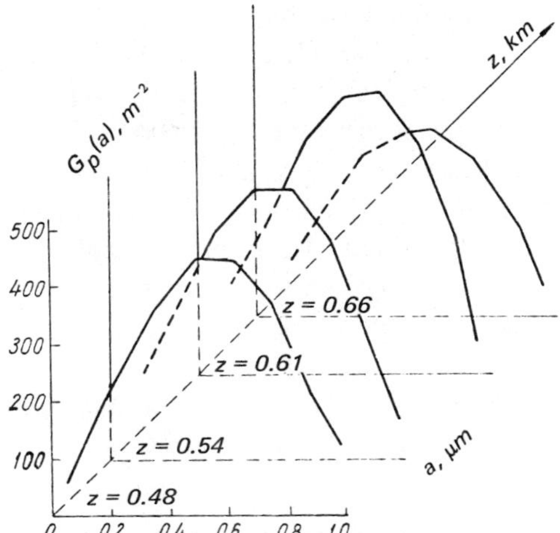



Fig. 7.28.

Recent attempts have been undertaken to utilize the fluorescence effect in laser monitoring of industrial aerosols, the majority of which have rather strong luminescence bands associated with the excitation of ultraviolet radiation [171–173]. Kaul' [174] has derived a lidar equation for a luminescent aerosol. Work in this area is really just beginning. However, it is already clear what kind of difficulty is involved in this method in connection with the need to consider overlapping of the broad fluorescence bands identified with different components of the aerosol matter. On the other hand, the large fluorescence cross sections of these components are extremely encouraging for the future development of this approach.

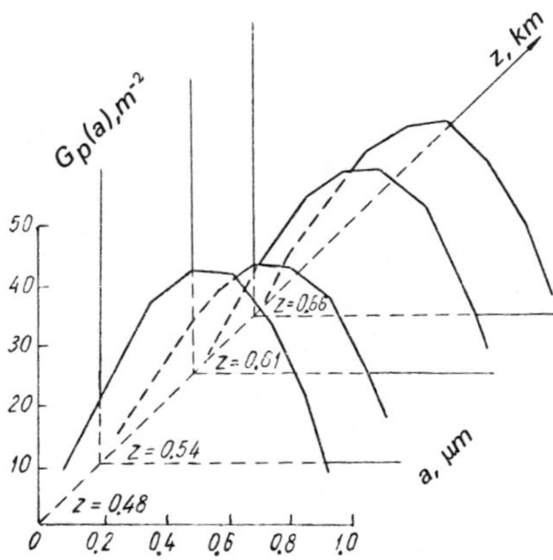



Fig. 7.29.

We conclude this section with a brief look at data obtained in our work [175] on the particle-size spectra of ground-layer aerosols in multifrequency laser monitoring with the use of algorithms for the solution of the inverse problem. Three wavelengths were used for monitoring ($\lambda_1 = 1.06$ $\mu$m; $\lambda_2 = 0.6943$ $\mu$m; $\lambda_3 = 0.53$ $\mu$m) in the autumn of 1975. The distributions of the particles by geometrical cross sections were reconstructed by the regularization algorithms described in Section 7.6. Example distributions of the geometrical cross sections of the particles in unit volume $G_p(a)$ at various distances from the lidar in the atmospheric ground layer are given in Figs. 7.28 and 7.29, illustrating the variation of the particle-size spectra with distance. We note that the total particle concentration differed by an order of magnitude in the two examples given of the results of determining $G_p(a)$.

## 7.9 Laser Monitoring of Aerosols in the Troposphere and Stratosphere

The first work on laser probing of the atmosphere was concerned with aerosol monitoring [1]. Since that time, the research in this area has grown from year to year, in part because of the unquestionable significance of the problem and in part because of the relative simplicity of the actual experimental operation when one thinks solely in terms of recording echo, or return, signals elicited by aerosol scattering and ignores the dilemma of their unambiguous interpretation.

The majority of published works on laser monitoring of atmospheric aerosols are tied in with the determination of the vertical profiles of the volume aerosol backscattering coefficient from the measured profile of the sum of the volume aerosol (particulate) backscattering and Rayleigh scattering coefficients [176–240]. In this work, the volume Rayleigh scattering coefficient was calculated from the standard model of the atmosphere. The resulting profiles give a good pictorial representation of the aerosol stratification structures, and the method itself enables us to analyze the dynamics of that stratification. For this reason, similar studies are continuing at the present time, particularly insofar as their capabilities have been significantly expanded through the use of airborne lidar systems [241–246].

Not long after publication of the first papers on laser monitoring of aerosols, it became clear that the accumulated volume of measurement data from single-frequency monostatic probing was decidedly insufficient for any quantitative interpretation of the monitoring results, even in terms of the profiles of the volume aerosol scattering coefficients, not to mention the microphysical parameters of aerosols. Consequently, in conjunction with lidars, researchers began to employ other methods that would significantly expand the possibilities for the interpretation of the laser echo pulses [246–265]. Some authors used radiosondes in parallel with laser monitoring, others resorted to direct measurements of the aerosol characteristics by the scooping method with the use of towers and aircraft, and a third group used radiometric or radar techniques.

The capabilities of laser aerosol-monitoring methods were greatly expanded by the use of bistatic probing configurations and analysis of the polarization characteristics of the echo signals [181, 266–269]. Finally, without a doubt the most promising trends in the laser monitoring of aerosols must be recognized as those in which the measurement information is of such a "quality" that the corresponding inverse problems are rendered solvable, either with recourse to substantiated *a priori* information or, most particularly, without such information. In this category we find multifrequency monitoring, either monostatic or bistatic, bistatic monitoring at different scattering angles, measurements of the polarization characteristics of echo signals, or any combination of these methods [270–282].

We have already discussed the theoretical problems of laser aerosol monitoring. In this section, therefore, we consider the most interesting results of experimental studies and their interpretation.

Figure 7.30 gives the results of laser monitoring of the vertical profiles of the ratio of the sum of the volume aerosol backscattering and Rayleigh

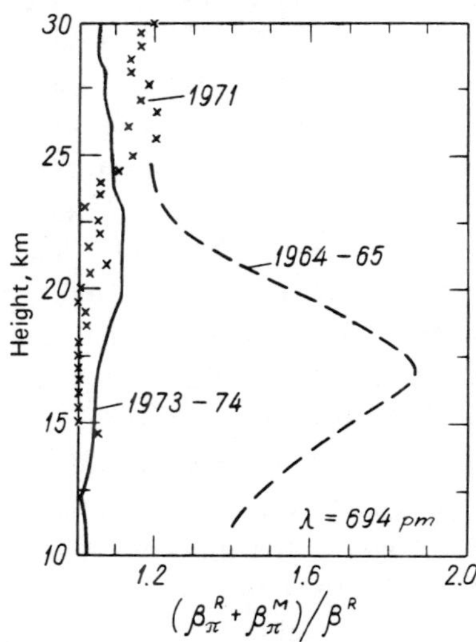


Fig. 7.30.

$$\left(\beta_\pi^R + \beta_\pi^M\right)/\beta^R$$

scattering coefficients to the volume Rayleigh backscattering coefficient for the lower stratosphere according to different authors at different times. The solid curve represents the averaging of 16 series of measurements performed in the period from June 1973 through March 1974 along the central California coastline of the Pacific Ocean [230] with the use of a ruby-laser lidar system (emission wavelength 0.69438 $\mu$m). The crosses represent averaged data obtained by Fox and others [243] with an airborne dye-laser lidar (wavelength 0.585 $\mu$m) and reduced to 0.69438 $\mu$m on the basis of assumptions concerning the validity of the relation $\alpha_M(\lambda) \sim \lambda^{-1}$, where $\alpha_M$ is the volume aerosol scattering coefficient. These data characterize the profile obtained by aircraft measurements over the Pacific Ocean in August 1971. Finally, the dashed curve represents the results of averaging of 66 profiles obtained during 1964–65 with the use of a ground-based ruby-laser lidar system in Massachusetts [189].

It is evident from Fig. 7.30 that a distinct maximum of the aerosol layer at heights of about 17 km was observed in the period 1964–65, whereas in prior years this maximum was much less pronounced and its height was greater than 20 km. This difference in the behavior of the vertical stratification profile of the aerosols in the lower stratosphere is attributable to the conspicuous volcanic activity present up through May 1970, most of all the eruption of the Agung Volcano in March 1963.

A powerful eruption of the Fuego Volcano in Guatemala occurred in October 1974, and soon after that event various scientific groups working with laser monitoring of the stratospheric aerosol registered a significant increase in the echo-signal intensity [230–235].

Figure 7.31 gives the results of observations [235] made by means of the same apparatus as was used to obtain the data in Fig. 7.30 discussed above. For comparison, the dashed curves give the average profile of the observations of this group of authors in the period from June 1973 through March 1974 (see Fig. 7.30). The 15 profiles in Fig. 7.31 were obtained in the period February–November 1975. The first observation was made four months after eruption of the volcano. The results indicate the presence of a strong narrow maximum of the aerosol layer at a height of about 20 km, along with a series of less-distinct layers at lower altitudes. In further observations, the stratification of the aerosol layers and their intensity gradually lose their definition in comparison with the first observation.

The results of systematic measurements of the ratio of the aerosol and Rayleigh scattering echo signals to the Rayleigh signal in the period from October 1974 to July 1976 at Hampton, Virginia, are given in Fig. 7.32 [283]. The values of the maximum of $R(r) - 1$ are plotted on the vertical

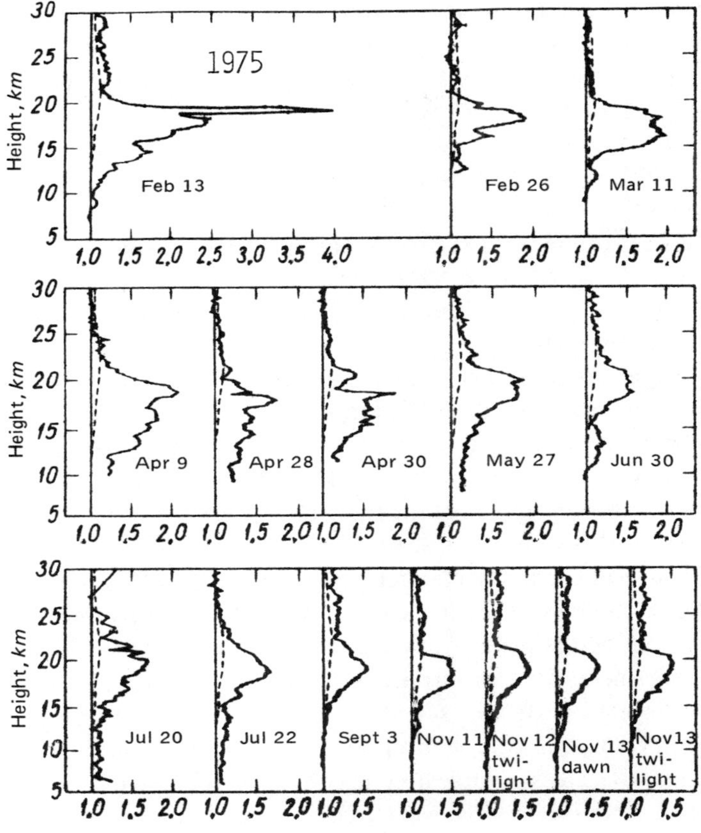


Fig. 7.31.



Fig. 7.32.

axis, where $R(r)$ is the indicated echo-signal ratio, and the time is plotted along the horizontal axis. It is important to note that the first observation was made October 10, 1974, several days after eruption of the Fuego Volcano. The value of $R(r)$ was equal to 1.3 in this case. The maximum value of $R(r)$, approximately equal to 5, was attained at the beginning of January 1975. Thereafter it was observed to decrease gradually for the remainder of the year.

The next example of laser monitoring of the stratospheric aerosols is the work of Fernald *et. al.* [256], who used an airborne lidar to obtain unique data on the spatial aerosol distribution at heights from about 10 to 27 km in a flight from Washington, D.C., to Madrid. To eliminate the influence of errors associated with imprecise determination of the echo-signal components due to Rayleigh scattering, those components were determined from radiosonde atmospheric-density data obtained at stations along the course of the aircraft and processed by a special technique. As a result of the flight, data were obtained on the stratospheric aerosols, characterizing their variability on a synoptic scale.

Considering the many illustrations of the results of aerosol monitoring in the troposphere in the earlier section devoted to investigation of the lidar ratio, we confine the present discussion to problems in the use of polarization measurements for the purpose of acquiring information on aerosols in the lower layers of the atmosphere. This topic is given the most complete coverage in [284]. The lidar used there was capable of measuring the linearly copolarized and cross-polarized components of echo signals at the fundamental and second-harmonic wavelengths of ruby laser emission. Measurements performed under various meteorological conditions near Toronto, Canada, disclosed a vast set of variations of the polarization characteristics of echo signals, particularly in the lower kilometer layer. Specifically, the degree of depolarization in this layer varied from one case to another in a range of values from close to 0 up through 0.5, although the most frequent values occurred between 0.05 and 0.2. Not one case was encountered in which the polarization characteristics of the echo signal in the lower kilometer layer were equal to the theoretical values for a Rayleigh atmosphere, even though such observations occurred repeatedly at heights of several kilometers. Unfortunately, the lidar studies in the cited paper were not accompanied by other aerosol measurements so the data cannot be interpreted from the point of view of comparing the polarization characteristics with a definite state of the aerosol atmosphere.

In conclusion, we discuss our own efforts aimed at extracting information on the microphysical parameters of the stratospheric aerosol from the results of two- and three-frequency laser monitoring on the basis of the algorithms developed by us and described in Section 7.6 for solution of the corresponding inverse problems [281, 282]. The measurements were carried out with a three-wave lidar ($\lambda_1 = 1.06$, $\lambda_2 = 0.59438$, $\lambda_3 = 0.53$ $\mu$m) in the vicinity of Tomsk for two stratospheric layers at heights from 13.5 to 15 km and from 15 to 16.5 km. The interval of heights for the wavelengths $\lambda_2$ and $\lambda_3$ ranged from 15 to 28 km.

As shown in Section 7.6, the three and, more so, two wavelengths at which the monitoring was performed were inadequate for the extraction of unambiguous data on the microphysical parameters of the aerosols without recourse to *a priori* information on their particle-size distribution and complex refractive index. Accordingly, in processing the monitoring results, the value of the complex refractive index of the particles was taken from published data, and gamma and Young distribution functions were used for the particle-size spectra.

Figure 7.33a gives two representative examples of the vertical profiles of the volume aerosol backscattering coefficients at $\lambda_2$ and $\lambda_3$. Assuming a gamma particle-size distribution, we used the optimal parametrization method to reconstruct from the indicated profiles the height variations of

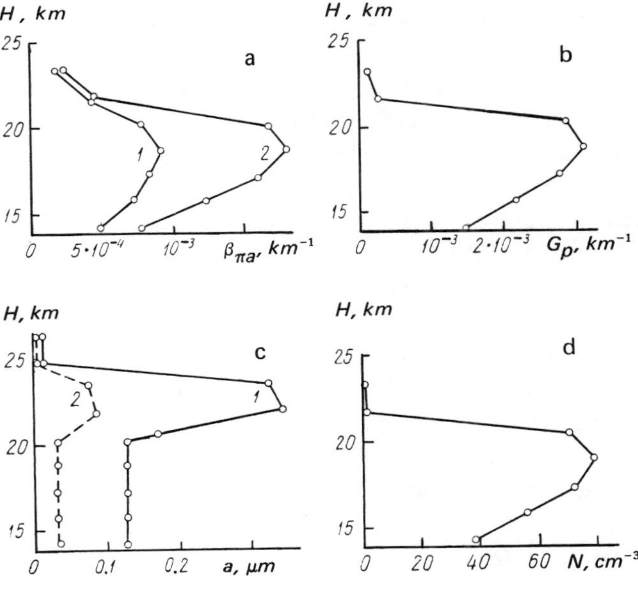

Fig. 7.33.

the total geometrical cross section of the particles in unit volume $G_p$, the modal radius $a_s$ in the distribution $G_p(a) = \pi a^2 n(a)$ (Figs. 7.33b and 7.33c), and, from the $G_p$ and $a$ data, the profile of the particle concentration $N$ (Fig. 7.33d), which exhibits satisfactory agreement with the existing data in the literature.

More comprehensive information on the microphysical parameters of the aerosol were obtained in three-frequency monitoring of the atmospheric layers from 13.5 to 15 km and from 15 to 16.5 km with the aid of the regularization method [281].


## 7.10. Determination of the Slant-Path Transmittance of the Atmosphere

Knowledge of the transmittance of the atmosphere in a given direction is equivalent to knowledge of the optical wave-energy losses in that direction. This fact accounts for the continual preoccupation of scientists and technicians with the problems of determining the transmittance of the atmosphere.

In general, the transmittance of the atmosphere in a particular direction is determined by the losses of optical wave energy due to absorption by atmospheric gases, molecular and aerosol (particulate) scattering, and a number of other less significant effects. In this section, we consider only the component of the transmittance associated with aerosol scattering. In other words, we are interested in methods of laser monitoring of the profiles of the volume aerosol scattering coefficients from which the profiles of the atmospheric transmittance can be readily obtained. We emphasize the fact that the determination of atmospheric transmittance by laser monitoring techniques has a powerful advantage over corresponding standard methods used to measure the transmittance in the ground layer. The data obtained by the latter approach are useful only in the case of a homogeneous atmosphere, whereas laser monitoring methods provide a picture of the transmittance profile with a high degree of spatial resolution for any atmosphere, no matter how inhomogeneous.

All methods for laser monitoring of the profiles of the volume aerosol scattering coefficient are based on Eq. (7.68) (see Section 7.7.1), which we write in the form

$$S(r) = Ab(r)\alpha(r)T^2(r) \qquad (7.123)$$

where $S(r)=P_r(r)r^2$ is the amplitude of the echo signal, corrected for the square of the distance $r$, $\alpha(r)$ is the volume aerosol scattering coefficient, $b(r)=\beta_\pi(r)/\alpha(r)$ is the lidar ratio, $\beta_\pi(r)$ is the volume aerosol backscattering coefficient, and $T(r)=\exp[-\int_0^r\alpha(r')\,dr']$ is the one-way transmittance of the atmospheric layer between the lidar and the monitored volume.

As mentioned earlier, Eq. (7.123) contains two unknowns, $b(r)$ and $\alpha(r)$, and cannot be solved in the case of single-frequency monostatic monitoring without the use of *a priori* information either about the properties of the monitored medium or about the values of $b(r)$. Below we give a concise analysis of the existing methods for the solution of Eq. (7.123) with regard for the nature of the recruited *a priori* information.

## 7.10.1 Methods Based on the Stratification Properties of the Atmosphere

### 7.10.1.1. Log-Derivative Method

As in cloud-probing applications (see Section 7.7.1.1), the log-derivative method is based on the hypothesis of a homogeneous atmosphere so that $b(r)=$const and $\alpha(r)=$const. In this case, we obtain directly from expression (7.123)

$$\alpha=\frac{1}{2}\frac{d}{dr}\ln[S(r)]\tag{7.124}$$

The method does not require absolute calibration of the lidar, but the underlying assumptions limit its applicability to crude estimates of the transmittance along horizontal and mildly slanting paths [96, 285, 286].

### 7.10.1.2. Slant-Path Method

In Section 7.7.1.2., we examined in detail algorithms for the slant-path method based on the assumption of horizontal homogeneity of the atmosphere. Despite its stability under the influence of multiple-scattering effects, the given method has limited applicability due to the assumptions on which it is based.

## 7.10.2. Numerical Methods

### 7.10.2.1. Method of Successive Layers

According to the method of successive layers, the monitoring path is partitioned into a sequence of sufficiently thin layers, within each of which the volume scattering coefficient and angular scattering function are considered to be constant. The lidar equation is written for each layer in this case, its solution requiring knowledge of $\alpha(r)$ at the beginning of the path and the profile of the lidar ratio in $b(r)$. Algorithms for this method are described in Section 7.7.1.3.

Algorithms are described in Section 7.7.1.4 for a modified successive-layer method proposed by us [104, 105], which has considerably greater stability under the influence of multiple-scattering effects.

### 7.10.2.2. Iterative Method

The iterative method is based on the following scheme for the solution of Eq. (7.123):

$$\beta_\pi^{(m)}(r) = \frac{S(r)}{A T^{(m-1)}(r)}$$

$$T^{(m)}(r) = \exp\left[-2\int_{r_1}^{r} \alpha^{(m)}(r')\, dr'\right] \qquad (7.125)$$

$$\alpha^{(m)}(r) = \frac{\beta_\pi^{(m)}(r)}{b(r)}$$

where $m$ is the iteration number.

The solution of (7.125) is initiated with a certain zeroth approximation, which can be taken as

$$T^0(r) = \exp(-2\bar{\alpha} r) \qquad (7.126)$$

where $\bar{\alpha}$ is the average value of the volume scattering coefficient along the monitoring path and can be determined either by some independent means or by specification on the basis of reasonable assumptions. Experience in the application of the given algorithm indicates that the solution converges after three or four iterations [73]. The method is applicable for monitoring of a slightly turbid atmosphere in the case of optical thicknesses $\tau \leqslant 0.5$.

### 7.10.3. Analytical Methods

### 7.10.3.1. Continuous-Update Method

The continuous-update method postulates a known profile of the lidar ratio along the monitoring path. Its algorithms and limits of applicability are discussed in Section 7.7.15. In Section 7.7.16, we describe algorithms for a parametric modification of the continuous-update method, greatly expanding its limits of applicability from the viewpoint of optical multiple-scattering effects.

### 7.10.3.2. Method of S Functions

The algorithms for the method of $S$ functions and for our proposed modification thereof are described in Section 7.7.1.7.

### 7.10.3.3. Asymptotic-Signal Method

The asymptotic-signal method does not require any assumptions as to the structure and nature of the scattering particles, provides a simple means for eliminating the influence of instrument errors and fluctuations of the coefficient $\beta_\pi$, and diminishes the role of multiple-scattering noise. The algorithms for the method are described in Section 7.7.1.8.

## 7.10.4. Methods Based on Measurements of the Temporal Characteristics of Echo Signals

### 7.10.4.1. Echo-Signal Distortion

When a transmitted probe pulse propagates through an aerosol medium, its echo (return) suffers distortion, which depends on the optical properties of the medium. Detailed experimental studies of this phenomenon by the author's working group with artifical fogs have indicated a dependence of the peak amplitude, width, and time shift of the echo signals on the volume aerosol-scattering coefficient when the values of the latter are less than 0.4 m$^{-1}$. Shuleikin [287] has used this method successfully for the laser monitoring of aerosols under natural conditions when the meteorological visibility range did not exceed 8 km.

### 7.10.4.2. Time Lag between the Polarized and Depolarized Echo-Signal Components

It has already been mentioned that the quality of the information obtained in single-frequency monostatic laser monitoring of aerosols improves significantly with the utilization of polarization effects. Thus, in measuring the intensities of the copolarized and cross-polarized components of echo signals returned from aerosol layers, along with the time shift between them, information can be extracted on the volume aerosol scattering coefficient [134, 135]. The following empirical relation between the volume aerosol scattering coefficient $\alpha$ and the separation of the maxima of the copolarized and cross-polarized components has been obtained by analysis of the experimental data:

$$\Delta L \cdot \alpha \approx 0.5 \qquad (7.127)$$

This relation is valid for the given experimental conditions.

### 7.10.4.3. Extraction of the Multiple-Scattering Signal

In all the methods discussed above, multiple scattering represents an interfering noise factor that limits the domain of their applicability. At the same time, multiple scattering can be used for laser monitoring of atmospheric transmittance profiles. It suffices in a number of instances to use the lidar equation in the double-scattering approximation [53, 54]. In experimental work, the multiple-scattering signal can be separated either by geometrical means (with the placement of an iris of appropriate size in the focal plane of the lidar receiving system) or on the basis of the depolarized component of the echo signal. The given approach is well suited to the probing of media with a volume aerosol scattering coefficient $\alpha \geqslant 1$ km$^{-1}$.

Common to all the methods of Section 7.10.4 is the fact that they do not require the use of *a priori* values of the lidar ratio.

## 7.10.5. Summary Remarks

We now summarize the results of analysis of the applicability of the foregoing methods of single-frequency laser monitoring of the atmospheric transmittance profile. First and foremost, it must be emphasized that none of these methods is universal. Moreover, they all depend in some measure on the quality of the *a priori* input information.

A method that is exempt from the need for *a priori* information on the scattering properties of the probed aerosols can be found among any laser atmospheric-monitoring techniques that yield data on the size spectra, concentration (number density), and complex refractive index of the aerosol particles. Representative of such methods is multifrequency monitoring or measurements of echo signals at several different scattering angles in a bistatic monitoring configuration. In these cases, the transmittance profiles can be obtained concurrently on the basis of suitable straightforward calculations according to familiar algorithms relating the values of the volume aerosol-scattering coefficients to the microphysical parameters of the particles. In this case as well, however, the precise value of the sought-after atmospheric transmittance profile can be obtained only for aerosols consisting of homogeneous spherical particles.

In practice, clearly, the most acceptable means of obtaining sufficiently accurate data on the transmittance profiles of the atmosphere is to use the above-investigated relations between the lidar ratio for the corresponding aerosol types and the relative humidity for the purpose of utilizing such information in one of the single-frequency methods discussed above.

In this case, the relative humidity is measured simultaneously with lidar measurements along the monitoring path. Also, if monitoring is performed in a coastal region, it is necessary to know the wind direction in order to be certain whether one is dealing with a marine or overland aerosol.


## 7.11. Laser Monitoring of Humidity and the Concentration of Gaseous Components of the Atmosphere

### 7.11.1. Differential Absorption Method

The basic idea underlying the differential absorption method is to probe the atmosphere with pulses at two wavelengths, one of which coincides with the center of the absorption line of the probed gas, while the second falls within an atmospheric window not too far from the first wavelength, so that the volume aerosol and molecular scattering coefficients can be regarded as identical for both wavelengths at the same clock time. In this case, a reasonably simple expression can be derived for the concentration profile of the probed gas if the emission lines of the probe pulses are sufficiently narrow.

The amplitude of the output signal of the lidar photodetector at time $t$ in probing with a pulse of frequency $\nu$ can be described by the expression

$$u_t(r) = \int_{\Delta\nu_1} q(\nu) P_r^{(t)}(\nu, r) \, d\nu \qquad (7.128)$$

in which $q(\nu)$ is the spectral sensitivity of the receiver (photodetector), $P_r^{(t)}(\nu, r)$ is the echo signal from the probe pulse at a lidar receiver situated at a distance $r$, and $\Delta\nu_1$ is the spectral width of the probe pulse.

The echo signal $P_r^{(t)}(\nu, r)$ is given by the atmospheric lidar equation (7.1), which we rewrite in a more practical form for the present situation:

$$P_r^{(t)}(\nu, r) = \eta(\nu) P_0(\nu) A r^{-2} \frac{c\tau}{2} \beta_\pi(\nu, r, t) T_a^2(\nu, r, t) T_s^2(\nu, r, t) \qquad (7.129)$$

where $T_a$ and $T_s$ are the components of the transmittance of the atmospheric layer between the lidar and the probed volume due to absorption by gas molecules and scattering by aerosols and molecules, respectively.

Substituting (7.129) into expression (7.128) and assuming that the coefficients $\eta(\nu)$, $\beta_\pi(\nu, r, t)$, $q(\nu)$, and $T_s(\nu, r, t)$ are constant within the band $\Delta\nu$, we obtain

$$u_t(r) = q\eta A r^{-2}\frac{c\tau}{2}\left[\beta_\pi^R(r,t) + \beta_\pi^M(r,t)\right]T_s^2\int_{\Delta\nu}P_0(\nu)T_a^2(\nu, r, t)\, d\nu$$

$$(7.130)$$

Writing expression (7.130) twice for a sequence of two probe pulses with wavelengths $\lambda_1$ and $\lambda_2$ and forming the ratio between them, we obtain

$$\frac{u_{t_1\lambda_1}(r)}{u_{t_2\lambda_2}(r)} = \frac{\beta_\pi^a(r,t_1) + \beta_\pi^M(r,t_1)}{\beta_\pi^R(r,t_2) + \beta_\pi^M(r,t_2)}\frac{T_s^2(r,t_1)}{T_s^2(r,t_2)}$$

$$\times\frac{\displaystyle\int_{\Delta\nu_1}P_0(\nu)T_a^2(\nu, r, t_1)\, d\nu}{\displaystyle\int_{\Delta\nu_2}P_0(\nu)T_a^2(\nu, r, t_2)\, d\nu}\tag{7.131}$$

Equation (7.131) incorporates the assumption that the volume coefficients of aerosol and molecular scattering have identical values for the wavelengths $\lambda_1$ and $\lambda_2$.

We assume that $t_2 - t_1 < t_a$, where $t_a$ is a characteristic time in which the scattering properties of the medium vary appreciably along the transmission path. We can then set the first two cofactors on the right-hand side of (7.131) equal to unity. We also assume that the half-width of the emission lines of the probe pulses is much smaller than the half-width of the absorption line of the probed gas (for example, $\gamma_{\text{em}} = 0.1\gamma_{\text{abs}}$). Now expression (7.131) can be rewritten in the form

$$\frac{u_{t_1\lambda_1}(r)}{u_{t_2\lambda_2}(r)} = \frac{P_0(\nu_1)}{P_0(\nu_2)}\frac{\exp\left[-2\int_0^r\sigma_a(\nu_1, r')N(r', t_1)\, dr'\right]}{\exp\left[-2\int_0^r\sigma_a(\nu_2, r')N(r', t_2)\, dr'\right]}\tag{7.132}$$

where

$$P_0(\nu_i) = \int_{\Delta\nu_i}P_0(\nu_i)\, d\nu_i, \qquad i = 1, 2.\tag{7.133}$$

Comparing the signals obtained for both wavelengths from distances $r$ and $r+dr$, we obtain the concentration of the unknown absorbing gas at a distance $r$ in the layer $\Delta r$ on the assumption that it is invariant in time $\Delta t = t_2 - t_1$:

$$N(r, \Delta r) = \frac{\ln\left[\dfrac{u_{\nu_1}(r)}{u_{\nu_1}(r+dr)}\right]}{\ln\left[\dfrac{u_{\nu_2}(r)}{u_{\nu_2}(r+dr)}\right]} \frac{1}{2\left[\sigma_a(\nu_1, r) - \sigma_a(\nu_2, r)\right]\Delta r} \tag{7.134}$$

For the calculation of $N(r)$ in this case, it is necessary to know the differential absorption cross section for the frequencies $\nu_1$ and $\nu_2$ along the probing path.

Equation (7.134) gives the concentration profile of the probed gas with spatial resolution $\Delta r$ or, more precisely, a histogram of the concentration distribution with step $\Delta r$. If we know the values of the differences $\sigma_a(\nu_1, r) - \sigma_a(\nu_2, r)$ for all points of the monitoring path and if all the assumptions underlying the derivation of this equation are valid, the determination of the profile of the gas concentration by the procedure described here will necessarily yield an unambiguous result, the accuracy of which depends, on the one hand, on the reliability of the underlying assumptions and, on the other hand, on the errors of the measurements and their processing. We now examine these problems in closer detail.

The errors of determination of the concentration of atmospheric gases by the differential absorption method can be classified into three groups: (1) errors induced by the atmosphere; (2) spectral errors; (3) instrument errors. The first group is attributable to the fact that both the scattering properties of the atmosphere and the concentration of the probed gas at any point along the monitoring path can vary in the period between probe-pulse transmissions $\Delta t = t_2 - t_1$. Also, the measurement results are drastically affected by atmospheric background noise. Spectral errors are associated with instability of the probe-pulse emission spectra, imprecise knowledge of the absorption coefficients and their behavior along the monitoring path, and failure to allow for the finite width of the probe-pulse emission line. Finally, instrument errors are caused by inherent noise in the photodetectors, instability in the operation of the recording instrumentation, and return-signal processing errors.

An analysis of the various types of errors of the differential absorption method has been carried out in several papers [13, 288–292]. Achmed [290] and Marichev and Mitsel' [291] have analyzed the dependence of the minimum detectable gas concentration on the total error of its determination on the basis of the expression

$$N_{min} = \frac{\ln[1+\Delta P_r]}{2[\sigma_a(\nu_1)-\sigma_a(\nu_2)]\Delta r} \tag{7.135}$$

in which $\Delta P_r$ is the relative variation of the ratio of the received signals at wavelengths $\lambda_1$ and $\lambda_2$, the minimum value of which is determined by the error $\delta(\Delta r)$ representing the sum of all types of errors.

It is evident from (7.135) that the minimum values of the detectable concentrations $N_{min}$ can be increased, for identical values of the total error $\delta(\Delta r)$, as a result of an increase in either $\Delta r$ or the difference $\sigma_a(\nu_1)-\sigma_a(\nu_2)$. In the first case, spatial resolution is sacrificed in the monitoring results, and in the second case there is a loss of observation range because return signals from the center of the absorption lines will be equal to zero from short distances due to strong absorption.

Expression (7.135) shows that a high concentration sensitivity and good spatial resolution can be obtained in monitoring the concentration of gases at short distances by working with the strong absorption lines of the monitored gas. Conversely, weak lines are preferable whenever data is required on the concentration distribution of a gas over long paths.

An analysis by Schotland [289] of the components of the total error in the determination of the concentration of a probed gas has shown that a major contribution to the sum-total effect is introduced by error associated with variation of the scattering properties of the atmosphere along the monitoring path. For example, the return from a height of 1 km in monitoring with a lidar using a ruby laser at a pulse firing rate of 1 sec$^{-1}$ has been found to vary by as much as 20%.

Investigations by Hinkley [292] led to the conclusion that the time in which the atmosphere can be regarded as "frozen" from the standpoint of its scattering properties is estimated to be of the order of $10^{-3}$ sec. Thus, to avoid the influence of variations of the scattering properties of the atmosphere, a sequence of two probe pulses must be transmitted not more than 1 msec apart. The technical implementation of this objective demands considerable effort.

It has been shown [289] that the spectral errors are far more attributable to instability in the reproducibility of the emission spectrum of the probe pulses than to instability in the determination of the differential absorption coefficient along the monitoring path due to temperature and pressure fluctuations.

The influence of instrument noise on the signal-reception range and sensitivity of the lidar system has been analyzed in detail [13]. In this work, in particular, an expression is given relating the energy of the probe pulse to the minimum detectable concentration at a distance $r$ for a given system signal-to-noise ratio.

The influence of the half-width of the probe-pulse emission line on the error of determination of the concentration of water vapor has been studied in detail [288] by means of appropriate numerical experiments. Calculations have been carried out for the water-vapor line with center $\lambda_0 = 6943.83$ Å, half-width $\gamma = 0.097$ cm$^{-1}$ atm$^{-1}$, and intensity $S_0 = 0.1616$ cm$\cdot$g$^{-1}$ [293] (in the vicinity of the ruby laser line) for summer and winter models of the midlatitude atmosphere [294]. The half-widths of the emission lines were taken equal to 0.048, 0.072, 0.097, 0.194, and 0.388 cm$^{-1}$. It turned out that the error in the determination of the absorption coefficient at the line center due to the finite width of the emission line for the summer and winter models of the atmosphere assumes respective sets of values 4, 15, 25, 38, 61% and 4, 11, 20, 29, 50% for the above-indicated five values of the emission line half-width. Similar calculations were carried out for different heights. Here we give one illustration. For the summer model and an emission line half-width of 0.097 cm$^{-1}$, the errors in the determination of the absorption coefficient at heights of 0, 5, and 10 km are approximately 11, 23, and 37%, respectively. Thus, neglect of the nonmonochromatic character of the probe-pulse emission can induce very substantial errors in the reconstruction of the concentration profile of the probed gas.

Consequently, despite the simplicity of the differential absorption method from the point of view of the underlying mathematical expressions, which ensure the unambiguous extraction of information on the profiles of the probed gases, its technical implementation poses an exceedingly complicated problem. It is for this reason that the practical utilization of the method has failed to gain much popularity. Below we give the main monitoring results obtained by the differential absorption method.

### 7.11.1.1. Humidity Monitoring

The first results of application of the differential absorption method were obtained by Schotland in 1964 [295] in monitoring of the humidity profile up to a height of about 2 km with the use of a ruby-laser lidar. The apparatus was subsequently improved, but the results of its application are not known.

Johnson and LaGrone [293] have proposed that two-frequency measurements be superseded by monitoring of the concentration of an absorbing gas according to measurements of the line intensity, which, of course, depends on the pressure. A ruby-laser lidar with an emission line half-width of 0.01 Å, adjusted for variations of the ruby temperature, was used to obtain the contour of the water-vapor line $\lambda_0 = 6943.83$ Å at a distance of 0.86 km (the pulse traveling a distance of 0.43 km from the lidar to the reflecting shield and back again) for a humidity of 17.2 $g \cdot m^{-3}$. The resulting line contour was satisfactorily described by the dispersion formula. Attempts to study the vertical profile of the total intensity of the water-vapor absorption line proved fruitless due to the marked scatter of the values of the volume backscattering coefficient during the measurements of the line contour.

In studies at the Institute of Optics of the Atmosphere of the Siberian Branch of the Academy of Sciences of the USSR (IOA SO AN SSR) [296–299], a number of techniques for laser monitoring of the humidity by the differential method were proposed with increased accuracy. In one of those techniques, it is proposed that the measurement of two-wavelength return signals be accompanied over the initial part of the monitoring path by simultaneous measurements of the humidity for normalization of the differential absorption coefficient in terms of the water-vapor concentration. In a second technique, the laser radiation passes through a spectrophone chamber, which is filled with a mixture of air and the probed gas, making it possible to determine the differential absorption cross section directly. By contrast with the first technique, the second one ensures monitoring not only along a horizontal path, but also in any direction of the irradiated hemisphere.

Marichev and others [298] have obtained water-vapor concentration profiles at distances up to 900 m along a horizontal path above rugged terrain. A spectrophone was used for calibration of the lidar. These results exhibit a startling attribute in connection with the fact that the humidity profiles emulate the irregularities of the underlying terrain. Zuev [299] has monitored the humidity along a horizontal path, using reflection from a topographical target situated at a distance of 980 m from the lidar. In the same work, we have proposed a method for locating water-vapor absorption lines with the use of probe pulses from a free-running laser (spiking regime), along with a number of techniques for improving the accuracy of determination of the concentration profile of the absorbing gas in monitoring with pulses having emission lines with half-widths of the order of the half-widths of the absorption lines of the probed gases.

Derr and others [300], using a tunable-wavelength dye laser capable of emitting two wavelengths simultaneously, have observed two relatively strong absorption lines for water vapor over a horizontal path, with centers at $\lambda_1 = 6475.1$ and $\lambda_2 = 6475.8$ Å, which can be used to monitor the humidity profiles with high spatial resolution in localized volumes. Of course, these data by no means exhaust the list of strong $H_2O$ lines even in the visible part of the spectrum, let alone the infrared. If we analyze the vibration–rotation absorption spectrum of water vapor, we readily deduce a proliferation of absorption lines that are suitable for the differential absorption method. Consequently, the principal obstacle to the application of this method is related to the problem of finding the necessary lasers.

### 7.11.1.2. *Monitoring of Nitrogen Peroxide*

The electron transitions in $NO_2$ produce a series of overlapping branches in the visible region of the spectrum, which have been investigated in detail [301–309]. These bands are in very propitious positions by virtue of a number of studies devoted to applications of the differential absorption method for investigation of the $NO_2$ concentration in the atmosphere.

O'Shea and Dodge [310] have used a tunable argon laser to monitor the concentration of $NO_2$ at its absorption lines with centers at $\lambda_1 = 496.5$ and $\lambda_2 = 501.7$ nm. The measurements were carried out near a highway at a distance of 2.6 km from the city of Atlanta. A laser beam was transmitted at a height of 30 m to a corner reflector mounted a distance of 3540 m from the lidar and returned to a receiver equipped for round-the-clock measurements. Three of the four experimentally obtained concentration maxima coincided with the observed peaks of the movement of the air mass. The minimum discernible $NO_2$ concentration over a 9050-m path was 0.01 ppm (parts per million).

Rothe and others [311, 312] have monitored the $NO_2$ concentration above the city of Cologne, using a tunable-wavelength dye laser. The maximum monitoring range realized in the experiments was 4 km with a minimum detectable concentration of 0.2 ppm. Each monitoring spatial gate had its own photon-counting channel for each of the two monitor wavelengths. The lidar had the following characteristics; pulse energy 1 J; pulse duration 300 nsec; firing rate 1 Hz; spectral width of pulse 1 Å; beam spread 0.1 Å; diameter of receiving antenna 0.6 m. The $NO_2$ concentration measured over the city fell in the interval from 5 to 10 ppm. It was observed to decrease with height and in lightly populated parts of the city. The concentration distribution of $NO_2$ was also obtained in a smokestack plume with an average value of 1170 ppm, which is consistent with the results of direct measurements.

Grant and others [313] have measured the $NO_2$ concentration in a cell located at a distance of 365 m from the lidar. A tunable dye laser was used for monitoring. The measurement wavelengths were 4418, 4448, 4465, and 4481 Å, for which the respective absorption cross sections are $(3.76, 6.33, 3.83, 6.70)\cdot 10^{-19}$ $cm^2$. The results exhibited good agreement with transmissometer measurements of the $NO_2$ concentration.

Tsuji and others [314], using the wall of a building as a reflecting shield and a lidar with a tunable dye laser over a path length of 1 km, obtained a minimum detectable $NO_2$ concentration equal to 3 ppb (parts per billion) with a measurement error of 0.2% for 1000 pairs of probe pulses. Other Japanese scientists [315] report the results of successful tests using a commercial lidar designed for the measurement of $NO_2$ and $SO_2$ concentrations by the differential absorption method.

### 7.11.1.3. Monitoring of Sulfur Dioxide and Ozone

Both sulfur dioxide (sulfurous anhydride) and ozone have strong (from the standpoint of the differential technique) electron absorption bands in the ultraviolet wavelength range from 260 to 320 nm. The most comprehensive data on the $SO_2$ absorption bands are reported by Thompson and others [316].

Remote measurements of the $SO_2$ and $O_3$ concentrations have been carried out [317] by means of a frequency-tunable dye laser and cells containing the investigated gas. The $SO_2$ concentration was monitored at wavelengths of 292.3 and 293.3 nm with corresponding absorption coefficients of 16 and 24 $cm^{-1}$ $atm^{-1}$. Wavelengths of 292.3 and 294 nm were used for $O_3$ monitoring, with corresponding absorption coefficients of 28 and 22 $cm^{-1} atm^{-1}$. The monitoring results were compared with the results of transmissometer measurements in order to estimate the concentration sensitivity, which turned out to be 0.6 and 1.2 ppm per 0.1 km probed atmospheric thickness for $SO_2$ and $O_3$, respectively. To enhance the sensitivity of the method, the authors of [317] propose the simultaneous application of two lasers tuned to the absorption line of the investigated gas and to a point in the weak absorption region. The following wavelengths are recommended for monitoring in this case:

$$SO_2: \lambda_1 = 299.5 \text{ nm} \quad \text{and} \quad \lambda_2 = 300.05 \text{ nm}, \qquad \Delta\sigma_a = 25.6 \text{ cm}^{-1}\text{atm}^{-1}$$

$$O_3: \lambda_1 = 292.3 \text{ nm} \quad \text{and} \quad \lambda_2 = 301.0 \text{ nm}, \qquad \Delta\sigma_a = 18 \text{ cm}^{-1}\text{atm}^{-1}$$

at which it is possible to attain the following sensitivities for a probed thickness of 100 m: 0.10 ppm for $SO_2$ and 0.13 ppm for $O_3$ for eight pairs of probe pulses with an energy of 15 mJ, an emission spectral width of 1 Å, a receiving mirror with an area of 0.056 $m^2$ and an interference filter with a bandwidth of 13 nm and 27% transmission at the peak.

We recall that a sensitivity of 3 ppb with an rms error of 0.2% was attained in the work cited above [315] for the transmission of 1000 pairs of pulses over a 1-km path. The monitoring wavelengths were 300.1 and 301.4 Å, and the probe pulses had a spectral width of 3 Å and an energy of the order of 0.1 mJ. The area of the receiving aperture was 0.196 $m^2$.

### 7.11.1.4. Summary Remarks

It is apparent from the foregoing examples that the differential absorption method has been developed for the visible and ultraviolet regions for two reasons. First, the return pulses associated with aerosol and molecular scattering are much stronger in the visible and ultraviolet regions; second, the most sensitive receivers are available for these ranges.

It is evident from the preceding discussion that the given method has the best concentration sensitivity of all the methods developed to date for the remote determination of the concentrations of the gaseous components of the atmosphere, although certainly not all of its potential capabilities have been fully exploited.

We now indicate the principal goals of researchers and designers in connection with further improving the concentration sensitivity of the method: (1) to preclude (minimize) the influence of temporal fluctuations of the scattering properties of the atmosphere along the monitoring path; (2) to increase the monochromaticity, power (energy), and frequency stability of the transmitted probe pulses; (3) to increase the accuracy of determination of the differential absorption cross sections for corresponding pairs of probe pulses; (4) to diminish receiving equipment noise and improve the accuracy of processing of the measurement data; (5) to enhance the potential of lidar in connection with the area of the receiving antenna and the quality of the monochromators or interference filters used.

There is no doubt that dramatic progress will be forthcoming in the near future toward further refinement of the differential absorption method in stride with the overall advancement of laser techniques and measurement techniques as well as with the growing engineering demands for data on the space–time distribution of the concentration of gaseous components of the atmosphere, including those of industrial origin.

### 7.11.2. *Spontanteous Raman Scattering Method*

The idea underlying the spontaneous Raman scattering (SRS) method is based on utilization of the spontaneous Raman scattering effect, which occurs, generally speaking, during the propagation of a laser probe pulse of any emission frequency in the atmosphere (see Chap. 3). Strictly speaking, a laser return pulse contains components corresponding to combination frequencies of all the gases. Because of the small values of the SRS cross sections, however, the application of this method is sensible only for gases such as $N_2, O_2, H_2O$, and $CO_2$ as well as the gases contained in industrial emissions, where their concentration is less than an order of magnitude greater than the ambient content. We examine the application of the SRS method in the example of humidity monitoring.

The SRS spectrum contains the excitation frequency of water molecules $\nu_{H_2O} = 3650$ cm$^{-1}$, i.e., this frequency is far enough from the frequency of the probe pulse in order to be able to discriminate the return signal associated with the combination excitation frequency of water vapor apart from the influence of the signal associated with aerosol and Rayleigh scattering of the probe pulse. The lidar equation for this echo signal has the form

$$P_{r\lambda_1}(r) = \eta \frac{P_0 c \tau A}{2r^2} \sigma_{\lambda_1}(r) N_1(r) T(r, \lambda_0) T(r, \lambda_1) \qquad (7.136)$$

where $\sigma_{\lambda_1}(r)$ is the Raman scattering cross section for water vapor molecules, $N_1(r)$ is the concentration (number density) of $H_2O$ molecules, and $T(r, \lambda_0)$ and $T(r, \lambda_1)$ are the transmittances of the atmospheric layer between the lidar and the probed volume at the wavelengths of the probe pulse and the $H_2O$ combination frequency. The rest of the notation is the same as before.

It is evident from expression (7.136) that if we know the value of $\sigma_{\lambda_1}(r)$ and the transmittances $T(r, \lambda_0)$ and $T(r, \lambda_1)$, we can determine the required concentration distribution of $H_2O$ molecules along the monitoring path directly from the results of monitoring. In practice, however, a different approach is customarily taken, namely, the return signals at the combination frequencies of water vapor and nitrogen or oxygen are measured simultaneously and then the ratio between these signals is determined. If, for example, we write the lidar equation for the combination frequency of $N_2$ and refer expression (7.136) to it, we obtain the simple expression

$$\frac{P_{r, \lambda_1}}{P_{r, \lambda_2}} = \frac{\sigma_{\lambda_1}(r)}{\sigma_{\lambda_2}(r)} \frac{N_1(r)}{N_2(r)} \frac{T(r, \lambda_1)}{T(r, \lambda_2)} \qquad (7.137)$$

The ratio $\sigma_{\lambda_1}/\sigma_{\lambda_2}$ is known from corresponding laboratory measurements or can be determined in the lidar calibration process. The concentration distribution of nitrogen molecules along the monitoring path is taken from the standard model of the atmosphere, the values of $T(r,\lambda_1)$ and $T(r,\lambda_2)$ are either determined by an independent method or are calculated on the basis of specific assumptions concerning the variation of the volume aerosol scattering coefficients and the known values of the volume Rayleigh scattering coefficients, or the ratio $T(r,\lambda_1)/T(r,\lambda_2)$ is taken equal to unity if the monitoring is conducted in very clear weather since the probe ceiling does not exceed 1–3 km and the indicated ratio is in fact very close to unity in this case.

All papers devoted to SRS humidity monitoring [318–324] report satisfactory agreement of the results with radiosonde data. The probe ceiling is usually not greater than 1 or 2 km.

Problems related to the influence of atmospheric transmittance on the accuracy of determination of humidity by the SRS method are discussed in detail in [325]. Arshinov and others [326] have derived an expression for determining the partial pressure of water vapor from SRS-return data when the values of the pressure and temperature are known at the corresponding heights.

We note in conclusion that the humidity-monitoring ceiling for the SRS method can be elevated somewhat by realizing a corresponding increase in the potential of lidar, but it is difficult to anticipate any significant elevation, considering the small SRS cross sections and concentration of water vapor. This conclusion also applies to other gaseous components of the atmosphere because the SRS cross sections of all known gases do not differ too appreciably from one another.

## 7.12. Laser Monitoring of the Temperature, Density, and Pressure

The temperature, density, and pressure are interrelated by the familiar ideal-gas equation of state, which is fully applicable to the atmospheric conditions of earth:

$$p=(\rho/M)RT \qquad (7.138)$$

where $p$ is the pressure, $\rho$ is the density, $T$ is the absolute temperature, $M$ is the molecular weight of the gas, and $R$ is the universal gas constant.

Equation (7.138) is applicable to each localized volume of the atmosphere so that if the profiles of any pair of variables $p$, $\rho$, and $T$ are known, the profile of the third is found automatically. On the other hand, the pressure profile is related to the density profile by the hydrostatic equation

$$p(z)=p_0\int_0^z g\rho(z')dz' \qquad (7.139)$$

In Eq. (7.139), $p(z)$ and $\rho(z)$ denote the pressure and density profiles, $p_0$ is the pressure at sea level, and $g$ is the acceleration of gravity.

Thus, to find the profiles $p$, $\rho$, and $T$, it is sufficient to know the profile of one of these quantities. Naturally, the error of determination of any one of a pair of quantities is related one-to-one with the error of determination of the third, for which the corresponding inverse problem is solved. Below we discuss methods for the laser monitoring of the atmospheric parameters covered in this section with the utilization of various processes of interaction of the probe pulse with the atmospheric medium.

### 7.12.1. Methods Based on Rayleigh Scattering

As mentioned, the volume Rayleigh backscattering coefficient is related one-to-one with the density of the atmosphere. Accordingly, the use of Rayleigh scattering to determine the density and, therefore, also the temperature and pressure appears highly promising. So far, however, this method has been used only for heights above 30 km. The latter restriction is imposed by the fact that in layers below 30 km the measured lidar return contains both a Rayleigh and an aerosol (particulate) component, and so the successful application of the given method requires solution of the problem of precise separation of those components. It will be shown presently that the required error limits in the determination of the component identified with Rayleigh scattering must not be greater than 1 or 2%. This kind of accuracy has been unattainable to date.

Numerous experiments in the laser probing of the atmosphere with the use of a ruby laser at heights of about 30 km indicate that the contribution of the aerosol component of the return signal can be disregarded in comparison with the Rayleigh part. Accordingly, the lidar can be calibrated, for example, by means of a radiosonde that measures the atmospheric density in ascensions to heights of about 30 km. In this calibration, the transmittance of the atmospheric layer up to 30 km and the volume aerosol backscattering coefficient in the lidar equation are automatically incorporated in the calibration constant.

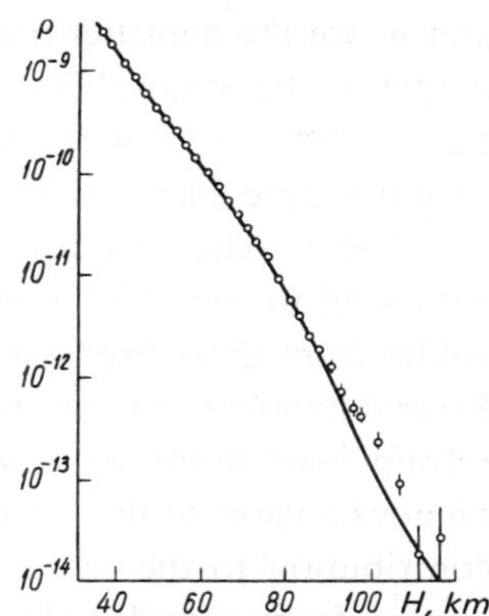

Fig. 7.34. Vertical profile of atmospheric density in the height interval 40–120 km.

If we now assume that the aerosol component of the return signal above 30 km is negligible in comparison with the Rayleigh component, we can obtain the density profiles for the corresponding interval of heights automatically from direct measurements of the return profiles. We illustrate the results of monitoring of the density of the upper layers of the atmosphere in certain examples obtained by the indicated method.

Figure 7.34 gives a vertical atmospheric–density profile obtained at Kingston, Jamaica, on March 25, 1969, at which time 300 probe pulses were transmitted in the time interval 0010–0235, March 25, 1969 [6]. The solid curve corresponds to the standard Rayleigh model of the atmosphere, the points correspond to the monitoring data, and the vertical strokes characterize the measurement errors. The same data are represented by the upper curve of Fig. 7.35 in coordinates of $\rho_m/\rho_c$ versus the height, where $\rho_m$

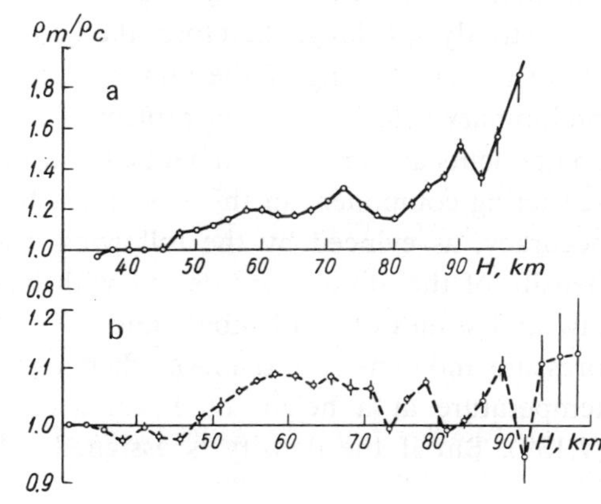

Fig. 7.35. Ratio of measured density $\rho_m$ to density $\rho_c$ calculated for standard atmosphere model, obtained at Kingston, Jamaica, with the use of a ruby laser. (a) 300 probe pulses during a 2.5-h period on Mar. 25, 1969; (b) 1500 probe pulses during one night, Apr. 7–8, 1970.

and $\rho_c$ are the densities measured and calculated according to the standard model of the atmosphere. The lower curve of this figure is plotted for the transmission of 1500 probe pulses during the one night of April 7–8, 1970, with the same lidar system.

The wavelike variation of the atmospheric density with height is clearly witnessed in Fig. 7.35 along with the appreciable deviation of its absolute values from those predicted by the standard model at heights above 50 km. Several hypotheses could be invoked to account for either fact, but we shall refrain from doing so in view of the impossibility of providing an unambiguous answer to the question of the corresponding role of aerosols, whose contribution to the return signal has been assumed to be negligible. It is known from a multitude of direct and indirect measurements, including those obtained by the twilight and rocket-probe methods, that aerosol layers are observed at all heights up to 500 km. Accordingly, the contribution of aerosol scattering to the return signals at heights above 30 km must be additionally and carefully analyzed. It is quite clear that single-frequency laser monitoring can yield information about the aerosol layers at any heights, simply by using laser wavelengths in the infrared region, where the Rayleigh component of the return signal can safely be neglected. This condition is completely satisfied, for example, by a fluorite–dysprosium laser with a wavelength of 2.36 $\mu$m. For monitoring in the visible portion of the spectrum, the question of the aerosol contribution to the return signal at heights above 30 km can be answered by means of the multifrequency probing method, or with the use of a bistatic configuration, or even by measuring the polarization characteristics of the return signals. Clearly, all of the indicated possibilities will eventually be exploited because the problem of the aerosol component of return signals at large heights is of considerable independent significance.

Strictly speaking, therefore, the application of the Rayleigh scattering effect for monitoring of the atmospheric density at any heights requires a preliminary solution of the problem of separating the return signal into its components associated with aerosol and molecular scattering. The Rayleigh scattering component in this case must be determined with extremely high accuracy, as evinced by the following example. If it is assumed that the density of the atmosphere decays with height according to an exponential law and values of 1013 mbars and $1.77 \times 10^{-3}$ g/cm$^3$ are adopted for the pressure and density at sea level, then a value of 295.6°K is obtained for the temperature at a height of 1 km according to expressions (7.138) and (7.139). But if the density is assigned values $\rho(z) + 0.01\rho(z)$ and $\rho(z) +$

$0.09\rho(z)$, we obtain respective temperature values of 292.3 and 268.2°K. Thus, a 1% error in the determination of the atmospheric density induces a 3.3°K error in the determination of the temperature in the given example.

## 7.12.2. Methods Based on the Spontaneous Raman Scattering (SRS) Effect.

It is well known that the primary atmospheric gases $N_2$ and $O_2$ are well intermixed in the atmosphere up to heights of 90–100 km. Consequently, the return profiles associated with SRS of the vibrational and rotational transitions in these molecules carry information about the density profiles of the atmosphere. Simultaneously, these return signals carry information about the temperature. The SRS of vibrational and rotational transitions has a highly specific character, and so we discuss the corresponding laser monitoring methods separately for the cases in which the pure rotational and the vibration–rotation SRS spectra are utilized.

### 7.12.2.1. Application of Pure Rotational SRS Spectra

When a laser probe pulse is transmitted into the atmosphere, its return exhibits both vibration–rotation and pure rotational SRS spectra. The lines of the pure rotational spectra in this case are situated near the probe emission line, whereas the vibration–rotation bands are situated much farther away. The proposal to use the pure rotational SRS spectra for laser monitoring of the temperature of the atmosphere was first advanced by Cooney [327, 328]. The method essentially entails the following.

The intensity of an individual line of the pure rotational SRS spectrum of linear molecules such as $N_2$ and $O_2$ is expressed by the equation [329]

$$I(J,T)=I_0 C \nu_J^4 g_I \frac{N_0 B}{kT}(2J+1)\exp\left[-\frac{B}{kT}J(J+1)\right]|H_{J'}^J|^2 \quad (7.140)$$

in which $I_0$ is the intensity of the incident radiation of frequency $\nu_0$, $C$ is a constant, $\nu_J = \nu_0 \mp \Delta\nu_J, |\Delta\nu_J| = 4B(J+3/2)$, $B$ is the rotational constant of the molecule, $I$ is the rotational quantum number, $g_I$ is the statistical weight associated with the nuclear spin of the molecule, $N_0$ is the total number density of the molecules, $k$ is the Boltzmann constant, $|H_{J'}^J|$ is the matrix element for transition of the molecule from state $J$ to state $J'$.

The product $(2J+1)|H_{J'}^J|^2$ for the Stokes lines is written in the form

$$(2J+1)|H_{J'}^J|^2 = \frac{3(J+1)(J+2)}{2(2J+3)} \quad (7.141)$$

and for the anti-Stokes lines, in the form

$$(2J+1)|H^J_{J'}|^2 = \frac{3}{2}\frac{J(J-1)}{2J-1} \tag{7.142}$$

Substituting (7.141) or (7.142) into (7.140), we readily isolate in the latter expression a factor depending only on the temperature; for a Stokes line, for example:

$$f(J,T)=\frac{(J+1)(J+2)}{(2J+3)T}\exp\left[-\frac{B}{kT}J(J+1)\right] \tag{7.143}$$

Investigations [330–332] of the intensities of various lines of the pure rotational SRS spectrum of nitrogen permit the expressions given above to be used for the extraction of information on the temperature profiles from the results of measurements of return signals from pure rotational SRS lines. We have previously discussed a number of procedures [333–337]. We now look at what are, from our point of view, the two most interesting procedures; in the first, it is proposed that return signals be measured at two rotational lines exhibiting opposite behaviors on the part of the temperature dependence of the intensity. The ratio of the return signals from two lines characterized by rotational quantum numbers $J_1$ and $J_2$ represents a quantity $F(r)$ depending on the distance $r$:

$$F(r)=G(J_1, J_2)\exp\left\{-\frac{B}{kT}\left[J_1(J_1+1)-J_2(J_2+1)\right]\right\} \tag{7.144}$$

Included in the quantity $G$ are the known factors from (7.143) containing $J_1$ and $J_2$. All other characteristics entering into the lidar equation describing the return signals $T_1(r)$ and $T_2(r)$ cancel out since they are identical, within very small error limits, for two probe wavelengths separated only by tens of $cm^{-1}$. Within the limits of such a spectral interval, the volume aerosol and Rayleigh scattering coefficients and their values in the backward direction may be considered invariant, and so the transmittance of the atmosphere may be regarded as constant.

From (7.144) we deduce the required expression for the temperature:

$$T=B\frac{J_1(J_1+1)-J_2(J_2+1)}{k\ln[G(J_1, J_2)F(r)]} \tag{7.145}$$

A drawback of this procedure is the need for very high-resolution spectral instrumentation in order to measure the return signals $F_1(r)$ and $F_2(r)$. Out of the total pure rotational SRS spectrum in this case, only a small fraction of the lines bearing information on the temperature of the lines is utilized. Moreover, certain $N_2$ lines overlap with $O_2$ lines.

The above-indicated shortcomings are remedied in the second procedure, whereby, rather than individual $N_2$ and $O_2$ lines, whole intervals with a uniform temperature dependence of the intensity of the lines included therein are isolated. An analysis of the problem has shown that within the temperature interval from 220 to 320°K molecular oxygen lines with values of $J$ from 1 to 9 and nitrogen lines with $J$ from 2 to 8 are included in one of the spectral intervals, while lines with $J > 10$ for nitrogen and $J > 11$ for oxygen are included in another interval. The ratio of the total return signals for these spectral intervals is given by the expression

$$F(r) = \frac{F_1(r)}{F_2(r)} = \frac{\Sigma_i \nu_{J_i}^4 g_I f_{N_2}(J_i, T) + (N_{O_2}/N_{N_2}) A \Sigma_i \nu_{J_i}^4 f_{O_2}(J_i, T)}{\Sigma_j \nu_{J_j}^4 g_I f_{N_2}(J_j, T) + (N_{O_2}/N_{N_2}) A \Sigma_j \nu_{J_j}^4 f_{O_2}(J_j, T)}$$

$$(7.146)$$

in which $N_{O_2}$ and $N_{N_2}$ are the number densities of oxygen and nitrogen molecules, $A$ is a constant determined by the cross sections of these gases, and $f_{N_2}$, $f_{O_2}$ are functions containing the temperature dependence of the intensities of the corresponding nitrogen and oxygen lines. It is clear that either the lidar temperature function must be calculated beforehand or the lidar must be calibrated.

Arshinov and others [336] describe a lidar that permits the given procedure to be used for temperature monitoring with separation of the SRS lines of $N_2$ and $O_2$. The most important component of this lidar is a special dual monochromator, which suppresses spurious return signals by 7 or 8 orders of magnitude. This lidar has been used to monitor the temperature along horizontal paths over distances up to 1 km. In the investigated temperature interval from 252 to 270°K, the method had a sensitivity close to the theoretical value characterized by the quantity $\partial F(T)/\partial T \cong 0.1$.

Salzman and Coney [338] have published data on temperature monitoring with the use of the pure rotational SRS spectrum. A temperature measurement error of $\pm 3°C$ was obtained in the transmission of 10 ruby laser pulses with a single-pulse energy of approximately 4 J. The probed volume was situated 100 m from the lidar, and the temperature in it varies from $-20$ to $+30°C$. It is essential to note, however, that interference filters were used to separate out the intervals of the SRS spectrum, an approach that could not help but inject errors into the interpretation of the data because it is well known that interference filters do not have contrast for the indicated purposes in discriminating the monitored parts of the spectrum relative to the spurious return signals. Two later studies by Cooney and Pina [339, 340] suffer from the same shortcoming. In [340], they report the first preliminary results of temperature monitoring in a vertical column of the atmosphere at heights from 500 to 1000 m.

In closing the discussion of methods for laser monitoring of the temperature of the atmosphere by means of the pure rotational SRS spectra of nitrogen and oxygen, we note that these methods will unquestionably come to enjoy practical utilization. It should not be forgotten that the SRS cross sections in this case are 2 or 3 orders of magnitude smaller than the Rayleigh scattering cross sections, so that these methods are suitable for temperature monitoring only in the lower layers of the atmosphere.

### 7.12.2.2. Application of Vibrational SRS Spectra

The possibility of using the vibrational SRS spectra of nitrogen and oxygen for laser temperature monitoring is explored in [341]. The intensity ratio between the Stokes and anti-Stokes components of the vibrational SRS spectrum has the form

$$\frac{I_{\mathrm{aSt}}}{I_{\mathrm{St}}} = \frac{(\nu_0 + \nu_1)^4}{(\nu_0 - \nu_1)^4} \exp\left(-\frac{h\nu_1}{kT}\right) \tag{7.147}$$

where $\nu_0$ is the probe pulse frequency and $\nu_1$ is the frequency of transition to the first vibrational level of the molecule.

The intensity of the anti-Stokes component depends strongly on the population of the first molecular vibrational level. At a temperature of 300°K, the population of this level for nitrogen molecules is $1.4 \times 10^{-5}$ part of all molecules, and for oxygen molecules it is $5.74 \times 10^{-4}$ part. Consequently, it is preferable to use the vibrational SRS spectrum of oxygen.

The populations of the first vibrational level of $O_2$ molecules at temperatures of 270, 240, and 225°K have been calculated to have respective values of $(2.6, 0.91, \text{ and } 0.49) \times 10^{-4}$ part of all molecules. Thus, the greatest obstacle to the implementation of this method in practice is the large disparity of the intensities between the Stokes and anti-Stokes components of the vibrational SRS spectra of nitrogen and oxygen. Also, the distance between these components in the spectrum is such that the corresponding difference between the volume aerosol and molecular scattering coefficients and so also the transmittance of the atmosphere must be taken into account. The latter consideration imposes additional difficulties in regard to the given method.

## 7.12.3. Method Based on the Doppler Effect

The method based on the Doppler effect was proposed by Fiocco and De Wolf [342] and is based on the fact that the return-signal components associated with Rayleigh and aerosol scattering have very different spectral widths. The return Doppler shift due to the directional motion of windborne aerosols is given by the simple expression

$$\Delta\nu \sim 2v_\perp/\lambda \tag{7.148}$$

where $v_\perp$ is the radial component of the wind velocity and $\lambda$ is the probe pulse wavelength. For $v_\perp = 10$ m/sec and $\lambda = 0.488$ $\mu$m, the shift $\Delta\nu \approx 41$ MHz or, roughly, $0.001$ cm$^{-1}$. The thermal velocities of the molecules are much greater than the wind velocity, so that their induced broadening of the probe pulse due to the Rayleigh component is also proportionately larger and its measurement is much more accessible.

In the case of noninteracting molecules, such that $l \sim \lambda/\sin(\theta/2)$, where $l$ is the mean free path and $\theta$ is the angle of observation, the spectrum of the Doppler-broadened return signal is in the shape of a Gaussian curve for a Maxwell velocity distribution. At higher pressures, such that $l \leqslant \lambda \sin(\theta/2)$, pressure fluctuations in the probed volumes invest the return signals with two shifted Mandel'shtam–Brillouin components.

The capabilities of the given method have been demonstrated in [343, 344]. An argon laser with a wavelength of 0.488 $\mu$m and power of 0.5 W and a receiving system with an antenna diameter of 0.5 m were used for the reception and analysis of return signals from distances of 3 to 5 km. The temperature measured at a height of 4 km was equal to 276°K. The temperature at the earth's surface was 303°K. The results of the measurements were in good agreement with theoretical predictions.

In conclusion, we stress the fact that the technical implementation of the given method is extremely complicated. It is possibly for this reason that it has not been developed any further to date for temperature monitoring in the troposphere.

Several authors [345–349] have investigated aspects of the application of the Doppler effect for temperature monitoring in the upper layers of the atmosphere on the basis of an analysis of the broadening of return signals due to resonance scattering by sodium vapor. The possibility of determining the temperature at heights of 80 to 100 km within 10–15% error limits has been demonstrated.

### 7.12.4. Method Based on the Differential Approach

The method based on the differential approach was proposed in [350–352] and is based on the different temperature dependences of the intensities of the rotational lines in the vibration–rotation absorption band of oxygen in the near-infrared region. Its basic concept is essentially to measure return signals at wavelengths corresponding to the centers of definite lines of the vibration–rotation absorption band where the values and temperature dependence of their intensities are known beforehand.

This method actually comprises a modification of the differential procedure discussed previously. Its implementation requires highly mono-chromatic lasers with a capacity for discrete or smooth tuning of the emission frequency and a high degree of stabilization in cases where the frequency of the laser emission line coincides with the center of the corresponding absorption line. Moreover, it is necessary to have sufficiently accurate data on the parameters of the corresponding lines and their temperature dependence. The parameters in question are the intensities, center positions, and half-widths of the lines.

Practical realization of the given method has yet to be achieved.

## 7.13. Laser Methods for the Determination of Wind Velocity

All methods for the determination of wind velocity by means of lasers rest on the assumption that all particles interacting with the transmitted radiation (atoms, molecules, and aerosol particles) are entrained by the wind. Appropriate estimates have indicated that this assumption is fully justified.

From the methodological point of view, all laser methods developed for the determination of wind velocity can be classified as Doppler and correla-tion methods. Below we analyze their capabilities.

### 7.13.1. Doppler Methods

The Doppler shift of the emission frequency due to the motion of particles interacting with the probe pulse in the optical wavelength range potentially has a number of advantages in comparison with the microwave range. The much higher frequencies of optical radiation induce considerably larger Doppler shifts. The small wavelengths ensure significantly better spatial resolution. The presence of a sufficient quantity of active optical scattering centers in the atmosphere and the thoroughly studied scattering mechanisms afford extensive possibilities for the application of Doppler methods.

The Doppler frequency shift $f_D$ is described by the simple expression

$$f_D = \frac{2}{\lambda} v \sin \frac{\theta}{2} \cos \varphi$$

in which $\lambda$ is the probe wavelength, $\theta$ is the scattering angle, and $\varphi$ is the angle between the direction of the wind velocity $v$ and the bisector of the angle between the transmitted and scattered beams. In monostatic probing, the Doppler shift $f_D$ is caused by the projection of the wind velocity onto the probing axis. Diverse methods are used to record the Doppler shifts.

### 7.13.1.1. *Spectral Analysis of Return Signals*

The spectral analysis of return signals method is best illustrated in the singular work of Fiocco's group [344, 353, 354]. Using a highly stabilized single-frequency argon laser ($\lambda = 0.488$ $\mu$m) with a power of 0.2 W, a lidar receiving mirror 0.5 m in diameter, and a Fabry–Perot scanning interferometer, the authors were able to perform a spectral analysis of return signals in the vicinity of 750 MHz (0.025 cm$^{-1}$). The Doppler shifts associated with the wind motion of aerosols fall well within this interval. To ensure the necessary spatial resolution of the monitoring results, the continuous output of the laser was modulated to provide a pulse duration of 10 $\mu$ sec and an off-duty factor equal to 6.5.

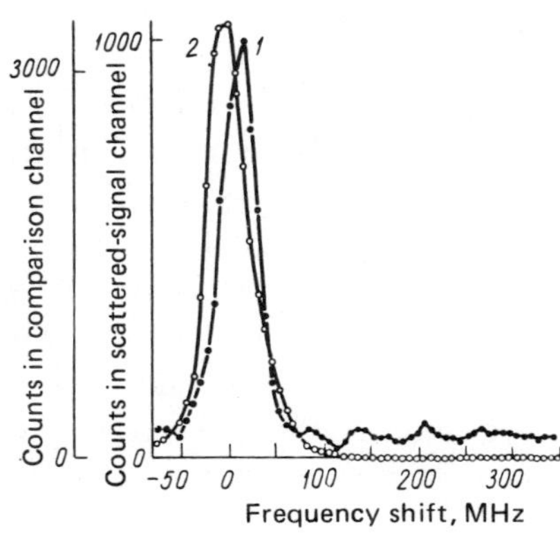


Fig. 7.36. Results of Fiocco from Doppler-effect monitoring of the radial component of the wind velocity. (1) Scattering signal; (2) primary signal.

Figure 7.36 gives the results of monitoring of the wind velocity in a volume corresponding to the pulse duration at a height of 750 m above the earth's surface. The shift of the return-pulse maximum from the probe-pulse maximum in the figure corresponds to a radial component of the wind velocity equal to 3.18 m/sec.

### 7.13.1.2. Heterodyning

The use of lasers with a large coherence time ensures the possibility of measuring the Doppler frequency shifts of transmitted radiation by the heterodyne method. In connection with continuously emitted radiation, localization of the probed volume is realized by focusing the laser beam at the investigated range for typical scattering volumes with scales on the order of a few centimeters in diameter and several tens of meters in length. The optimal results have been obtained using a stabilized $CO_2$ laser with a wavelength of 10.6 $\mu$m [355–357].

In view of the fact that the volume aerosol backscattering coefficients are small in the vicinity of a wavelength of 10.6 $\mu$m in a slightly turbid atmosphere, the lidar range cannot exceed a few hundred meters. It can attain a kilometer or more in a turbid atmosphere.

The lidar range can be extended substantially with the use of a pulsed laser, as noted in [358]. However, data have not yet been published to corroborate this assertion.

Future progress in the heterodyne method will depend largely on the concurrent advances made in the synthesis of laser sources.

### 7.13.1.3. Direct Photodetection

The direct photodetection method may be essentially summarized as follows. When two coherent laser beams intersect in an investigated volume of the atmosphere, a stationary interference pattern is created and the transport of aerosol particles across that pattern induces modulation of the scattered flux with a frequency proportional to the wind velocity. A separate detector records the dominant frequency of the spectrum of power fluctuations of the reflected radiation, and the wind velocity is then estimated from the result. When two mutually orthogonal systems of interference fringes are created on the basis of orthogonally polarized beams, it is possible to determine two components of the wind velocity and, hence, its direction.

Argon laser systems developed for the given method have made it possible to measure wind velocity up to heights of 100–150 m [359, 360]. Distortion of the interference pattern by atmospheric turbulence prevents the probe ceiling from being raised any further. Nonetheless, a certain increase in the monitoring height can be achieved by increasing the lidar potential. For example, Bartlett and She [361] have demonstrated the possibility of reaching a ceiling of 300 m through the use of a receiving device with a mirror diameter of 0.4 m and a 20-W argon laser.

### 7.13.1.4. Microwave Modulation of the Transmitted-Beam Intensity

The transmitted-beam intensity method was proposed by Belov and others [362]. It is based on the notion of performing measurements of the Doppler shift in the microwave range of the radiation modulating the transmitted beam. The best results should be expected in the investigation of dense aerosol layers of the cloud type.

## 7.13.2. Correlation Methods

Windborne aerosol inhomogeneities passing through a laser-illuminated scattering volume elicit return-signal fluctuations, which can be correlation analyzed to extract information on the characteristics of the wind velocity. The schematic configuration of the method is illustrated in Fig. 7.37. A splitting device directs the laser emission into the atmosphere as two beams. Two receiving systems delineate the investigated volumes from these beams. If the direction of the wind velocity coincides with the line joining those

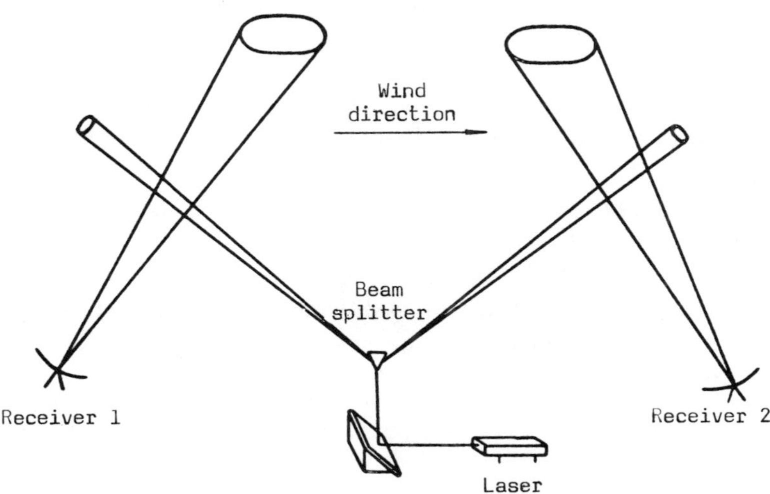


Fig. 7.37. Simplified schematic representation of laser monitoring of the horizontal component of the wind velocity.

volumes, then the same aerosol inhomogeneities will necessarily pass through both volumes in succession. By performing correlation analysis of the returns from both volumes with respect to the temporal shift of the maximum of the fluctuation cross-correlation function, it is possible to determine the wind velocity if the distance between the volumes is known.

The author and others [363–365] have investigated in detail the aerosol inhomogeneities of the atmosphere and their influence on laser return signals. These investigations have indicated a high degree of definition of the indicated inhomogeneities in the returns and, hence, the considerable promise of utilizing this effect in the laser monitoring of wind velocity. In the practical application of the method, however, it is essential to take into consideration the presence of transmittance fluctuations of the atmospheric layer between the lidar and the probed volume. It is quite clear that if these fluctuations exceed the fluctuations of the return signal from the investigated volume, it will be impossible to extract any useful information from that volume. This problem has been investigated in our work [366], in which we obtained the following condition for a negligibly small contribution of fluctuations of the square of the transmittance of the atmosphere in the return signal:

$$\bar{\alpha}_M (L \cdot l_0)^{1/2} \ll 0.5 \qquad (7.149)$$

where $\bar{\alpha}_M$ is the average value of the volume aerosol scattering coefficient, $l_0$ is the average scale of the aerosol inhomogeneities, and $L$ is the monitoring range. If we take $\bar{\alpha}_M = 0.1$ km$^{-1}$ and $l_0 = 0.02$ to 0.05 km for the maximum range, we obtain values in the interval $L_{\max} = 5$ to 12 km. It is clear that $L_{\max}$ will decrease for greater values of the turbidity. Consequently, correlation methods exhibit the best capabilities in a slightly turbid cloudless atmosphere.

Correlation methods have been tested in two variants: (1) information is recorded in several scattering volumes [363, 367]; (2) measurements are performed with recording of the instantaneous distributions of the inhomogeneities along the monitoring path at different times [366, 368]. It has been shown in observations of the random field of temporal inhomogeneities in two volumes separated by a distance $\Delta x$ that the velocity

$$v' = \Delta x (\tau')^{-1} \qquad (7.150)$$

is found from the time shift $\tau'$ of the maximum of the fluctuation cross-correlation function in the two volumes, where this velocity is related to the modulus of the wind velocity $v$ by the simple equation

$$v' = v/\cos\varphi \qquad (7.151)$$

in which $\varphi$ is the angle between the direction of the wind and the line joining the scattering volumes.

Expressions (7.150) and (7.151) show that both the magnitude and the direction of the wind velocity can be determined by varying the locations of the probed volumes and, hence, the angle $\varphi$. Measurements were performed with continuous lasers, from the beams of which the scattering volumes were delineated by means of receiving apertures. Variation of the angle $\varphi$ made it possible, on the basis of expressions (7.150) and (7.151), to acquire data on the modulus and direction of the wind velocity in the terrestrial layer of the atmosphere up to heights of 20–50 m. When lidars incorporating pulsed lasers are used and space is scanned with transmitted pulses of sufficiently high frequency, it is acknowledged that the described method will play an important role in the future. Corresponding algorithms for the processing of measurement data are described for this case in [369].

With the use of a lidar operating in a monostatic configuration, it is possible to record inhomogeneities along the monitoring path. The projection of the wind velocity onto the monitoring direction $v_x$ can be determined by transmitting pulses at time intervals $\tau_0$ and performing cross-correlation processing of the returns:

$$v_x = \Delta x'/\tau_0 \qquad (7.152)$$

where $\Delta x'$ is the spatial lag of the maximum of the cross-correlation function of the fluctuations of the volume backscattering coefficient of successive return signals.

Inasmuch as $v_x = v\cos\varphi$, where $\varphi$ is the angle between the wind direction and the monitoring direction, by determining $v_x$ for various angles $\varphi$ it is possible to find both the modulus and the direction of the wind velocity. A comparison of the values obtained in our measurements for the wind velocity according to the described procedure with the data of anemometric measurements indicates satisfactory agreement of those data [366].

A lidar with a range of 7–8 km has been used to determine the height profile of the wind velocity [368]. The atmosphere was probed at a 10° angle relative to the horizon. The total monitoring path was partitioned into 1-km intervals, corresponding to a height increment of about 100 m. In each interval, expression (7.152) was used to determine the velocity $v_x$ and thereby reconstruct the wind profile up to heights of 0.7–0.8 km. In some instances, it was possible to perform measurements up to heights of 1 km. Any further increase in the height requires a correspondingly greater enhancement of the lidar potential. From the practical standpoint, therefore, scanning (beam-slewing) systems are preferable.

Consequently, correlation methods provide a means for determining both the magnitude and the direction of the wind velocity. Their technical implementation, as in the case of Doppler methods, does not pose a simple task.

## 7.14. Laser Determination of the Turbulence Characteristics of the Atmosphere

Atmospheric turbulence effects, the laws of which are discussed in Chap. 4, create corresponding prerequisites for solving the inverse problems of turbulent-atmosphere optics. The feasibility of extracting information on the turbulence characteristics of the medium from the results of studies of the interaction of waves with the medium was first indicated by Obukhov [370]. Problems related to the application of incoherent light sources for the measurement of turbulence characteristics are discussed in Tatarskii's esteemed book [371].

Optical methods for determining the parameters of turbulence realized their greatest development after lasers were brought into service in this connection [372]. The methods that have gained reliable experimental confirmation are based on the irradiation of a particular investigated thickness of the atmosphere with a laser beam. The source and receiver in this case can be situated either at opposite ends of the path or at a single station. In the former case, we work with single one-way wave transmission through a layer of the atmosphere, and in the latter case wave propagation takes place according to an echo-location scheme, being reflected from a reflector with known properties at one end of the path. The fundamental parameter to be determined as a characteristic of the intensity of micro-fluctuations of the refractive index and, in the final analysis, the majority of statistical characteristics of the field of a laser beam in the atmosphere is the structural characteristic of the refractive index $C_n^2$.

The most common methods of determining $C_n^2$ are based on utilization of the loss of coherence of a wave propagating in a turbulent atmosphere. For example, the loss of coherence of a laser beam diminishes the average intensity on its axis. The ratio of the radiation flux $P_S$ transmitted through a narrow slit at the center of the focal spot of the receiving system to the total flux $P$ transmitted through the objective is written in the form [372]

$$\frac{P_S}{P} = \frac{2kR\Delta}{\pi^2 F} I(\mu) \tag{7.153}$$

where

$$I(\mu) = \frac{\pi^{3/2}\Phi(\mu^{3/5})}{4\mu^{3/5}} - \frac{1-(1/6\mu^{6/5})}{\mu^{6/5}} + \frac{\exp(-\mu^{6/5})\left[5-(1/6\mu^{6/5})\right]}{6\mu^{6/5}}$$

$$\tag{7.154}$$

$2R$ is the diameter of the receiving objective, $F$ is its focal length, $k=2\pi/\lambda$ is the wave number, $\Delta$ is the slit width,

$$\Phi(x) = \frac{2}{\sqrt{\pi}} \int_0^x \exp(-t^2)\,dt$$

is the error probability integral,

$$\mu = 1.45\tilde{C}_n^2 k^2 x (2R)^{5/3}$$

$$\tilde{C}_n^2(x) = \frac{1}{x}\int_0^x C_n^2(\xi) f_c(\xi)\,d\xi \tag{7.155}$$

$x$ is the path length, $\xi$ is the running coordinate along the path of the laser beam, and $f_c(\xi)$ is the filtering function, the form of which is determined in accordance with the measurement technique; in the given case, $f_c(\xi)=1$ and $f_c(\xi)=(\xi/x)^{5/3}$ for illumination of the receiving objective with, respectively, a plane wave (broad collimated beam) and a spherical wave (divergent beam).

An instrument designed according to the scheme described here [372] makes it possible to measure the fluxes $P_S$ and $P$ and yields their ratio in decibels, guaranteeing measurement error limits of $\pm 1.5$ dB.

In the case of scanning of a narrow slit in the focal plane of the receiving objective, we can form the distribution of the average intensity and measure its half-width $y_k$ at the level of half the peak value of the average intensity. The quantity $y_k$ in this case is related to $\tilde{C}_n^2$ by the simple expression [372]

$$\tilde{C}_n^2 = \frac{0.95}{2.91\,k^{1/3}x}\left(\frac{y_k}{2F}\right)^{5/3} \tag{7.156}$$

affording an additional possibility for determining the path-average value of the structural characteristic of the refractive index.

Belen'kii and others [373] have used the procedure described above to determine $\tilde{C}_n^2$ with the use of several laser sources situated at different heights on a mountain slope adjacent to a valley, making it possible to obtain the height distribution of the structural characteristic of the refractive index in a mountainous setting. The results of processing of the measurement data for individual paths are given in Fig. 7.38 in the form of height profiles of the structural characteristic of the index fluctuations $C_n^2$. A comparison of these data with those of corresponding measurements under flatland conditions indicates that the decay of $C_n^2$ with height in both the daytime and nighttime mountain environment is slower.

Subramanian [374] has used a method based on measurements of the variance of the intensity fluctuations of a laser beam reflected from a spherical mirror carried aloft by an aerostat in order to determine the height dependence of $C_n^2$. The measurement data obtained in [374] are interpreted in [375] (namely, an integral equation is presented) relating the measured optical characteristic to the behavior of $C_n^2$ with regard for two-way wave transmission along the path, a technique is proposed for solving this equation, and the measurement data are processed accordingly.

Aerostat measurements are quite time consuming. This drawback was removed in [376], in which the atmosphere was simultaneously irradiated with five laser beams, in which case it took about 2 min to determine a single $C_n^2(h)$ profile. The receivers were situated at different heights on a meteorological tower, and the authors obtained the variances of the fluctuations of the logarithm of the intensity $\sigma^2(h)$, which is related to the $C_n^2(h)$

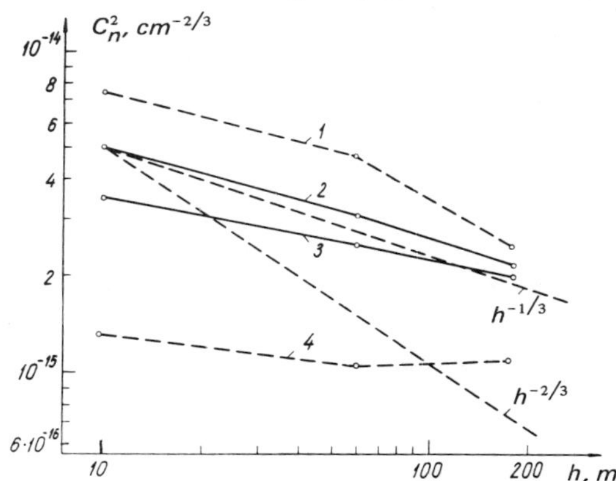


Fig. 7.38. Height profiles of sample average values of the parameter $C_n^2$. (2) Daytime conditions; (3) nighttime conditions; (1, 4) individual samples of $C_n^2(h)$ corresponding to maximum and minimum values of $C_n^2(10\ m)$.

profile by the integral equation

$$\sigma^2(h)=224k^{7/6}\left(\frac{h}{x}\right)^{-11/6}\int_0^h C_n^2(t)t^{5/6}\left(1-\frac{t}{h}\right)^{5/6}dt \qquad (7.157)$$

in which $h$ is the excess height of the receiver above the source.

From Eq. (7.157) we arrive at the important conclusion that the state of the turbulent atmosphere near the source and receiver scarcely affects the measured quantity $\sigma^2(h)$. The greatest contribution to $\sigma^2(h)$ is from layers situated midway along the path. It has been shown [375] that the solution of the system of algebraic equations equivalent to the integral equation (7.157) is stable. Accordingly, in the processing of the experimental data of [376], the solution of the system of algebraic equations without regularization made it possible to reconstruct the height profiles $C_n^2(h)$ within worst-case error limits of 0.25. The height profiles determined in this way and normalized to the value of $C_n^2$ at the point closest to the underlying surface (ground) are given in Fig. 7.39. Also shown in Fig. 7.39 for comparison are the corresponding data obtained for $C_n^2(h)$ by means of microthermometers under similar conditions in a flatland setting [377, 378].

The given method can be used successfully to measure the height profiles $C_n^2(h)$ by means of a helicopter because the atmospheric disturbances created by the latter, as we infer from (7.157), have scarcely any effect on the variance $\sigma^2(h)$ or, accordingly, on the error of determination of the function $C_n^2(h)$.

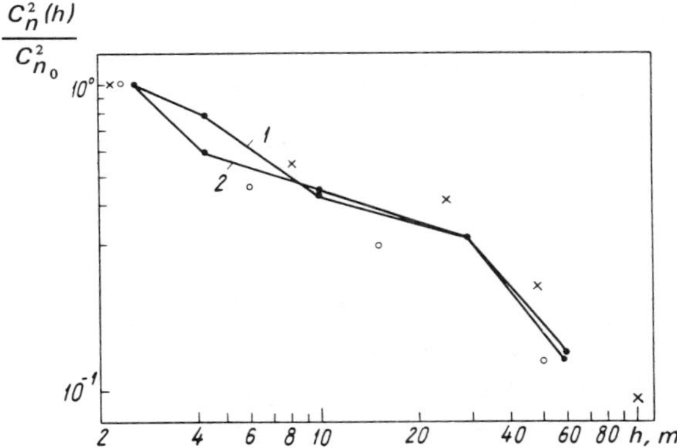

Fig. 7.39. Normalized height profiles of $C_n^2(h)/C_{n_0}^2$. (1, 2) Results of optical measurements (Tsimlyansk, USSR [376]); (1) time 1100 to 1530; (2) 0700 to 1100; ($\times$) results of [377] (Moscow environs, $C_{n_0}^2=4.35\times10^{-16}$ cm$^{-2/3}$, $h_{n_0}=2$ m); (O) data of [378] (Australia, $C_{n_0}^2=1.2\times10^{-14}$ cm$^{-2/3}$, $h_{n_0}=2$ m).

Along with measurements of the path-average values of $C_n^2$ and their height dependence, lasers can also be used to determine the functional form of the turbulence spectrum in the interval of dissipation of kinetic energy and in the energy interval [372]. Here the short wavelength of laser radiation makes it possible in principle to ascertain subtle details in the structure of atmospheric turbulence that have defied access by other, nonoptical techniques to date. It is also important to note that the optical sensor does not influence the measured characteristics, and in measurements of the spectra in a region of large space scales the path length is such as to ensure additional spatial averaging and stabilization of the acquired statistical data; these considerations are important in the investigation of locally homogeneous processes with stationary increments in short time intervals. The methods for reconstruction of turbulence spectra from appropriate laser measurements may be essentially summarized as follows.

If the spectrum of microfluctuations of the refractive index is written in the form

$$\Phi_n(\kappa) = 0.033 C_n^2(\kappa)^{-11/3} \varphi(\kappa l_0) \tag{7.158}$$

where $\kappa$ is the modulus of the wave vector and $l_0$ is the inner turbulence scale, then the function $\varphi(\kappa l_0)$ characterizing the deviation from a pure power-law spectrum in the dissipation interval is related to the normalized dimensionless spectrum $u(\chi, G) = \omega W_\chi(\omega)/2\pi(\chi^2)$ of the fluctuations of the logarithm of the intensity by an equation of the form [372]

$$u(\chi, G) =$$

$$\frac{2}{\pi} \frac{\chi \int_0^\infty dy \left\{ 1 - \left[ \sin(y^2 + x^2)/(y^2 + x^2) \right] \right\} (y^2 + x^2)^{-11/6} \varphi \left[ (y^2 + x^2)/G \right]^{1/2}}{\int_0^\infty dy \left[ 1 - (\sin y^2/y^2) \right] y^{-8/3} \varphi (y^2/G)^{1/2}}$$

$$\tag{7.159}$$

in which

$$\langle \chi^2 \rangle = \frac{1}{2\pi i} \int_0^\infty W_\chi(\omega) d\omega$$

is the variance of the fluctuations of the logarithm of the amplitude, $\chi = \omega(x/k)^{1/2}/v_\perp$ is the dimensionless frequency, $v_\perp$ is the component of the wind velocity perpendicular to the path, and $G = \kappa/kl_0$ is the wave parameter, calculated relative to the inner turbulence scale $l_0$.

Invoking the well-known model representations of the turbulence spectrum, we can compare the measured spectrum with the family of curves

$u(\chi, G)$ plotted for various values of the parameter $G$ and thereby determine the value of $l_0$ from the best fit between the experimental spectrum and the calculated version. If $\langle \chi^2 \rangle$ is known, then (7.159) becomes an integral equation relating the unknown function $\varphi(xl_0)$ to the measured function $u(\chi, G)$. The results of solving this equation by the statistical regularization method show that the spectrum measured by the given technique in the high-frequency range ($\kappa l_0 > 1$) will yield spectral density values higher than those obtained by means of microthermometers [372]. This discrepancy is conceivably the result of the distorting effect of microthermometers on the turbulence structure.

The high sensitivity of the spectrum of log-intensity fluctuations to the behavior of $\Phi_n(\kappa)$ at high frequencies was utilized in the above-described determinations of the spectrum $\Phi_n(\kappa)$. In determining the spectrum of index fluctuations in the energy interval ($\kappa L_0 = 1$), it is practical to make use of the sensitivity of the phase fluctuations of an optical wave field to the behavior of the spectrum $\Phi_n(\kappa)$ in this range. Pursuing this idea, Lukin and others [379, 380] have conducted measurements of the spatial correlation function of the phase of optical radiation, employing two identical spatially separated single-mode laser beams. The spectrum reconstructed from these measurements was compared with the model spectrum

$$\Phi_n(\kappa) = 0.033 C_n^2 \left( \kappa^2 + \kappa_0^2 \right)^{-11/6}$$

The comparison of the indicated spectra enabled the authors to obtain the value of the outer scale $L_0 = 1.3$ m, which roughly coincides with the height of the measurement path $h = 1.5$ m, consistent with existing notions about the value of $L_0$ in the ground layer [371].

Measurements of the variance of the phase difference in an optical wave with receiver spacings such that in one case the distance $\rho$ between receivers is commensurate with the inner scale $l_0$ and in another it is much greater, provide a means for determining the value of $l_0$ if a definite model is adopted for the high-frequency part of the spectrum: $\Phi_n(\kappa)$ [381].


## 7.15. Laser Probing of the Atmosphere from Space

Laser monitoring of the parameters of the atmosphere from outer space is highly significant in connection with the solution of many major problems, first and foremost such problems as long-term weather predictions and protection of the environment against contaminations by the products of industrial activity. The significance of this problem area stems from the possibility of obtaining space–time data arrays on the atmospheric parameters on a planetary scale.

The simplest problem of laser monitoring of the environment from space is the high-precision determination of the distance from a lidar-carrying space vehicle to the top of clouds or to the ground surface. Zakharov and Kostko [7] have published the results of calculations of the power of a ruby laser pulse in order to solve the stated problems successfully. The calculations were carried out for a lidar with the following parameters: diameter of the receiving mirror 25 cm; receiving system f.o.v. 2′; width of the interference filter 10 Å. The transmittance through a vertical slab of the atmosphere was assumed to be 68%. The background noise associated with the reflection of solar radiation from snow and low-level clouds for the given lidar is $6.5 \times 10^{-10}$ and $7.3 \times 10^{-10}$ W, respectively. Table 7.5 shows, for the indicated conditions and the lidar at a height of 500 km above the earth's surface, the values obtained for the minimum transmitted pulse power required for the correct detection, with probability 0.9999, of various clouds and underlying terrains. Here $A$ is the albedo of the underlying surface, $\alpha$ is the volume aerosol scattering coefficient, $h$ is the height, and $\Delta h$ is the vertical thickness of the clouds.

The fundamental possibilities of laser monitoring of the profiles of aerosols from space and the requirements on the corresponding instrumentation can be assessed on the basis of the results of calculations carried out by the author and others [382, 383].

Figure 7.40 illustrates the optical model of the atmosphere used in the calculations, describing the vertical profiles of the volume aerosol and

Table 7.5.

| Target | Probe-pulse power, MW |
|---|---|
| Grass, $A = 0.3$, clear sky | 2.1 |
| Snow, $A = 0.9$, clear sky | 0.7 |
| Low-level clouds, $\alpha = 10^{-2}\ \mathrm{m}^{-1}$, clear sky | 1.6 |
| Low-level clouds through $C_i$ at $h = 7$ and 13 km | 3.0 |
| Grass through $C_i$ at $h = 7$ and 13 km | 3.9 |
| Snow through $C_i$ at $h = 7$ and 13 km | 1.3 |
| Grass through $C_i$ at $h = 13$ km | 2.2 |
| Snow through $C_i$ at $h = 13$ km | 0.72 |
| $C_i$ at $h = 13$ km, $\alpha = 5 \times 10^{-1}\ \mathrm{m}^{-1}$, $\Delta h = 600$ m | 380 |
| $C_i$ at $h = 7$ km, $\alpha = 10^{-3}\ \mathrm{m}^{-1}$, $\Delta h = 600$ m | 20 |

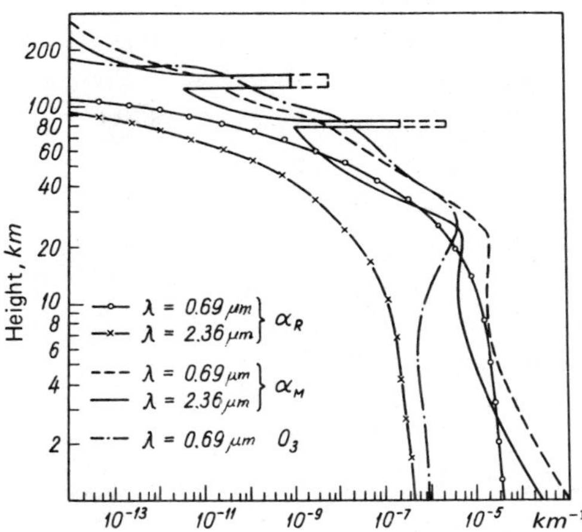


Fig. 7.40

Rayleigh scattering coefficients $\alpha_R(r)$ and $\alpha_M(r)$ for probe-pulse wavelengths of 0.69 and 2.36 $\mu$m as well as the profile of the volume absorption coefficient of ozone for a wavelength of 0.69 $\mu$m. The maxima of $\alpha_M$ for both wavelengths at heights between 80 and 90 km and between 100 and 200 km are associated with, respectively, noctilucent clouds and an aerosol layer of meteoric origin. The optical thicknesses of the noctilucent clouds and aerosol layer for $\lambda = 0.69$ and $\lambda = 2.36$ $\mu$m were taken equal to $6 \times 10^{-4}$, $5 \times 10^{-5}$ and $5 \times 10^{-5}$, $5 \times 10^{-5}$, respectively. The given model of the atmosphere was constructed on the basis of an analysis of pertinent data in the literature.

The results of calculations of histograms of the profiles of lidar returns at a wavelength of 0.69 $\mu$m for a lidar receiving mirror with a diameter of 30 cm set up at a height of 300 km with viewing angles of 180° and 40′ and a 1% receiver quantum efficiency are given in Fig. 7.41. The calculations were carried out for a terrain albedo $A = 0.65$. The vertical profiles obtained for the return signals are normalized to the energy of the probe pulse. The numbers along the horizontal axis indicate what fraction of the probe-pulse energy is recorded in the form of return signals. The left vertical axis represents the height and the right vertical axis the time between transmission of the probe pulse and arrival of the return signal from the corresponding height. The profiles below the surface of the earth are attributable to multiple-scattering effects.

It is evident from Fig. 7.41 that a lidar with the given analytical parameters is capable of receiving return signals from atmospheric layers having a vertical thickness (depth) of 5 km and situated at various heights

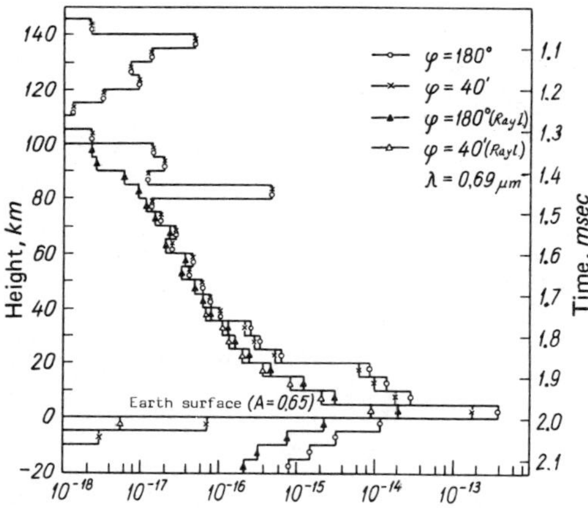


Fig. 7.41

with energies ranging from $\sim 10^{-13}$ to $10^{-18}$ times the energy of the probe pulse for the given model of the atmosphere. Thus, if the probe pulse contains $10^{19}$ photons, the minimum energy of the return signal can be recorded under such conditions, and so the entire histogram of the vertical profile of the return signal can be obtained under the same conditions at heights up to about 150 km.

If noctilucent clouds and the aerosol layer of meteoric origin, which are distinctly manifested in the histogram, are not present in the given optical model of the atmosphere, then the foregoing conclusions as to the possibility of aerosol detection at heights greater than 80 km under such conditions require additional substantiation. In regard to atmospheric layers below 80 km, their detection in single-pulse monitoring from a height of 300 km is fully realistic.

Similar conclusions can be deduced concerning the possibilities for the monitoring of aerosols from space with probe pulses having a wavelength of 2.36 $\mu$m. A remarkable attribute of this wavelength is the negligible contribution of Rayleigh scattering at all heights to the return signal in comparison with aerosol scattering. The energy of the Rayleigh component of the return signal at $\lambda = 2.36$ $\mu$m above 30 km is less than $10^{-18}$ times the energy of the probe pulse.

The results of calculations of histograms of the vertical profiles of return signals from probe pulses with wavelengths of 0.69 and 2.36 $\mu$m show that the bottom 5-km layer yields the strongest return signal, which at both wavelengths has an energy of the order of $10^{-13}$ times the probe-pulse energy. This means that when it arrives at the ground the probe pulse still has a considerable energy reserve, which can be utilized to determine the water transmittance from the energy of the return after the maximum corresponding to reflection from the ground surface.

The advances in laser monitoring of other parameters of the atmosphere, primarily the profiles of the gaseous components of the atmosphere, are dictated largely by current advances in the development of laser technology. This assertion refers to the application of lasers emitting highly stabilized monochromatic radiation at predetermined wavelengths in order to exploit the corresponding resonance effects effectively. For example, in probing from the surface of the earth, it is meaningless to use probe pulses with wavelengths occurring at the centers of strong vibration–rotation absorption bands of atmospheric gases because the absorption at the centers of strong lines can reach saturation after the first few centimeters or even millimeters of the path of the transmitted pulse in the atmosphere. In the case of probing from outer space, on the other hand, the stronger the lines with which the wavelength of the probe pulse coincides, the higher will be the frequency and the lower the concentrations of the corresponding gas that can be detected. A set of lines of different intensities for the same gas in combination with an appropriate set of probe wavelengths can ensure the possibility of determining the vertical profiles of the gaseous components of the atmosphere in a wide frequency range.

The practical demands for the acquisition of space–time arrays of data on various physical parameters of the atmosphere will doubtless encourage the concomitant development of laser technology and, at the same time, perfection of the methods of laser probing of the atmosphere from space.

## 7.16. Determination of the Concentrations of Atmospheric Gases by Laser-Spectroscopic Methods

### 7.16.1. Differential Absorption Methods

The generation of highly monochromatic frequency-tunable laser radiation, serving as the basis of high- and ultrahigh-resolution laser-spectroscopic methods, offers conceptually new possibilities for the spectral analysis of gases. The laser emission line can be aligned with the center of an absorption line with smooth tuning of the laser output. This possibility is not afforded by discrete wavelength adjustments. Even in this case, however, as will be shown presently, lasers can be used with reasonable success for analytical applications. With the use of both smoothly and discretely tuned laser emission to determine the concentration of atmospheric gases, the most popular approach is the differential absorption method, the basic notion of which is discussed in Section 7.11.1 in application to remote probing of the gaseous components of the atmosphere.

In this section, we discuss the differential method in application to long measurement paths, bearing in mind the following modifications: (1) the use of a spaced transmitter and receiver; (2) the use of an artificial reflector; (3) the use of a topographic target as a natural reflector.

In all situations, the measurements are performed with two wavelengths, one coinciding with an absorption line of a particular gas and the other occurring in the nearest atmospheric microwindow. In the first method, the source and receiver are located at opposite ends of the measurement path, while in the second and third methods they are set up next to one another. The wavelengths are spaced in such a way as to make their volume aerosol and Rayleigh scattering coefficients coincide within very narrow error limits. If $\gamma_L \ll \gamma_a$, where $\gamma_L$ is the half-width of the laser emission line and $\gamma_a$ is the half-width of the absorption line of the analyzed gas, then for a homogeneous measurement path we can write the following expression for the case of spaced transmitter and receiver:

$$P_{\nu_i}(L) = \eta P_{0\nu_i} \exp\left[-\alpha(\nu_i)L\right] \qquad (7.160)$$

where $P_{\nu_i}$ is the signal power at frequency $\nu_i$ recorded by the receiver, $P_{0\nu_i}$ is the signal power of the source at the same frequency, $\eta$ is the calibration constant of the instrument, $\alpha$ is the volume extinction coefficient representing the sum of the volume aerosol and Rayleigh scattering and molecular absorption coefficients, and $L$ is the path length.

Writing expression (7.160) for two wavelengths, expressing the volume molecular scattering coefficient $\sigma_a(\nu_i)$ in terms of the product of the concentration per unit volume $C$ of the gas and the absorption cross section $k'(\nu_i)$, and taking into account the assumptions made with regard to the volume aerosol and Rayleigh scattering coefficients, we obtain an expression for the concentration $C$:

$$C = \frac{1}{\Delta k'L} \ln\left[\frac{P_{\nu_2}(L)P_{0\nu_1}}{P_{\nu_1}(L)P_{0\nu_2}}\right] \qquad (7.161)$$

In cases where an artificial reflector and a topographic target are used, the right-hand side of Eq. (7.160) acquires additional factors, namely, the efficiency $\xi$ of an artificial reflector or, in the case of a topographic target, assuming the scattering of radiation by it obeys Lambert's law, the factor

$(\rho/\pi)(A/L^2)$, where $\rho$ is the reflectivity of the target and $A$ is the area of the receiving mirror. The quantities $\xi$ and $\rho$ may be regarded as identical for the frequencies $\nu_1$ and $\nu_2$ and, hence, for the concentration $C$. In these cases, we arrive once again at expression (7.161), but now with a different concentration sensitivity. It is substantially lower for the method of a topographic target.

The practical application of the differential absorption method in conjunction with long measurement paths has been realized in the last few years by many groups of researchers using continuously tunable semiconductor lasers or lasers with discrete frequency tuning. The most significant results of using continuously tuned semiconductor lasers have been obtained by Hinkley's group at MIT's Lincoln Laboratory [384–390]. The success of their work has been greatly abetted by the lasers built at this laboratory with an emission band up to $2\times10^{-6}$ cm$^{-1}$, frequency fluctuations between limits of $3\times10^{-4}$ cm$^{-1}$, and a pulse repetition rate of 10 kHz at the temperature of a closed cryogenic cooling unit [391, 392]. The set of lasers is capable of spanning a broad range of wavelengths in the infrared region of the spectrum.

The cited papers [384–390] include a comprehensive analysis of the absorption spectra of atmosphere-contaminating gases such as CO, NO, $O_3$, $SO_2$, and $C_2H_6$ from the point of view of selecting the most appropriate absorption lines, laboratory measurements of the parameters of those lines, and the synthesis of laboratory and field equipment for determining the concentration of CO and $H_2O$. Field studies are reported on the signal fluctuations induced by atmospheric conditions. A sensitivity of several ppb in the determination of the CO concentration over a path of 0.61 km in the atmosphere was attained. Figure 7.42 gives one of the traces of the CO concentration in the vicinity of Saint Louis University for a measurement path of 0.61 km. A sensitivity of 80 ppb was attained in measurements of the $C_2H_4$ concentration for a path length of 0.5 km. In several instances, $C_2H_4$ contained in the exhausts of individual automobiles was detected. Laboratory measurements of the absorption coefficients at the centers of nonoverlapping absorption lines of CO ($\lambda=4.74$ $\mu$m), $O_3$ (4.75 $\mu$m), NO (5.31 $\mu$m), $SO_2$ (5.88 $\mu$m), and $C_2H_4$ (10.54 $\mu$m) served as a basis for determining the minimum detectable concentrations of these gases over a path length of 2 km within 0.3% measurement error limits; the results were 1.5, 3.0, 1.5, 15, and 0.8 ppb, respectively.

Examples of the use of directly tuned lasers for the determination of the concentration of atmospheric gases by the differential method may be found in [310, 393–398]. The application of a $CO_2$ laser with a tunable

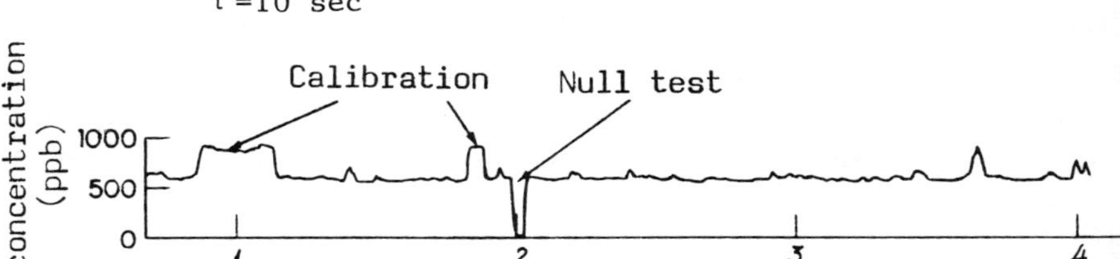


Fig. 7.42. Trace of the CO concentration near St. Louis University for a measurement path of
with some overlap.)

wavelength range of 9.1 to 10.9 $\mu$m looks highly promising in this regard. A
great many absorption lines of such gases and vapors as ozone, ammonia,
sulfur dioxide, ethylene, acetone, water vapor, carbon dioxide, formaldehyde, acetaldehyde, methyl mercaptan, benzene, diphenyl, nitric oxide, fall
within the indicated range. For example, Montgomery and Hill [399], using
a laser spectrometer with a resolution of 0.008 cm$^{-1}$ in the spectral interval
from 947.1 to 951.9 cm$^{-1}$, observed 169 absorption lines in the $\nu_7$ band of
ethylene. Patty and others [400] have obtained data on the absorption
coefficients of ozone, ammonia, and ethylene in mixtures with air for
various $CO_2$ laser emission lines. Analogous data for mixtures of ethylene,
acetone, sulfur dioxide, formaldehyde, and acetaldehyde with nitrogen may
be found in [401] and for ammonia, acetone, and methyl alcohol in [398].

Figure 7.43 gives the results of our measurements of the absorption
coefficients for various emission lines of a discretely tuned $CO_2$ laser in the
ground layer of the atmosphere over a path length of 2.1 km. The upper
curve corresponds to springtime measurements and the lower curve to
winter measurements. The concentrations of various gases were determined
from the measured values of the absorption coefficients for the following

Fig. 7.43

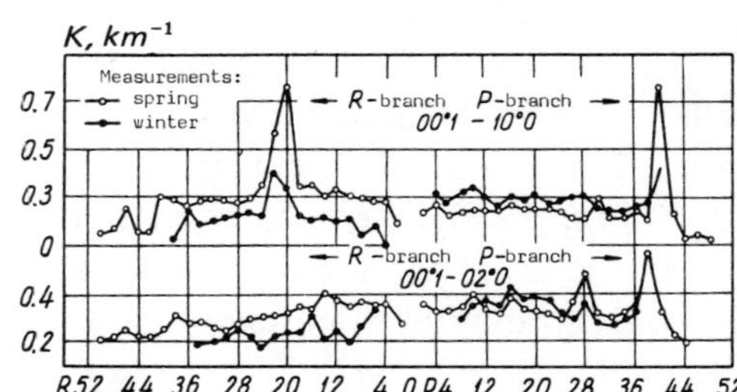

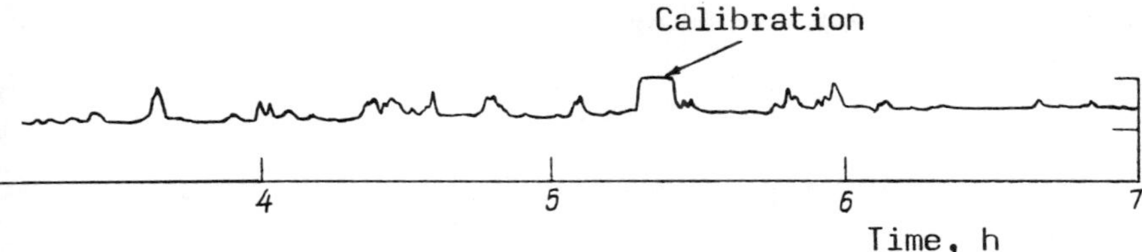



0.61 km. (Note that, for the sake of clarity, the two halves of the figure are reproduced here

pairs of $CO_2$ laser emission lines: (1) ozone: $P_{(22)}$, $P_{(24)}$; $P_{(28)}$, $P_{(24)}$; $P_{(24)}$, $P_{(14)}$, $00^0 1 - 02^0 0$ band; (2) ammonia: $P_{(34)}$, $P_{(28)}$, $00^0 1 - 10^0 0$ band; (3) ethylene: $P_{(14)}$, $P_{(12)}$; $P_{(14)}$, $P_{(20)}$, $00^0 1 - 10^0 0$ band. The measured concentrations of ozone, ammonia, and ethylene fall within the limits $6.7 \times 10^{-8}$ to $6.3 \times 10^{-7}$ atm; $3 \times 10^{-9}$ to $8.5 \times 10^{-8}$ atm; $1.1 \times 10^{-8}$ to $5.2 \times 10^{-8}$ atm, respectively.

The conspicuous maxima of the absorption coefficients for the $CO_2$ laser lines $R(20)$ and $P(40)$ of the $00^0 1 - 10^0 0$ band (see Fig. 7.43) are attributable to water vapor [402]. The results of our measurements of the absorption coefficients for the indicated laser lines at various humidities and temperatures enabled us to obtain the following simple relation between the absolute humidity $a(g/m^3)$ and the difference between the absorption coefficients $\Delta\sigma_a(km^{-1})$ at the water-vapor absorption line and far from it:

$$\Delta\sigma_a = \alpha_{1,2} a \qquad (7.162)$$

The proportionality factor $\alpha_1 = (0.084 \pm 0.012)$ m$^3$/g km for the line $P(40)$ and $\alpha_2 = (0.072 \pm 0.013)$ m$^3$/g km for the line $R(20)$.

Figure 7.44 gives the results of measurements of the dependence of $\Delta\sigma$ on $a$ for the line $P(40)$. The standard deviations given in the figure are associated with the fact that the humidity was measured at one or two

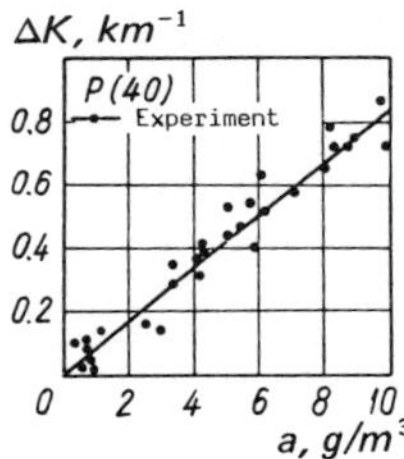



Fig. 7.44

points along the path, whereas the absorption coefficients were measured over the entire path. Expression (7.162) and the data of Fig. 7.44 support the feasibility of using the indicated lines of water vapor for the real-time determination of humidity.

## 7.17. The Outlook for Future Research and Development

The application of lasers for exploration of the atmosphere has made enormous progress in recent years through the advances of laser technology and concurrent progress in the solution of inverse problems, both in laser probing of the atmosphere and in the laser spectroscopy of atmospheric gases.

The greatest strides have been made to date in regard to the problems of laser monitoring of aerosols, including their microphysical characteristics. Such important practical problems as the real-time determination of the slant visibility range, the bottom and water content of clouds, and the spatial distribution of the mass concentration of aerosols have now been brought to a state where their realization rests mainly with industry rather than with scientists.

Future advancement in the development of laser methods for investigation of the atmosphere presents specific demands for the synthesis of special lasers, needed primarily for utilization of a broad range of resonance phenomena in the interaction of radiation with the medium. The development and construction of such lasers remains one of the most serious problems. We need lasers with high monochromaticity, a controllable variation of the wavelength, and an adequately high radiated power at durations that will ensure high spatial resolution of the monitoring results.

Together with the development of laser technology, developments of new probing techniques will necessarily play an important part in the future progress realized in the solution of the problem of remote monitoring of the parameters of the atmosphere by means of lasers. For example, there are definite expectations for the widespread utilization of effects of nonlinear interaction of laser radiation with the atmosphere as an absorbing, scattering, randomly inhomogeneous medium, although currently existing notions and methods in the linear optics of the atmosphere have by no means been exhausted.

# References

## Chapter 1


1. K. V. Kazanskii, *Terrestrial Refraction over Vast Water Surfaces* [in Russian], Gidrometeoizdat, Leningrad (1966).
2. I. G. Kolchinskii, *Light Refraction in the Earth's Atmosphere* [in Russian], Naukova Dumka, Kiev (1967).
3. A. I. Nefed'eva, *Izv. Astron. Obs. im. Éngel'gardta*, No. 36, p. 3 (1968).
4. I. F. Kushtin, *Refraction of Light Rays in the Atmosphere* [in Russian], Nedra, Moscow (1971).
5. V. Numerova, *Byull. Astron. Inst.*, No. 35 (1934).
6. F. Link and Z. Sekera, *Dioptrische Tabeln der Erdatmosphäre*, Przaske Hvesdarny, Prague (1940).
7. F. Link and L. Neuzil, *Dioptrické Tabulky Zemskè Atmosfery*, Česk. Akad. Véd., Astron. Ústav, Prague (1965).
8. I. F. Kushtin, *Izv. Vyssh. Uchebn. Zaved., Geod. Kartogr.*, No. 11 (1966); No. 1 (1966).
9. A. A. Dmitrievskii and V. N. Koshevoi, *Fundamentals of the Theory of Rocket Flight* [in Russian], Voenizdat, Moscow (1964).
10. *Pulkovo Observatory Refraction Tables* [in Russian], Izd. AN SSSR, Moscow–Leningrad (1956).
11. B. M. Fannin and K. H. Jehn, *IRE Trans. Antennas Propag.*, AP-5:71 (1957).
12. V. E. Zuev, *Laser Scans the Sky* [in Russian], Zap.–Sib. Knizhn. Izd. (1972).
13. V. E. Zuev, *The Laser Meteorologist* [in Russian], Gidrometeoizdat, Leningrad (1974).
14. E. D. Hinkley, S. H. Melfi, V. E. Zuev, *et al.*, *Laser Monitoring of the Atmosphere*, Springer, Berlin–Heidelberg–New York (1976).
15. A. A. Izotov and L. P. Pellinen, *Tr. TsNIIGAiK*, No. 102 (1955).
16. D. I. Maslich, *Geod. Kartogr. Aéros"emka*, No. 9, p. 33 (1969).
17. V. A. Krat, in *Proc. Conf. Investigation of the Scintillation of Stars* [in Russian], Izd. AN SSSR, Moscow–Leningrad (1959).
18. P. Beckmann, *J. Res. Natl. Bur. Stand., Sec. D*, 69(4):629 (1965).
19. H. Hodara, "Laser wave propagation through the atmosphere," *Proc. IEEE*, 54(3) (1966).
20. V. N. Genin and S. S. Khmelevtsov, *Izv. Vyssh. Uchebn. Zaved., Fiz.*, No. 11 (1967).
21. *The Geodesist's Handbook* [in Russian], Nedra, Moscow (1966).
22. *Geophysics Handbook* [in Russian], Nauka, Moscow (1965).
23. I. L. Zel'manovich and A. I. Serbin, *Tr. Gl. Geofiz. Obs.*, No. 183, p. 56 (1966).
24. K. V. Kazanskii, *Izv. Akad. Nauk SSSR, Geofiz.*, No. 2, p. 332 (1959).

25. G. V. Rozenberg and I. G. Mel'nikova, *Izv. Akad. Nauk SSSR*, *Ser. Fiz. Atm. Okeana*, 7(10):1053 (1971).

26. I. A. Khvostikov, *Dokl. Akad. Nauk SSSR*, 51(5):343 (1946).

27. I. T. Prilepin, *Izv. Vyssh. Uchebn. Zaved.*, *Geod. Aérofotos"emka*, No. 3, p. 3 (1970).

28. M. P. Dolukhanov, *Propagation of Radio Waves* [in Russian], Svyaz', Moscow (1972).

29. L. N. Korsunskii, *Radio-Wave Propagation in Connection with Artifical Earth Satellites* [in Russian], Sov. Radio, Moscow (1971).

30. F. B. Chernyi, *Propagation of Radio Waves* [in Russian], Sov. Radio, Moscow (1972).

31. V. N. Genin and N. F. Nelyubin, in *Propagation and Refraction of Optical Waves in the Atmosphere* [in Russian], Inst. Opt. Atm. Sib. Otd. Akad. Nauk SSSR, Tomsk (1976), p. 141.

32. V. D. Reshetov, *Variability of Meteorological Elements in the Atmosphere* [in Russian], Gidrometeoizdat, Leningrad (1973).

33. G. S. Tyuterev, in *Oscillations of the Latitudes and Movement of the Poles of Earth* [in Russian], Nauka, Moscow (1965), p. 50.

34. N. F. Nelyubin, in *Scattering and Refraction of Optical Waves in the Atmosphere* [in Russian], Inst. Opt. Atm. Sib. Otd. Akad. Nauk SSSR, Tomsk (1976), p. 153.

35. M. V. Zavarina, *Tr. NIU GUGMS*, Ser. 1, No. 21 (1946).

36. O. A. Drozdov and A. A. Shipelevskii, *Tr. NIU GUGMS*, Ser. 1, No. 13 (1946).

37. N. A. Vasilenko, in *Astrometry and Astrophysics* [in Russian], No. 17, Naukova Dumka, Kiev (1972), p. 91.

38. V. V. Kirichuk, *Izv. Vyssh. Uchebn. Zaved.*, *Geod. Aérofotos"emka*, No. 3, p. 67 (1971).

39. V. Kh. Buinitskii, *Probl. Arktiki*, 72(3) (1949).

40. V. G. Fesenkov, *Russk. Astron. Zh.*, 4:37 (1927).

41. G. M. Clemens, *Astron. J.*, 56:1193 (1951).

42. V. N. Genin, M. V. Kabanov, and N. F. Nelyubin, in *Abstr. Fourth All-Union Symp. Propagation of Laser Radiation in the Atmosphere* [in Russian], Inst. Opt. Atm. Sib. Otd. Akad. Nauk SSSR, Tomsk (1977), p. 72.

43. V. A. Yakovlev, in *Abstr. Fourth All-Union Symp. Propagation of Laser Radiation in the Atmosphere* [in Russian], Inst. Opt. Atm. Sib. Otd. Akad. Nauk SSSR, Tomsk (1977), p. 78.

44. A. E. Fedorishchev, in *Abstr. Fourth All-Union Symp. Propagation of Laser Radiation in the Atmosphere* [in Russian], Inst. Opt. Atm. Sib. Otd. Akad. Nauk SSSR, Tomsk (1977), p. 83.

45. I. F. Kushtin, in *Abstr. Fourth All-Union Symp. Propagation of Laser Radiation in the Atmosphere* [in Russian], Inst. Opt. Atm. Sib. Otd. Akad. Nauk SSSR, Tomsk (1977), p. 88.

46. V. P. Nelyubina and N. F. Nelyubin, in *Abstr. Fourth All-Union Symp. Propagation of Laser Radiation in the Atmosphere* [in Russian], Inst. Opt. Atm. Sib. Otd. Akad. Nauk SSSR, Tomsk (1977), p. 74.

47. A. V. Alekseev, V. N. Genin, and M. V. Kabanov, in *Scattering and Refraction of Optical Waves in the Atmosphere* [in Russian], Inst. Opt. Atm. Sib. Otd. Akad. Nauk SSSR, Tomsk (1976), p. 165.

48. A. S. Monin and A. M. Yaglom, *Statistical Fluid Mechanics* [in Russian], Part 1, Nauka, Moscow (1967).

49. L. Z. Rumshinskii, *Elements of Probability Theory* [in Russian], Nauka, Moscow (1976).

50. V. D. Gabrielyan and R. G. Manucharyan, in *Abstr. Fourth All-Union Symp. Propagation of Laser Radiation in the Atmosphere* [in Russian], Inst. Opt. Atm. Sib. Otd. Akad. Nauk SSSR, Tomsk (1977), p. 70.

51. D. N. Maslich, B. T. Tlustyak, and N. I. Kravtsov, in *Abstr. Fourth All-Union Symp. Propagation of Laser Radiation in the Atmosphere* [in Russian], Inst. Opt. Atm. Sib. Otd. Akad. Nauk SSSR, Tomsk (1977), p. 93.

52. A. V. Alekseev, in *Scattering and Refraction of Optical Waves in the Atmosphere* [in Russian], Inst. Opt. Atm. Sib. Otd. Akad. Nauk SSSR, Tomsk (1978), p. 179.

53. D. I. Maslich, *Geod. Kartogr. Aérofotos"emka*, No. 5, p. 52 (1966).
54. B. T. Tlustyak, *Geod. Kartogr. Aérofotos"emka*, No. 20, p. 86 (1974).
55. B. T. Tlustyak, A. Ya. Timoshik, and I. O. Voznyak, *Geod. Kartogr.*, No. 5, p. 21 (1975).
56. B. T. Tlustyak, *Geod. Kartogr. Aérofotos"emka*, No. 22, p. 78 (1975).

## Chapter 2

1. V. E. Zuev, *Propagation of Visible-Light and Infrared Waves in the Atmosphere* [in Russian], Sov. Radio, Moscow (1970).
2. V. E. Zuev, in *Laser Monitoring of the Atmosphere*, Springer, Berlin–New York (1976).
3. G. Traving, *Über die Theorie der Druckverbreiterung von Spectrallinien*, Braun, Karlsruhe (1960).
4. R. G. Breen, *The Shift and Shape of Spectral Lines*, Pergamon, Oxford–London–New York–Paris (1961).
5. I. I. Sobel'man, *Usp. Fiz. Nauk*, 54:551 (1954).
6. S. Y. Chen and M. Takeo, *Rev. Mod. Phys.*, 29:20 (1957).
7. C. J. Tsao and B. Curnutte, *J. Quant. Spectrosc. Radiat. Transfer*, 2:41 (1962).
8. I. I. Sobel'man, *Introduction to the Theory of Atomic Spectra* [in Russian], Fizmatgiz, Moscow (1963).
9. S. G. Rautian and I. I. Sobel'man, *Usp. Fiz. Nauk*, 90:209 (1966).
10. R. M. Goody, *Atmospheric Radiation*, Clarendon, Oxford (1964).
11. H. A. Lorentz, *Proc. R. Acad. Sci.* (Amsterdam), 8:591 (1906).
12. P. W. Anderson, *Phys. Rev.*, 76:647 (1949).
13. I. Ward, I. Cooper, and E. M. Smith, *J. Quant. Spectrosc. Radiat. Transfer*, 14:555 (1974).
14. R. H. Dicke, *Phys. Rev.*, 89:472 (1953); I. P. Wittke and R. H. Dicke, *Phys. Rev.*, 103:620 (1956).
15. S. G. Rautian, *Tr. Fiz. Inst. Akad. Nauk SSSR*, No. 43 (1968).
16. V. A. Alekseev, T. L. Andreeva, and I. I. Sobel'man, *Zh. Éksp. Teor. Fiz.*, 62:614 (1972).
17. P. R. Berman, *Comment. At. Mol. Phys.*, 5:19 (1975).
18. B. W. Fowler and C. C. Sung, *J. Opt. Soc. Am.*, 65:949 (1975).
19. F. de Martini, *Nota Interna, Inst. Fis., G. Marconi-Univ. Roma*, No. 345 (1971).
20. R. L. Armstrong, *Appl. Opt.*, 14:56 (1975).
21. A. D. May, I. C. Stryland, and G. Varghese, *Can. J. Phys.*, 48:2331 (1970).
22. L. I. Nesmelova, S. D. Tvorogov, and V. V. Fomin, *Spectroscopy of the Wings of Lines* [in Russian] (V. E. Zuev, ed.), Nauka, Novosibirsk (1977).
23. B. N. Winters, S. S. Silverman, and W. S. Benedict, *J. Quant. Spectrosc. Radiat. Transfer*, 4:527 (1964).
24. D. E. Burch, D. A. Gryvnak, R. R. Patty, and C. E. Bartky, *J. Opt. Soc. Am.*, 59:267 (1969).
25. P. Varanasi, *J. Quant. Spectrosc. Radiat. Transfer*, 12:1283 (1972).
26. L. Traffton, *Icarus*, 15:27 (1971).
27. L. Traffton, *J. Quant. Spectrosc. Radiat. Transfer*, 13:821 (1973).
28. T. E. Walsh, *J. Opt. Soc. Am.*, 59:261 (1969).
29. W. L. France and D. Williams, *J. Opt. Soc. Am.*, 56:70 (1966).
30. L. L. Abels and L. M. De Ball, *J. Quant. Spectrosc. Radiat. Transfer*, 13:663 (1973).
31. W. S. Benedict, R. Herman, G. E. Moore, and S. Silverman, *Astrophys. J.*, 135:295 (1962).
32. K. Bignell, F. Saiedy, and P. A. Sheppard, *J. Opt. Soc. Am*, 53:466 (1963).
33. V. Ya. Ryadov and N. I. Furashov, *Izv. Vyssh. Uchebn. Zaved., Radiofiz.*, 11:1138 (1968).
34. J. H. McCoy, D. B. Rensch, and R. K. Long, *Appl. Opt.*, 8:1471 (1969).
35. K. J. Bignell, *Q. J. R. Meteorol. Soc.*, 96:390 (1970).

36. V. Ya. Ryadov and N. I. Furashov, *Izv. Vyssh. Uchebn. Zaved., Radiofiz.*, 15:1469 (1972).
37. V. Ya. Ryadov and N. I. Furashov, in *Abstr. Tenth All-Union Conf. Radio-Wave Propagation* [in Russian], Nauka, Moscow (1972), p. 48.
38. A. C. Lee, *Q. J. R. Meteorol. Soc.*, 99:409 (1973).
39. N. I. Moskalenko, *Izv. Akad. Nauk SSSR, Ser. Fiz. Atm. Okeana*, 10:999 (1974).
40. V. N. Aref'ev, V. I. Dianov-Klokov, and N. I. Sizov, *Tr. Inst. Éksp. Meteorol.*, 61(4) (1976).
41. A. V. Povarov, V. Ya. Ryadov, B. A. Sverdlov, and N. I. Furashov, *Izv. Vyssh. Uchebn. Zaved.*, (4):529 (1976).
42. N. H. Schwendeman and V. W. Laurie, *Tables of Line Strengths for Rotational Transmissions of Asymmetric Rotor Molecules*, Pergamon, New York (1958).
43. P. L. Kelley, R. A. McClatchey, R. K. Long, and A. Suelson, *Opt. Quantum Electron.*, 8:117 (1976).
44. S. R. Drayson, *Appl. Opt.*, 5:385 (1966).
45. V. I. Dianov-Klokov, *Opt. Spektrosk.*, 16:409 (1964).
46. J. C. Hardwick and J. C. D. Brand, *Can. J. Phys.*, 54:80 (1976).
47. J. A. Hodgeson, E. E. Silbert, and R. F. Curl, *J. Chem. Phys.*, 67:2833 (1963).
48. W. H. Kirchhoff, *J. Mol. Spectrosc.*, 41:333 (1972).
49. K. Ramaswany and S. Jayaraman, *Z. Phys. Chem.* (Leipzig), 249:188 (1972).
50. A. J. van Straten and W. M. A. Smit, *J. Mol. Spectrosc.*, 62:297 (1976).
51. I. Ozier, *Phys. Rev. Lett.*, 27:1329 (1971).
52. K. Fox, *Phys. Rev. Lett.*, 27:233 (1971).
53. K. Fox, *Phys. Rev. A*, 6:907 (1972).
54. A. Rosenberg, I. Ozier, and A. K. Kundian, *J. Chem. Phys.*, 57:568 (1972).
55. A. K. Cole and F. R. Honey, *J. Mol. Spectrosc.*, 55:492 (1975).
56. M. M. Shapiro and H. P. Gush, *Can. J. Phys.*, 44:949 (1966).
57. D. R. Bosomworth and H. P. Gush, *Can. J. Phys.*, 43:751 (1965).
58. E. B. Wilson and J. B. Howard, *J. Chem. Phys.*, 4:260 (1936).
59. M. A. El'yashevich, *Tr. Gos. Opt. Inst.*, No. 106, p. 1 (1938).
60. B. T. Darling and D. M. Dennison, *Phys. Rev.*, 57:128 (1940).
61. B. J. Howard and R. E. Moss, *Mol. Phys.*, 20:147 (1971).
62. B. J. Howard and R. E. Moss, *Mol. Phys.*, 19:433 (1970).
63. Yu. S. Makushkin, *Opt. Spektrosk.*, 37:662 (1974).
64. Yu. S. Makushkin and O. N. Ulenikov, *Opt. Spektrosk.*, 36:1091 (1974).
65. Yu. S. Makushkin and O. N. Ulenikov, *Izv. Vyssh. Uchebn. Zaved., Fiz.*, No. 8, p. 54 (1975).
66. Yu. S. Makushkin and O. N. Ulenikov, *J. Mol. Spectrosc.*, 68:1 (1977).
67. H. H. Nielsen, *Rev. Mod. Phys.*, 23:90 (1961).
68. A. A. Kiselev, *Opt. Spektrosk.*, 22:193 (1967).
69. A. A. Kiselev, *J. Phys. B: At. Mol. Phys.*, 3:904 (1970).
70. J. K. G. Watson, *Mol. Phys.*, 15:479 (1968).
71. M. Goldsmith, G. Amat, and H. H. Nielsen, *J. Chem. Phys.*, 24:1178 (1956).
72. Yu. S. Makushkin, Vibration–Rotation Energy Spectrum of Type $XY_2$ Nonlinear Molecules (Candidates Dissertation), Tomsk (1967).
73. L. Henry and G. Amat, *J. Mol. Spectrosc.*, 5:319 (1960).
74. S. Maes, *Cah. Phys.*, 14:125 (1960).
75. A. Sayvetz, *J. Chem. Phys.*, 7:383 (1939).
76. J. T. Hougen, *J. Chem. Phys.*, 36:519 (1962).
77. W. H. Shaffer and H. H. Nielsen, *J. Chem. Phys.*, 9:847 (1941).
78. J. K. G. Watson, *Mol. Phys.*, 19:465 (1970).
79. A. N. Petelin and A. A. Kiselev, *Intern. J. Quant. Chem.*, 6:701 (1972).
80. H. H. Nielsen, *Phys. Rev.*, 66:282 (1944).

81. Yu. I. Polyakov, *Opt. Spektrosk.*, 39:253 (1975).
82. M. Born and R. Oppenheimer, *Ann. Phys.* (Leipzig), 84:457 (1927).
83. W. Kolos and L. Wolniewicz, *J. Chem. Phys.*, 41:3663 (1964).
84. W. Kolos and L. Wolniewicz, *Rev. Mod. Phys.*, 35:473 (1963).
85. R. T. Pack and J. O. Hirschfelder, *J. Chem. Phys.*, 49:4009 (1968).
86. P. R. Bunker, *J. Mol. Spectrosc.*, 42:478 (1972).
87. P. R. Bunker, *J. Mol. Spectrosc.*, 28:422 (1968).
88. P. R. Bunker, *J. Mol. Spectrosc.*, 39:90 (1971).
89. J. L. Dunham, *Phys. Rev.*, 41:721 (1932).
90. J. K. G. Watson, *J. Mol. Spectrosc.*, 45:99 (1973).
91. A. E. Bolonkin and Yu. S. Makushkin, *Opt. Spektrosk.*, 32:264 (1972).
92. A. E. Bolonkin and Yu. S. Makushkin, *Opt. Spektrosk.*, 33:844 (1972).
93. A. E. Bolonkin and Yu. S. Makushkin, *Opt. Spektrosk.*, 35:82 (1973).
94. Yu. S. Makushkin and O. N. Ulenikov, *Izv. Vyssh. Uchebn. Zaved., Fiz.*, No. 7, p. 120 (1975).
95. M. R. Aliev and V. T. Aleksanyan, *Opt. Spektrosk.*, 24:520 (1968).
96. W. H. Shaffer, H. H. Nielsen, and L. H. Thomas, *Phys. Rev.*, 56:885 (1939).
97. J. H. Van Vleck, *Phys. Rev.*, 33:467 (1929).
98. W. H. Shaffer, H. H. Nielsen, and L. H. Thomas, *Phys. Rev.*, 56:1051 (1939).
99. R. C. Herman and W. H. Shaffer, *J. Chem. Phys.*, 16:453 (1948).
100. G. Amat, M. Goldsmith, and H. H. Nielsen, *J. Chem. Phys.*, 27:838 (1957).
101. G. Amat and H. H. Nielsen, *J. Chem. Phys.*, 27:845 (1957); G. Amat and H. H. Nielsen, *J. Chem. Phys.*, 29:665 (1958); G. Amat and H. H. Nielsen, *J. Chem. Phys.*, 36:1859 (1962).
102. M. R. Aliev and V. T. Aleksanyan, *Opt. Spektrosk.*, 24:695 (1968).
103. M. R. Aliev and V. T. Aleksanyan, *Dokl. Akad. Nauk SSSR*, 173:302 (1967).
104. M. R. Aliev and V. T. Aleksanyan, *Opt. Spektrosk.*, 24:388 (1968).
105. M. R. Aliev, *Pis'ma Zh. Eksp. Teor. Fiz.*, 14:600 (1971).
106. Yu. S. Makushkin and Vl. G. Tyuterev, *Phys. Lett. A*, 47:128 (1974).
107. Yu. S. Makushkin and Vl. G. Tyuterev, in *Propagation of Optical Waves in the Atmosphere* [in Russian], Nauka, Novosibirsk (1975), p. 129.
108. Vl. G. Tyuterev, Method and Certain Results of an Investigation of Vibration–Rotation Interactions in Molecules (Candidates Dissertation), Tomsk (1974).
109. Yu. S. Makushkin and Vl. G. Tyuterev, *Izv. Vyssh. Uchebn. Zaved., Fiz.*, No. 7, p. 75 (1977).
110. Yu. S. Makushkin and Vl. G. Tyuterev, in *Proc. Second All-Union Symp. Molecular Spectroscopy* [in Russian] (1974), p. 40.
111. Yu. S. Makushkin and Vl. G. Tyuterev, *Opt. Spektrosk.*, 35:439 (1973).
112. Yu. S. Makushkin and Vl. G. Tyuterev, *Opt. Spektrosk.*, 37:59 (1974).
113. Vl. G. Tyuterev, in *High- and Ultrahigh-Resolution Molecular Spectroscopy* [in Russian], Nauka, Novosibirsk (1976), p. 93.
114. Yu. S. Makushkin and Vl. G. Tyuterev, *Abstr. Seventeenth All-Union Congr. Spectroscopy* [in Russian], Minsk (1971), p. 167.
115. Vl. G. Tyuterev, in *Intramolecular Interactions and Infrared Spectra of Spherical-Atom Gases* [in Russian], Tomsk (1975), p. 3.
116. H. M. Hanson, H. H. Nielsen, W. H. Shaffer, and J. Waggoner, *J. Chem. Phys.*, 27:40 (1957).
117. H. M. Hanson and H. H. Nielsen, *J. Mol. Spectrosc.*, 4:468 (1960).
118. H. M. Hanson and A. R. Cook, *J. Mol. Spectrosc.*, 16:130 (1965).
119. H. M. Hanson, *J. Mol. Spectrosc.*, 23:287 (1967).
120. C. Secroun, A. Barbe, and P. Jouve, *J. Mol. Spectrosc.*, 45:1 (1973).
121. H. H. Nielsen, *Intern. J. Quant. Chem.*, 1:217 (1967).

122. Y. Y. Kwan, *J. Mol. Spectrosc.*, 49:27 (1974).
123. H. Primas, *Helv. Phys. Acta*, 34:331 (1961).
124. H. Primas, *Rev. Mod. Phys.*, 35:710 (1963).
125. L. M. Sverdlov, *Dokl. Akad. Nauk SSSR*, 78:1115 (1951).
126. E. B. Wilson, Jr., J. C. Decius, and P. C. Cross, *Molecular Vibrations: The Theory of IR and Raman Vibrational Spectra*, McGraw-Hill, New York (1955).
127. O. Redlich, *Z. Phys. Chem., Abt. B*, 28:371 (1935).
128. L. M. Sverdlov, *Dokl. Akad. Nauk SSSR*, 85:513 (1952).
129. L. M. Sverdlov, *Dokl. Akad. Nauk SSSR*, 94:451 (1954).
130. L. M. Sverdlov, *Opt. Spektrosk.*, 8:36 (1960).
131. S. Brodersen, *J. Mol. Spectrosc.*, 3:450 (1959).
132. J. Heicklen, *J. Chem. Phys.*, 36:721 (1962).
133. L. M. Sverdlov, *Dokl. Akad. Nauk SSSR*, 88:249 (1953).
134. W. E. Smyth, *Austral. J. Phys.*, 12:109 (1959).
135. V. T. Aleksanyan, A. P. Aleksandrov, and M. R. Aliev, *Opt. Spektrosk.*, 26:526 (1969).
136. A. P. Aleksandrov, M. R. Aliev, and V. T. Aleksanyan, *Opt. Spektrosk.*, 29:1064 (1970).
137. Yu. S. Makushkin and O. N. Ulenikov, *Opt. Spektrosk.*, 39:629 (1975).
138. Yu. S. Makushkin and O. N. Ulenidov, *Opt. Spektrosk.*, 40:452 (1976).
139. Yu. S. Makushkin, A. V. Terent'ev, and O. N. Ulenikov, *Opt. Spektrosk.*, 40:989 (1976).
140. Yu. S. Makushkin and O. N. Ulenikov, *Opt. Spektrosk.*, 42:276 (1977).
141. Yu. S. Makushkin and O. N. Ulenikov, *Opt. Spektrosk.*, 41:198 (1976).
142. Yu. S. Makushkin and O. N. Ulenikov, *Opt. Spektrosk.*, 40:938 (1976).
143. N. Jacobi, *J. Chem. Phys.*, 52:2694 (1970).
144. M. T. Emerson and D. F. Eggers, *J. Chem. Phys.*, 37:251 (1962).
145. Y. Ben-Aryeh, *J. Opt. Soc. Am.*, 60:1469 (1970).
146. J. Braslawsky and Y. Ben-Aryeh, *J. Chem. Phys.*, 51:2233 (1969).
147. F. Legay, *Cah. Phys.*, 12:416 (1958).
148. C. Camy-Peyret and J.-M. Flaud, *Mol. Phys.*, 32:523 (1976).
149. O. K. Voitsekhovskaya and Yu. S. Makushkin, *Opt. Spektrosk.*, 33:32 (1975).
150. O. K. Voitsekhovskaya, Yu. S. Makushkin and O. N. Sulakshina, *Izv. Vyssh. Uchebn. Zaved., Fiz.*, No. 11, p. 152 (1976).
151. I. I. Ippolitov and Yu. S. Makushkin, *Izv. Vyssh. Uchebn. Zaved., Fiz.*, No. 10, p. 19 (1970).
152. I. I. Ippolitov and Yu. S. Makushkin, *Izv. Vyssh. Uchebn. Zaved., Fiz.*, No. 3, p. 101 (1970).
153. O. K. Voitsekhovskaya, I. I. Ippolitov, and Yu. S. Makushkin, *Opt. Spektrosk.*, 35:42 (1973).
154. O. K. Voitstekhovskaya, I. I. Ippolitov, and Yu. S. Makushkin, *Opt. Spektrosk.*, 33:78 (1972).
155. O. K. Voitsekhovskaya, V. E. Zuev, and I. I. Ippolitov, *Zh. Prikl. Spektrosk.*, 17:164 (1972).
156. O. K. Voitsekhovskaya and Yu. S. Makushkin, *Opt. Spektrosk.*, 41:40 (1976).
157. O. K. Voitsekhovskaya, I. I. Ippolitov, and Yu. S. Makushkin, in *Proc. Tenth All-Union Conf. Radio-Wave Propagation* [in Russian], Nauka, Irkutsk (1972).
158. O. K. Voitsekhovskaya, I. I. Ippolitov, and Yu. S. Makushkin, in *Abstr. Seventeenth All-Union Congr. Spectroscopy* [in Russian], Minsk (1971).
159. A. Ben-Reuven, *Phys. Rev.*, 141:34 (1966).
160. A. D. Bykov, Yu. S. Makushkin, and M. R. Cherkasov, *Opt. Spektrosk.*, 39:880 (1975).
161. M. Baranger, *Phys. Rev.*, 112:855 (1958).
162. A. C. Kolb and H. Griem, *Phys. Rev.*, 111:514 (1958).
163. U. Fano, *Phys. Rev.*, 131:259 (1963).
164. A. Ben-Reuven, *Phys. Rev.*, 145:7 (1966).

165. J. Fiutak, *Acta Phys. Pol.*, 27:753 (1965).

166. A. Ben-Reuven, *Phys. Rev. Lett.*, 14:349 (1965).

167. A. I. Burshtein, M. L. Strekalov, and S. I. Temkin, *Zh. Éksp. Teor. Fiz.*, 66:894 (1974).

168. V. A. Alekseev and I. I. Sobel'man, *Acta Phys. Pol.*, 34:579 (1968).

169. B. Bleaney and J. H. N. Loubser, *Proc. Phys. Soc. London*, 63:483 (1960).

170. A. H. Nethercot, J. A. Klein, J. H. N. Loubser, and C. H. Townes, *Nuovo Cimento*, 9:358 (1952).

171. A. Lightman and A. Ben-Reuven, *J. Chem. Phys.*, 50:351 (1969).

172. A. Ben-Reuven and A. Lightman, *J. Chem. Phys.*, 46:2429 (1967).

173. M. P. Cherkasov, *Formalism of the Liouville Quantum-Mechanical Operator in Calculations of Relaxation Parameters*, Preprint No. 4 [in Russian], Inst. Opt. Atm. Sib. Otd. Akad. Nauk SSSR, Tomsk (1975).

174. M. R. Cherkasov, *Opt. Spektrosk.*, 40:7 (1976).

175. M. R. Cherkasov, *VINITI Abstract No. 4281-77* [in Russian], Vses. Inst. Nauch. Tekh. Inform. (1977).

176. M. R. Cherkasov, *VINITI Abstract No. 4278-77* [in Russian], Vses. Inst. Nauch. Tekh. Inform. (1977).

177. R. L. Legan, J. A. Roberts, E. A. Rinehart, and C. C. Lin, *J. Chem. Phys.*, 43:4337 (1965).

178. P. L. Hewitt and R. W. Parsons, *Phys. Lett. A*, 45:21 (1973).

179. S. Gierszal, J. Galica, J. Stankowski, and W. Prussak, *Acta Phys. Pol. A*, 50:255 (1976).

180. K. N. Rao and C. W. Mathews (eds.), *Molecular Spectroscopy: Modern Research*, Academic Press, New York–London (1972).

181. G. Amat, H. H. Nielsen, and G. Torrago, *Rotation–Vibration of Polyatomic Molecules*, M. Dekker, New York (1971), p. 488.

182. A. Chedin and Z. Cihla, *J. Mol. Spectrosc.*, 45:475 (1973).

183. Z. Cihla and A. Chedin, *J. Mol. Spectrosc.*, 40:337 (1971).

184. Z. Cihla and A. Chedin, *J. Mol. Spectrosc.*, 47:531 (1973).

185. D. B. Keck and C. D. Hause, *J. Mol. Spectrosc.*, 26:163 (1968).

186. A. Chedin, Thesis, Univ. Paris, Cent. Nat. Rech. Sci. (1971).

187. G. Amat and M. Pimbert, *J. Mol. Spectrosc.*, 16:278 (1965).

188. A. P. Gal'tsev and V. M. Osipov, *Opt. Spektrosk.*, 30:674 (1971).

189. V. M. Osipov, Theoretical Study of the IR Spectrum of $CO_2$ at High Temperatures (Candidates Dissertation), Leningrad (1971).

190. C. P. Courtoy, *Ann. Soc. Sci. Bruxelles*, 73:5 (1959).

191. R. Overly, K. N. Rao, L. H. Jones, and M. Goldblatt, *J. Mol. Spectrosc.*, 40:357 (1971).

192. J. Moret-Bailly, *J. Mol. Spectrosc.*, 15:344 (1965).

193. K. T. Hecht, *J. Mol. Spectrosc.*, 5:390 (1960).

194. F. Michelot, J. Moret-Bailly, and K. Fox., *J. Chem. Phys.*, 60:2606 (1974).

195. J. Moret-Bailly, *Cah. Phys.*, 15:237 (1961).

196. J. Pliva, *J. Mol. Spectrosc.*, 27:461 (1968).

197. K. T. Hecht, *J. Mol. Spectrosc.*, 5:355 (1960).

198. I. Ozier, *Phys. Rev. Lett.*, 27:1329 (1971).

199. R. F. Curl, J. T. Oka, and D. S. Smith, *J. Mol. Spectrosc.*, 46:518 (1973).

200. R. F. Curl, *J. Mol. Spectrosc.*, 48:165 (1973).

201. C. W. Holb, M. C. L. Gerry, and I. Ozier, *Phys. Rev. Lett.*, 31:1033 (1973).

202. K. Fox, *Phys. Rev. Lett.*, 27:233 (1971).

203. J. K. G. Watson, *J. Mol. Spectrosc.*, 40:536 (1971).

204. A. J. Dorney and J. K. G. Watson, *J. Mol. Spectrosc.*, 42:135 (1972).

205. M. R. Aliev, *Pis'ma Zh. Éksp. Teor. Fiz.*, 14:600 (1971).

206. G. Tarrago, M. Dang-Nhu, and G. Poussique, *J. Mol. Spectrosc.*, 49:322 (1974).

207. G. Amat, *Energy Levels of Polyatomic Molecules*, Final Report, Contract AF-61(052)-369, Paris (1966).

208. K. Fox, *Phys. Rev. A*, 6:907 (1972).

209. G. Herzberg, *Molecular Spectra and Molecular Structure, Vol. 2: Infrared and Raman Spectra of Polyatomic Molecules*, Van Nostrand, New York (1945).

210. G. N. Zhizhin (ed.), *High-Resolution Infrared Spectroscopy* [in Russian], Mir, Moscow (1972).

211. V. E. Zuev, V. P. Lopasov, and M. M. Makogon, *Dokl. Akad. Nauk SSSR*, 199:1041 (1971).

212. A. N. Zaidel', G. V. Ostrovaskaya, and Yu. I. Ostrovskii, *Techniques and Practice of Spectroscopy* [in Russian], Nauka, Moscow (1972).

213. T. P. Belikova, B. K. Dorofeev, É. A. Sviridenkov, and A. F. Suchdov, *Kvantovaya Élektron.* (Moscow), 2:1325 (1975).

214. W. G. Planet, J. R. Aronson, and J. F. Butler, *J. Mol. Spectrosc.*, 54:331 (1975).

215. R. S. Eng, A. R. Calawa, T. C. Harman, P. L. Kelley, and A. Javan, *Appl. Phys. Lett.*, 21:303 (1972).

216. A. S. Pine, *J. Mol. Spectrosc.*, 54:132 (1975).

217. F. S. Stauffer and H. Sakai, *Appl. Opt.*, 7:61 (1968).

218. R. N. Hager and R. C. Anderson, *J. Opt. Soc. Am.*, 60:1444 (1970).

219. R. T. Ku, E. D. Hinkley, and J. O. Sample, *Appl. Opt.*, 14:854 (1975).

220. G. A. Antcliffe and J. S. Wrobel, *Appl. Opt.*, 11:1548 (1972).

221. R. S. Smith, *Rev. Sci. Instrum.*, 34:296 (1963).

222. V. S. Letokhov, *Usp. Fiz. Nauk.*, No. 2, pp. 118–199 (1976).

223. L. B. Kreuzer, *J. Appl. Phys.*, 42:2934 (1971).

224. E. L. Kerr and J. G. Atwood, *Appl. Opt.*, 7:915 (1968).

225. C. W. Bruce, B. S. Soika, E. S. Hurd, W. Watkins, K. White, and Z. Dersko, *Appl. Opt.*, 15:2976 (1970).

226. S. Gregory, G. Yach, and S. Hayden, *Chem. Phys. Lett.*, 39:146 (1976).

227. M. S. Shumate, R. T. Menzies, J. S. Margolis, and L. G. Rosengren, *Appl. Opt.*, 15:2480 (1976).

228. R. T. Menzies and M. S. Shumate, *Appl. Opt.*, 15:2025 (1976).

229. B. A. Antipov, V. E. Zuev, D. P. Pyrsikova, and V. A. Sapozhnikova, *Opt. Spektrosk.*, 38:681 (1975).

230. B. G. Ageev, A. B. Antipov, A. A. Pomeshchenko, and Yu. N. Ponomarev, *Opt. Spektrosk.*, 40(3) (1976).

231. A. B. Antipov and V. A. Kapitanov, in *Proc. Regional Sci.-Pract. Conf. Young Scientists and Specialists of the National Economy* [in Russian], Inst. Opt. Atm. Sib. Otd. Akad. Nauk SSSR, Tomsk (1977).

232. T. P. Belikova, E. A. Sviridenkov, A. F. Suchkov, L. V. Titova, and S. S. Churilov, *Zh. Éksp. Teor. Fiz.*, 62:2060 (1972).

233. B. I. Stepanov, A. N. Rubinov, and M. V. Belokon', *Zh. Prikl. Spektrosk.*, 24:423 (1976).

234. A. P. Godlevskii, V. P. Lopasov, and S. F. Luk'yanenko, *Kvantovaya Élektron.* (Moscow), 2:701 (1975).

235. T. W. Hänsch, A. L. Schawlow, and P. E. Toschek, *IEEE J. Quantum Electron.*, QE-8:802 (1972).

236. S. A. Batishche, V. A. Mostovnikov, and A. N. Rudinov, *Kvantovaya Élektron.* (Moscow), 3:2516 (1976).

237. C. Chackerian and M. F. Weisbach, *J. Opt. Soc. Am.*, 63:342 (1973).

238. V. M. Baev, E. A. Sviridenkov, V. Ya. Gulov, and M. P. Frolov, *Kvantovaya Élektron.* (Moscow), 2:1328 (1975).

239. L. N. Sinitsa, "Intraresonator neodymium-glass laser spectrometer with a dispersive resonator," *Kvantovaya Élektron.* (Moscow), 4(1):148 (1977).

240. P. Connes and G. Michel, *Appl. Opt.*, 14(9):2067 (1975).

241. J. Connes, in *Aspen Intern. Conf. Fourier Spectroscopy*, AFCRL Spec. Rep. 114 (1971), p. 83.

242. J. Dowling, in *Aspen Intern. Conf. Fourier Spectroscopy*, AFCRL Spec. Rep. 114 (1971), p. 55.
243. R. J. Bell, *Introductory Fourier Transform Spectroscopy*, Academic Press, New York (1972).
244. H. Sakai, G. A. Vanasse, and M. L. Forman, *J. Opt. Soc. Am.*, 58(1):84 (1968).
245. R. A. McClatchey, W. S. Benedict, S. A. Clough, D. E. Burch, R. F. Calfee, K. Fox, L. S. Rothman, and J. S. Garing, *Atmospheric Absorption Line Parameters Compilation*, AFCRL-TR-73-0096, Environmental Research Papers, No. 434 (1976).
246. W. S. Benedict, and R. F. Calfee, *Line Parameters for the 1.9 and 6.3 Micron Water Vapor Bands*, ESSA Professional Paper 2 (June 1967), U. S. Government Printing Office, Washington, DC (1967).
247. D. E. Burch, D. A. Gryvnak, R. R. Patty, and C. Bartky, *The Shapes of Collision-Broadened $CO_2$ Absorption Lines*, Aeronutronic Rep. U-3203, Contract No. 23560(00) (1968).
248. R. F. Calfee and W. S. Benedict, *Carbon Dioxide Spectral Line Positions and Intensities Calculated for the 2.05 and 2.7 Micron Regions*, Nat. Bur. Stand. Tech. Note 332 (1966).
249. S. R. Drayson and C. Young, *The Frequencies and Intensities of Carbon Dioxide Absorption Lines between 12 and 18 Microns*, Univ. Michigan Tech. Rep. 08183-1-T (1967).
250. D. M. Gates, R. F. Calfee, D. W. Hanson, and W. W. Benedict, *Line Parameters and Computed Spectra for Water Vapor Bands at 27 $\mu m$*, Nat. Bur. Stand. Monogr. 71 (1964).
251. V. G. Kunde, *Tables of Theoretical Line Positions and Intensities for the $v = 1$, $v = 2$, and $v = 3$ Vibration–Rotation Bands of $C^{12}O^{16}$, $C^{13}O^{16}$*, NASA TMX-63182 (1967).
252. T. G. Kyle, *Line Parameters of the Infrared Methane Bands*, AFCRL-68-0521 (1968).
253. V. E. Zuev, *Izv. Vyssh. Uchebn. Zaved., Fiz.*, No. 3, p. 138 (1967).
254. V. E. Zuev, *Izv. Vyssh. Uchebn. Zaved., Fiz.*, No. 10, p. 53 (1967).
255. V. E. Zuev, V. V. Pokasov, Yu. A. Pkhalagov, A. V. Sosnin, and S. S. Khmelevtsov, *Izv. Akad. Nauk SSSR, Fiz. Atm. Okeana*, 4:63 (1968).
256. B. A. Antipov, V. E. Zuev, and V. A. Sapozhnikova, *Izv. Vyssh. Uchebn. Zaved., Fiz.*, No. 7, p. 142 (1967).
257. B. A. Antipov, V. E. Zuev, and V. A. Sapozhnikova, *Izv. Vyssh. Uchebn. Zaved., Fiz.*, No. 6, p. 152 (1967).
258. V. E. Zuev, A. V. Sosnin, and S. S. Khmelevtsov, *Izv. Akad. Nauk SSSR, Fiz. Atm. Okeana*, 5:201 (1969).
259. S. I. Vavilov, *Microstructure of Light* [in Russian] (1950).
260. V. E. Zuev, V. P. Lopasov, and Yu. N. Ponomarev, *Dokl. Akad. Nauk SSSR*, 231:1106 (1976).
261. V. E. Zuev, V. P. Lopasov, and Yu. N. Ponomarev, in *Proc. First All-Union Conf. Atmospheric Optics* [in Russian], Part 1, Tomsk (1976), p. 56.
262. A. B. Antipov, and Yu. N. Ponomarev, *Kvantovaya Élektron.* (Moscow), 1:1345 (1974).
263. O. R. Wood, P. L. Gordon, and S. E. Schwarz, *IEEE Quantum Electron.*, QE-5(10):502 (1969).
264. V. S. Letokhov, A. A. Makarov, and E. A. Ryabov, *Dokl. Akad. Nauk SSSR*, 212:75 (1973).
265. N. Djeu and G. J. Wolga, *J. Appl. Phys.*, 42:3226 (1971).
266. E. A. Ryabov, *Kvantovaya Élektron.* (Moscow), 2:138 (1975).
267. J. H. Kostkowski and A. M. Bass, *J. Opt. Soc. Am.*, 46:1060 (1956).
268. R. F. Calfee, *J. Quant. Spectrosc. Radiat. Transfer*, 6:221 (1966).

## Chapter 3

1. V. E. Zuev, *The Laser Meteorologist* [in Russian], Gidrometeoizdat, Leningrad (1974).
2. L. Elterman, *Atmospheric Attenuation Model in the Ultraviolet, Visible, and Infrared Regions for Altitudes to 50 km*, Rep. AFCRL-64-740, ERPN 46, AFCRL, Bedford, MA (1964).

3. R. Penndorf, *J. Opt. Soc. Am.*, 47:176 (1957).
4. V. E. Zuev, *Propagation of Visible-Light and Infrared Waves in the Atmosphere* [in Russian], Sov. Radio, Moscow (1970).
5. S. D. Tvorogov, *Izv. Vyssh. Uchebn. Zaved., Fiz.*, No. 3, p. 147 (1965).
6. K. S. Shifrin, *Light Scattering in a Turbid Medium* [in Russian], Gostekhizdat, Moscow-Leningrad (1951).
7. H. C. Van de Hulst, *Light Scattering by Small Particles*, Wiley, New York–London (1957).
8. S. D. Tvorogov, *Izv. Vyssh. Uchebn. Zaved., Fiz.*, No. 1, p. 87 (1961).
9. K. S. Shifrin, *Tr. Gl. Geofiz. Obs.*, No. 26, p. 83 (1951).
10. K. S. Shifrin and I. L. Zel'manovich, *Light-Scattering Tables, Vol. 1* [in Russian], Gidrometeoizdat, Leningrad (1966).
11. K. S. Shifrin and I. L. Zel'manovich, *Light-Scattering Tables, Vol. 2: Tables of Scattering Matrices and Scattered-Field Components* [in Russian], Gidrometeoizdat, Leningrad (1968).
12. A. P. Prishivalko and E. K. Naumenko, [no title], Inst. Fiz. Akad. Nauk B. SSR, Minsk (1972).
13. R. Penndorf, *Research in Aerosol Scattering in the Infrared*, Sci. Rep. 5, Tech. Rep. RAD-TR-61-32, Off. Tech. Serv., U. S. Dept. Commerce (1961).
14. M. Kerker, *The Scattering of Light and Other Electromagnetic Radiation*, Academic Press, New York (1969).
15. W. J. Pangonis and W. Heller, *Angular Scattering Function for Spherical Particles*, Wayne State Univ. Press, Detroit (1960).
16. H. H. Denman, et al., *Angular Scattering Function for Spheres*, Wayne State Univ. Press, Detroit (1966).
17. R. H. Giese et al., *Tables Related to Scattering Functions and Scattering Cross Sections of Particles According to the Mie Theory*, Abh. Dtsch. Akad. Wiss., Kl. Math. Phys. Tech., No. 6, Berlin (1961).
18. D. Deirmendjian, *Tables of Mie Scattering Cross Sections and Amplitudes*, Rep. R-407-PR, Rand Corp., Santa Monica, CA (1963), p. 107.
19. L. M. Levin, *Investigations in the Physics of Coarse-Disperse Aerosols* [in Russian], Izd. AN SSSR, Moscow (1961).
20. D. Deirmendjian, *Q. J. Roy. Meteorol. Soc.*, 86:371 (1960).
21. J. C. Johnson and J. R. Terrell, *J. Opt. Soc. Am*, 45:451 (1955).
22. R. Penndorf, *J. Opt. Soc. Am.*, 52:402 (1962).
23. F. Volz, *Ber. Dtsch. Wetterdienstes*, 2 (1954).
24. L. L. Foldy, *Phys. Rev.*, 67:107 (1945).
25. M. Lax, *Rev. Mod. Phys.*, 23:287 (1951); *Phys. Rev.*, 85:621 (1952).
26. P. C. Waterman and R. Truell, *J. Math. Phys.*, 2:512 (1961).
27. V. Twersky, *J. Math. Phys.*, 3:700 (1962).
28. Yu. N. Gnedin and A. Z. Dolginov, *Astron. Zh.*, 43(4):800 (1966); *Zh. Eksp. Teor. Fiz.*, 45(4):1136 (1963).
29. A. G. Borovoi, *Izv. Vyssh. Uchebn. Zaved., Fiz.*, No. 2, p. 175 (1966); No. 6, p. 50 (1966); No. 4, p. 97 (1967); No. 5, p. 7 (1967).
30. G. V. Rozenberg, *Usp. Fiz. Nauk*, 56(1):77 (1955).
31. V. S. Malkova, *Izv. Akad. Nauk SSSR, Fiz. Atm. Okeana*, 1:109 (1965).
32. R. Eiden, *Appl. Opt.*, 5:569 (1966).
33. D. Deirmendjian, *Electromagnetic Scattering on Spherical Polydispersions*, Am. Elsevier, New York (1969).
34. A. P. Prishivalko, in *Proc. Third All-Union Symp. Propagation of Laser Radiation in the Atmosphere* [in Russian], Inst. Opt. Atm. Sib. Otd. Akad. Nauk SSSR, Tomsk (1975), p. 6.
35. L. S. Ivlev and S. I. Popova, *Izv. Akad. Nauk SSSR, Fiz. Atm. Okeana*, 9:1034 (1973).
36. G. I. Gorchakov and G. V. Rozenberg, *Izv. Akad. Nauk SSSR, Fiz. Atm. Okeana*, 1:1279 (1965).

37. G. I. Gorchakov, *Izv. Akad. Nauk SSSR, Fiz. Atm. Okeana*, 2:595 (1966).
38. G. I. Gorchakov and G. V. Rozenberg, *Izv. Akad. Nauk SSSR, Fiz. Atm. Okeana*, 3:611 (1967).
39. G. V. Rozenberg and G. I. Gorchakov, *Izv. Akad. Nauk SSSR, Fiz. Atm. Okeana*, 3:699 (1967).
40. G. V. Rozenberg, *Usp. Fiz. Nauk*, 95:159 (1968).
41. G. I. Gorchakov, *Izv. Akad. Nauk SSSR, Fiz. Atm. Okeana*, 9:204 (1973); 10:1317 (1974).
42. B. S. Pritchard and W. G. Elliott, *J. Opt. Soc. Am.*, 50(3):191 (1960).
43. Yu. S. Georgievskii, *Izv. Akad. Nauk SSSR, Fiz. Atm. Okeana*, 5:388 (1969).
44. V. L. Filippov and S. O. Mirumyants, *Izv. Akad. Nauk SSSR, Fiz. Atm. Okeana*, 8:818 (1971).
45. M. V. Kabanov, A. A. Pershin, Yu. A. Pkhalagov, and S. M. Sakerin, in *Proc. Third All-Union Symp. Propagation of Laser Radiation in the Atmosphere* [in Russian], Inst. Opt. Atm. Sib. Otd. Akad. Nauk SSSR, Tomsk (1975), p. 19.
46. M. V. Kabanov, A. A. Pershin, Yu. A. Pkhalagov, and V. N. Uzhegov, in *Problems of Remote Sensing of the Atmosphere* [in Russian], Inst. Opt. Atm. Sib. Otd. Akad. Nauk SSSR, Tomsk (1975), p. 189.
47. S. D. Andreev, V. E. Zuev, L. S. Ivlev, M. V. Kabanov, and Yu. A. Pkhalagov, *Izv. Akad. Nauk SSSR, Fiz. Atm. Okeana*, 8:2161 (1972).
48. V. E. Zuev, L. A. Ivlev, and K. Ya. Kondrat'ev, *Izv. Akad. Nauk SSSR, Fiz. Atm. Okeana*, 9:371 (1973).
49. M. V. Kabanov, in *Actinometry and Optics of the Atmosphere* [in Russian], Nauka, Moscow (1964), p. 85.
50. M. V. Kabanov and Yu. A. Pkhalagov, in *Light Scattering in the Earth's Atmosphere* [in Russian], Inst. Fiz. Nauk, Akad. Nauk K. SSR, Alma-Ata, p.177 (1972).
51. R. W. Wilson and A. A. Penzias, *Nature*, 211:1081 (1966).
52. J. Rössler, *Meteorol. Rundschau*, 21:26 (1968).
53. T. S. Chu and D. C. Hogg, *Bell Syst. Tech. J.*, 47:723 (1968).
54. A. V. Sokolov, *Radiotekh. Elektron.*, 15:2463 (1970).
55. M. V. Kabanov and Yu. A. Pkhalagov, *Izv. Akad. Nauk SSSR, Fiz. Atm. Okeana*, 6:213 (1970).
56. V. V. Sobolev, *Radiative Energy Transfer in the Atmospheres of Stars and Planets* [in Russian], Gostekhizdat, Moscow (1956).
57. M. V. Kabanov, *Izv. Vyssh. Uchebn. Zaved., Fiz.*, No. 8, p. 26 (1967).
58. G. I. Marchuk and G. A. Mikhailov, *Izv. Akad. Nauk SSSR, Fiz. Atm. Okeana*, 3:258 (1967).
59. G. N. Glazov and G. A. Titov, *Izv. Vyssh. Uchebn. Zaved., Fiz.*, No. 9, p. 103 (1977).
60. V. V. Belov, G. M. Krekov, and G. A. Titov, in *Problems of Remote Probing of the Atmosphere* [in Russian], Inst. Opt. Atm. Sib. Otd. Akad. Nauk SSSR, Tomsk (1975), p. 103.
61. V. V. Belov and G. M. Krekov, *Izv. Vyssh. Uchebn. Zaved., Fiz.*, No. 11, p. 129 (1976).
62. G. M. Krekov and G. A. Titov, *Izv. Vyssh. Uchebn. Zaved., Radiofiz.*, 17:1678 (1974).
63. G. M. Krekov, *Izv. Vyssh. Uchebn. Zaved., Fiz.*, No. 6, p. 28 (1969).
64. G. M. Krekov, *Izv. Vyssh. Uchebn. Zaved., Fiz.*, No. 6, p. 74 (1969).
65. G. I. Marchuk, G. A. Mikhailov, M. A. Nazaraliev, *et al.*, *The Monte Carlo Method in Atmospheric Optics* [in Russian], Nauka, Novosibirsk (1976).
66. B. A. Kargin and G. A. Mikhailov, *Zh. Vychisl. Mat. Mat. Fiz.*, 12:150 (1972).
67. G. A. Mikhailov, *Zh. Vychisl. Mat. Mat. Fiz.*, 13:574 (1973).
68. A. A. Gershun, *Selected Works on Photometry and Optical Engineering* [in Russian], Fizmatgiz, Moscow (1958).
69. R. B. Penndorf, *J. Opt. Soc. Am.*, 52:797 (1962).

70. A. P. Ivanov and A. Ya. Khairullina, *Izv. Akad. Nauk SSSR, Fiz. Atm. Okeana*, 2:721 (1966).
71. A. Ya. Khairullina and A. P. Ivanov, *Zh. Prikl. Spektrosk.*, 7:255 (1967).
72. G. D. Gilbert and J. C. Pernicka, *Appl. Opt.*, 6:741 (1967).
73. M. V. Kabanov, B. A. Savel'ev, and I. V. Samokhvalov, *Izv. Akad. Nauk SSSR, Fiz. Atm. Okeana*, 4:1116 (1968).
74. V. A. Donchenko, I. V. Samokhvalov, and G. G. Matvienko, *Izv. Akad. Nauk SSSR, Fiz. Atm. Okeana*, 7:1183 (1971).
75. P. Ya. Ganich and A. P. Ivanov, *Zh. Prikl. Spektrosk.*, 12:280 (1970).
76. I. N. Minin, *Theoretical and Applied Light-Scattering Problems* [in Russian], Nauka i Tekhnika, Minsk (1971).
77. L. M. Romanova, *Theoretical and Applied Light-Scattering Problems* [in Russian], Nauka i Tekhnika, Minsk (1971).
78. A. P. Ivanov, *Optics of Scattering Media* [in Russian], Nauka i Tekhnika, Minsk (1969).
79. J. R. Kerr, P. J. Titterton, and C. M. Brown, *Appl. Opt.*, 8:2233 (1969).
80. G. M. Krekov, *Izv. Vyssh. Uchebn. Zaved., Fiz.*, 6:68 (1969).
81. I. L. Katsev and A. P. Ivanov, *Izv. Akad. Nauk B. SSR, Ser. Fiz.-Mat. Nauk*, No. 4, p. 102 (1968).
82. A. L. Skrelin, A. P. Ivanov, and I. I. Kalinin, *Izv. Akad. Nauk SSSR, Fiz. Atm. Okeana*, 6:889 (1970).
83. R. T. Brown, Jr., in *Proc. Twelfth Conf. Radar Meteorology, Norman, OK* (1966), p. 105.
84. R. T. Brown, Jr., in *Proc. Thirteenth Conf. Radar Meteorology, Montreal, 1968*, Am. Meteorol. Soc., Boston (1968), p. 524.
85. A. P. Ivanov, I. I. Kalinin, V. D. Kozlov, A. L. Skrelin, and I. D. Sherbakh, *Izv. Akad. Nauk SSSR, Fiz. Atm. Okeana*, 5:212 (1969).
86. M. V. Kabanov and I. V. Samokhvalov, *Izv. Vyssh. Uchebn. Zaved., Fiz.*, No. 3, p. 80 (1969).
87. G. M. Krekov, M. M. Krekova, and I. V. Samokhvalov, *Izv. Vyssh. Uchebn. Aved., Fiz.*, No. 5, p. 150 (1969).
88. V. E. Zuev, G. M. Krekov, and A. I. Popkov, *Izv. Vyssh. Uchebn. Zaved., Fiz.*, No. 2, p. 50 (1973).
89. V. E. Zuev, G. M. Krekov, and A. I. Popkov, *Izv. Vyssh. Uchebn. Zaved., Fiz.*, No. 10, p. 126 (1973).
90. D. Deirmendjian, *Electromagnetic Scattering on Spherical Polydispersions*, Am. Elsevier, New York (1969).
91. L. W. Carrier, G. A. Cato, and K. J. von Essen, *Appl. Opt.*, 6:1209 (1967).
92. V. A. Donchenko and I. V. Samokhvalov, *Izv. Vyssh. Uchebn. Zaved., Fiz.*, No. 10, p. 150 (1971).
93. V. A. Donchenko, M. V. Kabanov, G. G. Matvienko, and I. V. Samokhvalov, *Izv. Vyssh. Uchebn. Zaved., Fiz.*, No. 11, p. 61 (1973).
94. E. A. Bucher and R. M. Lerner, *Appl. Opt.*, 12:2401 (1973).
95. V. A. Donchenko, M. V. Kabanov, and I. V. Samokhvalov, *Izv. Vyssh. Uchebn. Zaved., Fiz.*, No. 4, p. 95 (1974).
96. A. P. Ivanov, *Physical Fundamentals of Fluid Optics* [in Russian], Nauka i Tekhnika, Minsk (1975).
97. O. D. Barteneva, E. N. Dovgyalo, and E. A. Polyakova, *Tr. Gl. Geofiz. Obs.*, No. 220 (1967).
98. B. N. Denchik, M. V. Kabanov, B. A. Savel'ev, and B. V. Goryachev, *Izv. Vyssh. Uchebn. Zaved., Fiz.*, No. 1, p. 144 (1971).
99. B. V. Goryachev, B. N. Denchik, and B. A. Savel'ev, *Izv. Vyssh. Uchebn. Zaved., Fiz.*, No. 2, p. 116 (1973).

100. M. V. Kabanov, Yu. A. Pkhalagov, and V. E. Gologuzov, *Izv. Akad. Nauk SSSR, Fiz. Atm. Okeana*, 7:804 (1971).
101. M. V. Kabanov, Yu. A. Pkhalagov, and N. M. Ontikova, in *Proc. Tenth All-Union Conf. Radio-Wave Propagation* [in Russian], Sec. 4, Nauka, Moscow (1972), p. 165.
102. A. S. Gurvich and V. V. Pokasov, *Izv. Akad. Nauk SSSR, Fiz. Atm. Okeana*, 8:878 (1972).
103. K. S. Shifrin, B. Z. Moroz, and A. N. Sakharov, *Dokl. Akad. Nauk SSSR*, 199:589 (1971).
104. E. L. O'Neill, *Introduction to Statistical Optics*, Addison-Wesley, Reading, MA (1963).
105. M. V. Kabanov and V. A. Krutikov, *Izv. Vyssh. Uchebn. Zaved., Fiz.*, No. 3, p. 37 (1974).
106. J. W. Goodman, *Introduction to Fourier Optics*, McGraw-Hill, New York (1968).
107. M. M. Savelli and J. G. Solera, *C. R. Acad. Sci.*, 244:2020 (1957).
108. V. E. Zuev, *Transmittance of the Atmosphere for Visible and Infrared Rays in the Atmosphere* [in Russian], Sov. Radio, Moscow (1966).
109. K. Ya. Kondrat'ev, O. B. Vasil'ev, L. S. Ivlev, *et al.*, *Influence of Aerosol on Radiative Transfer: Possible Climatic Aftereffects* [in Russian], Leningr. Univ., Leningrad (1973).
110. V. E. Zuev, V. F. Belov, and G. M. Krekov, *Physics of the Mesosphere and Mesospheric Clouds* [in Russian], Nauka, Moscow (1975), p. 69.
111. L. Elterman, *UV, Visible, and IR Attenuation for Altitudes to 50 km*, Rep. AFCRL-68-0153, ERP No. 285, Bedford, MA (1968).
112. J. S. Curcio, G. L. Knestrick, and T. H. Cosden, *Atmospheric Scattering in the Visible and Infrared*, Rep. 5567, Washington, DC (1961).
113. R. A. McClatchey, R. W. Fenn, J. E. A. Selby, E. E. Volz, and J. S. Garing, *Optical Properties of the Atmosphere* (3rd ed.), *Environ. Res. Pap.* No. 411 AFCRL, Bedford, MA (1972).
114. V. E. Zuev, L. S. Ivlev, G. M. Krekov, and R. F. Rakhimov, *Izv. Vyssh. Uchebn. Zaved., Fiz.*, No. 11, p. 128 (1974).
115. V. E. Zuev and M. V. Kabanov, *Transfer of Optical Signals in the Earth's Atmosphere* (under Interference Conditions) [in Russian], Sov. Radio, Moscow (1977).

# Chapter 4

1. V. E. Zuev, *Propagation of Visible-Light and Infrared Waves in the Atmosphere* [in Russian], Sov. Radio, Moscow (1970).
2. V. I. Klyatskin and V. I. Tatarskii, *Izv. Vyssh. Uchebn. Zaved., Radiofiz.*, 15:1433 (1972).
3. A. M. Prokhorov, F. V. Bunkin, K. S. Gochelashvili, and V. I. Shishov, *Usp. Fiz. Nauk*, 114:415 (1974).
4. A. S. Gurvich, A. I. Kon, V. L. Mironov, and S. S. Khmelevtsov, *Laser Radiation in a Turbulent Atmosphere* [in Russian], Nauka, Moscow (1976).
5. A. N. Kolmogorov, *Dokl. Akad. Nauk SSSR*, 30:299 (1941).
6. A. M. Obukhov, *Izv. Akad. Nauk SSSR, Ser. Geogr. Geofiz.*, 13:58 (1949).
7. M. A. Kallistratova and D. F. Timanovskii, *Izv. Akad. Nauk SSSR, Fiz. Atm. Okeana*, 7:73 (1971).
8. A. S. Gurvich, B. M. Koprov, L. R. Tsvang, and A. M. Yaglom, *Atmospheric Turbulence and Propagation of Radio Waves* [in Russian], Nauka, Moscow (1967).
9. Yu. A. Volkov, V. P. Kukharets, and L. R. Tsvang, *Izv. Akad. Nauk SSSR, Fiz. Atm. Okeana*, 4:1026 (1968).
10. F. Ya. Voit, E. E. Kornienko, V. P. Kukharets, S. B. Khusid, and L. R. Tsvang, *Izv. Akad. Nauk SSSR, Fiz. Atm. Okeana*, 9:451 (1973).

11. N. L. Byzova and É. E. Vyal'tseva, *Izv. Akad. Nauk SSSR, Fiz. Atm. Okeana*, 6:1209 (1970).

12. Yu. N. Barabanenkov, Yu. A. Kravtsov, S. M. Rytov, and V. I. Tatarskii, *Usp. Fiz. Nauk*, 102:3 (1970).

13. F. V. Bunkin and K. S. Gochelashvili, *Izv. Vyssh. Uchebn. Zaved., Radiofiz.*, 13:1039 (1970).

14. V. I. Tatarskii, *Propagation of Short Waves in a Medium Containing Random Inhomogeneities in the Approximation of a Markov Stochastic Process*, Preprint [in Russian], Otd. Okeanol. Fiz. Atm. Geogr. Akad. Nauk SSSR, Moscow (1970).

15. W. P. Brown, *J. Opt. Soc. Am.*, 61(8):1051 (1971).

16. A. I. Kon, V. L. Mironov, and V. V. Nosov, *Izv. Vyssh. Uchebn. Zaved., Radiofiz.*, 17:1501 (1974).

17. A. L. Buck, *Appl. Opt.*, 6(4):706 (1967).

18. M. A. Kallistratova and V. V. Pokasov, *Izv. Vyssh. Uchebn. Zaved., Radiofiz.*, 14:1200 (1971).

19. V. Ya. S"edin and S. S. Khmelevtsov, *Izv. Vyssh. Uchebn. Zaved., Fiz.*, No. 3, p. 91 (1972).

20. M. A. Kallistratova and A. I. Kon, *Izv. Vyssh. Uchebn. Zaved., Radiofiz.*, 15:545 (1972).

21. I. A. Starobinets, *Izv. Vyssh. Uchebn. Zaved., Radiofiz.*, 15:738 (1972).

22. V. L. Mironov and S. S. Khmelevtsov, *Izv. Vyssh. Uchebn. Zaved., Radiofiz.*, 15:743 (1972).

23. A. I. Kon, V. L. Mironov, and V. E. Tseitlin, *Izv. Vyssh. Uchebn. Zaved., Fiz.*, No. 11, p. 149 (1973).

24. V. A. Banakh, V. L. Mironov, and T. V. Myshkina, *Izv. Akad. Nauk SSSR, Fiz. Atm. Okeana*, 9:539 (1973).

25. A. I. Kon and V. I. Tatarskii, *Izv. Vyssh. Uchebn. Zaved., Radiofiz.*, 15:1547 (1972).

26. M. Born and E. Wolf, *Principles of Optics* (2nd ed.), Pergamon, New York (1964).

27. A. V. Artem'ev and A. S. Gurvich, *Izv. Vyssh. Uchebn. Zaved., Radiofiz.*, 14:734 (1971).

28. H. T. Yura, *Appl. Opt.*, 11(6):1399 (1972).

29. V. A. Banakh, G. M. Krekov, and V. L. Mironov, in *Abstr. Tenth All-Union Conf. Radio-Wave Propagation* [in Russian], Sec. 4, Nauka, Moscow (1972), p. 191.

30. R. L. Fante, *Proc. IEEE*, 62(11):1604 (1974).

31. M. S. Belen'kii and V. L. Mironov, in *Abstr. Third All-Union Symp. Propagation of Laser Radiation in the Atmosphere* [in Russian], Tomsk (1975), p. 202.

32. M. S. Belen'kii, A. I. Kon, and V. L. Mironov, *Kvantovaya Élektron.* (Moscow), 4:517 (1977).

33. M. S. Belen'kii, V. V. Boronoev, N. Ts. Gomboev, and V. L. Mironov, in *Abstr. Fourth All-Union Symp. Propagation of Laser Radiation in the Atmosphere* [in Russian], Tomsk (1977), p. 42.

34. V. I. Tatarskii, *Wave Propagation in a Turbulent Atmosphere* [in Russian], Nauka, Moscow (1967).

35. A. I. Kon, *Izv. Vyssh. Uchebn. Zaved., Radiofiz.*, 13:61 (1970).

36. V. I. Klyatskin and A. I. Kon, *Izv. Vyssh. Uchebn. Zaved., Radiofiz.*, 15:1381 (1972).

37. A. I. Kon, *Izv. Vyssh. Uchebn. Zaved., Radiofiz.*, 15:533 (1972).

38. É. I. Gel'fer, A. I. Kon, and A. M. Cheremukhin, *Izv. Vyssh. Uchebn. Zaved., Radiofiz.*, 16:245 (1973).

39. V. L. Mironov and V. V. Nosov, *Izv. Vyssh. Uchebn. Zaved., Radiofiz.*, 17:247 (1974).

40. V. L. Mironov and V. V. Nosov, *Izv. Vyssh. Uchebn. Zaved., Radiofiz.*, 18:990 (1975).

41. R. L. Cook, *J. Opt. Soc. Am.*, 65(8):942 (1975).

42. A. I. Kon, V. L. Mironov, and V. V. Nosov, *Izv. Vyssh. Uchebn. Zaved., Radiofiz.*, 19:1015 (1976).

43. V. L. Mironov and V. V. Nosov, *J. Opt. Soc. Am.*, 67(8):1073 (1977).

44. V. A. Banakh and V. L. Mironov, *Opt. Lett.*, 1(5):172 (1977).

45 M. A. Kallistratova and V. V. Pokasov, *Izv. Vyssh. Uchebn. Zaved., Radiofiz.*, 14:1200 (1971).

46. É. I. Gel'fer, N. I. Murav'ev, S. E. Finkel'shtein, and A. M. Cheremukhin, *Izv. Vyssh. Uchebn. Zaved., Radiofiz.*, ., 14:1838 (1971).

47. M. A. Kallistratova and V. V. Pokasov, *Izv. Vyssh. Uchebn. Zaved., Radiofiz.*, 15:723 (1972).

48. A. C. Drofa, in *Abstr. Fourth All-Union Symp. Propagation of Laser Radiation in the Atmosphere* [in Russian], Tomsk (1977), p. 45.

49. L. A. Chernov, *Waves in Randomly Inhomogeneous Media* [in Russian], Nauka, Moscow (1975).

50. E. Brookner, *IEEE Trans. Commun.* COM-18(4):396 (1970).

51. R. S. Lawrence and J. W. Strohbehn, *Proc. IEEE*, 58(10):1523 (1970).

52. V. I. Shishov, *Tr. Fiz. Inst. Akad. Nauk SSSR*, 38:171 (1967).

53. V. I. Tatarskii, *Zh. Éksp. Teor. Fiz.*, 56:2106 (1969).

54. L. A. Chernov, *Akust. Zh.*, 15:559 (1969).

55. V. I. Klyatskin and V. I. Tatarskii, *Izv. Vyssh. Uchebn. Zaved., Radiofiz.*, 13:1061 (1970).

56. J. E. Molyneux, *J. Opt. Soc. Am.*, 61(2):248 (1971).

57. V. I. Klyatskin, *Statistical Description of Dynamic Systems with Fluctuating Parameters* [in Russian], Nauka, Moscow (1975).

58. V. I. Shishov, *Izv. Vyssh. Uchebn. Zaved., Radiofiz.*, 14:85 (1971).

59. V. I. Shishov, *Zh. Éksp. Teor. Fiz.*, 61:1397 (1971).

60. V. I. Shishov, *Izv. Vyssh. Uchebn. Zaved., Radiofiz.*, 15:904 (1972).

61. K. S. Gochelashvili [Gochelashvily] and V. I. Shishov, *Opt. Acta*, 18(4):313 (1971).

62. K. S. Gochelashvili [Gochelashvily] and V. I. Shishov, *Opt. Acta*, 18(10):767 (1971).

63. K. S. Gochelashvili and V. I. Shishov, in *Abstr. Second All-Union Symp. Propagation of Laser Radiation in the Atmosphere* [in Russian], Tomsk (1973), p. 216.

64. K. S. Gochelashvili and V. I. Shishov, *Zh. Éksp. Teor. Fiz.*, 66:1237 (1974).

65. K. S. Gochelashvili, V. G. Pevgov, and V. I. Shishov, *Kvantovaya Élektron.* (Moscow), 1:1156 (1974).

66. K. S. Gochelashvili, *Izv. Vyssh. Uchebn. Zaved., Radiofiz.*, 14:592 (1971).

67. K. S. Gochelashvili [Gochelashvily], *Opt. Acta*, 20(3):193 (1973).

68. K. S. Gochelashvili, *Kvantovaya Élektron.* (Moscow), 1:848 (1974).

69. R. L. Fante, *Radio Sci.*, 10(1):77 (1975).

70. R. L. Fante, *J. Opt. Soc. Am.*, 65(5):548 (1975).

71. R. L. Fante, *IEEE Trans. Antennas Propag.*, AP-23(3):382 (1975).

72. R. L. Fante, *Proc. IEEE*, 63(12):1669 (1975).

73. I. G. Yakushkin, *Izv. Vyssh. Uchebn. Zaved., Radiofiz.*, 18:1660 (1975).

74. V. I. Zavorotnyi, V. I. Klyatskin, and V. I. Tatarskii, *Zh. Éksp. Teor. Fiz.*, 23:481 (1977).

75. V. A. Banakh, G. M. Krekov, and V. L. Mironov, *Izv. Vyssh. Uchebn. Zaved., Radiofiz.*, 17:252 (1974).

76. V. A. Banakh, G. M. Krekov, V. L. Mironov, S. S. Khmelevtsov, and R. Sh. Tsvyk [Tsvik], *J. Opt. Soc. Am.*, 64(4):516 (1974).

77. V. A. Banakh, A. F. Zhukov, V. L. Mironov, and R. Sh. Tsvyk, *Izv. Vyssh. Uchebn. Zaved., Fiz.*, No. 2, p. 33 (1975).

78. V. A. Banakh and V. L. Mironov, *Kvantovaya Élektron.* (Moscow), 2:2163 (1975).

79. Z. I. Feizulin and Yu. A. Kravhtsov, *Izv. Vyssh. Uchebn. Zaved., Radiofiz.*, 10:68 (1967).

80. Yu. A. Kravhtsov and Z. I. Feizulin, *Izv. Vyssh. Uchebn. Zaved., Radiofiz.*, 12:886 (1969).

81. I. G. Yakushkin, *Izv. Vyssh. Uchebn. Zaved., Radiofiz.*, 19:384 (1976).

82. G. I. Marchuk, G. A. Mikhailov, M. A. Nazaraliev, R. A. Darbinyan, B. A. Kargin, and B. S. Elepov, *The Monte Carlo Method in Atmospheric Optics* [in Russian], Nauka, Novosibirsk (1976).

83. D. J. Fried and J. B. Seidman, *J. Opt. Soc. Am.*, 57(2):181 (1967).

84. S. S. Khmelevtsov and R. Sh. Tsvyk, *Izv. Vyssh. Uchebn. Zaved., Radiofiz.*, 13:146 (1970).

85. M. E. Gracheva, A. S. Gurvich, and M. A. Kallistratova, *Radiotekh. Élektron.*, 15:1290 (1970).

86. V. A. Banakh and V. L. Mironov, *Kvantovaya Élektron.* (Moscow), 5:1535 (1978).

87. M. E. Gracheva, A. S. Gurvich, S. S. Kashkarov, and Vl. V. Pokasov, Preprint [in Russian], Otd. Okeanol. Fiz. Atm. Geogr. Akad. Nauk SSSR (1973).

88. M. E. Gracheva, A. S. Gurvich, and Vl. V. Pokasov, *Zh. Éksp. Teor. Fiz.*, 67:2035 (1974).

89. A. S. Gurvich and V. I. Tatarskii, *Radio Sci.*, 10(1):3 (1975).

90. A. S. Gurvich and S. S. Kashkarov, *Izv. Vyssh. Uchebn. Zaved., Radiofiz.*, 18:69 (1975).

91. V. A. Banakh, V. V. Boronoev, Ch. Ts. Gomboev, É. V. Zubritskii, V. L. Mironov, and Ch. Ts. Tsydypov, in *Abstr. Fourth All-Union Symp. Laser Probing of the Atmosphere* [in Russian], Tomsk (1976), p. 337.

92. V. L. Mironov and G. Ya. Patrushev, *Izv. Vussh. Uchebn. Zaved., Radiofiz.*, 15:865 (1972).

93. V. L. Mironov, G. Ya. Patrushev, and L. I. Shchavlev, in *Abstr. Second All-Union Symp. Propagation of Laser Radiation in the Atmosphere* [in Russian], Tomsk (1973), p. 242.

94. V. L. Mironov and G. Ya. Patrushev, *Izv. Vyssh. Uchebn. Zaved., Radiofiz.*, 18:450 (1975).

95. A. F. Zhukov, A. V. Efremov, S. S. Khmelevtsov, and R. Sh. Tsvyk, *Izv. Vyssh. Uchebn. Zaved., Fiz.*, No. 11, p. 122 (1975).

96. V. Ya. S"edin, S. S. Khmelevtsov, and R. Sh. Tsvyk, *Izv. Vyssh. Uchebn. Zaved., Radiofiz.*, 15:798 (1972).

97. A. S. Gurvich and I. A. Starobinets, *Izv. Vyssh. Uchebn. Zaved., Radiofiz.*, 14:1834 (1971).

98. J. R. Kerr and J. R. Dunphy, *J. Opt. Soc. Am.*, 63(1):1 (1973).

99. É.I. Gel'fer, M. M. Knyazev, T. A. Postnikova, and A. M. Cheremykhin, *Izv. Vyssh. Uchebn. Zaved., Radiofiz.*, 17:710 (1974).

100. M. S. Belen'kii and V. L. Mironov, *Izv. Vyssh. Uchebn. Zaved., Radiofiz.*, 17:1050 (1974).

101. N. Ts. Gomboev, É. V. Zubritskii, G. F. Malygina, V. L. Mironov, and S. S. Khmelevtsov, *Kvantovaya Élektron.* (Moscow), 2:1262 (1975).

102. A. Ishimaru, *Proc. IEEE*, 57(4):407 (1969).

103. A. S. Gurvich and N. S. Time, *Radiotekh. Élektron.*, 15:812 (1970).

104. N. S. Time, *Izv. Vyssh. Uchebn. Zaved., Radiofiz.*, 14:1195 (1971).

105. V. L. Mironov and L. I. Shchavlev, *Radiotekh. Élektron.*, 20:413 (1975).

106. A. G. Vinogradov and Yu. A. Kravtsov, in *Summar. Sixth All-Union Symp. Wave Diffraction and Propagation* [in Russian], Vol. 1, Moscow (1973), p. 294.

107. M. S. Belen'kii and V. L. Mironov, *Kvantovaya Élektron.* (Moscow), 1:2253 (1974).

108. V. P. Aksenov, V. A. Banakh, and V. L. Mironov, *Kvantovaya Élektron.* (Moscow), 3:2297 (1976).

109. M. H. Lee, J. F. Holmes, and J. R. Kerr, *J. Opt. Soc. Am.*, 66(11):1164 (1976).

110. M. S. Belen'kii and V. L. Mironov, in *Abstr. Fourth All-Union Symp. Propagation of Laser Radiation in the Atmosphere* [in Russian], Tomsk (1977), p. 149.

111. V. P. Aksenov, V. A. Banakh, and V. L. Mironov, in *Abstr. Fourth All-Union Symp. Propagation of Laser Radiation in the Atmosphere* [in Russian], Tomsk (1977), p. 154.

112. A. S. Gurvich, M. A. Kallistratova, and N. S. Time, *Izv. Vyssh. Uchebn. Zaved., Radiofiz.*, 11:1360 (1968).

113. G. R. Ochs and R. S. Lawrence, *J. Opt. Soc. Am.*, 59(2):226 (1969).

114. M. W. Fitzmaurice, J. L. Bufton, and P. O. Minott, *J. Opt. Soc. Am.*, 59(1):7 (1969).

115. P. H. Deitz and N. J. Wright, *J. Opt. Soc. Am.*, 59(5):527 (1969).

116. M. E. Gracheva, A. S. Gurvich, and M. A. Kallistratova, *Izv. Vyssh. Uchebn. Zaved., Radiofiz.*, 13:56 (1970).

117. R. H. Kleen and G. R. Ochs, *J. Opt. Soc. Am.*, 60(12):1695 (1970).

118. V. Ya. S"edin, S. S. Khmelevtsov, and M. F. Nebol'sin, *Izv. Vyssh. Uchebn. Zaved., Radiofiz.*, 13:44 (1970).
119. M. I. Mordukhovich, *Izv. Vyssh. Uchebn. Zaved., Radiofiz.*, 13:275 (1970).
120. J. R. Kerr, *J. Opt. Soc. Am.*, 62(9):1040 (1972).
121. S. S. Khmelevtsov and R. Sh. Tsvyk, *Izv. Vyssh. Uchebn. Zaved., Fiz.*, No. 6, p. 130 (1973).
122. S. S. Khmelevtsov, *Appl. Opt.*, 12(10):2421 (1973).
123. S. S. Khmelevtsov and R. Sh. Tsvyk, *Izv. Vyssh. Uchebn. Zaved., Fiz.*, No. 9, p. 108 (1973).
124. H. Raidt and D. H. Höhn, *Appl Opt.*, 12(1):103 (1973).
125. G. R. Ochs, R. R. Bergman, and J. R. Snyder, *J. Opt. Soc. Am.*, 59(2):231 (1969).
126. G. A. Andreev, É.I. Gel'fer, V. A. Zverev, and V. A. Tseitlin, *Izv. Vyssh. Uchebn. Zaved., Radiofiz.*, 14:276 (1971).
127. M. E. Gracheva, A. S. Gurvich, and A. S. Khrupin, *Izv. Vyssh. Uchebn. Zaved., Radiofiz.*, 17:155 (1974).
128. N. N. D'yachenko, V. Ya. S"edin, and S. S. Khmelevtsov, *Izv. Vyssh. Uchebn. Zaved., Fiz.*, No. 7, p. 132 (1974).
129. M. S. Belen'kii, A. F. Zhukov, V. L. Mironov, S. S. Khmelevtsov, and R. Sh. Tsvyk, in *Propagation of Optical Waves in the Atmosphere* [in Russian], Nauka, Novosibirsk (1975), p. 72.
130. N. S. Time, *Izv. Akad. Nauk SSSR, Fiz. Atm. Okeana*, 8:90 (1972).
131. A. S. Gurvich and Vl. V. Pokasov, *Izv. Vyssh. Uchebn. Zaved., Radiofiz.*, 16:913 (1973).
132. A. S. Gurvich, R. A. Kazaryan, K. P. Pogosyan, and V. V. Pokasov, *Izv. Vyssh. Uchebn. Zaved., Radiofiz.*, 18:610 (1975).
133. I. G. Yakushkin, in *Summar. Seventh All-Union Symp. Wave Diffraction and Propagation* [in Russian], Vol. 1 (1977), p. 326.
134. M. E. Gracheva, A. S. Gurvich, S. O. Lomadze, V. V. Pokasov, and A. S. Khrupin, *Izv. Vyssh. Uchebn. Zaved., Radiofiz.*, 17:105 (1974).
135. D. H. Höhn, *Appl. Opt.*, 5(9):1427 (1966).
136. P. O. Minott, *J. Opt. Soc. Am.*, 62(7):885 (1972).
137. D. S. Fried, G. E. Mevers, and M. P. Keister, *J. Opt. Soc. Am.*, 57(6):787 (1967).
138. R. A. Kazaryan, R. G. Manucharyan, and S. S. Gasparyan, *Experimental Studies of Intensity Fluctuations of Laser Radiation in the Atmosphere and Their Averaging by the Receiving Aperture*, Preprint 72-06 [in Russian], Inst. Fiz. Issled., Akad. Nauk Arm. SSR, Erevan (1972).
139. F. V. Bunkin and K. S. Gochelashvili, *Izv. Vyssh. Uchebn. Zaved., Radiofiz.*, 11:1864 (1968).
140. F. V. Bunkin and K. S. Gochelashvili, *Izv. Vyssh. Uchebn. Zaved., Radiofiz.*, 12:875 (1969).
141. Yu. I. Khramtsov, *Izv. Vyssh. Uchebn. Zaved., Radiofiz.*, 17:1175 (1974).
142. Yu. I. Khramtsov, *Izv. Vyssh. Uchebn. Zaved., Radiofiz.*, 18:453 (1975).
143. V. P. Aksenov, K. S. Gochelashvili [Gochelashvily], and V. I. Shishov, *Appl. Opt.*, 15(5):1172 (1976).
144. É. I. Gel'fer, A. S. Gurvich, and A. M. Cheremukhin, *Izv. Vyssh. Uchebn. Zaved., Radiofiz.*, 14:1208 (1971).
145. A. I. Kon, *Izv. Vyssh. Uchebn. Zaved., Radiofiz.*, 12:149 (1969).
146. V. L. Mironov and Yu. A. Pkhalagov, *Izv. Vyssh. Uchebn. Zaved., Fiz.*, No. 1, p. 145 (1972).
147. S. S. Khmelevtsov and R. Sh. Tsvyk, *Izv. Vyssh. Uchebn. Zaved., Fiz.*, No. 2, p. 52 (1970).
148. N. Ts. Gomboev, É. V. Zubritskii, V. V. Boronoev, S. S. Khmelevtsov, and R. Sh. Tsvyk, in *Abstr. Tenth All-Union Conf. Radio-Wave Propagation* [in Russian], Sec. 4, Nauka, Moscow (1972), p. 216.

149. É. S. Vartanyan, S. E. Voskanyan, R. A. Kazaryan, and R. G. Manucharyan, *Dokl. Akad. Nauk Arm. SSR. Fizika.* 1:86 (1970).

150. A. I. Kon and V. I. Tatarskii, *Izv. Vyssh. Uchebn. Zaved., Radiofiz.,* 8:870 (1965).

151. R. A. Schmeltzer, *Q. Appl. Math.,* 24(4):339 (1967).

152. A. Ishimaru, *Radio Sci.,* 4(4):295 (1969).

153. V. P. Lukin, V. V. Pokasov, and S. S. Khmelevtsov, in *Proceedings of the Commemorative Conference of the Radiophysics Faculty of Tomsk State University* [in Russian], Tomsk. Univ. (1973).

154. R. F. Lutomirski and H. T. Yura, *J. Opt. Soc. Am.,* 61(4):482 (1971).

155. A. Consortini and L. Rouchi, *Lett. Nuovo Cimento,* 3(13):571 (1972).

156. V. P. Lukin, V. L. Mironov, V. V. Pokasov, and S. S. Khmelevtsov, *Radiotekh. Elektron.,* 20:1064 (1975).

157. V. V. Pokasov and S. S. Khmelevtsov, *Izv. Vyssh. Uchebn. Zaved., Fiz.,* No. 5, p. 82 (1968).

158. M. Bertolotti, M. Carnevale, L. Muzii, and D. Sette, *Appl. Opt.,* 7(11):2246 (1968).

159. T. I. Arsen'yan, F. F. Pashkov, A. A. Semenov, A. A. Tishchenko, and N. I. Rimskii, *Izv. Vyssh. Uchebn. Zaved., Radiofiz.,* 15:1228 (1972).

160. R. Buser and J. J. Kainz, *Appl. Opt.,* 8(12):1495 (1969).

161. V. P. Lukin, V. V. Pokasov, and S. S. Khmelevtsov, *Izv. Vyssh. Uchebn. Zaved., Radiofiz.,* 15:1861 (1972).

162. S. F. Clifford, J. M. B. Bouricius, and J. R. Ochs, *J. Opt. Soc. Am.,* 61(10):1279 (1971).

163. S. Lawrence, *Appl. Opt.,* 14(11):2750 (1975).

164. V. P. Lukin, *Kvantovaya Elektron.* (Moscow), 4:923 (1977).

165. R. L. Fante, *J. Opt. Soc. Am.,* 66(7):730 (1976).

166. V. P. Lukin and I. P. Lukin, *Kvantovaya Élektron.* (Kiev) 14:116 (1977).

167. V. P. Lukin, *Kvantovaya Élektron.* (Moscow), 5:1124 (1978).

168. J. E. Pearson, *Appl. Opt.,* 15(5):622 (1976).

169. W. B. Bridges, P. J. Brunner, S. P. Lazzara, T. A. Nussmeier, T. R. O'Meara, J. A. Sanguinet, and W. P. Brown, *Appl Opt.,* 13(2):291 (1974).

170. D. P. Greenwood and D. L. Fried, *J. Opt. Soc. Am.,* 66(3):193 (1976).

171. J. E. Pearson and S. Hansen, *J. Opt. Soc. Am.,* 67(3):325 (1977).

172. R. Hudgin, *J. Opt. Soc. Am.,* 67(3):375 (1977).

173. R. F. Lutomirski, W. L. Woodle, and R. G. Buser, *Appl. Opt.,* 16(3):665 (1977).

174. V. Wang and C. R. Giuliano, in *Program 1977 CLEA IEE/OSA Conf. Laser Engineering and Applications,* Washington, D.C. (1977), p. 38.

175. P. A. Bakut, N. D. Ustinov, I. N. Troitskii, and K. I. Sviridov, *Zarubezhn. Radioelektron.,* No. 7, p. 15 (1976); No. 9, p. 3 (1976); No. 1, p. 3 (1977).

176. V. L. Mironov and V. V. Nosov, in *Abstr. Fourth All-Union Symp. Propagation of Laser Radiation in the Atmosphere* (Section on Propagation of Laser Radiation in a Turbulent Atmosphere) [in Russian], Tomsk (1977), p. 61.

177. V. P. Aksenov and V. L. Mironov, in *Abstr. Fourth All-Union Symp. Propagation of Laser Radiation in the Atmosphere* (Section on Propagation of Laser Radiation in a Turbulent Atmosphere) [in Russian], Tomsk (1977), p. 110.

178. A. B. Aleksandrov and V. A. Loginov, in *Abstr. Fourth All-Union Symp. Propagation of Laser Radiation in the Atmosphere* (Section on Propagation of Laser Radiation in a Turbulent Atmosphere) [in Russian], Tomsk (1977), p. 115.

179. G. Ya. Patrushev, in *Abstr. Fourth All-Union Symp. Propagation of Laser Radiation in the Atmosphere* (Section on Propagation of Laser Radiation in a Turbulent Atmosphere) [in Russian], Tomsk (1977), p. 123.

180. S. I. Tuzova, in *Abstr. Fourth All-Union Symp. Propagation of Laser Radiation in the Atmosphere* (Section on Propagation of Laser Radiation in a Turbulent Atmosphere) [in Russian], Tomsk (1977), p. 131.

181. M. S. Belen'kii, A. A. Makarov, V. L. Mironov, and V. V. Pokasov, in *Abstr. Fourth All-Union Symp. Propagation of Laser Radiation in the Atmosphere* (Section on Propagation of Laser Radiation in a Turbulent Atmosphere) [in Russian], Tomsk (1977), p. 136.

182. V. P. Aksenov, N. Ts. Gomboev, É. V. Zubritskii, G. F. Malygina, V. L. Mironov, and É. A. Trubacheev, in *Abstr. Fourth All-Union Symp. Propagation of Laser Radiation in the Atmosphere* (Section on Propagation of Laser Radiation in a Turbulent Atmosphere) [in Russian], Tomsk (1977), p. 139.

183. A. A. Makarov and V. V. Pokasov, in *Abstr. Fourth All-Union Symp. Propagation of Laser Radiation in the Atmosphere* (Section on Propagation of Laser Radiation in a Turbulent Atmosphere) [in Russian], Tomsk (1977), p. 179.

184. M. A. Belov and V. M. Orlov, in *Abstr. Fourth All-Union Symp. Propagation of Laser Radiation in the Atmosphere* (Section on Propagation of Laser Radiation in a Turbulent Atmosphere) [in Russian], Tomsk (1977), p. 118.

185. I. P. Lukin, in *Abstr. Fourth All-Union Symp. Propagation of Laser Radiation in the Atmosphere* (Section on Propagation of Laser Radiation in a Turbulent Atmosphere) [in Russian], Tomsk (1977), p. 214.

## Chapter 5

1. V. E. Zuev, *Propagation of Visible-Light and Infrared Waves in the Atmosphere* [in Russian], Sov. Radio, Moscow (1970).

2. Yu. P. Raizer, *Laser Spark and Propagation of Discharges* [in Russian], Nauka, Moscow (1974).

3. J. F. Ready, *Effects of High-Power Laser Radiation*, Academic Press, New York (1971).

4. Yu. P. Raizer, *Usp. Fiz. Nauk*, 87(1):29 (1965).

5. Yu. P. Raizer, *Usp. Fiz. Nauk*, 108(3):429 (1972).

6. I. P. Shkarofsky, *RCA Rev.*, 35:48 (1974).

7. V. P. Ageev, A. I. Barchukov, F. V. Bunkin, V. I. Konov, S. M. Mitev, A. S. Silenok, and N. I. Chapliev, *Izv. Vyssh. Uchebn. Zaved., Fiz.*, No. 11, p. 34 (1977).

8. I. K. Krasyuk, P. P. Pashinin, and A. M. Prokhorov, *Zh. Éksp. Teor. Fiz.*, 58(5):1606 (1970).

9. A. J. Alcock and M. C. Richardson, *Phys. Rev. Lett.*, 21:667 (1968).

10. F. V. Bunkin and V. V. Savranskii, *Zh. Éksp. Teor. Fiz.*, 65(6):2185 (1973).

11. M. V. Aleshin, S. I. Anisimov, A. M. Bonch-Bruevich, Ya. A. Imas, and V. L. Komolov, *Zh. Éksp. Teor. Fiz.*, 70(4):1214 (1976).

12. F. V. Bunkin, I. K. Krasyuk, V. M. Marchenko, P. P. Pashinin, and A. M. Prokhorov, *Zh. Éksp. Teor. Fiz.*, 60(4):1326 (1971).

13. V. A. Volkov, F. V. Grigor'ev, V. V. Kalinovskii, S. B. Kormer, L. M. Lavrov, Yu. V. Maslov, V. D. Urlin, and V. P. Tsudinov, *Zh. Éksp. Teor. Fiz.*, 69(1):115 (1975).

14. D. E. Lencioni, *Appl. Phys. Lett.*, 23:12 (1973).

15. G. A. Askar'yan, M. S. Rabinovich, M. M. Savchenko, and A. D. Smirnova, *Pis'ma Zh. Éksp. Teor. Fiz.*, 1(1):9 (1965).

16. G. A. Askar'yan, M. S. Rabinovich, A. D. Smirnova, and V. B. Studenov, *Pis'ma Zh. Éksp. Teor. Fiz.*, 2(11):503 (1965).

17. G. A. Askar'yan, M. S. Rabinovich, M. M. Savchenko, and V. K. Stepanov, *Pis'ma Zh. Éksp. Teor. Fiz.*, 3(12):465 (1966).

18. Yu. P. Raizer, *Zh. Éksp. Teor. Fiz.*, 48(5):1508 (1965).

19. R. V. Ambartsumyan, N. G. Basov, V. A. Boiko, V. S. Zuev, O. N. Krokhin, P. G. Kryukov, Yu. V. Senatskii, and Yu. Yu. Stoilov, *Zh. Éksp. Teor. Fiz.*, 48(6):1583 (1965).

20. F. V. Bunkin, V. I. Konov, A. M. Prokhorov, and V. B. Fedorov, *Pis'ma Zh. Éksp. Teor. Fiz.*, 9(11):609 (1969).

21. D. C. Smith and M. C. Fowler, *Appl. Phys. Lett.*, 22:500 (1973).

22. A. I. Barchukov, F. V. Bunkin, V. I. Konov, and A. M. Prokhorov, *Pis'ma Zh. Éksp. Teor. Fiz.*, 17(8):413 (1973).

23. A. I. Burchukov, F. V. Bunkin, V. I. Konov, and A. A. Lyubin, *Zh. Éksp. Teor. Fiz.*, 66:965 (1974).

24. F. V. Bunkin and A. M. Prokhorov, *Usp. Fiz. Nauk*, 119(3):425 (1976).

25. V. P. Ageev, A. I. Barchukov, F. V. Bunkin, V. I. Konov, A. S. Silenok, and N. I. Chapliev, *Kvantovaya Élektron. (Kiev)*, No. 2, p. 310 (1977).

26. L. D. Landau and E. M. Lifshits, *Continuum Electrodynamics* [in Russian], Gostekhizdat, Moscow (1957).

27. P. A. Apanasevich, *Aspects of Nonlinear Spectroscopy* [in Russian], Nauka i Tekhnika, Minsk (1974), p. 301.

28. R. Z. Vitlina and A. V. Chaplik, *Zh. Éksp. Teor. Fiz.*, 70(6):2127 (1976).

29. B. F. Gordiets, A. I. Osipov, E. V. Stupochenko, and L. A. Chelepin, *Usp. Fiz. Nauk*, 108(4):655 (1972).

30. S. G. Rautian, *Tr. Fiz. Inst. Akad. Nauk SSSR*, 43:3 (1968).

31. O. R. Wood, P. L. Gordon, and S. E. Schwarz, *IEEE J. Quantum Electron.*, QE-5:502 (1969).

32. V. S. Letokhov, A. A. Makarov, and E. A. Ryabov, *Dokl. Akad. Nauk SSSR*, 212(1):75 (1973).

33. N. Djeu and G. J. Wolga, *J. Appl. Phys.*, 42:3226 (1971).

34. E. A. Ryabov, *Kvantovaya Élektron. (Moscow)*, 2(1):138 (1975).

35. V. E. Zuev, V. P. Lopasov, and Yu. N. Ponomarev, *Dokl. Akad. Nauk SSSR*, 231(5):1106 (1976).

36. V. E. Zuev, V. P. Lopasov, and Yu. N. Ponomarev, in *Proc. First All-Union Conf. Atmospheric Optics* [in Russian], Part 1, Inst. Opt. Atm., Sib. Otd. Akad. Nauk SSSR, Tomsk (1976), p. 56.

37. A. B. Antipov and Yu. N. Ponomarev, *Kvantovaya Elektron. (Moscow)*, 1(6):1345 (1974).

38. A. M. Bonch-Bruevich and V. A. Khodovoi, *Usp. Fiz. Nauk*, 93(1):71 (1967).

39. A. L. Golger, V. S. Letokhov, and S. P. Fedoseev, *Kvantovaya Élektron. (Moscow)*, 3(7):1457 (1976).

40. V. S. Lisitsa and S. I. Yakovlenko, *Zh. Éksp. Teor. Fiz.*, 68(1):479 (1975).

41. P. A. Apanasevich and A. P. Nizovtsev, *Kvantovaya Élektron. (Moscow)*, 2(8):1654 (1975).

42. P. G. Kryukov and V. S. Letokhov, *Usp. Fiz. Nauk*, 99(2):169 (1969).

43. É. G. Pestov and S. G. Rautian, *Zh. Éksp. Teor. Fiz.*, 64(6):2032 (1973).

44. V. P. Kochanov, S. G. Rautian, and A. M. Shalagin, in *Proc. Eighth All-Union Conf. Nonlinear Optics* [in Russian], Tbilisi (1975), p. 260.

45. E. Wietz and G. Flynn, *Ann. Rev. Phys. Chem.*, 25:275 (1974).

46. A. E. Kaplan, *Zh. Éksp. Teor. Fiz.*, 65:1416 (1973).

47. L. M. Frantz and J. S. Nodvih, *J. Appl. Phys.*, 34:2346 (1963).

48. R. V. Ambartsumyan, N. G. Basov, V. S. Zuev, P. G. Sryukov, and V. S. Letokhov, *IEEE J. Quantum Electron.*, QE-2:436 (1966).

49. R. V. Ambartsumyan, N. G. Basov, V. S. Zuev, G. G. Kryukov, and V. S. Letokhov, in *Nonlinear Optics* [in Russian], Nauka, Novosibirsk (1968).

50. A. C. Selden, *Br. J. Appl. Phys.*, 18:743 (1967).

51. C. K. N. Patel and R. F. Slusher, *Phys. Rev. Lett.*, 19:1019 (1967).

52. V. P. Lopasov, S. Yu. Nechaev, and Yu. N. Ponomarev, in *Proc. Siberian Symp. Laser Spectroscopy* [in Russian], Krasnoyarsk (1973), p. 29.

53. S. Yu. Nechaev and Yu. N. Ponomarev, *Kvantovaya Élektron. (Moscow)*, 2(2):440 (1975).

54. S. A. Akhmanov, V. M. Gordienko, and V. Ya. Panchenko, *Izv. Vyssh. Uchebn. Zaved., Fiz.*, No. 11, p. 14 (1977).

55. R. C. C. Leite, R. S. Moore, and J. R. Whinnery, *Appl. Phys. Lett.*, 5:141 (1964).
56. J. R. Gordon, R. C. C. Leite, R. S. Moore, S. P. S. Porto, and J. R. Whinnery, *J. Appl. Phys.*, 35:3 (1965).
57. K. E. Rieckhoff, *Appl. Phys. Lett.*, 9:87 (1966).
58. S. A. Akhmanov, D. P. Krindach, A. P. Sukhorukov, and R. V. Khokhlov, *Pis'ma Zh. Éksp. Teor. Fiz.*, 6(2):509 (1967).
59. S. A. Akhmanov, D. P. Krindach, A. V. Migulin, and A. P. Sukhorukov, *IEEE J. Quantum Electron.*, QE-4:568 (1968).
60. H. Inaba and H. Ito, *IEEE J. Quantum Electron.*, QE-4:45 (1968).
61. D. S. Smith, *IEEE J. Quantum Electron.*, QE-5:600 (1969).
62. G. A. Askar'yan and V. B. Studenov, *Pis'ma Zh. Éksp. Teor. Fiz.*, 10(3):113 (1969).
63. G. A. Askar'yan, V. G. Mikhalevich, V. B. Studenov, and G. P. Shupilo, *Zh. Éksp. Teor. Fiz.*, 59(6):1917 (1970).
64. S. A. Armand, Preprint No. 14 [in Russian], Inst. Radioelektron. Akad. Nauk SSSR (1973).
65. Yu. P. Raizer, *Zh. Éksp. Teor. Fiz.*, 52(2):470 (1967).
66. P. B. Ulrich and J. Wallace, *J. Opt. Soc. Am.*, 63:8 (1973).
67. P. J. Berger, P. B. Ulrich, J. T. Ulrich, and F. G. Gebhardt, *Appl. Opt.*, 16:345 (1977).
68. V. A. Aleshkevich, S. A. Akhmanov, V. M. Gordienko, A. V. Migulin, A. P. Sukhorukov, and É. N. Shumilov, in *Abstr. Eleventh All-Union Conf. Radio-Wave Propagation* [in Russian], Kazan' (1976), p. 54.
69. J. Wallace and M. Camac, *J. Opt. Soc. Am.*, 60:1587 (1970).
70. L. C. Bradley and J. Herrmann, *J. Opt. Soc. Am.*, 61:668 (1971).
71. J. N. Hayes and P. B. Ulrich, *Appl. Opt.*, 11:257 (1972).
72. P. B. Ulrich, J. N. Hayes, and A. H. Aitken, *J. Opt. Soc. Am.*, 62:298 (1972).
73. V. V. Vorob'ev, Yu. V. Grebenyuk, A. S. Gurvich, and F. É. Martvel', in *Proc. Seventh All-Union Conf. Coherent and Nonlinear Optics* [in Russian], Tashkent (1974), p. 123.
74. V. A. Petrishchev, N. M. Sheropova, and V. E. Yashin, in *Proc. Seventh All-Union Conf. Coherent and Nonlinear Optics* [in Russian], Tashkent (1974), p. 128.
75. V. A. Aleshkevich and A. P. Sukhorukov, *Pis'ma Zh. Éksp. Teor. Fiz.*, 12(2):112 (1970).
76. G. A. Askar'yan and I. L. Chistyi, *Zh. Éksp. Teor. Fiz.*, 58(1):133 (1970).
77. G. A. Askar'yan and V. A. Pogosyan, *Zh. Éksp. Teor. Fiz.*, 60(4):1295 (1971).
78. F. G. Gebhardt and D. C. Smith, *Appl. Phys. Lett.*, 14:52 (1969).
79. D. C. Smith and F. G. Gebhardt, *Appl. Phys. Lett.*, 16:275 (1970).
80. R. J. Hull and P. L. Kelly, *Appl. Phys. Lett.*, 17:539 (1970).
81. F. G. Gebhardt and D. C. Smith, *IEEE J. Quantum Electron.*, QE-7:63 (1971).
82. P. M. Livingston, *Appl. Opt.*, 10:426 (1971).
83. F. G. Gebhardt and D. C. Smith, *Appl. Opt.*, 11:244 (1972).
84. J. N. Hayes, *Appl. Opt.*, 13:2072 (1974).
85. R. T. Brown and D. C. Smith, *Appl. Phys. Lett.*, 25:500 (1974).
86. T. G. Miller, R. G. Polk, F. P. Gibson, and J. Wallace, *J. Opt. Soc. Am.*, 65:1191 (1975).
87. V. V. Vorob'ev, in *Abstr. Third All-Union Symp. Propagation of Laser Radiation in the Atmosphere* [in Russian], Tomsk (1975), p. 80.
88. V. V. Vorob'ev, *Kvantovaya Élektron.* (*Moscow*), 3(3):605 (1976).
89. J. Wallace and J. Parciak, *Appl. Opt.*, 15:218 (1976).
90. J. E. Pearson, C. Jeh, and W. P. Brown, Jr., *J. Opt. Soc. Am.*, 66:1384 (1976).
91. J. A. Fleck and J. R. Morris, *Appl. Phys.*, 10:129 (1976).
92. F. G. Gebhardt, *Appl. Opt.*, 15:1479 (1976).
93. V. V. Vorob'ev, *Izv. Vyssh. Uchebn. Zaved., Fiz.*, No. 11, p. 61 (1977).
94. A. P. Sukhorukov and É. N. Shumilov, in *Abstr. Fourth All-Union Symp. Propagation of Laser Radiation in the Atmosphere* (Nonlinear Effects in the Propagation of Laser Radiation in the Atmosphere) [in Russian], Tomsk (1977), p. 160.

95. Yu. M. Sorokin, in *Abstr. Fourth All-Union Symp. Propagation of Laser Radiation in the Atmosphere* (Absorption and Scattering of Laser Radiation by Gases in Atmospheric Aerosols) [in Russian], Tomsk (1977), p. 79.

96. J. R. Whinnery, *IEEE J. Quantum Electron.*, QE-3:382 (1967).

97. R. A. Chodzko and S. C. Lin, *Appl. Phys. Lett.*, 16:434 (1970).

98. J. R. Kenemuth, C. B. Hogge, and P. V. Avizonis, *Appl. Phys. Lett.*, 17:220 (1970).

99. J. N. Hayes, *Appl. Opt.*, 11:455 (1972).

100. R. W. Buser and R. S. Rohde, *Appl. Opt.*, 12:205 (1973).

101. A. H. Aitken, J. N. Hayes, and P. B. Ulrich, *Appl. Opt.*, 12:193 (1973).

102. A. V. Lykov and B. M. Berkovskii, *Convection and Thermal Waves* [in Russian], Energiya, Moscow (1974).

103. B. P. Gerasimov, V. M. Gordienko, and A. P. Sukhorukov, Preprint No. 59 [in Russian], Inst. Prikl. Mat. Akad. Nauk SSSR, Moscow (1974).

104. B. P. Gerasimov, V. M. Gordienko, and A. P. Sukhorukov, Preprint No. 131 [in Russian], Inst. Prikl. Mat. Akad. Nauk SSSR, Moscow (1974).

105. V. A. Petrishchev, N. M. Sheronova, and V. E. Yashin, *Izv. Vyssh. Uchebn. Zaved., Radiofiz.*, 18(7):963 (1975).

106. V. A. Petryshchev and V. I. Talanov, *Kvantovaya Élektron.* (*Moscow*), No. 6, p. 35 (1971).

107. S. A. Akhmanov, A. P. Sukhorukov, and R. V. Khokhlov, in *Nonlinear Optics* [in Russian], Nauka, Novosibirsk (1968), p. 348.

108. A. V. Kuzikovskii and S. S. Khmelevtsov, *Izv. Akad. Nauk SSSR, Fiz. Atm. Okeana*, 4(3):363 (1968).

109. A. V. Kuzikovskii, *Izv. Vyssh. Uchebn. Zaved., Fiz.*, No. 5, p. 89 (1970).

110. A. P. Sukhorukov, R. V. Khokhlov, and É. N. Shumilov, *Pis'ma Zh. Éksp. Teor. Fiz.*, 14(4):245 (1971).

111. A. P. Sukhorukov and É. N. Shumilov, *Zh. Tekh. Fiz.*, 18(5):1029 (1973).

112. D. E. Svetogorov, *Kvantovaya Élektron.* (*Moscow*), No. 1(13), p. 63 (1973).

113. V. E. Zuev, V. I. Bukatyi, A. V. Kuzikovskii, and S. S. Khmelevtsov, *Dokl. Akad. Nauk SSSR*, 217(1):52 (1974).

114. V. E. Zuev, V. I. Bukatyi, A. V. Kuzikovskii, M. F. Nebol'sin, and S. S. Khmelevtsov, *Dokl. Akad. Nauk SSSR*, 218(3):558 (1974).

115. K. S. Shifrin and Zh. K. Zolotova, *Izv. Akad. Nauk SSSR, Fiz. Atm. Okeana*, 2(12):1311 (1966).

116. V. I. Bukatyi and V. A. Pogodaev, *Izv. Vyssh. Uchebn. Zaved., Fiz.*, No. 1, p. 141 (1970).

117. A. V. Kuzikovskii, V. A. Pogodaev, and S. S. Khmelevtsov, *Inzh.-Fiz. Zh.*, 20(1):21 (1971).

118. V. K. Rudash, V. P. Bisyarin, N. M. Il'in, A. V. Sokolov, and G. M. Strelkov, *Kvantovaya Élektron.* (*Moscow*), 17(5):21 (1973).

119. Yu. N. Grachev and G. M. Strelkov, *Kvantovaya Élektron.* (*Moscow*), 1(10):2192 (1974).

120. Yu. N. Grachev and G. M. Strelkov, *Izv. Vyssh. Uchebn. Zaved., Fiz.*, No. 11, p. 27 (1975).

121. V. V. Barinov and S. A. Sorokin, *Kvantovaya Élektron.* (*Moscow*), 14(2):5 (1973).

122. V. E. Zuev, A. V. Kuzikovskii, V. A. Pogodaev, S. S. Khmelevtsov, and L. K. Chistyakova, *Dokl. Akad. Nauk SSSR*, 205(5):1069 (1972).

123. A. V. Korotin, L. P. Semenov, and P. N. Svirkunov, *Tr. Inst. Éksp. Meteorol.*, 54(11):24 (1975).

124. G. A. Askar'yan and E. M. Moroz, *Zh. Éksp. Teor. Fiz.*, 43(6):2319 (1962).

125. G. A. Askar'yan, M. S. Rabinovich, M. M. Savchenko, V. K. Stepanov, and V. B. Studenov, *Pis'ma Zh. Éksp. Teor. Fiz.*, 5(8):258 (1967).

126. V. I. Bukatyi, Yu. D. Kopytin, V. A. Pogodaev, S. S. Khmelevtsov, and L. K. Chistyakova, *Izv. Vyssh. Uchebn. Zaved., Fiz.*, No. 3, p. 41 (1972).

127. K. S. Shifrin and I. L. Zel'manovich, *Opt. Spektrosk.*, 17:313 (1964).

128. A. V. Kats, *Izv. Vyssh. Uchebn. Zaved., Radiofiz.*, 18(4):566 (1975).

129. V. I. Bukatyi and Yu. D. Kopytin, *Izv. Vyssh. Uchebn. Zaved., Fiz.*, No. 6, p. 91 (1971).

130. E. V. Ivanov, M. P. Kolomeev, N. K. Kraskovskii, P. M. Svirkunov, and L. P. Semenov, *Tr. Inst. Éksp. Meteorol.*, 54(11):19 (1975).

131. A. V. Kuzikovskii and S. S. Khmelevtsov, *Izv. Akad. Nauk SSSR, Fiz. Atm. Okeana*, 11(4):362 (1975).

132. M. P. Kolomeev and L. P. Semenov, *Tr. Inst. Éksp. Meteorol.*, 58(13):3 (1976).

133. A. V. Korotin and A. A. Semenov, *Tr. Inst. Éksp. Meteorol.*, No. 10, p. 65 (1972).

134. V. K. Rudash, A. V. Sokolov, and G. M. Strelkov, in *Proc. First All-Union Conf. Atmospheric Optics* [in Russian], Part 2, Inst. Opt. Atm. Sib. Otd. Akad. Nauk SSSR, Tomsk (1976), p. 175.

135. A. A. Manenkov, *Dokl. Akad. Nauk SSSR*, 190(6):1315 (1970).

136. Yu. K. Danileiko, A. A. Manenkov, V. S. Nechitailo, and V. Ya. Khaimov-Mal'kov, *Zh. Éksp. Teor. Fiz.*, 59(4):1083 (1970); 60(4):1245 (1971).

137. G. A. Askar'yan, V. G. Mikhalevich, and G. P. Shipulo, *Zh. Éksp. Teor. Fiz.*, 60(4):1270 (1971).

138. V. I. Bukatyi, Yu. D. Kopytin, and S. S. Khmelevtsov, *Kvantovaya Élektron. (Moscow)*, No. 1(13), p. 70 (1973).

139. V. I. Bukatyi, Yu. D. Kopytin, S. S. Khmelevtsov, and D. P. Chaporov, in *Elements and Devices of Radioelectronics* [in Russian], Tomsk. Univ., Tomsk (1974), p. 138.

140. Yu. D. Kopytin and S. S. Khmelevtsov, *Kvantovaya Élektron. (Moscow)*, 1(4):806 (1974).

141. V. I. Bukatyi, Yu. D. Kopytin, and S. S. Khmelevtsov, *Izv. Vyssh. Uchebn. Zaved., Fiz.*, No. 1, p. 113 (1974).

142. Yu. D. Kopytin and S. S. Khmelevtsov, in *Propagation of Optical Waves in the Atmosphere* [in Russian], Nauka, Novosibirsk (1974), p. 84.

143. Yu. D. Kopytin and S. S. Khmelevtsov, *Pis'ma Zh. Éksp. Teor. Fiz.*, 21(1):45 (1975).

144. V. I. Bukatyi, Yu. D. Kopytin, S. S. Khmelevtsov, and D. P. Chaporov, *Izv. Vyssh. Uchebn. Zaved., Fiz.*, No. 3, p. 33 (1976).

145. V. I. Bukatyi, Yu. D. Kopytin, S. S. Khmelevtsov, and D. P. Chaporov, Preprint No. 12 [in Russian], Inst. Opt. Atm. Sib. Otd. Akad. Nauk SSSR, Tomsk (1976).

146. Yu. D. Kopytin and S. S. Khmelevtsov, in *Propagation of Optical Waves in Inhomogeneous Media* [in Russian], Inst. Opt. Atm. Sib. Otd. Akad. Nauk SSSR, Tomsk (1976), p. 86.

147. V. E. Zuev and Yu. D. Kopytin, *Izv. Vyssh. Uchebn. Zaved., Fiz.*, No. 11, p. 79 (1977).

148. G. S. Romanov and V. K. Pustovalov, *Zh. Prikl. Spektrosk.*, 19(2):332 (1973).

149. F. A. Williams, *Intern. J. Heat Mass Trans.*, 8:575 (1965).

150. P. N. Svirkunov and L. P. Semenov, *Tr. Inst. Éksp. Meteorol.*, No. 30, p. 54 (1972).

151. A. P. Prishivalko and L. G. Astaf'eva, *Zh. Prikl. Spektrosk.*, 16:344 (1972).

152. A. P. Prishivalko and L. G. Astaf'eva, *Dokl. Akad. Nauk B. SSR*, 16(4):305 (1972).

153. A. P. Prishivalko and L. G. Astaf'eva, *Dokl. Akad. Nauk B. SSR*, 16(5);404 (1972).

154. N. V. Bukzdorf, *Izv. Vyssh. Uchebn. Zaved., Fiz.*, No. 3, p. 114 (1973).

155. L. G. Astaf'eva, *Zh. Prikl. Spektrosk.*, 18(3):469 (1973).

156. A. P. Prishivalko and N. G. Kondrat'ev, in *Proc. First All-Union Conf. Atmospheric Optics* [in Russian], Part 2, Tomsk (1976), p. 172.

157. V. P. Skripov, *Metastable Liquids* [in Russian], Nauka, Moscow (1972).

158. K. S. Shifrin, in *Investigation of Clouds, Precipitations, and Thunderstorm Electricity* [in Russian], Gidrometeoizdat, Leningrad (1957), p. 19.

159. G. M. Strelkov and Yu. N. Grachev, Preprint No. 27(139) [in Russian], Inst. Radio-elektron. Akad. Nauk SSSR, Moscow (1973).

160. L. K. Chistyakova, Dynamics of the Motion and Breakup of Liquid Droplets in Strong Optical Fields, Dissertation for Candidate of Physicomathematical Sciences, Tomsk (1977).

161. A. I. Ioffe, N. A. Mel'niko, K. A. Naugol'nykh, and V. A. Upadyshev, *Zh. Prikl. Mekh.*

*Tekh. Fiz.*, No. 3, p. 125 (1970).

162. M. P. Felox and A. T. Ellis, *Appl. Phys. Lett.*, 19:484 (1971).

163. A. V. Butenin and B. Ya. Kogan, *Kvantovaya Élektron.* (*Moscow*), No. 5, p. 143 (1971).

164. L. D. Landau and E. M. Lifshits, *Continuum Mechanics* [in Russian], Gostekhizdat, Moscow (1953).

165. V. E. Zuev and A. V. Kuzikovskii, *Izv. Vyssh. Uchebn. Zaved., Fiz.*, No. 11, p. 106 (1977).

166. G. W. Sutton, *AIAA Journal*, 8:1907 (1970).

167. M. P. Gordin and G. M. Strelkov, *Kvantovaya Élektron.* (*Moscow*), 2(3):559 (1975).

168. O. A. Volkovitskii, E. V. Ivanov, M. G. Kolomeev, N. K. Kraskovskii, and L. P. Semenov, *Izv. Akad. Nauk SSSR, Fiz. Atm. Okeana*, 11(8):361 (1975).

169. G. A. Askar'yan, A. M. Prokhorov, G. F. Chanturiya, and G. N. Shipulo, *Zh. Éksp. Teor. Fiz.*, 44(6):2180 (1963).

170. G. A. Askar'yan, *Zh. Éksp. Teor. Fiz.*, 45(3):810 (1963).

171. Yu. K. Danileiko, A. A. Manenkov, V. S. Nechitailo, and V. Ya. Khaimov-Mal'kov, *Zh. Eksp. Teor. Fiz.*, 60(4):1245 (1971).

172. G. A. Askar'yan, V. G. Mikhalevich, and G. P. Shipulo, *Zh. Éksp. Teor. Fiz.*, 60(4):1270 (1971).

173. V. I. Tatarskii, *Wave Propagation in a Turbulent Atmosphere* [in Russian], Nauka, Moscow (1967).

174. Yu. N. Barabanenkov, Yu. A. Kravtsov, S. M. Rytov, and V. I. Tatarskii, *Usp. Fiz. Nauk*, 102(1):3 (1970).

175. V. I. Bukatyi, Yu. D. Kopytin, S. S. Khmelevtsov, and D. P. Chaporov, in *Abstr. Third All-Union Symp. Propagation of Laser Radiation in the Atmosphere* [in Russian], Inst. Opt. Atm. Sib. Otd. Akad. Nauk SSSR, Tomsk (1975), p. 111.

176. V. I. Bespalov, A. G. Litvik, and V. I. Talanov, in *Nonlinear Optics* [in Russian], Nauka, Novosibirsk (1968), p. 428.

177. D. R. Skinner, *Opt. Commun.*, 1(2):57 (1969).

178. V. V. Vorob'ev, *Izv. Vyssh. Uchebn. Zaved., Radiofiz.*, 13(7):1053 (1970).

179. S. N. Vlasov, V. A. Petrishchev, and V. I. Talanov, Preprint No. 8 [in Russian], Nauchn.-Issled. Inst. Radiofiz., Gor'kii (1970).

180. V. A. Petrishchev, *Izv. Vyssh. Uchebn. Zaved., Radiofiz.*, 14(9):1416 (1971).

181. V. V. Vorob'ev, *Izv. Vyssh. Uchebn. Zaved., Radiofiz.*, 14(8):1283 (1971); 14(6):865 (1971).

182. S. A. Armand, *Radiotekh. Élektron.*, 16:2151 (1971).

183. V. V. Vorob'ev, *Kvantovaya Élektron.* (*Moscow*), No. 7, p. 5 (1972).

184. A. G. Muradyan, O. G. Martynenko, A. A. Baranov, V. L. Kolpashchikov, and A. F. Yakubov, *Radiotekh. Élektron.*, 18:2398 (1973).

185. F. G. Gebhardt, D. C. Smith, R. G. Buser, and R. S. Rohde, *Appl. Opt.*, 12:1794 (1973).

186. R. Alferness, *J. Opt. Soc. Am.*, 64:1645 (1974).

187. V. V. Vorob'ev and V. V. Shemetov, *Kvantovaya Élektron.* (*Moscow*), 2:1428 (1975).

188. Yu. D. Kopytin, in *Proc. First All-Union Conf. Atmospheric Optics* [in Russian], Part 2, Tomsk (1976), p. 222.

189. A. A. Zemlyanov, A. V. Kuzikovskii, and S. S. Khmelevtsov, *Izv. Vyssh. Uchebn. Zaved., Fiz.*, No. 10, p. 13 (1976).

190. A. G. Arutyunyan, V. M. Gordienko, and V. G. Tunkin, in *Proc. Sixth All-Union Conf. Nonlinear Optics* [in Russian], Minsk (1972), p. 10.

191. F. G. Gebhardt, D. C. Smith, R. G. Buser, and R. Rohde, *J. Opt. Soc. Am.*, 62:924 (1972).

192. F. G. Gebhardt, D. C. Smith, R. G. Buser, and R. S. Rohde, *Appl. Opt.*, 12:1794 (1973).

193. S. A. Akhmanov, A. P. Sukhorukov, and R. V. Khokhlov, *Usp. Fiz. Nauk*, 93(1):19 (1976).

194. V. N. Lugovoi and A. M. Prokhorov, *Usp. Fiz. Nauk*, 111(2):203 (1973).

195. G. A. Askar'yan, *Usp. Fiz. Nauk*, 111(2):249 (1973).
196. G. A. Pasmanik and V. I. Talanov, in *Abstr. Eleventh All-Union Conf. Radio-Wave Propagation* [in Russian], Kazan' (1975), p. 57.
197. Yu. E. D'yakov, in *Nonlinear Processes in Optics* [in Russian], Nauka, Novosibirsk (1970), p. 135.
198. A. A. Betin, G. A. Pasmanik, and L. V. Piskunov, *Kvantovaya Élektron.* (*Moscow*), 2:2403 (1975).
199. V. I. Bespalov, A. M. Kubarev, and G. A. Pasmanik, *Izv. Vyssh. Uchebn. Zaved., Radiofiz.*, 13:1433 (1970).
200. P. V. Elyutin, *Opt. Spektrosk.*, 30(2):248 (1971).
201. O. Yu. Nosach, V. I. Popovichev, V. V. Ragul'skii, and F. S. Faizullov, *Pis'ma Zh. Éksp. Teor. Fiz.*, 16:617 (1972).
202. A. A. Betin and G. A. Pasmanik, *Kvantovaya Élektron.* (*Moscow*), No. 4, p. 60 (1973).
203. G. A. Pasmanik, *Zh. Éksp. Teor. Fiz.*, 66:490 (1974).
204. B. Ya. Zel'dovich, V. I. Popovichev, V. V. Ragul'skii, and F. S. Faizullov, *Pis'ma Zh. Éksp. Teor. Fiz.*, 15:160 (1972).
205. V. S. Averbakh, A. I. Makarov, and V. I. Talanov, *Kvantovaya Élektron.* (*Moscow*), 2:2207 (1975).


# Chapter 6

1. V. E. Zuev and M. V. Kabanov, *Transfer of Optical Signals in the Earth's Atmosphere* (*under Interference Conditions*) [in Russian], Sov. Radio, Moscow (1977).
2. K. Ya. Kondrat'ev (ed.), *Actinometry* [in Russian], Gidrometeoizdat, Leningrad (1965).
3. K. Ya. Kondrat'ev (ed.), *Radiation Characteristics of the Atmosphere and Earth's Surface* [in Russian], Gidrometeoizdat, Leningrad (1969).
4. V. I. Kushpil', *Daytime Clear-Sky Luminance* (*Experimental Data*) [in Russian], Gos. Opt. Inst., Leningrad (1971).
5. K. L. Coulson, J. Dave, and Z. Sekera, *Tables Related to Radiation Emerging from a Planetary Atmosphere with the Rayleigh Scattering*, Univ. California Press, Berkeley–Los Angeles (1960).
6. G. Sh. Lifshits, *Scattered Light in the Daytime Sky* [in Russian], Nauka, Alma-Ata (1973).
7. V. N. Glushko, A. I. Ivanov, G. Sh. Lifshits, *et al.*, *Scattering of Infrared Radiation in the Cloudless Atmosphere* [in Russian], Nauka, Alma-Ata (1974).
8. O. P. Kuznechik, in *Light Scattering in the Earth's Atmosphere* [in Russian], Nauka, Alma-Ata (1972), p. 263.
9. O. P. Kuznechik, *Dokl. Akad. Nauk B. SSR*, 13(10):896 (1969).
10. G. V. Rozenberg, *Twilight* [in Russian], Fizmatgiz, Moscow (1963).
11. V. K. Pyldmaa and R. G. Timanovskaya, *Izv. Akad. Nauk SSSR, Fiz. Atm. Okeana*, 5(5):457 (1969).
12. G. A. Kostyanoi and L. A. Pakhomova, *Tr. Tsentr. Aérol. Obs.*, No. 66, p. 63 (1965).
13. M. I. Allenov and Yu. A. Shuba, *Izv. Akad. Nauk SSSR, Fiz. Atm. Okeana*, 7(9):956 (1971).
14. Yu.-A. R. Mullamaa, M. A. Sulev, and V. K. Pyldmaa, in *Radiation and Cloudiness* [in Russian], Inst. Fiz. Astron. Akad. Nauk É. SSR, Tartu (1969), p. 130.
15. O. P. Kuznechik and G. K. Afanas'ev, in *Light Scattering in the Earth's Atmosphere* [in Russian], Nauka, Alma-Ata (1972), p. 258.
16. Yu.-A. R. Mullamaa, M. A. Sulev, and V. K. Pyldmaa, *Stochastic Structure of the Cloudiness and Radiation Fields* [in Russian], Inst. Fiz. Astron. Akad. Nauk É. SSR, Tartu (1972).

17. Kh. Niilisk, Yu.-A. R. Mullamaa, and M. A. Sulev, in *Radiation in the Atmosphere* [in Russian], Inst. Fiz. Astron. Akad. Nauk É. SSR, Tartu (1969), p. 38.

18. K. Ya. Kondrat'ev, *Radiative Heat Transfer in the Atmosphere* [in Russian], Gidrometeoizdat, Leningrad (1956).

19. K. Ya. Kondrat'ev, O. A. Avaste, *et al.*, *Radiation Field of the Earth as a Planet* [in Russian], Gidrometeoizdat, Leningrad (1967).

20. I. A. Khvostikov, *The Night Airglow* [in Russian], Izd. Akad. Nauk SSSR, Moscow–Leningrad (1948).

21. J. W. Chamberlain, *Physics of the Aurora and Airglow*, Academic Press, New York (1961).

22. S. I. Isaev and M. I. Pudovkin, *The Aurorae and Processes in the Earth's Magnetosphere* [in Russian], Nauka, Leningrad (1972).

23. R. A. Young, "The airglow," *Sci. Am.*, 214(3):103 (1966).

24. R. M. Goody, *Atmospheric Radiation*, Clarendon, Oxford–New York (1964).

25. H. Philipps, *Gerl. Beitr. Geophys.*, 56(3):229 (1940).

26. M. I. Allenov, V. D. Bokii, and Yu. A. Shuba, in *Proc. All-Union Conf. Light Scattering* [in Russian], Astrofiz. Inst. Akad. Nauk K. SSR (1972), p. 184.

27. M. I. Allenov, L. G. Chubakov, and Yu. A. Shuba, in *Abstr. Second All-Union Symp. Propagation of Laser Radiation in the Atmosphere* [in Russian], Inst. Opt. Atm. Sib. Otd. Akad. Nauk SSSR. Tomsk (1973), p. 106.

28. R. A. Gafuri, *Izv. Akad. Nauk SSSR, Fiz. Atm. Okeana*, 4(8):891 (1968).

29. Yu. A Ryzhov and V. V. Tamoikin, *Izv. Vyssh. Uchebn. Zaved., Radiofiz.*, 13(3):356 (1970).

30. A. Omholt, *Optical Aurora*, Springer, Berlin–New York (1971).

31. A. I. Nefed'eva, *Izv. Astron. Obs. im. Éngel'gardta*, No. 36, p. 3 (1968).

32. Yu. G. Andrianov, I. I. Karavaev, and Yu. P. Safronov, *Infrared Spectra of the Earth's Radiation in Space* [in Russian], Sov. Radio, Moscow (1973).

33. Kh. Yu. Niilisk and R. Yu. Noorma, in *Investigation of the Radiation Environment of the Atmosphere* [in Russian], Inst. Fiz. Astron. Akad. Nauk É. SSR, Tartu (1967).

34. L. C. Block and A. S. Zachor, *Appl. Opt.*, 3:209 (1964).

35. G. V. Rozenberg, *Optics of Thin-Film Coatings* [in Russian], Gostekhizdat, Moscow (1958).

36. Yu.-A. R. Mullamaa, *Atlas of Optical Characteristics of the Rough Sea Surface* [in Russian], Inst. Fiz. Astron. Akad. Nauk É. SSR, Tartu (1964).

37. E. L. Krinov, *Spectral Reflectivity of Natural Formations* [in Russians], Izd. Akad. Nauk SSSR, Moscow (1974).

38. Yu. A. Zaitsev and L. A. Mukhin, *Geological Applications of Color and Spectrozonal Aerial Photography* [in Russian], Mosk. Univ., Moscow (1966).

39. D. A. Yanusht and Yu. K. Yutsevich (eds.), *Investigation of the Optical Properties of Natural Objects and Their Aerial-Photographic Images* [in Russian], Nauka, Leningrad (1970).

40. K. Ya. Kondrat'ev, Z. F. Mironova, and A. N. Otto, *Probl. Fiz. Atm.*, No. 3, p. 24 (1965).

41. E. M. Feigel'son, *Radiative Heat Transfer and Clouds* [in Russian], Gidrometeoizdat, Leningrad (1970).

42. G. I. Marchuk, G. A. Mikhailov, M. A. Nazaraliev, *et al.*, *Solution of Direct and Certain Inverse Problems of Atmospheric Optics by the Monte Carlo Method* [in Russian], Nauka, Novosibirsk (1968).

43. B. D. Borisov, *Spectral Reflectivity of Certain Natural Objects and Materials in the Range 2.2–3.7 $\mu m$*, VINITI Abstr. No. 2216-75 [in Russian], Vses. Inst. Nauchn. Tekh. Inform. (1975).

44. V. I. Korzov and L. B. Krasil'shchikov, *Tr. Gl. Geofiz. Obs.*, No. 183, p. 27 (1966).

45. M. A. Kropotkin and B. P. Kozyrev, *Opt. Spektrosk.*, 17(2):259 (1964).

46. D. I. Kalinenko, P. N. Kokhanenko, and V. K. Sonchik, *Izv. Vyssh. Uchebn. Zaved., Fiz.*, No. 6, p. 116 (1974).

47. M. V. Kabanov and A. A. Pershin, *Izv. Vyssh. Uchebn. Zaved., Fiz.*, No. 4, p. 74 (1972).

## Chapter 7


1. G. Fiocco and L. D. Smullin, *Nature (London)*, 199:1275 (1963).
2. G. G. Goyer and R. Watson, *Bull. Am. Meteorol. Soc.*, 44:564 (1963).
3. E. W. Barrett and D. Ben-Dov, *J. Appl. Meteorol.*, 6:500 (1967).
4. O. K. Kostko, *Tr. Tsentr. Aérol. Obs.*, No. 77, p. 67 (1967).
5. R. T. H. Collis, *Lidar: Atmospheric Exploration by Remote Probes*, *Vol.* 2, Nat. Acad. Sci. and Nat. Res. Council (1969), p. 147.
6. G. S. Kent and R. W. H. Wright, *J. Atm. Terr. Phys.*, 32:917 (1970).
7. V. M. Zakharov and O. K. Kostko, *Lasers and Meteorology* [in Russian], Gidrometeoizdat, Leningard (1972).
8. V. E. Zuev, *Laser Scans the Sky* [in Russian], Zapad.-Sib. Knizhn. Izd. (1972).
9. V. E. Zuev, "Laser probing of the atmosphere," *Priroda*, No. 10, p. 86 (1972).
10. V. E. Zuev, *The Laser Meteorologist* [in Russian], Gidrometeoizdat, Leningrad (1974).
11. F. F. Hall, Jr., *Laser Appl.*, 2:161 (1974).
12. O. K. Kostko, *Kvantovaya Élektron. (Moscow)*, 2(10):2133 (1975).
13. R. L. Byer, *Opt. Quantum Electron.*, 7:147 (1975).
14. V. M. Zakharov, O. K. Kostko, V. A. Torgovichev, and É. A. Chayanova, *Laser Methods of Investigation of the Polluted Atmosphere* [in Russian], Vses. Nauchn.-Issled. Inst. Gidrometeoinform., Inform. Tsentr, Obninsk (1976).
15. V. E. Zuev, G. M. Krekov, I. É. Naats, and V. N. Skorinov, *Izv. Akad. Nauk SSSR, Fiz. Atm. Okeana*, 11:1326 (1975).
16. V. E. Zuev, G. M. Krekov, I. É. Naats, and V. N. Skorinov, in *Laser Probing of the Atmosphere* [in Russian], Nauka, Moscow (1976), p. 46.
17. R. G. Strauch and A. Cohen, *Remote Sensing of the Troposhere* (V. E. Derr, ed.), U. S. Dept. Commerce, NOAA, Washington, D. C. (1972), p. 23.
18. A. Cohen and V. E. Derr, in *Conf. Atmospheric Radiation, Fort Collins, CO*, Am. Meteorol. Soc., Boston (1972), p. 301.
19. A. Cohen and M. Graber, in *Proc. IAMAP/IAPSO Comb. First Spec. Assembly*, Intern. Assoc. Meteorol. Atm. Phys. and Intern. Assoc. Phys. Sci. Ocean, Melbourne (1974).
20. V. M. Zakharov, O. K. Kostko, and V. S. Portasov, *Meteorol. Gidrol.*, No. 4, p. 80 (1974).
21. V. M. Zakharov, O. K. Kostko, and V. S. Portasov, in *Abstr. Second All-Union Symp. Propagation of Laser Radiation in the Atmosphere* [in Russian], Inst. Opt. Atm. Sib. Otd. Akad. Nauk SSSR, Tomsk (1973), p. 131.
22. V. M. Zakharov, O. K. Kostko, and V. S. Portasov, in *Abstr. Third All-Union Symp. Laser Probing of the Atmosphere* [in Russian], Inst. Opt. Atm. Sib. Otd. Akad. Nauk SSSR, Tomsk (1974), p. 24.
23. Yu. S. Balin, V. P. Galileiskii, V. N. Goryshin, and I. V. Samokhvalov, in *Abstr. Third All-Union Symp. Laser Probing of the Atmosphere* [in Russian], Inst. Opt. Atm. Sib. Otd. Akad. Nauk SSSR, Tomsk (1974), p. 24.
24. Yu. S. Balin and I. V. Samokhvalov, in *Abstr. Fourth All-Union Symp. Laser Probing of the Atmosphere* [in Russian], Inst. Opt. Atm. Sib. Otd. Akad. Nauk SSSR, Tomsk (1976), p. 59.
25. T. P. Toropova and A. P. Ten, in *Abstr. Fourth All-Union Symp. Laser Probing of the Atmosphere* [in Russian], Inst. Opt. Atm. Sib. Otd. Akad. Nauk SSSR, Tomsk (1976), p. 53.
26. L. S. Ivlev, B. V. Kaul', I. V. Samokhvalov, and V. S. Shamanaev, in *Problems of Remote Sensing of the Atmosphere* [in Russian], Inst. Opt. Atm. Sib. Otd. Akad. Nauk SSSR, Tomsk (1975), p. 16.
27. I. P. Polovina, I. V. Samokhvalov, and V. S. Shamanaev, *Izv. Akad. Nauk SSSR, Fiz. Atm. Okeana*, 11:760 (1975).

28. Yu. S. Balin, I. V. Samokhvalov, G. G. Matvienko, A. I. Grishin, and Yu. M. Vorevodin, in *Problems of Remote Sensing of the Atmosphere* [in Russian], Inst. Opt. Atm. Sib. Otd. Akad. Nauk SSSR, Tomsk (1975), p. 23.

29. Yu. S. Balin, Yu. M. Vorevodin, A. I. Grishin, I. V. Samokhvalov, and G. G. Matvienko, in *Radiophysical Studies of the Atmosphere* [in Russian], Gidrometeoizdat, Leningrad (1977), p. 66.

30. I. V. Samokhvalov and V. S. Shamanaev, *Izv. Vyssh. Uchebn. Zaved., Fiz.*, No. 7, p. 126 (1975).

31. V. S. Shamanaev, in *Abstr. Fourth All-Union Symp. Laser Probing of the Atmosphere* [in Russian], Inst. Opt. Atm. Sib. Otd. Akad. Nauk SSSR, Tomsk (1976), p. 155.

32. I. V. Samokhvalov and V. S. Shamanaev, *Izv. Akad. Nauk SSSR, Fiz. Atm. Okeana*, 12:208 (1976).

33. Yu. S. Balin, G. G. Matvienko, I. V. Samokhvalov, and Yu. S. Shamanaev, in *Abstr. Fourth All-Union Symp. Laser Probing of the Atmosphere* [in Russian], Inst. Opt. Atm. Sib. Otd. Akad. Nauk SSSR, Tomsk (1976), p. 63.

34. M. A. Gol'dberg, *Tr. Nauchn.-Issled. Inst. Gidrometeorol. Priborostr.*, No. 8, p. 61 (1968).

35. G. M. Krekov, R. F. Rakhimov, and T. P. Toropova, in *Abstr. Third All-Union Symp. Laser Probing of the Atmosphere* [in Russian], Inst. Opt. Atm. Sib. Otd. Akad. Nauk SSSR, Tomsk (1974), p. 95.

36. P. M. Hamilton, *Philos. Trans. R. Soc. London, Ser. A*, 265:153 (1969).

37. G. I. Gorchakov and G. V. Rozenberg, *Izv. Akad. Nauk SSSR, Fiz. Atm. Okeana*, 3:611 (1967).

38. K. S. Shifrin and E. A. Chayanova, *Izv. Akad. Nauk SSSR, Fiz. Atm. Okeana*, 3:274 (1967).

39. B. G. Andreev, *Izv. Akad. Nauk SSSR, Fiz. Atm. Okeana*, 3:979 (1967).

40. R. R. Alan and D. A. Bateman, in *Abstr. Seventh Intern. Laser Radar Conf.*, Stanford Res. Inst., Menlo Park, CA (1975), p. 84.

41. V. E. Zuev, G. M. Krekov, and M. M. Krekova, *Kvantovaya Élektron. (Moscow)*, 4(11) (1977).

42. B. M. Golubitskii, T. M. Zhad'ko, and M. V. Tantashev, *Izv. Akad. Nauk SSSR, Fiz. Atm. Okeana*, 8:1226 (1972).

43. J. A. Weinman, *J. Atm. Sci.*, 33:1763 (1976).

44. K. E. Kunkel and J. A. Weinman, *J. Atm. Sci.*, 33:1772 (1976).

45. B. V. Kaul', G. M. Krekov, and M. M. Krekova, *Kvantovaya Élektron. (Moscow)*, 4:2408 (1977).

46. N. L. Kuo, *J. Atm. Sci.*, 28:20 (1971).

47. E. W. Eloranta, in *Abstr. Fourth Conf. Laser Radar Studies of the Atmosphere*, Tucson, AZ (1972), p. 25.

48. E. W. Eloranta, in *Abstr. Fifth Conf. Laser Radar Studies of the Atmosphere*, Williamsburg, VA (1973), p. 21.

49. B. V. Kaul' and I. V. Samokhvalov, in *Abstr. Third All-Union Symp. Propagation of Laser Radiation in the Atmosphere* [in Russian], Inst. Opt. Atm. Sib. Otd. Akad. Nauk SSSR, Tomsk (1975), p. 56.

50. A. Cohen and M. Graber, *Opt. Quantum Electron.*, 7:221 (1975).

51. V. E. Zuev, B. V. Kaul', and I. V. Samokhvalov, in *Abstr. Seventh Intern. Laser Radar Conf.*, Stanford Res. Inst., Menlo Park, CA (1975), p. 103.

52. B. V. Kaul' and I. V. Samokhvalov, in *Abstr. Fourth All-Union Symp. Laser Probing of the Atmosphere* [in Russian], Inst. Opt. Atm. Sib. Otd. Akad. Nauk SSSR, Tomsk (1976), p. 83.

53. G. M. Krekov, M. M. Krekova, and A. I. Popkov, in *Abstr. Fourth All-Union Symp. Laser Probing of the Atmosphere* [in Russian], Inst. Opt. Atm. Sib. Otd. Akad. Nauk SSSR, Tomsk (1976), p. 151.

54. B. V. Kaul' and I. V. Samokhvalov, *Izv. Vyssh. Uchebn. Zaved., Fiz.*, No. 8, p. 109 (1975).
55. B. V. Kaul' and I. V. Samokhvalov, *Izv. Vyssh. Uchebn. Zaved., Fiz.*, No. 1, p. 80 (1976).
56. I. É. Naats, *Opt. Spektrosk.*, 35:966 (1973).
57. É. V. Makienko and I. É. Naats, in *Abstr. Second All-Union Symp. Propagation of Laser Radiation in the Atmosphere* [in Russian], Inst. Opt. Atm. Sib. Otd. Akad. Nauk SSSR, Tomsk (1973), p. 148.
58. B. S. Kostin, É. V. Makienko, and I. É. Naats, in *Propagation of Optical Waves in the Atmosphere* [in Russian], Nauka, Novosibirsk (1974), p. 208.
59. É. V. Makienko and I. É. Naats, *Izv. Akad. Nauk SSSR, Fiz. Atm. Okeana*, 10:543 (1974).
60. É. V. Makienko and I. É. Naats, in *Atmospheric Optics* [in Russian], Nauka, Moscow (1974), p. 186.
61. I. É. Naats, in *Problems of Remote Sensing of the Atmosphere* [in Russian], Inst. Opt. Atm. Sib. Otd. Akad. Nauk SSSR, Tomsk (1975), p. 35.
62. I. É. Naats, in *Propagation of Optical Waves in the Atmosphere* [in Russian], Nauka, Novosibirsk (1975), p. 202.
63. É. V. Makienko and I. É. Naats, in *Problems of Remote Sensing of the Atmosphere* [in Russian], Inst. Opt. Atm. Sib. Otd. Akad. Nauk SSSR, Tomsk (1975), p. 49.
64. B. S. Kostin and I. É. Naats, in *Problems of Remote Sensing of the Atmosphere* [in Russian], Inst. Opt. Atm. Sib. Otd. Akad. Nauk SSSR, Tomsk (1975), p. 61.
65. I. É. Naats, in *Problems in Laser Probing of the Atmosphere* [in Russian], Nauka, Novosibirsk (1976), p. 74.
66. V. V. Veretennikov, B. S. Kostin, and I. É. Naats, in *Problems in Laser Probing of the Atmosphere* [in Russian], Nauka, Novosibirsk (1976), p. 82.
67. B. S. Kostin and I. É. Naats, in *Problems in Laser Probing of the Atmosphere* [in Russian], Nauka, Novosibirsk (1976), p. 104.
68. É. V. Makienko and I. É. Naats, in *Problems in Laser Probing of the Atmosphere* [in Russian], Nauka, Novosibirsk (1976), pp. 115, 121.
69. I. É. Naats, in *Laser Probing of the Atmosphere* [in Russian], Nauka, Moscow (1976), p. 3.
70. É. V. Makienko and I. É. Naats, in *Laser Probing of the Atmosphere* [in Russian], Nauka, Moscow (1976), p. 11.
71. V. V. Veretennikov and I. É. Naats, in *Laser Probing of the Atmosphere* [in Russian], Nauka, Moscow (1976), p. 20.
72. B. S. Kostin and I. É. Naats, in *Laser Probing of the Atmosphere* [in Russian], Nauka, Moscow (1976), p. 94.
73. V. V. Veretennikov, I. É. Naats, I. V. Samokhvalov, and V. S. Shamanaev, in *Laser Probing of the Atmosphere* [in Russian], Nauka, Moscow (1976), p. 98.
74. D. Deirmendjian, *Electromagnetic Scattering on Spherical Polydispersions*, Am. Elsevier, New York (1969).
74a. C. D. Rodgers, *J. Quant. Spectros. Radiat. Transfer* 11:767 (1971).
75. A. N. Tikhonov, *Dokl. Akad. Nauk SSSR*, 151:501 (1963).
76. A. N. Tikhonov, *Dokl. Akad. Nauk SSSR*, 153:49 (1963).
77. A. N. Tikhonov and V. B. Glasko, *Zh. Vychisl. Mat. Mat. Fiz.*, 4:564 (1964).
78. A. N. Tikhonov and V. B. Glasko, *Zh. Vychisl. Mat. Mat. Fiz.*, 5:463 (1965).
79. V. V. Badaev, Yu. S. Lyubovtseva, and L. S. Turovpeva, *Izv. Akad. Nauk SSSR, Fiz. Atm. Okeana*, 9:1044 (1973).
80. V. V. Veretennikov and I. É. Naats, in *Problems of Remote Sensing of the Atmosphere* [in Russian], Inst. Opt. Atm. Sib. Otd. Akad. Nauk SSSR, Tomsk (1975), p. 69.
81. D. L. Phillips, *J. Assoc. Comput. Mach.*, 9:84 (1962).
82. D. K. Faddeev and V. N. Faddeeva, *Zh. Vychisl. Mat. Mat. Fiz.*, 1:412 (1961).
83. B. M. Herman, S. R. Browning, and J. A. Reagan, *J. Atm. Sci.*, 28:763 (1971).
84. E. R. Westwater and A. Cohen, *Appl. Opt.*, 12:1340 (1973).

85. V. E. Zuev, G. M. Krekov, M. M. Krekova, and I. É. Naats, in *Problems in Laser Probing of the Atmosphere* [in Russian], Nauka, Novosibirsk (1976), p. 3.

86. R. T. H. Collis, *Science*, 149:978 (1965).

87. R. T. H. Collis, F. G. Fernald, and J. E. Alder, *J. Appl. Meteorol.*, 7:227 (1968).

88. E. G. Shvidkovskii, V. M. Zakharov, V. M. Orlov, V. A. Torgovichev, É. A. Chayanova, and V. P. Fadina, *Izv. Akad. Nauk SSSR, Fiz. Atm. Okeana*, 7:404 (1971).

89. V. E. Zuev, G. M. Krekov, G. G. Matvienko, and A. I. Popkov, in *Laser Probing of the Atmosphere* [in Russian], Nauka, Moscow (1976), p. 29.

90. G. V. Rozenberg (ed.), *Searchlight Beams in the Atmosphere* [in Russian], Nauka, Moscow (1961).

91. M. H. Horman, *J. Opt. Soc. Am.*, 51:681 (1961).

92. I. V. Samokhvalov, in *Light Scattering in the Earth's Atmosphere* [in Russian], Nauka, Alma-Ata (1972), p. 194.

93. É. P. Zege, A. P. Ivanov, B. A. Kargin, and I. L. Katsev, *Izv. Akad. Nauk SSSR, Fiz. Atm. Okeana*, 7:750 (1971).

94. W. Viezee, J. Oblanas, and R. T. H. Collis, Rep. AFCRL-72-01730, Bedford, MA (1972), p. 57.

95. R. T. Brown, *J. Appl. Meteorol.*, 12:698 (1972).

96. V. E. Zuev, I. V. Samokhvalov, and Yu. S. Balin, *Izv. Vyssh. Uchebn. Zaved., Fiz.*, No. 5, p. 125 (1972).

97. M. Kano, *Pap. Meteorol. Geophys. (Tokyo)*, 19:121 (1968).

98. C. S. Kent, B. R. Clemesha, and R. W. Wright, *J. Atm. Terr. Phys.*, 29:169 (1967).

99. R. T. H. Collis, *J. Spacecr. Rockets*, 3:599 (1966).

100. E. G. Shvidkovskii and O. K. Kostko, *Dokl. Akad. Nauk SSSR*, 194:1316 (1970).

101. E. G. Shvidkovskii, V. M. Zakharov, O. K. Kostko, V. M. Orlov, B. A. Torgovichev, É. A. Chayanova, and V. P. Fadina, *Izv. Akad. Nauk SSSR, Fiz. Atm. Okeana*, 7:404 (1971).

102. V. E. Zuev, G. M. Krekov, and A. I. Popkov, *Izv. Vyssh. Uchebn. Zaved., Fiz.*, No. 10, p. 126 (1973).

103. V. E. Zuev, G. M. Krekov, and M. M. Krekova, *Izv. Vyssh. Uchebn. Zaved., Fiz.*, No. 8, p. 13 (1974).

104. V. E. Zuev, G. M. Krekov, M. M. Krekova, É. V. Makienko, and I. É. Naats, in *Radiophysical Studies of the Atmosphere* [in Russian], Gidrometeoizdat, Leningrad (1977), p. 6.

105. V. E. Zuev, G. M. Krekov, M. M. Krekova, É. V. Makienko, and I. É. Naats in *Proc. IAMAP/IAPSO Comb. First Spec. Assembly*, Intern. Assoc. Meteorol. Atm. Phys. and Intern. Assoc. Phys. Sci. Ocean, Melbourne (1974), p. 24.

106. F. G. Fernald, M. B. Herman, and J. A. Reagan, *J. Appl. Meteorol.*, 11(6):482 (1972).

107. N. B. Stevens, M. H. Horman, and E. E. Dodd, Rep. AFCRL-57-201, Riverside, CA (1957), p. 82.

108. Yu. S. Balin, I. V. Samokhvalov, and V. S. Shamanaev, in *Abstr. Second All-Union Symp. Propagation of Laser Radiation in the Atmosphere* [in Russian], Inst. Opt. Atm. Sib. Otd. Akad. Nauk SSSR, Tomsk (1973), p. 176.

109. A. L. Skrelin, I. S. Khutko, and L. V. Nikolaev, in *Abstr. Third All-Union Symp. Laser Probing of the Atmosphere* [in Russian], Inst. Opt. Atm. Sib. Otd. Akad. Nauk SSSR, Tomsk (1974), p. 112.

110. G. M. Krekov, I. É. Naats, and A. I. Popkov, in *Abstr. Third All-Union Symp. Laser Probing of the Atmosphere* [in Russian], Inst. Opt. Atm. Sib. Otd. Akad. Nauk SSSR, Tomsk (1974), p. 39.

111. R. T. H. Collis, in *Advances in Geophysics* (H. E. Landsberg and J. van Mieghem, eds.), Vol. 13, Academic Press, New York (1969), p. 113.

112. W. Viezee, J. Oblanas, and R. T. H. Collis, Rep. 1 AFCRL-TR-73-0146 (1973).

113. W. Viezee, J. Oblanas, and R. T. H. Collis, Final Rep. AFCRL-TR-73-0052 (1973).
114. W. Viezee, J. Oblanas, and R. T. H. Collis, Final Rep., Parts 1 and 2, AFCRL-TR-73-0708, Stanford Res. Inst., Menlo Park, CA (1973).
115. W. Viezee, E. Uthe, and R. T. H. Collis, *J. Appl. Meteorol.*, 8:971 (1969).
116. P. A. Davis, *Appl. Opt.*, 8:2099 (1969).
117. V. A. Kovalev, *Tr. Gl. Geofiz. Obs.*, 255:125 (1970).
118. V. A. Kovalev, "Inventors Certificate No. 309338," *Otkrytiya Izobret. Prom. Obraztsy Tov. Znaki*, No. 22, p. 181 (1971).
119. V. A. Kovalev, *Tr. Gl. Geofiz. Obs.*, 279:194 (1972).
120. V. A. Kovalev, *Tr. Gl. Geofiz. Obs.*, 312:128 (1973).
121. V. E. Zuev, G. M. Krekov, M. M. Krekova, É. V. Makienko, and I. É. Naats, in *Abstr. Fifth Conf. Laser Radar Studies of the Atmosphere*, Williamsburg, VA (1973), p. 100.
122. L. Jánossy, *Theory and Practice of the Evaluation of Measurements*, Clarendon, Oxford–New York (1964).
123. V. E. Zuev, G. M. Krekov, M. M. Krekova, É. V. Makienko, and I. É. Naats, in *Propagation of Optical Waves in the Atmosphere* [in Russian], Nauka, Novosibirsk (1975), p. 196.
124. V. E. Zuev, and G. M. Krekov, in *Physics of Mesospheric Clouds* [in Russian], Izd. Tomsk. Univ., Tomsk (1971), p. 7.
125. K.-N. Liou, *J. Atm. Sci.*, 28:824 (1971).
126. K.-N. Liou, *J. Atm. Sci.*, 29:1000 (1972).
127. K.-N. Liou, and R. M. Schotland, *J. Atm. Sci.*, 28:772 (1971).
128. S. R. Pal and A. I. Carswell, *Appl. Opt.*, 12:1530 (1973).
129. K.-N. Liou and H. Lahore, *J. Appl. Meteorol.*, 13:257 (1974).
130. A. Cohen, *Appl. Opt.*, 14:2873 (1975).
131. R. W. L. Thomas and A. C. Holland, in *Abstr. Seventh Intern. Laser Radar Conf.*, Stanford Res. Inst., Menlo Park, CA (1975), p. 105.
132. J. V. Winstanley and C. Wigmore, in *Abstr. Seventh Intern. Laser Radar Conf.*, Stanford Res. Inst., Menlo Park, CA (1975), p. 156.
133. Yu. S. Balin, G. O. Zadde, V. E. Zuev, G. G. Matvienko, I. V. Samokhvalov, and V. S. Shamanaev, in *Proc. IAMAP/IAPSO Comb. First Spec. Assembly*, Intern. Assoc. Meteorol. Atm. Phys. and Intern. Assoc. Phys. Sci. Ocean, Melbourne (1974), p. 186.
134. Yu. S. Balin, G. O. Zadde, G. G. Matvienko, I. V. Samokhvalov, and V. S. Shamanaev, in *Propagation of Optical Waves in the Atmosphere* [in Russian], Nauka, Novosibirsk (1975), p. 183.
135. Yu. S. Balin, G. G. Matvienko, and V. S. Shamanaev, "Inventors Certificate No. 473143," *Otkrytiya Izobret. Prom. Obraztsy Tov. Znaki*, No. 21, p. 123 (1975).
136. K. Sassen, *J. Appl. Meteorol.*, 13:923 (1974).
137. A. B. Shupyatskii, V. I. Shlyakhov, V. V. Kravets, and A. E. Tyabotov, *Meteorol. Gidrol.*, No. 2, p. 104 (1967).
138. A. E. Tyabotov, V. I. Shlyakhov, and A. B. Shupyatskii, *Izv. Akad. Nauk SSSR, Fiz. Atm. Okeana*, 5:192 (1969).
139. A. I. German, A. P. Tikhonov, and A. E. Tyabotov, in *Abstr. Third All-Union Symp. Laser Probing of the Atmosphere* [in Russian], Inst. Opt. Atm. Sib. Otd. Akad. Nauk SSSR, Tomsk (1974), p. 133.
140. A. E. Tyabotov, in *Abstr. Third All-Union Symp. Laser Probing of the Atmosphere* [in Russian], Inst. Opt. Atm. Sib. Otd. Akad. Nauk SSSR, Tomsk (1974), p. 139.
141. A. E. Tyabotov, V. I. Shlyakhov, and A. B. Shupyatskii, *Tr. Tsentr. Aérol. Obs.*, No. 109, p. 44 (1975).
142. A. I. German, A. P. Tikhonov, and A. E. Tyabotov, *Tr. Tsentr. Aérol. Obs.*, No. 109, p. 51 (1975).

143. A. E. Tyabotov, in *Abstr. Fourth All-Union Symp. Laser Probing of the Atmosphere* [in Russian], Inst. Opt. Atm. Sib. Otd. Akad. Nauk SSSR, Tomsk (1976), p. 123.

144. V. S. Pshonkin, A. E. Tyabotov, V. I. Shlyakhov, and A. B. Shupyatskii, *Tr. Tsentr. Aérol. Obs.*, No. 105, p. 57 (1973).

145. R. T. H. Collis, *Proc. Thirteenth Radar Meteorology Conf.*, McGill Univ., Montreal, August 20–23, 1968, Am. Meteorol. Soc., Boston (1968).

146. R. T. H. Collis, *J. Spacecr. Rockets*, 3:599 (1966).

147. R. T. H. Collis, *Q. J. R. Meteorol. Soc.*, 92:220 (1966).

148. R. T. H. Collis, *Bull. Am. Meteorol. Soc.*, 49:918 (1968).

149. R. T. H. Collis, *Microwaves*, 8:94 (1969).

150. E. E. Uthe and P. B. Russell, Preprint, *IAMAP Symp. Radiation in the Atmosphere*, Garmisch-Partenkirchen, GFR (1976), p. 242.

151. A. I. Carswell, A. K. McQuillan, and W. R. McNeil, *Can. Aerospace J.*, 17:419 (1971).

152. A. I. Carswell, J. D. Houston, W. R. McNeil, and S. Sizgoric, *Can. Aerospace J.*, 18:335 (1972).

153. A. I. Carswell, S. R. Pal, and J. S. Ryan, in *Abstr. Seventh Intern. Laser Radar Conf.*, Stanford Res. Inst., Menlo Park, CA (1975), p. 95.

154. V. N. Smiley, J. A. Warburton, and B. M. Morley, in *Abstr. Seventh Intern. Laser Radar Conf.*, Stanford Res. Inst., Menlo Park, CA (1975), p. 89.

155. E. Y. Moroz and G. A. Travers, in *Abstr. Seventh Intern. Laser Radar Conf.*, Stanford Res. Inst., Menlo Park, CA (1975), p. 151.

156. V. E. Zuev, I. V. Samokhvalov, and V. S. Shamanaev, in *Abstr. Seventh Intern. Laser Radar Conf.*, Stanford Res. Inst., Menlo Park, CA (1975), p. 92.

157. G. P. Zhukov, V. A. Korshunov, and N. P. Romanov, in *Abstr. Fourth All-Union Symp. Laser Probing of the Atmosphere* [in Russian], Inst. Opt. Atm. Sib. Otd. Akad. Nauk SSSR, Tomsk (1976), p. 137.

158. V. E. Zuev, B. V. Kaul', and I. V. Samokhvalov, in *Abstr. Fifth Conf. Laser Radar Studies of the Atmosphere*, Williamsburg, VA (1973), p. 81.

159. V. E. Zuev, B. V. Kaul', and I. V. Samokhvalov, in *Proc. IAMAP/IAPSO First Spec. Assembly*, Intern. Assoc. Meteorol. Atm. Phys. and Intern. Assoc. Phys. Sci. Ocean, Melbourne (1974).

160. V. E. Zuev, B. V. Kaul', O. A. Krasnov, G. M. Krekov, R. F. Rakhimov, and I. V. Samokhvalov, *Abstr. Sixth Conf. Laser Radar Studies of the Atmosphere*, Sendai, Japan (1974), p. 89.

161. B. V. Kaul', O. A. Krasnov, G. M. Krekov, and I. V. Samokhvalov, in *Problems in Remote Sensing of the Atmosphere* [in Russian], Inst. Opt. Atm. Sib. Otd. Akad. Nauk SSSR, Tomsk (1975), p. 3.

162. V. E. Zuev, B. V. Kaul', and I. V. Samokhvalov, in *Propagation of Optical Waves in the Atmosphere* [in Russian], Nauka, Novosibirsk (1975), p. 160.

163. B. V. Kaul' and I. V. Samokhvalov, in *Radiophysical Studies of the Atmosphere* [in Russian], Gidrometeoizdat, Leningrad (1977), p. 62.

164. R. T. H. Collis and E. E. Uthe, *Opto-Electron.*, 4:87 (1972).

165. W. B. Johnson, *J. Air Pollution Control Assoc.*, 19:176 (1969).

166. W. B. Johnson, *J. Appl. Meteorol.*, 8:443 (1969).

167. E. E. Uthe and W. B. Johnson, Final Rep. SRI Project 7929, AEC Contract AT(04-3)-115 (1971).

168. W. B. Johnson and E. E. Uthe, *Atm. Environ.*, 5:703 (1971).

169. E. E. Uthe and C. E. Lapple, Final Rep. SRI Project 8730, Contract CPA 70-173, Environ. Protection Agency, Stanford Res. Inst. Menlo Park, CA (1972).

170. E. E. Uthe, *Bull. Am. Meteorol. Soc.*, 53:358 (1972).

171. J. Gelbwachs and M. Birnbaum, *Appl. Opt.*, 12:2442 (1973).

172. B. P. Kashentsev, V. F. Krivolapov, Yu. A. Palatov, and V. A. Torgovichev, in *Abstr. Fourth All-Union Symp. Laser Probing of the Atmosphere* [in Russian], Inst. Opt. Atm. Sib. Otd. Akad. Nauk SSSR, Tomsk (1976), p. 10.

173. G. P. Zhukov, N. P. Romanov, and V. S. Shuklin, in *Abstr. Fourth All-Union Symp. Laser Probing of the Atmosphere* [in Russian], Inst. Opt. Atm. Sib. Otd. Akad. Nauk SSSR, Tomsk (1976), p. 134.

174. B. V. Kaul', in *Abstr. Fourth All-Union Symp. Laser Probing of the Atmosphere* [in Russian], Inst. Opt. Atm. Sib. Otd. Akad. Nauk SSSR, Tomsk (1976), p. 86.

175. V. E. Zuev, Yu. S. Balin, B. S. Kostin, I. É. Naats, and I. V. Samokhvalov, in *Abstr. Fourth All-Union Symp. Laser Probing of the Atmosphere* [in Russian], Inst. Opt. Atm. Sib. Otd. Akad. Nauk SSSR, Tomsk (1976), p. 147.

176. R. T. H. Collis and M. G. H. Ligda, *Nature (London)*, 203:508 (1964).

177. R. T. H. Collis, F. G. Fernald, and M. G. H. Ligda, *Nature (London)*, 203:1274 (1964).

178. G. Fiocco and G. Grams, *J. Atm. Sci.*, 21:323 (1964).

179. G. Fiocco and G. Colombo, *J. Geophys. Res.*, 69:1795 (1964).

180. G. Fiocco, *J. Geophys. Res.*, 70:2213 (1965).

181. K. Nishikori, T. Ishida, K. Uchikura, *et. al.*, *J. Radio Res. Lab. (Jpn.)*, 12:213 (1965).

182. W. C. Bain and M. C. W. Sandford, *J. Atm. Terr. Phys.*, 28:543 (1966).

183. G. Fiocco and G. Grams, *Tellus, Q. J. Geophys.*, 18:34 (1966).

184. M. P. McCormick, S. K. Poultney, U. Van Wijk, C. O. Alley, R. T. Bettinger, and J. A. Perschy, *Nature (London)*, 209:798 (1966).

185. B. R. Clemesha, G. S. Kent, and R. W. H. Wright, *Nature (London)*, 209:184 (1966).

186. R. T. H. Collis and M. G. H. Ligda, *J. Atm. Sci.*, 23:255 (1966).

187. B. R. Clemesha, G. S. Kent, and R. W. H. Wright, *Nature (London)*, 214:261 (1967).

188. B. R. Clemesha, G. S. Kent, and R. W. H. Wright, *J. Appl. Meteorol.*, 6:386 (1967).

189. G. Grams and G. Fiocco, *J. Geophys. Res.*, 72:3523 (1967).

190. G. S. Kent, B. R. Clemesha, and R. W. H. Wright, *J. Atm. Terr. Phys.*, 29:169 (1967).

191. P. D. McCormick, E. C. Silverberg, S. K. Poultney, U. Van Wijk, C. O. Alley, and R. T. Bettinger, *Nature (London)*, 215:1262 (1967).

192. M. C. W. Sandford, *J. Atm. Terr. Phys.*, 29:1657 (1967).

193. J. W. Oblanas and R. T. H. Collis, *Lidar Observations of the Pre-Gondola I Cloud*, U. S. Army Eng. Nuclear Cratering Group, Rep. PNE-1100 (1967).

194. E. C. Silverberg and S. K. Poultney, *Optical Radar Backscattering from the Mesopause Region During July and August 1967*, Dept. Phys. Astron., Univ. Maryland, College Park (1967), p. 35.

195. G. G. Boyer and R. D. Watson, *Bull. Am. Meteorol. Soc.*, 49:890 (1968).

196. J. D. Lawrence, Jr., M. P. McCormick, S. H. Melfi, and D. P. Woodman, in *Abstr. Fifth Symp. Remote Sensing of the Environment*, Ann Arbor, MI (1968), p. 609.

197. J. D. Lawrence, Jr., M. P. McCormick, S. H. Melfi, and D. P. Woodman, *Appl. Phys. Lett.*, 12:72 (1968).

198. R. T. H. Collis and W. E. Evans, *SPIE Journal*, 8:38 (1970).

199. G. E. Ashwell and J. A. Lane, *Nature (London)*, 222:464 (1969).

200. B. R. Clemesha, in *Atmospheric Exploration by Remote Probes*, Vol. 2, Nat. Acad. Sci. and Nat. Res. Council (1969), p. 201.

201. G. Fiocco and G. Grams, *J. Geophys. Res.*, 74:2453 (1969).

202. P. D. McCormick, E. C. Silverberg, S. K. Poultney, R. T. Bettinger, and C. O. Alley, *J. Atm. Terr. Phys.*, 31:185 (1969).

203. R. T. H. Collis, "Lidar," in *Advances in Geophysics* (H. E. Landsberg and J. van Mieghem, eds.), Vol. 13, Academic Press, New York (1969), p. 113.

204. W. E. Viezee and J. W. Oblanas, *J. Appl. Meteorol.*, 9:916 (1970).

205. G. W. Grams, *J. Atm. Terr. Phys.*, 32:729 (1970).

206. P. B. Russell, W. Viezee, R. D. Hake, Jr., and R. T. H. Collis, in *Proc. Fourth Conf. Climatic Impact Assessment Program* (1975).

207. F. F. Hall, Jr., *Opt. Spectrosc.*, 4:67 (1970).

208. B. G. Schuster, in *Laser Applications in Geosciences* (J. Gauger and F. F. Hall, Jr., eds.), Western Periodicals, North Hollywood, CA (1970), p. 33.

209. B. G. Schuster, *J. Geophys. Res.*, 75:3123 (1970).

210. K. Bartusek, D. J. Gambling, and W. G. Elford, *J. Atm. Terr. Phys.*, 32:1535 (1970).

211. B. R. Clemesha, *J. Appl. Meteorol.*, 10:171 (1971).

212. J. A. Lane, G. E. Ashwell, and A. Dagnall, *Atm. Environ.*, 5:49 (1971).

213. G. Witt and A. Lundin, Rep. AP-2, Inst. Meteorol., Univ. Stockholm (1971), p. 78.

214. B. R. Clemesha and S. N. Rodrigues, *J. Atm. Terr. Phys.*, 33:1119 (1971).

215. G. S. Kent, M. C. W. Sandford, and W. Keenliside, *J. Atm. Terr. Phys.*, 33:1257 (1971).

216. G. S. Kent, P. Sandland, and R. W. H. Wright, *J. Appl. Meteorol.*, 10:443 (1971).

217. E. E. Uthe, *Bull. Am. Meteorol. Soc.*, 53:358 (1972).

218. R. D. Hake, Jr., D. E. Arnold, D. W. Jackson, W. E. Evans, B. P. Ficklin, and R. A. Long, *J. Geophys. Res.*, 77:6839 (1972).

219. E. E. Uthe and J. H. S. Keolcha, *Lidar Observations of the Aerosol Structure over St. Louis, Missouri, during Metromex 1971, Final Rep., NSF Grant GA-30435*, Stanford Res. Inst., Menlo Park, CA (1972).

220. G. S. Kent, W. Keenliside, M. C. W. Sandford, and R. W. H. Wright, *J. Atm. Terr. Phys.*, 34:373 (1972).

221. V. M. Zakharov, O. K. Kostko, and V. S. Portasov, in *Abstr. Second All-Union Symp. Propagation of Laser Radiation in the Atmosphere* [in Russian], Inst. Opt. Atm. Sib. Otd. Akad. Nauk SSSR, Tomsk (1973), p. 131.

222. P. B. Russell, W. Viezee, and R. D. Hake, Jr., *Lidar Measurements of Stratospheric Aerosols over Menlo Park, California, October 1972–March 1974, Final Rep. SRI Project 2217*, Stanford Res. Inst., Menlo Park, CA (1974).

223. P. B. Russell, W. Viezee, R. D. Hake, Jr., and R. T. H. Collis, in *Abstr. 1974 Intern. Laser Radar Conf.—Sixth Conf. Laser Atmospheric Studies*, Sendai, Japan (1974), p. 118.

224. V. M. Zakharov, O. K. Kostko, and V. S. Portasov, in *Abstr. Sixth Conf. Laser Atmospheric Studies*, Sendai, Japan (1974), p. 180.

225. V. M. Zakharov, O. K. Kostko, and V. S. Portasov, in *Meteorology and Hydrology* [in Russian] (1974), p. 80.

226. V. M. Zakharov, O. K. Kostko, and V. S. Portasov, in *Abstr. Third All-Union Symp. Laser Probing of the Atmosphere* [in Russian], Inst. Opt. Atm. Sib. Otd. Akad. Nauk SSSR, Tomsk (1974), p. 6; p. 12.

227. A. I. German, V. M. Zakharov, O. K. Kostko, V. S. Portasov, V. E. Rokotyan, and E. A. Chayanova, in *Proc. IAMAP/IAPSO Comb. First Spec. Assembly, Intern. Assoc. Meteorol. Atm. Phys. and Intern. Assoc. Phys. Sci. Ocean*, Melbourne (1974).

228. M. P. McCormick, in *Abstr. 1974 Intern. Laser Radar Conf.—Sixth Conf. Laser Atmospheric Studies*, Sendai, Japan (1974); *Appl. Opt.*, 14:797 (1975).

229. S. A. Young and W. G. Elford, *J. Atm. Terr. Phys.* (1975).

230. P. M. McCormick, W. H. Fuller, Jr., W. P. Chu, and T. J. Swissler, in *Abstr. Seventh Intern. Laser Radar Conf.*, Stanford Res. Inst., Menlo Park, CA (1975), p. 40.

231. F. G. Fernald and C. Frush, in *Abstr. Seventh Intern. Laser Radar Conf.*, Stanford Res. Inst., Menlo Park, CA (1975), p. 42.

232. P. B. Russell, W. Viezee, and R. D. Hake, Jr., in *Abstr. Seventh Intern. Laser Radar Conf.*, Stanford Res. Inst., Menlo Park, CA (1975), p. 44.

233. J. A. Reagan, D. M. Byrne, B. L. Peck, and B. M. Herman, in *Abstr. Seventh Intern. Laser Radar Conf.*, Stanford Res. Inst., Menlo Park, CA (1975), p. 45.

234. M. Hirono, M. Fujiwara, and T. Itabe, in *Abstr. Seventh Intern. Laser Radar Conf.*, Stanford Res. Inst., Menlo Park, CA (1975), p. 47.

235. P. B. Russell, R. D. Hake, Jr., and W. Viezee, Preprint, *IAMAP Symp. Radiation in the Atmosphere*, Garmisch-Partenkirchen, GFR (1976), p. 141.

236. P. B. Russell *et al.*, *Q. J. R. Meteorol. Soc.*, 102:619 (1976).

237. I. P. Doktorov, V. A. Donchenko, V. E. Zuev, V. V. Kostin, I. V. Samokhvalov, and G. I. Tyul'kov, in *Laser Probing of the Atmosphere* [in Russian], Nauka, Moscow (1976), p. 111.

238. Yu. P. Dyabin, V. D. Marusyak, S. O. Mirumyants, and M. V. Tantashev, in *Abstr. Fourth All-Union Symp. Laser Probing of the Atmosphere* [in Russian], Inst. Opt. Atm. Sib. Otd. Akad. Nauk SSSR, Tomsk (1976), p. 7.

239. A. P. Ivanov, A. N. Kozhevnikov, V. S. Korneev, V. M. Orlov, F. P. Osipenko, I. S. Khutko, and A. P. Chaikovskii, in *Abstr. Fourth All-Union Symp. Laser Probing of the Atmosphere* [in Russian], Inst. Opt. Atm. Sib. Otd. Akad. Nauk SSSR, Tomsk (1976), p. 40.

240. V. P. Dugin and S. O. Mirumyants, in *Abstr. Fourth All-Union Symp. Laser Probing of the Atmosphere* [in Russian], Inst. Opt. Atm. Sib. Otd. Akad. Nauk SSSR, Tomsk (1976), p. 103.

241. R. T. H. Collis and J. W. Oblanas, *Airborne Lidar Observations — Pre-Gondola II*, U. S. Army Eng. Nuclear Cratering Group, Rep. PNE-1119 (1968).

242. R. T. H. Collis, in *Abstr. Fourteenth Radar Meteorology Conf.*, Tucson, AZ (1970), p. 265.

243. R. J. Fox, G. W. Grams, B. G. Schuster, and J. A. Weinman, *J. Geophys. Res.*, 78:7789 (1973).

244. F. G. Fernald, C. L. Frush, and B. G. Schuster, in *Proc. Third Conf. Climatic Impact Assessment Program*, Springfield, VA (1974), p. 318.

245. I. V. Samokhvalov and V. S. Shamanaev, in *Abstr. Fourth All-Union Symp. Laser Probing of the Atmosphere* [in Russian], Inst. Opt. Atm. Sib. Otd. Akad. Nauk SSSR, Tomsk (1976), p. 44.

246. A. I. German, A. P. Tikhonov, and A. E. Tyabotov, in *Radiophysical Studies of the Atmosphere* [in Russian], Gidrometeoizdat, Leningrad (1977), p. 36.

247. D. A. Lea, J. L. Karney, and C. A. Knudsen, in *Proc. Twelfth Conf. Radar Meteorology*, Norman, OK, Am. Meteorol. Soc., Boston (1966), p. 98.

248. S. Pilipowskyj, J. A. Weinman, B. R. Clemesha, G. S. Kent, and R. W. Wright, *J. Geophys. Res.*, 73:7553 (1968).

249. W. Viezee and J. Oblanas, *J. Appl. Meteorol.*, 8:369 (1969).

250. W. Viezee, J. Oblanas, and N. Nielsen, *Joint Radar and Lidar Observations of the Marine Layer at Point Loma, San Diego*, Rep., Contract No. 0244-72-C-0552, *SRI Project 1572*, Stanford Res. Inst., Menlo Park, CA (1972).

251. M. P. McCormick, S. H. Melfi, L. E. Olssen, W. L. Tuft, W. P. Elliott, and R. Egami, *Mixing-Height Measurement by Lidar, Particle Counter, and Rawinsonde in the Willamette Valley, Oregon*, NASA Tech. Note D-7103 (1972).

252. G. B. Northam, J. M. Rosen, S. H. Melfi, T. J. Pepin, M. P. McCormick, D. J. Hofmann, and W. H. Fuller, Jr., *Appl. Opt.*, 13:2416 (1974).

253. P. B. Russell and R. D. Hake, *J. Atm. Sci.*, 34:163 (1977).

254. V. R. Noonkester, D. R. Jensen, J. H. Richter, W. Viezee, and R. T. H. Collis, *J. Appl. Meteorol.*, 13:249 (1974).

255. E. E. Remsberg and G. B. Northam, *Proc. Fourth Conf. Climatic Impact Assessment Program*, Cambridge, MA (1975), p. 509.

256. F. G. Fernald, B. G. Schuster, E. F. Danielson, and D. G. Deaven, *Opt. Quantum Electron.*, 7:141 (1975).

257. J. D. Spinhirne, B. M. Herman, and J. A. Reagan, in *Abstr. Seventh Intern. Laser Radar Conf.*, Stanford Res. Inst., Menlo Park, CA (1975), p. 66.

258. J. A. Reagan, J. D. Spinhirne, D. M. Byrne, and R. L. Peck, in *Abstr. Seventh Intern. Laser Radar Conf.*, Stanford Res. Inst., Menlo Park, CA (1975), p. 68.

259. J. Mamane, R. Pena, and D. W. Thomson, in *Abstr. Seventh Intern. Laser Radar Conf.*,

Stanford Res. Inst., Menlo Park, CA (1975), p. 70.

260. P. B. Russell and E. E. Uthe, in *Abstr. Seventh Intern. Laser Radar Conf.*, Stanford Res. Inst., Menlo Park, CA (1975), p. 72.

261. E. M. Patterson, F. G. Fernald, C. L. Frush, and G. W. Grams, in *Abstr. Seventh Intern. Laser Radar Conf.*, Stanford Res. Inst., Menlo Park, CA (1975), p. 74.

262. J. L. McElroy, in *Abstr. Seventh Intern. Laser Radar Conf.*, Stanford Res. Inst., Menlo Park, CA (1975), p. 76.

263. V. E. Zuev, Yu. M. Vorevodin, A. I. Grishin, G. G. Matvienko, I. V. Samokhvalov, and N. I. Yurga, in *Abstr. Seventh Intern. Laser Radar Conf.*, Stanford Res. Inst., Menlo Park, CA (1975), p. 80.

264. J. A. Reagan, D. M. Byrne, and B. M. Herman, Preprint, *IAMAP Symp. Radiation in the Atmosphere*, Garmisch-Partenkirchen, GFR (1976), p. 165.

265. J. A. Reagan, J. D. Spinhirne, and B. M. Herman, Preprint, *IAMAP Symp. Radiation in the Atmosphere*, Garmisch-Partenkirchen, GFR (1976), p. 113.

266. J. A. Reagan and B. M. Herman, in *Proc. Fourteenth Conf. Radar Meteorology*, Tucson, AZ, Am. Meteorol. Soc., Boston (1970), p. 275.

267. J. A. Reagan, B. M. Herman, and R. J. Spiegel, in *Proc. 1970 Southwest IEEE Conf.*, SWIEEE Rec., Dallas, TX (1970), p. 526.

268. W. Graj, K. M. Cushing, R. D. McPeters, and A. E. S. Green, *Appl. Opt.*, 12:2585 (1973).

269. J. A. Reagan, D. M. Byrne, B. M. Herman, and R. L. Peck, in *Abstr. Seventh Intern. Laser Radar Conf.*, Stanford Res. Inst., Menlo Park, CA (1975), p. 67.

270. P. M. McCormick, *Proc. Electro-Optics Intern. Conf.*, Brighton, England (1971).

271. F. G. Fernald, B. M. Herman, and J. A. Reagan, *J. Appl. Meteorol.*, 11:482 (1972).

272. P. B. Russell, W. Viezee, and R. D. Hake, *Semiann. Rep.*, SRI Contract NAS2-7261, Stanford Res. Inst., Menlo Park, CA (1973).

273. M. Fujiwara, M. Hirono, T. Itabe, and O. Uchino, in *Abstr. Sixth Conf. Laser Atmospheric Studies*, Sendai, Japan (1974), p. 112.

274. M. Hirono, M. Fujiwara, O. Uchino, and T. Itabe, *Can. J. Chem.*, 26:1560 (1974).

275. J. D. Spinhirne, B. M. Herman, and J. A. Reagan, in *Abstr. Sixth Conf. Laser Atmospheric Studies*, Sendai, Japan (1974), p. 151.

276. R. E. W. Pettifer, P. G. Healey, J. Convery, and G. J. Jenkins, in *Abstr. Seventh Intern. Laser Radar Conf.*, Stanford Res. Inst., Menlo Park, CA (1975), p. 49.

277. B. V. Kaul', I. V. Samokhvalov, N. V. Kozlov, and V. N. Kuznetsov, in *Problems of Remote Sensing of the Atmosphere* [in Russian], Inst. Opt. Atm. Sib. Otd. Akad. Nauk SSSR, Tomsk (1975), p. 30.

278. Yu. S. Balin, V. P. Galileiskii, I. V. Samokhvalov, and V. S. Shamanaev, in *Problems in Laser Probing of the Atmosphere* [in Russian], Nauka, Novosibirsk (1976), p. 34.

279. Yu. M. Vorevodin, G. O. Zadde, G. G. Matvienko, and I. V. Samokhvalov, in *Problems in Laser Probing of the Atmosphere* [in Russian], Nauka, Novosibirsk (1976), p. 45.

280. V. N. Deev, B. V. Kaul', N. V. Kozlov, V. N. Kuznetsov, and I. V. Samokhvalov, in *Abstr. Fourth All-Union Symp. Laser Probing of the Atmosphere* [in Russian], Inst. Opt. Atm. Sib. Otd. Akad. Nauk SSSR, Tomsk (1976), p. 28.

281. V. E. Zuev, N. V. Kozlov, É. V. Makienko, I. É. Naats, and I. V. Samokhvalov, in *Abstr. Fourth All-Union Symp. Laser Probing of the Atmosphere* [in Russian], Inst. Opt. Atm. Sib. Otd. Akad. Nauk SSSR, Tomsk (1976), p. 142.

282. V. E. Zuev, N. V. Kozlov, É. V. Makienko, I. É. Naats, and I. V. Samokhvalov, in *Abstr. Fourth All-Union Symp. Laser Probing of the Atmosphere* [in Russian], Inst. Opt. Atm. Sib. Otd. Akad. Nauk SSSR, Tomsk (1976), p. 160.

283. M. P. McCormick, T. J. Swissler, and W. P. Chu, in *Abstracts on Atmospheric Aerosols: Their Optical Properties and Effects*, NASA Langley Res. Cent., Williamsburg, VA (1976), p. MB7-1.

284. W. R. McNeil and A. I. Carswell, *Appl. Opt.*, 14:2158 (1975).
285. A. D. Egorov and V. D. Stepanenko, in *Radiophysical Studies of the Atmosphere* [in Russian], Gidrometeoizdat, Leningrad (1977), p. 43.
286. É. P. Zege, A. P. Ivanov, B. A. Kargin, and I. L. Katsev, *Izv. Akad. Nauk SSSR, Fiz. Atm. Okeana*, 7:750 (1971).
287. V. N. Shuleikin, in *Abstr. Fourth All-Union Symp. Laser Probing of the Atmosphere* [in Russian], Inst. Opt. Atm. Sib. Otd. Akad. Nauk SSSR, Tomsk (1976), p. 24.
288. O. K. Voitsekhovskaya, Yu. S. Makushkin, V. N. Marichev, A. A. Mitsel', I. V. Samokhvalov, and A. V. Sosnin, *Izv. Vyssh. Uchebn. Zaved. SSSR, Fiz.*, No. 1, p. 62 (1977).
289. R. M. Schotland, *J. Appl. Meteorol.*, 13:71 (1974).
290. S. A. Achmed, *Appl. Opt.*, 12:901 (1973).
291. V. N. Marichev and A. A. Mitsel', in *Abstr. Fourth All-Union Symp. Laser Probing of the Atmosphere* [in Russian], Inst. Opt. Atm. Sib. Otd. Akad. Nauk SSSR, Tomsk (1976), p. 175.
292. E. D. Hinkley, *Opto-Electron.*, 4:69 (1972).
293. M. M. Johnson and A. H. LaGrone, *Radio Sci.*, 8:407 (1973).
294. R. A. McClatchey, R. W. Fenn, J. E. A. Selby, F. E. Volz, and J. S. Garing, *Optical Properties of the Atmosphere*, AFCRL 71-0279 (1971).
295. R. M. Schotland, in *Proc. Third Symp. Remote Sensing of the Environment*, Univ. Michigan, Ann Arbor, MI (1964), p. 215.
296. N. V. Marichev, A. V. Sosnin, and G. S. Khmel'nitskii, in *Abstr. Third All-Union Symp. Laser Probing of the Atmosphere* [in Russian], Inst. Opt. Atm. Sib. Otd. Akad. Nauk SSSR, Tomsk (1974), p. 220.
297. V. N. Marichev, I. V. Samokhvalov, and A. V. Sosnin, in *Problems of Remote Sensing of the Atmosphere* [in Russian], Inst. Opt. Atm. Sib. Otd. Akad. Nauk SSSR, Tomsk (1975), p. 126.
298. V. N. Marichev, I. V. Samokhvalov, and A. V. Sosnin, in *Proc. All-Union Symp. Radiophysical Methods of Atmospheric Research* [in Russian], Gl. Geofiz. Obs., Leningrad (1975), p. 77.
299. V. E. Zuev, Paper Presented at the Second Special Assembly of IAMAP, Seattle, WA (1977).
300. V. E. Derr, M. Post, R. L. Schwiesow, R. F. Calfee, and L. T. McNice, *A Theoretical Analysis of the Information Content of Lidar Atmospheric Returns*, NOAA Tech. Rep. ERL 296-WPL 29, Boulder, CO (1974).
301. J. K. Dixon, *J. Chem. Phys.*, 8:157 (1940).
302. G. W. Robinson, M. McCarty, Jr., and Mary C. Keelty, *J. Chem. Phys.*, 27:972 (1957).
303. W. H. Fink, *J. Chem. Phys.*, 49:5054 (1968).
304. L. Burnelle, A. M. Maj, and R. A. Gangi, *J. Chem. Phys.*, 49:561 (1968).
305. L. Burnelle and K. P. Dressler, *J. Chem. Phys.*, 51:2758 (1969).
306. R. W. B. Pearse and A. C. Gaydon, *The Identification of Molecular Spectra* (2nd ed. rev.), Vol. XI, Sec. 61, Chapman and Hall, London (1950), p. 276.
307. P. A. Leighton, *Photochemistry of Air Pollution*, Academic Press, New York–London (1961).
308. P. L. Hanst, in *Advances in Environmental Science and Technology*, Vol. 2 (1971), p. 91.
309. A. E. Douglas and K. P. Huber, *Can. J. Phys.*, 43:74 (1965).
310. D. C. O'Shea and L. G. Dodge, *Appl. Opt.*, 13:1481 (1974).
311. K. W. Rothe, U. Brinkmann, and H. Walther, *Appl. Phys.*, 3(2):115 (1974).
312. K. W. Rothe, U. Brinkmann, and H. Walther, *Appl. Phys.*, 4(2):181 (1974).
313. W. B. Grant, R. D. Hake, Jr., E. M. Liston, R. C. Robbins, and E. K. Proctor, Jr., *Appl. Phys. Lett.*, 24:550 (1974).

314. T. Tsuji, Y. Higuchi, and H. Kimura, in *Abstr. Sixth Intern. Laser Radar Conf.*, Sendai, Japan (1974), p. 103.

315. H. Inomata and T. Igarashi, *Jpn. J. Appl. Phys.*, 14:1751 (1975).

316. R. T. Thompson *et al.*, *J. Appl. Phys.*, 46:3040 (1975).

317. W. B. Grant and R. D. Hake, *J. Appl. Phys.*, 46:3019 (1975).

318. S. H. Melfi, J. D. Lawrence, Jr., and M. P. McCormick, *Appl. Phys. Lett.*, 15:295 (1969).

319. J. A. Cooney, *J. Appl. Meteorol.*, 9:182 (1970).

320. J. A. Cooney, *J. Appl. Meteorol.*, 10:301 (1971).

321. S. H. Melfi, *Appl. Opt.*, 11:1605 (1972).

322. J. A. Cooney, *J. Appl. Meteorol.*, 12:888 (1973).

323. J. A. Cooney, *J. Atm. Sci.*, No. 6, p. 7 (1974).

324. O. K. Kostko, V. U. Khattatov, G. A. Krikunov, and N. D. Smirnov, *Meteorol. Gidrol.*, No. 12, p. 95 (1975).

325. Yu. F. Arshinov and S. A. Danichkin, *Izv. Akad. Nauk SSSR, Fiz. Atm. Okeana*, 11:414 (1975).

326. Yu. F. Arshinov, S. A. Danichkin, V. E. Zuev, and I. V. Samokhvalov, in *Abstr. Second All-Union Symp. Propagation of Laser Radiation in the Atmosphere* [in Russian], Inst. Opt. Atm. Sib. Otd. Akad. Nauk SSSR, Tomsk (1973), p. 162.

327. J. A. Cooney, *Bull. Am. Phys. Soc.*, 16:524 (1971).

328. J. A. Cooney, *J. Appl. Meteorol.*, 11:108 (1972).

329. M. M. Sushinskii, *Raman Scattering Spectra of Molecules and Crystals* [in Russian], Nauka, Moscow (1969).

330. Yu. F. Arshinov and S. A. Danichkin, in *Propagation of Optical Waves in the Atmosphere* [in Russian], Nauka, Novosibirsk (1975), p. 169.

331. M. E. Hillard and A. R. Ban-Duny, *Appl. Spectrosc.*, 27:421 (1973).

332. M. A. Buldakov, Yu. T. Dashchuk, I. I. Matrosov, and T. N. Popova, in *Abstr. Eleventh Sci.-Tech. Conf. Young Specialists of the State Optical Institute* [in Russian], Leningrad (1975), p. 9.

333. V. E. Zuev, G. M. Krekov, I. É. Naats, and V. N. Skorinov, in *Abstr. Third All-Union Symp. Laser Probing of the Atmosphere* [in Russian], Inst. Opt. Atm. Sib. Otd. Akad. Nauk SSSR, Tomsk (1974), p. 72.

334. G. M. Krekov, I. É. Naats, and V. N. Skorinov, in *Problems in Laser Probing of the Atmosphere* [in Russian], Nauka, Novosibirsk (1976), p. 69.

335. Yu. F. Arshinov and S. A. Danichkin, in *Proc. Sib. Symp. Laser Spectroscopy* [in Russian], Inst. Fiz. Sib. Otd. Akad. Nauk SSSR, Krasnoyarsk (1973), p. 70.

336. Yu. F. Arshinov, S. M. Bobrovnikov, and S. A. Danichkin, in *Abstr. Fourth All-Union Symp. Laser Probing of the Atmosphere* [in Russian], Inst. Opt. Atm. Sib. Otd. Akad. Nauk SSSR, Tomsk (1976), p. 189.

337. Yu. F. Arshinov, S. A. Danichkin, S. M. Bobrovnikov, and I. V. Samokhvalov, in *Abstr. Fourth All-Union Symp. Laser Probing of the Atmosphere* [in Russian], Inst. Opt. Atm. Sib. Otd. Akad. Nauk SSSR, Tomsk (1976), p. 172.

338. J. A. Salzman and T. A. Coney, in *Abstr. Fifth Conf. Laser Radar Studies of the Atmosphere*, Williamsburgh, VA (1973), p. 49.

339. J. Cooney and M. Pina, in *Abstr. Sixth Conf. Laser Atmospheric Studies*, Sendai, Japan (1974), p. 52.

340. J. Cooney and M. Pina, *Appl. Opt.*, 15:602 (1976).

341. B. M. Urin, *Tr. Tsentr. Astrofiz. Inst.*, No. 106, p. 54 (1973).

342. G. Fiocco and J. B. De Wolf, *J. Atm. Sci.*, 25:488 (1968).

343. G. Fiocco, G. Benedetti-Michelangeli, K. Maischberger, and E. Madonna, *Nature*, 229:78 (1971).

344. G. Benedetti-Michelangeli, F. Congedutti, and G. Fiocco, in *Abstr. Fourth Conf. Laser Radar Studies of the Atmosphere*, Tucson, AZ (1972), p. 39.

345. J. E. Blamont, M. L. Chamin, and G. Megie, *Ann. Geophys.*, 28:833 (1972).

346. G. Megie, J. E. Blamont, and M. L. Chamin, *Proc. COSPAR Symp. Methods of Measurement and Results on the Lower Ionosphere Structure*, Lake Constance, GFR, Berlin (1973), p. 287.

347. G. Megie, Paper Presented at the Sixteenth General Assembly of IUGG, Grenoble (1976).

348. O. K. Kostko and G. A. Krikunov, in *Abstr. Second All-Union Symp. Propagation of Laser Radiation in the Atmosphere* [in Russian], Inst. Opt. Atm. Sib. Otd. Akad. Nauk SSSR, Tomsk (1973), p. 128.

349. O. K. Kostko and G. A. Krikunov, *Tr. Tsentr. Astrofiz., Obs.*, No. 109, p. 16 (1975).

350. M. Hirono and O. Uchino, *Mem. Fac. Sci. Kyushu Univ. B*, 4:119 (1972).

351. J. B. Mason, in *Abstr. Fifth Conf. Laser Radar Studies of the Atmosphere*, Williamsburg, VA (1973), p. 63.

352. J. B. Mason, *Appl. Opt.*, 14:76 (1975).

353. G. Benedetti-Michelangeli, F. Congedutti, and G. Fiocco, *J. Atm. Sci.*, 29:906 (1972).

354. G. Benedetti-Michelangeli, F. Congedutti, and G. Fiocco, *Atm. Environ.*, 8:793 (1974).

355. R. A. Brandewie and W. C. Davis, *Appl. Opt.*, 11:1526 (1972).

356. R. M. Huffaker, *Appl. Opt.*, 9:1026 (1970).

357. T. R. Lawrence, *Q. J. R. Meteorol. Soc.*, 80:174 (1972).

358. "Laser satellite systems due in '75," *Electronics*, 45(19):34 (1972).

359. W. M. Farmer and D. B. Broyton, *Appl. Opt.*, 10:2319 (1971).

360. P. J. Bourke and C. G. Brown, *Opt. Lasers Technol.*, 3:23 (1971).

361. K. G. Bartlett and C. Y. She, *Appl. Opt.*, 15:1980 (1976).

362. V. V. Belov, G. N. Glazov, and G. M. Krekov, in *Abstr. Second All-Union Symp. Propagation of Laser Radiation in the Atmosphere* [in Russian], Inst. Opt. Atm. Sib. Otd. Akad. Nauk SSSR, Tomsk (1973), p. 153.

363. V. E. Zuev, G. G. Matvienko, and I. V. Samokhvalov, in *Radiophysical Studies of the Atmosphere* [in Russian], Leningrad (1977), p. 67.

364. G. O. Zadde, G. G. Matvienko, and V. I. Rubtsov, in *Propagation of Optical Waves in the Atmosphere* [in Russian], Nauka, Novosibirsk (1975), p. 180.

365. Yu. M. Vorevodin, G. O. Zadde, G. G. Matvienko, and I. V. Samokhvalov, in *Problems in Laser Probing of the Atmosphere* [in Russian], Nauka, Novosibirsk (1976), p. 45.

366. V. E. Zuev, G. G. Matvienko, and I. V. Samokhvalov, *Izv. Akad. Nauk SSSR, Fiz. Atm. Okeana*, 12:1243 (1976).

367. V. E. Zuev, G. G. Matvienko, and I. V. Samokhvalov, in *Abstr. Seventh Intern. Laser Radar Conf.*, Stanford Res. Inst., Menlo Park, CA (1976), p. 53.

368. E. W. Eloranta, J. M. King, and J. A. Weinman, *J. Appl. Meteorol.*, 14:1485 (1975).

369. G. O. Zadde, V. E. Zuev, V. P. Tarasenko, and N. I. Yurga, in *Propagation of Optical Waves in the Atmosphere* [in Russian], Nauka, Novosibirsk (1975), p. 174.

370. A. M. Obukhov, *Izv. Akad. Nauk SSSR, Geofiz.*, No. 2, p. 155 (1975).

371. V. I. Tatarskii, *Wave Propagation in a Turbulent Atmosphere* [in Russian], Nauka, Moscow (1967).

372. A. S. Gurvich, A. I. Kon, V. L. Mironov, and S. S. Khmelevtsov, *Laser Radiation in a Turbulent Atmosphere* [in Russian], Nauka, Moscow (1976).

373. M. S. Belen'kii, V. V. Borovoi, N. Ts. Gomboev, É. V. Zubritskii, V. L. Mironov, and S. S. Khmelevtsov, *Optical Measurements of the Profiles of Refractive Index Fluctuations of the Atmosphere in Mountain Zones*, Preprint No. 2 [in Russian], Inst. Opt. Atm. Sib. Otd. Akad. Nauk SSSR, Tomsk (1975).

374. M. Subramanian, *J. Opt. Soc. Am.*, 62:677 (1972).

375. M. S. Belen'kii and V. L. Mironov, *Kvantovaya Élektron. (Moscow)*, 1:2253 (1974).

376. M. S. Belen'kii, A. A. Makarov, V. L. Mironov, and V. V. Pokasov, *Kvantovaya Élektron. (Moscow)*, 3:2051 (1976).

377. N. L. Byzova and É. E. Vyal'tseva, *Izv. Akad. Nauk SSSR, Fiz. Atm. Okeana*, 6:1209 (1970).

378. C. E. Coulman, *Solar Phys.*, 7:122 (1969).

379. V. P. Lukin, V. L. Mironov, V. V. Pokasov, and S. S. Khmelevtsov, *Izv. Akad. Nauk SSSR, Fiz. Atm. Okeana*, 12:550 (1976).
380. V. P. Lukin and V. V. Pokasov, *Izv. Vyssh. Uchebn. Zaved. SSSR, Radiofiz.*, No. 11, p. 1726 (1973).
381. V. P. Lukin, V. L. Mironov, V. V. Pokasov, and V. M. Sazonovich, *Izv. Akad. Nauk SSSR, Fiz. Atm. Okeana*, 12:1317 (1976).
382. V. E. Zuev, G. M. Krekov, and A. I. Popkov, Paper Presented at the Twenty-Third Astronautical Congress, Brussels (1971).
383. V. E. Zuev, G. M. Krekov, and I. É. Naats, *Acta Astronaut.*, 1:93 (1974).
384. E. D. Hinkley, *Appl. Phys. Lett.*, 16:351 (1970).
385. E. D. Hinkley and P. L. Keeley, *Science*, 171:635 (1971).
386. E. D. Hinkley, *Opto-Electron.*, 4:69 (1972).
387. E. D. Hinkley and R. T. Ku, *Ann. Rep. MIT Lincoln Lab.*, Lexington, MA (1974).
388. R. T. Ku, E. D. Hinkley, and J. O. Sample, *Appl. Opt.*, 14:854 (1975).
389. R. T. Ku and E. D. Hinkley, in *Applications of Laser Spectroscopy, Technical Digest* (Spring Conf., March 19–21, 1975), Paper FA4-1, Anaheim, CA (1975).
390. E. D. Hinkley, *Opt. Quantum Electron.*, 8:155 (1976).
391. J. C. Hill and G. P. Montgomery, Jr., *Appl. Opt.*, 15:748 (1976).
392. A. Mooradian, in *Proc. IEEE Region Six Conf.* (*Western U. S.*), Albuquerque, NM, 1974, New York (1974), p. 79.
393. P. L. Hanst, *Appl. Spectrosc.*, 24:161 (1970).
394. L. B. Kreuzer, N. D. Kenyon, and C. K. N. Patel, *Science*, 177:347 (1972).
395. R. T. Menzies and M. S. Shumate, *Science*, 184:570 (1974).
396. E. R. Murray, L. E. Van der Laan, and J. G. Hawley, *Appl. Opt.*, 15:3140 (1976).
397. A. V. Sosnin and G. S. Khmel'nitskii, in *Problems of Remote Sensing of the Atmosphere* [in Russian], Inst. Opt. Atm. Sib. Otd. Akad. Nauk SSSR, Tomsk (1975), p. 131.
398. V. E. Zuev, I. V. Samokhvalov, A. V. Sosnin, and G. S. Khmel'nitskii, in *Abstr. Intern. Symp. Radiation in the Atmosphere*, Garmisch-Partenkirchen, GFR (1976).
399. G. P. Montgomery and J. C. Hill, *J. Opt. Soc. Am.*, 65:379 (1975).
400. R. R. Patty, G. M. Russwurm, W. A. McClenny, and D. R. Morgan, *Appl. Opt.*, 13:2850 (1974).
401. J. W. Robinson and J. D. Dake, *Spectrosc. Lett.*, 6:569 (1973).
402. H. Walter, Jr., and D. Flanigan, *Appl. Opt.*, 14:1423 (1975).